CONTEMPORARY
CHINESE MEDICINE *and*
ACUPUNCTURE

MEDICAL GUIDES TO
Complementary & Alternative Medicine

CONTEMPORARY CHINESE MEDICINE *and* ACUPUNCTURE

CLAIRE MONOD CASSIDY, PhD, Dipl Ac, LAc, FNAAOM

Paradigms Found Consulting
Bethesda, Maryland;
Windpath Healing Works
Silver Spring, Maryland

Series Editor **MARC S. MICOZZI**, MD, PhD

Executive Director
The College of Physicians of Philadelphia
Adjunct Professor of Medicine and Rehabilitation Medicine
University of Pennsylvania
Philadelphia, Pennsylvania

with 71 illustrations

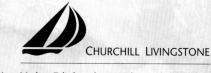

CHURCHILL LIVINGSTONE

New York   Edinburgh   London   Philadelphia

CHURCHILL LIVINGSTONE

The Curtis Center
Independence Square West
Philadelphia, Pennsylvania 19106-3399

Publishing Director: John A. Schrefer
Associate Editor: Kellie F. Conklin
Associate Developmental Editor: Jennifer L. Watrous
Project Manager: Karen Edwards
Design: Renée Duenow

CONTEMPORARY CHINESE MEDICINE AND ACUPUNCTURE   ISBN 0-443-06589-6

Contributors

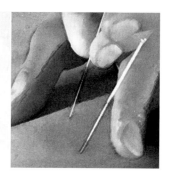

JOHN J. B. ALLEN, PhD
Assistant Professor
Department of Psychology
University of Arizona
Tucson, Arizona

W. JUMBÉ ALLEN, LAc
Private Practice
Oakland, California

STEPHEN BIRCH, PhD, LAc (USA), FNAAOM
President
Stichting (Foundation) for the Study of
    Traditional Asian Medicine (STEAM)
Amsterdam, The Netherlands

JUNE BRAZIL, Dipl Ac, PDM, LAc, FNAAOM
Deceased

ZOE BRENNER, MAc, LAc, Dipl Ac, Dipl CH,
    FNAAOM
Faculty
Traditional Acupuncture Institute
Columbia, Maryland

JAMES C. BUTLER-ARKOW, MA, Dipl Ac, LAc
Private Practice
Arlington, Virginia

BRYN CLARK, MAc, LAc, Dipl Ac, Dipl CH, CMT,
    FNAAOM
Faculty, Herb Program
Academy for Five Element Acupuncture
Halendale, Florida;
Herb Program
Traditional Acupuncture Institute
Columbia, Maryland;
Secretary, Association for Professional Acupuncture
Philadelphia, Pennsylvania

SUSAN CUSHING, LAc
Asari Acupuncture Clinic
Reedsburg, Wisconsin

DAVID L. DIEHL, MD, FACP
Clinical Associate Professor of Medicine
Department of Medicine
Division of Gastroenterology
NYU School of Medicine
New York, New York

PETER ECKMAN, MD, PhD, MAc (UK), FNAAOM
Private Practice
San Francisco, California

JEAN EDELEN
Management Consultant
Freelance Writer
Alexandria, Virginia

MITRA C. EMAD, PhD
Assistant Professor
Cultural Studies Program, Department
    of Sociology/Anthropology
University of Minnesota—Duluth
Duluth, Minnesota

ROBERT L. FELT, BA
Publisher
Paradigm Publications
Brookline, Massachusetts

JINGYUN GAO, BS, OMD, LAc
Chairperson
Department of Acupuncture
Maryland Institute of Traditional Chinese Medicine
Bethesda, Maryland;
Private Practice
Washington, DC

ALISON GOULD, MSc
Northern College of Acupuncture
York, England
United Kingdom

JANE A. GRISSMER, MAc
Senior Faculty
Tai Sophia Institute
Columbia, Maryland;
Director,
Crossings: A Center for the Healing Traditions
Takoma Park, Maryland

RICHARD HAMMERSCHLAG, PhD
Research Director
Oregon College of Oriental Medicine
Portland, Oregon

MARTHA HARE, PhD
Senior Health Research Scientist
Centers for Public Health Research and Evaluation
Battelle Memorial Institute
Arlington, Virginia

PAULETTE C. HILL, MD, MPH, MAc
Primary Care Physician and Acupuncturist
Sinai Hospital Addiction and Recovery Program
Baltimore, Maryland

LONNY S. JARRETT, MAc, LAc, FNAAOM
Private Practice
Spiritpasspress.com
Stockbridge, Massachusetts

KIM A. JOBST, MB, BS, MA, DM, MFHom, MRCP
Consultant Physician and Medical Homeopath
Visiting Professor of Healthcare and Integrated Medicine
Oxford Brooks University
Oxford, England
United Kingdom

CAROL KARI, RN, MAc, LAc
Traditional Acupuncture
Bethesda, Maryland

DAN KENNER, PhD, LAc
Board of Directors
Meiji College of Oriental Medicine
Berkeley, California

HAIYANG LI, LAc, OMD
Faculty
Maryland Institute of Traditional Chinese Medicine
Bethesda, Maryland

PAULETTE McMILLAN, LAc, Dipl Ac, Dipl CH, RD, LN
Faculty
Maryland Institute of Traditional Chinese Medicine;
Center for Acupuncture and Complementary Healing
Bethesda, Maryland

BARBARA B. MITCHELL, JD, LAc
Executive Director
Acupuncture and Oriental Medicine Alliance;
Co-Chair,
North American Council of Acupuncture and Oriental Medicine
Olalla, Washington

MARGARET A. NAESER, PhD, LAc, Dipl Ac
Neuroimaging/Aphasia Research
VA Boston Healthcare System;
Research Professor of Neurology
Boston University School of Medicine
Boston, Massachusetts

MICHAEL A. PHILLIPS, MAc, LAc
Faculty
Traditional Acupuncture Institute
Columbia, Maryland

ROSA N. SCHNYER, Dipl Ac, LAc
Senior Research Associate
Department of Psychology
University of Arizona
Tucson, Arizona

MICHAEL O. SMITH, MD, Dr Ac
Director
Lincoln Hospital Recovery Center
Bronx, New York;
Assistant Clinical Professor
Department of Psychiatry
Cornell Medical College
New York, New York

VALENTIN TUREANU, MD
Obstetrician/Gynecologist
Toronto, Ontario

LUMINITA TUREANU, MD
Obstetrician/Gynecologist
Toronto, Ontario

TAO WANG, BM, PhD, LAc
Manager, Clinical Development
Otsuka American Pharmaceutical, Inc
Rockville, Maryland;
Clinical Faculty
Maryland Institute of Traditional Chinese Medicine
Bethesda, Maryland

GRANT ZHANG
Assistant Professor
Complementary Medicine Program
University of Maryland School of Medicine
Baltimore, Maryland;
Faculty
Maryland Institute of Traditional Chinese Medicine
Bethesda, Maryland

To the memory of my parents

Hélène Lucile Monod

Frederic Gomes Cassidy

and to John and Julie
PS Don't forget to SMILE :)

"From wonder into wonder, existence opens"

Lao Tzu

Series Introduction

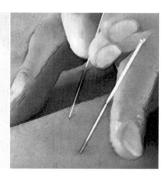

The aim of this Series is to provide clear and rational guides for health care professionals and students so they have current knowledge about:

- Therapeutic medical systems currently labeled as complementary medicine
- Complementary approaches to specific medical conditions
- Integration of complementary therapy into mainstream medical practice

Each text is written specifically with the needs and questions of a health care audience in mind. Where possible, basic applications in clinical practice are explored.

Complementary medicine is being rapidly integrated into mainstream health care largely in response to consumer demand, as well as in recognition of new scientific findings that are expanding our view of health and healing—pushing against the limits of the current biomedical paradigm.

Health care professionals need to know what their patients are doing and what they believe about complementary and alternative medicine. In addition, a basic working knowledge of complementary medical therapies is a rapidly growing requirement for primary care, some biomedical specialties, and the allied health professions. These approaches also expand our view of the art and science of medicine and make important contributions to the intellectual formation of students in health professions.

This Series provides a survey of the fundamentals and foundations of complementary medical systems currently available and practiced in North America and Europe. Each topic is presented in ways that are *understandable* and that provide an important *understanding* of the intellectual foundations of each system—with translation between the complementary and conventional medical systems where possible. These explanations draw appropriately on the social and scientific foundations of each system of care.

Rapidly growing contemporary research results are also included where possible. In addition to providing evidence indicating where complementary medicines may be of therapeutic benefit, guidance is also provided about when complementary therapies should not be used.

This field of health is rapidly moving from being considered *alternative* (implying exclusive use of one medical system or another) to *complementary* (used as an adjunct to mainstream medical care) to *integrative medicine* (implying an active, conscious effort by mainstream medicine to incorporate alternatives on the basis of rational clinical and scientific information and judgment).

Likewise, health care professionals and students must move rapidly to learn the fundamentals of complementary medical systems in order to better serve their patients' needs, protect the public health, and expand their scientific horizons and understandings of health and healing.

MARC S. MICOZZI
Philadelphia, Pennsylvania
1997

Series Editor's Preface

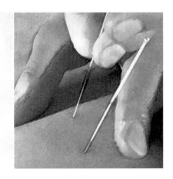

Traditional medicine of China can be thought of as an empirical tradition of systematic correspondences that make reference to five cosmic elements and extend back to approximately 3000 BCE. For comparative purposes, Chinese medicine is often viewed as a homogeneous monolithic structure; however, this view neglects the changing interpretations of basic paradigms offered by Chinese medicine through the ages and the synchronic plurality of differing opinions and ideas over thousands of years.

Chinese medicine presents other options for healing with a wide spectrum of alternative therapeutic modalities. We might compare Chinese medicine with the following characteristics of contemporary Western biomedicine:

1. Materialist focus on the body in a mechanical model vs energetic model
2. Emphasis on the physical body vs nonphysical realms of healing
3. Focus on the disease (or disease agent) vs the person ("le terrain" or host)
4. Taxonomy on disease types vs types of healing
5. Perception of high technology as having more healing power
6. Represents the most invasive therapies on the healing spectrum
7. Emphasis on acute, trauma, and end-of-life care vs wellness and prevention
8. High cost

The sheer power of modern biomedicine can be overwhelming. Although we tend to link this power to the ability to deliver "comprehensive" care, a balanced comparison of similarities and differences with Chinese medicine reveals that each system may be more comprehensive than the other, depending on which domain of healing is chosen for comparison. In fact, taken as a whole, modern Western biomedicine and ancient Chinese medicine might be considered quite complementary.

In theoretical terms, we have many choices in healing. In practical terms, the sheer cost, size, scale, and complexity of the health care system led to its regulation by "third parties," such as the government and the insurance industry. The introduction of "third parties" into the traditional doctor-patient relationship indirectly or directly (as in Oregon) leads to rationing of health care. So the success of biomedicine has ultimately contributed to health care rationing. Most Americans do not want to see necessities such as food and medicine rationed.

In China, far fewer resources are devoted to health care. There has been a recent reliance on the "barefoot doctor" in an attempt to address the minimal health care needs of the people in the Peoples' Republic of China. Much of what the traditional Chinese medical practitioner does is thought to influence the flow or balance of the body's energy called "Qi." In my view, the Chinese concept of Qi, which is translated as energy, bioenergy, or vital energy, has a metabolic quality because the Chinese character for Qi may be described as vapor or steam rising over rice. The term *rice* has a specific quality that we associate with a specific food, but it also has the generic meaning of "food" or foodstuff. For example, the character "rice hall" is used to describe a restaurant in Chinese. The elusive meaning of Qi may therefore be likened more to living metabolism (the "vital energy" of the 19th century) than to the energy that we associate today with electricity or electromagnetic radiation.

Energy or Qi also has the dynamic qualities of "flow" and "balance." Because flow and balance are dynamic, they might be described in changing terms from one patient to the next or in the same patient from one day to the next (not using static, fixed pathological diagnostic categories). Such concepts present great challenges in translation to the biomedical model.

Acupuncture is a major modality for the manipulation of Qi. Clinical observations of efficacy are increasing, and some biomedical explanations focuson the physiological effects of skin puncture and/or modulation of neurotransmitter substances. Some experiments indicate that the acupuncture needle may have the same effect when it is merely held in place over the appropriate point (without puncturing the skin), leading to bioenergetic explanations for mechanism of action.

As we look across the history and heritage of health and healing, through this book series, *Medical Guides to Complementary & Alternative Medicine,* it is clear that health is not solely about a given medical system or tradition. It is about the mind and the body, and how they work, and how they heal. Formulary approaches (to acupuncture, herbalism, and homeopathy for example) may work because they appear to affect the body in some of the same ways both within and without their cultural contents. These formulary approaches provide evidence that empirical cultural healing traditions may have discovered truths about human physiology and encoded them into cultural belief systems. Chinese civilization, which has made so many discoveries in science and technology over the centuries, surely holds promise for uncovering some of the still held secrets of the art and science of medicine.

MARC S. MICOZZI, MD, PhD
Philadelphia, Pennsylvania
March 2001

Preface

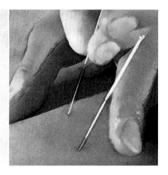

In just 30 short years Chinese, or Oriental, medicine has moved from a rare curiosity in the West to a well-known and widely available medicine ready for integration with biomedicine, chiropractic, massage therapy, naturopathy, and other medical practices. This remarkable transformation of attention and viewpoint originally owed much to politics and economic demand, but after 30 years it is eminently clear that traditional Chinese medical practices are clinically effective. This point is supported by the rapid growth of the profession—for a profession cannot grow unless patients demand its services, students attend its schools, and legal entities mandate its use. And though scientific research has been running to catch up—research was not originally part of the tradition—its results are increasingly providing not only statistical support for clinical effectiveness, but by using the energetic insights of the medicine, also opening new doors to understanding the physiology of the human body.

Considering how little was publicly known of this medicine outside of Asia even in the early 1970s, this growth has been nothing less than spectacular. James Reston reported using acupuncture for analgesia after surgery in 1971, sparking fascination as people realized Chinese medicine offered at least one avenue of release from the economic pressures associated with practicing the highly technological biomedicine. Hunger for this medicine was acute; by 1975 several pioneering schools were already training Oriental medicine practitioners in the United States, using teachers trained mostly in Asia or Europe. Today, there are over 40 accredited schools, well-developed professional and legal support systems, thousands of professional practitioners, and thousands of students who spend at least 3 years learning acupuncture, plus one or two more to learn herbology. Research interest was high from the outset, but success was slowed by factors such as the lack of a bioscience theoretical foundation that could subsume the energetic arguments of Chinese medicine, of physiological understandings of what was "happening" during acupuncture treatments, and of research designs that could accurately measure the effects of acupuncture, herbs, tuina massage, or Qi gong. The US National Institutes of Health (NIH) National Center for Complementary and Alternative Medicine (previously the NIH Office of Alternative Medicine formed in 1992), supported clinical research on OM from the outset. In the early 1990s a series of workshops sponsored by the US Food and Drug Administration (FDA) and the NIH focused on developing appropriate research methodologies for alternative medicine. Based on data concerning its safety and utility, the acupuncture needle was reclassified from "experimental" to "medical devices for general use" by trained professionals by the FDA in 1996. In 1997 the NIH hosted an Acupuncture Consensus Conference during which the newest clinical trials research data was presented. The consensus panel concluded that acupuncture was effective and listed a series of conditions for which the best research data existed. These data and much more are reviewed in this text.

Despite this growth, public and medical practitioner knowledge of the field remains limited. Although many new textbooks and popular introductions exist, to date there has been no introduction aimed at health care providers, researchers, and lay readers who want an in-depth yet nontechnical presentation. *Contemporary Chinese Medicine and Acupuncture* fills this gap and remedies this situation. This book is scholarly yet readable, offering enough detailed information to help readers appreciate both the complexity and clinical power of Oriental medicine as currently practiced in the West by professional acupuncturists and herbalists.

Part I begins with a review of Oriental medicine theory and interventive modalities. In Part II, actual practice is placed in context through discussions of the differing philosophies of care in biomedicine and Chinese medicine, and practitioners speak through case histories and brief autobiographies. Then in Part III, the current state of research on acupuncture is reviewed in multiple chapters on physiology, epidemiology, and clinical care. These chapters include analyses that can guide both referring clinicians and potential researchers. Finally, Part IV offers another approach to context by explaining how Chinese medicine practitioners are trained and how each US state licenses professional practitioners (with guidance for finding the laws that control practice in other parts of the world). The book ends with a special chapter on referral aimed at health care providers. This brief chapter discusses circumstances under which referral is likely to be helpful and explains how to meet and assess Chinese medicine professionals.

I chose to present this wide range of topics to offer a complete image of practice of this emerging (in the West) health care system, to demonstrate its high level of professionalism, and to support what I hope will be an increasingly informed, friendly, and effective integration of care among medical systems. I decided to include not only theory and interventive modalities (the topics of most texts) but also data on practice, research, and legal mandate when it became clear to me that many people, especially other health care practitioners, lacked useful knowledge of Chinese medicine and that some people labored under a number of prejudices. I hope this book will improve both knowledge and communication among patients, students, professional health care providers, and researchers.

ACKNOWLEDGMENTS

Many people contributed to this book, both actively and indirectly by their inspiration. First, I would like to thank each of the authors of the chapters and sidebars, who spent many hours not only working on their own contributions but also editing them later so that they would flow smoothly with all the other chapters. To these I say: wonderful work!

To my editors, Marc Micozzi, Inta Ozols, Kellie Conklin, and Jennifer Watrous, thanks for your patience and perception! Thanks also to my teachers, from Lao Tzu whose powerful words have guided untold lives for more than 2000 years to those of today, my fellow Chinese medicine practitioners, who inspired me to change my career. You are many in my heart.

I offer a special bow of acknowledgment for their insight and healing ways to Carol Kari and Richard Hammerschlag. Finally, I thank my parents for making me and my husband and daughter for succoring me day to day. To each and all of you, *metaqiesen*.

CLAIRE MONOD CASSIDY

Contents

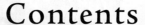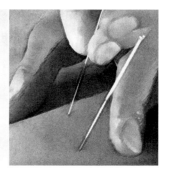

xvii

CONTEMPORARY CHINESE MEDICINE *and* ACUPUNCTURE

I

THE THEORY AND MODALITIES
OF CHINESE MEDICINE

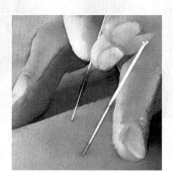

Only 25 to 30 years ago the average Westerner knew of Chinese or Oriental medicine only as an echo of something strange and distant and certainly esoteric. Today, this same medicine is so popular and so readily available that some call it mainstream. Health care practitioners need to understand enough about Oriental Medicine (OM) to recognize when it may benefit their own patients. This book provides that guidance.

Chapter 1 offers an overall introduction to the text and its intentions. It prepares the reader for the distinct character of Chinese medicine, and includes an important discussion of terminology and ways to access updated information via the Internet.

From there we move into the body of the text, starting with discussions of the theory and modalities of OM. To understand these, it is important to know that the theory of OM is quite different from the materialistic models common in Western medicines. OM is based on different perceptions, for example, that health is present when the Qi of the body is flowing smoothly and there is a sufficiency but not an excess. This definition is physiological, homeostatic, and nonmaterial. It does not mention "diseases" because OM is not focused on disease theory but on modulating dynamic change within the body.

Which brings us back to Qi . . . but what *is* Qi? In truth, this Chinese word has never yielded to translation. Some call it "breath," and it has been compared to "prana" and "vital spirit," but most commonly it is translated as "energy." This translation often is confusing because Western people tend to think of "energy" as a capacity for vigorous action and as something measurable as in physics. But Qi is much more than these: it is both what makes the body and what makes the body go; it is simultaneously both material and nonmaterial, single and multiple. Indeed, Qi has degrees of materiality, which are given different names in OM, and it also has different locations with different functions depending on location.

Understanding Qi is at the core of Chinese medicine. All the remainder of the theory of Chinese medicine and its subdivisions grows from this perception, which is based on detailed observation of life in process. In Chapter 2, Peter Eckman, MD, who is also a professional OM practitioner and historian of current practices, offers a model for understanding Qi and organizing the details of OM and comparing them with the details of biomedicine. His chapter forms the foundation on which the other chapters are built; readers can return to this chapter for guidance whenever theoretical assumptions in later chapters become puzzling.

Chapter 3 offers an introduction to diagnosis by Zoe Brenner, a long-time practitioner and student of the Chinese classics. Some of the processes she describes are familiar, but characteristically, Chinese medicine has developed diagnostic procedures, such as tongue or pulse analysis, in immense detail, and this allows for fine distinctions to be made even while remaining at the surface of the body. Traditionally, Chinese medicine has not entered the body to diagnose—traditional practitioners do not take blood, analyze urine, or image the interior organs with technology. Precision can still be achieved, and the cost and technological complexity of diagnosis markedly reduced.

Chapters 4, 5, and 6 introduce the major modalities of OM. The modality most familiar to Western readers, acupuncture, is discussed in Chapter 4 by Grant Zhang, who is an Oriental medical doctor and physiological researcher. While the subject is immense, Dr. Zhang provides just enough detail to explain without teaching exact technique. In the next chapter, Tao Wang, an Oriental medical doctor and pharmacologist, writes on the subject of herbs, which is another immense topic. Dr. Wang focuses on the theory of use and offers a special discussion of herb and pharmaceutical interactions. Chapter 6 is divided into three brief discussions of the remaining major modalities. First, Paulette McMillan, acupuncturist, herbalist, and registered dietitian, discusses Chinese dietetic models and methods. This is followed by a discussion of bodywork techniques by Bryn Clark, an acupuncturist and Chinese massage specialist. The chapter ends with a discussion of Qi gong and related moving meditation techniques that are used both to maintain health and to treat illness by Jean Edelin, a journalist with a specialty in martial arts. Each section includes recommended readings for those who want more detail on these important OM modalities. ∾

A Selection of Supplementary Readings

Popular Texts

Beinfield H, Korngold E: *Between heaven and earth: a guide to Chinese medicine,* New York, 1991, Ballantine Books.

Cohen MR: *The Chinese way to healing: many paths to wholeness,* New York, 1996, Berkeley Publishing Group.

Hicks A: *Principles of Chinese medicine,* London, 1996, Thorsons.

Kaptchuk TP: *The web that has no weaver: understanding Chinese medicine,* New York, 1992, Congdon & Weed.

Classics in Translation

Flaws B: *The classic of difficulties (Nan Jing),* Boulder, Colo, 1999, Blue Poppy Press.

Larre C, translator: *The way of heaven: Neijing suwen,* Cambridge, 1994, Monkey Press.

Nan Jing: *The classic of difficult issues* (translated by PU Unschuld), Berkeley, 1986, University of California Press.

Ni M: *The yellow emperor's classic of internal medicine (Neijing Suwen),* Boston, 1995, Shambala Press.

Spirit and axis (Ling Shu Jing), Beijing, 1981, People's Health Publishing House.

Unschuld PU: *Medicine in China: a history of ideas,* Berkeley, 1985, University of California Press.

Veith I, translator: *The yellow emperor's classic of internal medicine (Neijing Suwen),* Berkeley, 1949, University of California Press.

Dictionaries

Wiseman N, Ye F: *A practical dictionary of Chinese medicine,* ed 2, Brookline, Mass, 1999, Paradigm Publications.

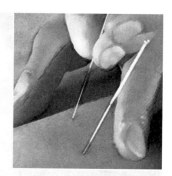

Introduction

CLAIRE M. CASSIDY

GOALS OF THIS BOOK

This book about Oriental medicine is written especially for biomedical health care specialists. Focused on contemporary practice in English-speaking nations, its intent is to help health care practitioners understand enough about this Asian medicine that is sweeping the West to be able to judge its utility for their own patients and learn how to develop collegial relationships with professional practitioners of Chinese medicine.

What Chinese/Oriental Medicine Is

Chinese, or Oriental, medicine is a vast and complex medicine with a long history and many variants of practice. These features make it difficult to summarize in a single introductory text, yet that is our task. As readers can imagine, with a history of practice by people of many cultural backgrounds dating back 2500 years—a history that was certainly preceded by a prehistory of greater length—this medicine emerges as an amalgam of assumptions, ideas, theories, modalities, and practices. It is indeed highly heterogeneous. We can speak of "a medicine," however, because its complexity is built on a few distinctive foundational ideas—as of Qi,* Yin and Yang, Five Phases, acupoints, and Meridians. These have been richly developed, examined, tested, manipulated, and modified over long use among uncounted billions of human beings and animals. Today, its practitioners understand that no one

---

*Pronounced chee; also spelled Chi, ch'i, ki in different sources.

Naming the Medicine

It is not easy to choose a "best" name for the medicine that is the topic of this book. If we call it "Chinese," we honor the land of its birth, where historical records date it to at least 4000 BP. However, this medicine long ago travelled outside of China, reaching Korea in the 8th century, Japan in the 9th century, Tibet in the 11th century, the Middle East by at least the 13th century, Europe starting in the 17th century, and North America by the early 19th century. Because it became widely established and continued to develop in Asia, many prefer to call it "Oriental," and it is this term that is honored in the names of many professional organizations in the United States and Europe. Either of these terms can have unwanted connotations, and many other names have been offered, such as "East Asian" medicine, "meridian" medicine, and so forth. Indeed, no single name suits all users, and in this book each contributor has been encouraged to use the term he or she prefers.

An important sidenote: although this medicine is the "traditional" medicine of China, Korea, and Japan in contrast to recently introduced medicines such as homeopathy or allopathy (biomedicine), it is not the only "traditional" medicine in these countries. To add to the complexity, the term *traditional* has been annexed for use in describing specific subpractices, or styles, and cannot be applied to the whole medicine. Finally, traditional implies, for many, a sense of "unchanging," which is certainly not characteristic of Chinese medicine.

In sum, in this book,

A whole practice of medicine is referred to as a medicine, whereas a subpractice within this medicine is referred to as a style.

We use the terms Chinese or Oriental medicine (CM or OM) interchangeably to refer to the whole practice of this medicine.

We reserve the term traditional to refer to particular styles of practice, specifically the modern practice known familiarly as "traditional Chinese medicine" (TCM), an approach developed in post-1949 China (see Chapter 2).

On "Western" Medicine: Biomedicine, Allopathy

The particular medicine that is usually signalled by the term *Western* is biomedicine, also called allopathy, in which the dominant practitioner earns the MD degree or an equivalent (e.g., DO, DMD). Clearly, the term Western is too broad because there are many Western practices (homeopathy, naturopathy, chiropractic, Christian Science, and so on), and practices from other world regions are also practiced in the West. Other popular names such as "conventional," "modern," "contemporary," "scientific," and "traditional" do not serve in that they reflect a limited and sometimes judgmental point of view (i.e., conventionality depends, after all, on both the country of one's residence and the historical time period; all medicines are contemporary or modern if they are presently practiced; and many medicines are scientific). Of course, some object to the term biomedicine because (they say) it implies that only this medicine understands biology or life, and others object to allopathy because many medicines accept opposing symptoms as a treatment guideline. Nevertheless, for the purposes of this text, we use biomedicine or allopathy interchangeably as the most neutral available names for the currently dominant medicine of Eurocentric nations.

can hope to master the whole of this medicine within one lifetime.

Taking a comparative view, we can also say that Oriental medicine is one of the handful of world medicines that is properly termed "comprehensive." In other words, this medicine takes on, and attempts to treat, all forms of malfunction, and offers a variety of interventive modalities. In addition, it attempts to maintain health both through wise self-care and through environmental quality control. Only a few other medicines offer an equally comprehensive view and set of techniques. These include ayurveda (India), unani (Pakistan, Afghanistan, Iran, etc), Tibetan medicine, and the dominant medicine of Western countries, biomedicine or allopathy.

At present, only Oriental medicine has developed a sufficient infrastructure as to be widely available outside Asia and thus able to stand in parallel with biomedicine, offering both complement and alternative to biomedical care. Oriental medicine today provides Western biomedical practitioners with a powerful and safe option to recommend when caring for patients who either have not responded to biomedical care, or can benefit from supplemental care of the kind Oriental medicine offers.

Finding Additional Information

Although Oriental medicine made its way onto the European and North American stages several times in the past, its recent reemergence starting in the 1970s has been without previous parallel. Today there are not only many schools, non-Asian practitioners, and patients demanding care, but also a rapidly enlarging corpus of information both of classics in translation from Asian languages and new works written in European languages. References to English-language texts and professional journals are found throughout this book, including those in the Supplementary Reading Lists found at the end of many chapters. Considerable material is also available on the Internet. Readers can use a keyword approach to find data on virtually any aspect of Oriental medicine. Some useful sites include the following:

- Acupuncture Research and Resources Centre: arrc@exeter.ac.uk
- American Association of Oriental Medicine: http://www.aaom.org
- Health Information Library, Acupuncture: http://www.americanwholehealth.com/library/acupuncture/tcm.htm
- Medical Matrix: http://www.medmatrix.org
- National Acupuncture and Oriental Medicine Alliance: http://www.acuall.org
- Society for Acupuncture Research: http://www.acupunctureresearch.com
- Summary of Controlled Clinical Studies Demonstrating the Effectiveness of Acupuncture Treatment for Various Conditions: http://www.halcyon.com/dember/studies.html

- U.S. National Library of Medicine. Current Bibliographies in Medicine: Acupuncture: http://www.nlm.gov/puls/cbm/acupuncture.html
- U.S. National Institutes of Health National Center for Complementary and Alternative Medicine, Acupuncture Information and Resources: http://nccam.nih.gov
- Finally, a site aimed at the layperson: http://www.healingpeople.com

ORGANIZATION OF THIS BOOK

This book differs from others on Oriental medicine in several important ways. First, in addition to covering theory of practice as other books do, it also provides a "feel" for what the patient experiences when he or she consults a Chinese medicine specialist, reviews current research on acupuncture (with additional data on herbs and medical Qi gong research), reviews educational and legal guidelines for practice, and provides guidance for biomedical practitioners on locating Oriental medicine professional colleagues for the purpose of establishing referral relationships.

Second, each chapter has been written with the biomedical reader in mind. Specialist language and biomedical detail are offered beyond that to be expected in a layperson's introduction to Chinese medicine. Similarities and differences in approach to the body in health and disease, and to health care delivery, are developed comparatively to help biomedical readers understand the rationale behind Oriental medicine practices that might otherwise appear foreign or perhaps "old-fashioned."

Finally, each chapter has been written by a specialist. Represented among the authors are acupuncturists, herbalists, and Oriental medical doctors, biomedical practitioners, and researchers specialized in the study of Oriental medicine, and at least one journalist. The Editor has a combined background in human biological and anthropological research, and Chinese medicine research and practice.

The book is divided into four Parts. Part I introduces the basic theory, diagnostic procedures, and major interventive modalities of Chinese medicine. Chapter 2 provides a model that guides the reader through a presentation of Chinese medical theory and practice, and also permits immediate comparison with the same issues in biomedicine. Several variant practices, called *styles* in this book, are described, helping to contextualize data later in the book.

Chapter 3 summarizes the most common diagnostic procedures in Oriental medicine, including the famous analyses of tongue and multiple pulse positions. The author clearly links diagnosis to theory, and explains why observation, rather than measurement or "looking inside the body," is core to Oriental medicine assessment.

Chapters 4, 5, and 6 summarize the five most important modalities of Chinese medicine, including acupuncture (with moxibustion, cupping, and related techniques), herbology, diet therapy, bodywork therapy, and moving meditation (Qi gong and similar techniques).

It is interesting to note that although there are five major modalities, only one is widely known outside the profession in Western countries. This situation is so characteristic of the Western knowledge base that many people simply say "acupuncture" when they mean the whole medicine. In contrast, in China herbal therapy is the most important interventive modality. Herbal therapy is gaining attention rapidly in Western nations, but faces several challenges. First, these nations are accustomed to pharmaceutical drugs and have well-developed pharmaceutical delivery and social support systems, but lack similar support for herbalism.* Second, research concerning herbs is in its infancy, and yet it is well understood that misused herbs can be dangerous (certainly more so than acupuncture needles), and that potential exists for harmful interactions with pharmaceuticals. In this text, the Western primacy of acupuncture is revealed in the fact that acupuncture care is featured in most sections or chapters, and that most research data concern acupuncture. This pattern will change; it is already changing as monies for research on the other modalities of Chinese medicine increase, but for the moment, and in this book, readers should be aware that acupuncture receives "more than its fair share" of attention.

Part II contextualizes theory in practice. It begins

with a discussion of the conceptual and philosophical differences between Oriental medicine and biomedicine, embedded in a description of an office visit. The differences in perspective between Oriental medicine and biomedicine are not slight, for Oriental medicine focuses on the flow of Qi throughout the person-body, whereas biomedicine focuses on local malformation and malfunction of the physical body. Thus biomedicine is an anatomical and materialist system, organ- and cell-based, with its major modalities consisting of pharmaceutical drugs and surgery. Chinese medicine, in contrast, is a physiological system that emphasizes homeostasis, feedback, and the interdependency of parts. These differences bring in turn many other differences, developed further in Chapter 7.

Chapter 8 brings the reader into the treatment room and into the minds of several practitioners as they contemplate medical problems and treat particular patients. In most cases, both the patient and the patient's medical doctor also speak, providing rich case histories that demonstrate the healing potential of Oriental medicine.

In Chapter 9, we follow an anthropologist into three Chinese medicine clinics specialized in the treatment of substance abuse. Focusing on the organization of the clinic, and how this enhances the healing potential, the author underlines the point (see Chapter 12) that sociality is a crucial aspect of the delivery of Oriental medical care in the West.

Chapter 10, "A Day in the Life," features practitioners reflecting on their lives as specialists in Oriental medicine. Each piece is personal, well flavored, and insightful, helping readers to develop an enhanced appreciation of Oriental medicine practitioners as people and as healers.

Finally, Part II offers a photo essay showing aspects of the delivery of Oriental medical care. Because pictures are worth a thousand words, we refer readers directly to this section without further discussion.

Part III moves into a technical section reviewing research on Oriental medicine. The primary question to answer in this Part is "Does it work?" This seemingly simple question actually demands a multiplicity of approaches, including the epidemiological, social, physiological, biochemical, and clinical. To date, most research has focused on acupuncture and on physiological and clinical research, as reflected in this section.

The section begins with a tour de force reviewing physiological research on acupuncture (Chapter 11).

---

*Herbology is much better developed in Europe than in North America. The herbs used are mainly from European sources; use of Chinese herbs demands numerous changes in viewpoint and the addition of new herbal resources. For a fascinating crossover text analyzing European herbs from an Oriental medicine viewpoint, see Kenner D, Requena Y: *Botanical medicine: a European professional perspective,* Brookline, Mass, 1996, Paradigm Publications.

Important points to be taken from this chapter include (1) acupuncture affects the nervous system measurably, and probably (as we increasingly understand) by affecting production of neurotransmitters, and (2) the aspect of classical theory that states that acupuncture returns the body-person to "balance," and that needling the same point can remedy either excess or deficiency conditions, is borne out in physiological research and can be summarized under the rubrics of "homeostasis" and "the bimodal effect."

Chapter 12 reviews epidemiological data and patient opinion collected in surveys of American users of Oriental medicine. These surveys show the wide range of complaints of real patients who seek care and analyze the reasons why patients like the care, find it effective, and are generally willing to pay for it out of their own pockets.

Chapters 13 through 19 examine clinical research data on Oriental medicine, especially acupuncture care, for a range of complaints. Each chapter considers a large topic—pain, substance abuse, respiratory disease, digestive disease, women's reproductive health, depression, or central nervous system dysfunction—for which there is a reasonably large corpus of research data available for review. A similar format is used in each chapter, including a general introduction of the Oriental medicine approach to the problem, a review of the available research, a statement about which biomedical disorders within the larger category are most likely to reward Oriental medicine care, and referral suggestions. In addition, the chapters on pain, respiratory disease, and depression provide discussions of the problems involved in doing clinical research on acupuncture. Each chapter includes a generous bibliography.

Numerous potential topics—conditions regularly treated clinically—are not discussed in this Part, either because little research has yet been done on the subject or simply because an introductory text cannot cover all topics. However, to help fill the gap for interested readers, the list of supplementary readings in the beginning of Part III includes some research references to topics not otherwise covered.

Part IV completes the book with just two chapters. Chapter 20 develops discussions on how Oriental medical practitioners are trained, the process of professionalization, and how the different states in the United States license practice; the sidebar in Chapter 20 on p. 385 offers guidance for finding similar data for other nations. Finally, Chapter 21 offers guidance

How Did They Know?

Traditional acupoints have specific uses. How did the ancient Chinese figure this out? We do not know, but using today's technology, we can sometimes show that what the ancients discovered clinically is borne out in the laboratory. Using brain imaging technology, such as positron emission tomography (PET), single photon-emission computed tomography (SPECT), functional magnetic resonance imaging (fMRI), researchers have measured neural activity associated with needling of acupoints, and their findings are striking. For example, a point on the outer edge of the nail of the fifth toe (UB 67) is traditionally used to treat the eyes. Neural imaging studies show that when it is stimulated, the ocular region in the occiput "lights up" just as it does if the brain is stimulated by a flash of light. The same region is also activated when a point on another meridian used to treat the eyes is needled—GB 37, located anterior to the fibula on the lower leg. But when GB 43, a point on the top of the foot, is stimulated, the auditory region of the brain "lights up." We should not be too surprised to learn that GB 43 is traditionally used to treat the ears and improve hearing. As yet, however, we do not know how these points—distant from the eyes and ears, and located on two different meridians—do their work. In short, although we can "map" the points and the meridians, and are beginning to be able to technologically trace the effects of needling, we as yet know little about the landscape behind the map. (For more on this subject, see Stux R, Hammerschlag, editors: *Clinical acupuncture: scientific basis*, Berlin, 2001, Springer.) ∾

on referring patients and for developing collegial relationships between biomedical and Oriental medical practitioners. After Part V is a glossary and an appendix, which contains the complete text of the NIH consensus conference conclusions on acupuncture.

TERMINOLOGY ISSUES

The issue of "what to call things" or "how to represent ideas" looms large in the study of Chinese medicine because the theory of the medicine, the language(s) in which it is expressed, and the orthography of Chinese are so different from their European counterparts. These issues are deeply interconnected.

In Chinese languages, most words have only one syllable, and the meaning of the syllable is modified by changing the tone of the voice. Additionally, the distinction between nouns and verbs is blurred. These features result in a spoken language that depends heavily on context, and is extremely flexible and capable of creating multiple meanings in almost any utterance. Writing with ideographs, which are made up of segments each of which also has meaning, supports the spoken language by also permitting great multiplicity of meaning. Together, these features mean that "translating" written texts, especially ancient texts, presents special problems even when both base languages are Chinese. Translating into European languages, which demand so many more specifications, presents great challenges.

As one example, although the idea of "energy flowing" is easy to express in Chinese, is indeed implied by the structure of the language, and is deeply embedded in the unconscious of speakers of this flexible language, it is difficult both to express and even to think in European languages. Eurocentric speakers seek specificity—what does that word mean? What is really happening here? Many are impatient with a disvalued function, "ambiguity," whereas the very structure of Chinese makes ambiguity, or flexibility, inevitable. For the Chinese, this is not a problem; if life is dynamic and constantly changing, little can be specified outside of the moment, and that is in the nature of things. Chinese medicine, for example, does not deal in definable stand-alone "diseases" but in people-who-are-now-expressing-malfunction-of-a-recognizable-pattern. The Eurocentric thinker, however, wants to know, preferably now, and tends to shape reality in oppositional and judgmental opposites: right/wrong, on time/late, good/bad, modern/old-fashioned, present/absent, sick/well.

Within the field of Oriental medicine, these sorts of issues have led to many arguments about how to represent various ideas in Chinese medicine. When the problem is broadened—how to represent Chinese ideas to practitioners of a different medicine—the need for an appropriate terminology looms even larger. For the purposes of this book, we have established certain usages. These are summarized in Box 1-1, and while they

BOX 1-1

Terminological Standards and Codes Used in This Text

Capitalized	*Not Capitalized*
Chinese physiological concepts	Western physiological concepts
Functional organs	Anatomical organs

Italicized
Chinese terms not widely known in Western countries

Acupoint Terminology
Organ Code with Number (Chinese name, English name[s])

will serve us here, readers should not be surprised if in referring to another book on Oriental medicine they find other standards in use.

Major Chinese physiological concepts such as Qi, Yin and Yang (complementary opposites), Blood (a fairly material expression of Qi, not the same thing as the blood of bioscience), Mind, Shen (usually translated as Spirit), and Meridians/Channels are all capitalized to signal their special meanings and distinctive link to Chinese medicine. However, some concepts, such as "balance" and "stress" are not capitalized because they are Western attempts to translate more or less shared concepts from the Chinese.

The names of many of the body's organs are very similar in Chinese medicine and in biomedicine, that is, they *sound* similar but, in fact, *mean* quite different things. We distinguish these concepts by referring to the localized, solid, material organs of Western anatomy as "anatomical organs," and to the dynamic complex organ systems of Chinese medicine as "functional Organs." We signal the difference in writing by using a capital letter for functional Organs (i.e., Heart, Kidney). Although the differences will be further developed in Chapter 2 and elsewhere, a brief comment will make the need for a special signal clear. The Heart in Chinese medicine subsumes not only the beating pump in the middle of the chest, but also all the blood vessels, and both the Mind and Spirit *(Shen)*. However, it does not subsume Blood, which is shared among several functional Organ systems. The Kidney subsumes not only the bean-shaped anatomical organs in the lumbar region but also the Essence inherited from one's ancestors, the Marrow (which makes up the substance of the spinal cord and brain as well as the centers of bones), the bones, ears, and what biomedicine specifies as the endocrinological and immune systems. If this combination of features seems surprising now, we hope that by the end of the book it will make good sense. The names of the Meridians (also called Channels) are also capitalized, thus Urinary Bladder Channel, Chong Meridian (or *Mai*).

Several concepts common in the practice of Chinese medicine have been popularized in the West, such as Qi and Yin and Yang. However, other concepts remain mysterious to most, and these usually are treated as foreign words, that is, *italicized*. Some examples in this book include the three *jiaos* (the three-part division of the trunk into upper, middle, and lower "burners"), the *jing* (Essence, inherited from one's ancestors), and *zhi* (Will, stored in the Kidneys). Notice that the English term, such as Will, is capitalized to help signal its distinct conceptualization in Oriental medicine.

Every acupoint has a specific name in Chinese. In an effort to simplify learning for Western people, and to improve interlanguage communication, all these points have today been given code names consisting of an abbreviation of the Organ followed by the number of the point. Thus St-36 means Stomach point number 36, called in Chinese Zu San Li and translated in English as Leg Three Miles. In this book, the numerical name is usually listed with the Chinese name in parentheses, thus St-36 *(Zu San Li)*.

One more terminology issue demands attention before we can move into the body of this book. Oriental medicine is practiced in the West "in translation," and it is not surprising that different scholars interpret Chinese (or Korean or Japanese) terms somewhat differently. The arguments in support of one or another translation are too technical for this text. However, it is important for readers to know that certain terms are more or less synonymous, or represent the same sort of finding or action by practitioners. Contributors have been encouraged to use the terminology that they prefer.

Some Organs and Meridians are known by more than one name. Thus Triple Heater, Triple Burner, and San Jiao all refer to the same Organ, one that does not have an anatomical counterpart but is concerned with water metabolism throughout the body. Similarly, authors may refer to the Ren or Conception Vessel, the Du or Governing Vessel, the Colon or Large Intestine, the Pericardium or Heart Protector.

Given the focus on "balance" in Chinese medicine, with a major goal of medical care being to "bring the patient back into balance," most expressions of malfunction also are framed in terms of balance. The words chosen to express the need and the process of amelioration vary considerably.

For example, if the patient seems to be unbalanced in the direction of too much, terms such as excess, stagnation, overacting, repletion, stuckness, and the like are used, and the appropriate treatment might require that the excess be drained, sedated, controlled, or coursed. In reading such terms, it should be noted that these are English efforts to translate Chinese concepts that do not translate easily. For example, if a person or a point is "sedated," the observer or reader should not expect that the patient becomes sleepy or excessively calm. The therapeutic task is merely to release the excess, to return the patient to homeostasis, not to push the patient in the opposite direction.

If the patient seems to be unbalanced in the direction of too little, terms such as deficiency, depletion, vacuity, and the like are used. Treatment aims to tonify, reinforce, supplement, fortify, and so forth.

ENVOI

Listing differences reinforces that the medicine you will read about is not a strange version of biomedicine but a completely different medicine with a long-separate history. Today both medicines work side by side, a situation that demands an understanding and appreciation of both. Why? Because despite differences of perception and vocabulary, both systems are effective at treating malfunction and sickness and in relieving suffering. Because this is so, it is worthwhile to try to understand Chinese medicine . . . on its own terms.

A journey of a thousand miles begins with the first step.

TRADITIONAL CHINESE SAYING

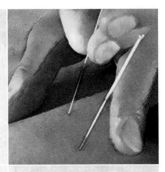

The Theory of Oriental Medicine

PETER ECKMAN

Acupuncture and Oriental medicine (OM) are based on a different paradigm than biomedicine, and although this chapter elaborates on the implications of starting from an alternative paradigm, it is important to stress that neither paradigm (nor its corresponding medical system) is more correct than the other. They are complementary rather than contradictory world views. Indeed, there are certain therapeutic procedures that are shared by both systems. A good example is the virtual identity of Western trigger point therapy, which uses dry needling of sensitive spots, and the treatment of Ah Shi or "ouch" points in traditional acupuncture. There also are many gray areas where both biomedi-

cine and OM thought have contributed to hybrid types of therapy. For example, scalp acupuncture uses the Western neuroanatomical mapping of the various functional regions of the cerebral cortex and other parts of the brain to select zones on the overlying scalp for acupuncture stimulation. It was originated by Dr. Jiao in 1965.[1] The Chinese government has explicitly recognized this unprecedented situation by proclaiming the "Three Roads Policy" whereby both biomedicine and OM are encouraged to continue to develop according to their unique paradigms, while those interested in fostering an integration of biomedicine and OM practices are likewise given equal encouragement.[2]

A BRIEF HISTORY OF ACUPUNCTURE AND ORIENTAL MEDICINE

But is acupuncture (and for the moment, this term is used as a shorthand for the unwieldy "acupuncture and OM") a uniquely Chinese phenomenon? For the novice reader, a very brief history is presented first; it should be noted that a proper understanding of the following chapters, culminating in Chapter 21, is impossible outside of the historical context. The standard texts on the history of acupuncture are those written by Lu and Needham[3] and Unschuld.[2] Recently, Eckman[4] incorporated the history of acupuncture's spread throughout the Orient, and subsequently to the West.

The practice of acupuncture can be traced back to neolithic times, and archaeological relics testifying to the antiquity of its practice have been found in both China and Korea.[3,5,6] For centuries, if not millennia, it was transmitted as an oral tradition, and the first book to systematically describe its practice, *The Yellow Emperor's Inner Classic,* or *Nei Jing* in Chinese, was probably compiled around 100 BCE.[2,3] From these oral and written traditions, acupuncture and its allied practices experienced two kinds of growth. First and foremost, successive generations of practitioners and theoreticians elaborated many new developments, but these were added onto the existing structure rather than replacing older ideas as is typical of new developments in biomedicine. The second growth pattern was geo-graphical, with acupuncture spreading first throughout Asia and subsequently to Europe and the Western hemisphere, so that today it is practiced in virtually every country throughout the world. As would be expected, regional differences in approach developed with its geographical spread, so that in addition to the layers of traditional teachings that have accumulated over time, there are also various relatively distinct styles of practice including the previously mentioned Western medical and hybrid approaches.

How is one to make sense of such a complex field without devoting an enormous amount of time to its study? The following models may be of some help. The first is simply a classification scheme whereby the various styles of practice are grouped into three categories: traditional, Western, and mixed (Table 2-1).

Because this book is primarily about the traditional styles of practice (which are defined by their common adherence to the vitalistic paradigm, i.e., a concept that the flow of Life Energy can be altered therapeutically), before discussing those it is appropriate to mention a few points about the other categories of acupuncture practice. Auriculotherapy, developed by Dr. Paul Nogier in France, uses needling or other stimulation of points on the ear as its sole therapeutic intervention.[7] Nogier's treatise on auriculotherapy was first published in 1969. The Chinese began incorporating ear acupuncture as a common practice only after acknowledging Nogier's discoveries. A more up-to-date account of Nogier's work is cited in the bibliography.[7] Although it was developed empirically,

TABLE 2-1

Styles of Acupuncture and Oriental Medicine Practice

Traditional styles	Western styles	Mixed styles
TCM, China MT, Japan	Auriculotherapy, France Trigger point therapy, United States	Scalp acupuncture, China Ryodoraku, Japan
Eight Constitutions (KCA), Korea		Electroacupuncture according to Voll (EAV), Germany
KHA, Korea SEL, France Five Element (LA), England		

Adapted from Eckman P: *In the footsteps of the Yellow Emperor: tracing the history of traditional acupuncture,* San Francisco, 1996, Cypress Book Co., p. xiv.
TCM, Traditional Chinese medicine; *MT,* Meridian therapy; *KCA,* Korean constitutional acupuncture; *KHA,* Korean hand acupuncture; *SEL,* six energetic levels; *LA,* Leamington acupuncture.

and uses Western medical concepts of anatomy, physiology, and pathology to guide the selection of points for treatment, it was subsequently incorporated into the practice of traditional Chinese medicine (TCM, the contemporary style of acupuncture most widely practiced in China) and now almost all TCM texts include information on ear acupuncture. Chapter 14 discusses drug detoxification protocols using acupuncture, which are essentially applications of auriculotherapy. The other example cited in Table 2-1 of a Western style of "acupuncture" is trigger point therapy, a procedure that was developed in the 20th century independent of any Oriental vitalistic theory. Trigger point therapy was mainly developed by Travell and Simons[8] between 1950 and 1983. Baldry's text[9] is an excellent presentation of the relationship of acupuncture and trigger point therapy, and the historical background of the latter. Interestingly, however, its methodology was described 1300 years ago by Sun Simiao in China as the treatment of "Ah Shi" or "ouch" points, which are now classified as one of the eight most commonly used points in TCM acupuncture.[10] The mixed styles of acupuncture share aspects of Oriental theory by definition. Scalp acupuncture, however, relies heavily on Western neuroanatomy, whereas the other two styles cited in Table 2-1 incorporate measurement of the electrical potential or conductivity at points on the skin, and this information is then used in choosing points for treatment.

ARE ACUPUNCTURE AND ORIENTAL MEDICINE SCIENTIFIC?

All of these styles of acupuncture practice have demonstrated their efficacy empirically—clinically—but there is a unique aspect of the traditional styles that accounts for their special appeal to those who believe that there is something lacking in the materialist conceptualization that provides the paradigm for biomedicine. It has been argued that Western medicine is the only "scientific" medical system for this very reason; however, some highly respected historians of science and sinologists have concluded that OM has also developed as a science, although it has developed from idealist as opposed to materialist axioms. For example, Needham[11] described the inductive methodology typical of Oriental medical thought as an expression of correlative thinking, a way of looking at the universe in which "conceptions are not subsumed under one another, but placed side by side in a pattern, and in which things influence one another not by acts of mechanical causation but by a kind of inductance." Learning to think inductively, to look for patterns rather than causal agents, is one of the major tasks in mastering traditional acupuncture. This task involves a kind of cognitive shift that can be difficult for those accustomed to Western scientific culture. Although a staunch believer in Western science himself, Needham observed that, "Chinese coordinative thinking was not primitive thinking in the sense that it was an alogical or pre-logical chaos in which anything could be the cause of anything else . . . it was a picture of an extremely and precisely ordered universe in which things 'fitted' so exactly that you could not insert a hair between them." As early as 1974 Porkert[12] carried this reasoning one step further in characterizing Chinese medicine as a "science" that "defines data on the basis of the inductive and synthetic mode of cognition." In 1995, Porkert[13] concluded that "Acu-moxi-therapy constitutes a rational method of therapy within the system of scientific Chinese medicine. Clearly Oriental "science" is different from Western "science"; the former is inductive and synthetic, whereas the latter is deductive and analytic. However, together they provide complementary rather than antagonistic explanations. What OM gives up in forfeiting explanations based on anatomy and physiology, for example, it recoups in addressing those areas of human experience most poorly understood in Western scientific terms (e.g., the realm of mental and spiritual life to which it attaches great significance). In Western medical thought, spirituality is in the domain of religion, which is outside the realm of science, whereas in OM these are seen more as opposite poles of a single continuum. Another way of phrasing this is that in OM there is no Cartesian mind-body split.

THE CIRCLE MODEL

If OM is to be given serious consideration as being scientific, then it must share some common attributes with the scientific biomedical system. Table 2-2 introduces a model, called the "Circle model," as one attempt to specify the structures or components necessary to any scientific medical system. The Circle model elaborates ideas first proposed by Liu Yanchi.[14] An early version of the model appeared in Kutchins and

TABLE 2-2

The Circle Model

Categories	Western medicine	Oriental medicine
1. Axioms and laws (Paradigm)	Physics and chemistry (materialism)	Energetics (Vitalism)
2. Essential functions	Physiology	12 Officials or organ systems
3. Essential structures	Anatomy	Meridian theory
4. Causes of illness	Etiology	Causal mechanisms
5. Nature of disharmony	Pathology	Exogenous and endogenous pathogens
6. Clinical investigation	Examination	Four-part traditional examination
7. Case analysis	Diagnosis	Pattern differentiation
8. Treatment	Therapy—various	Acupuncture, herbal prescription, diet, exercise, massage, meditation . . .

Adapted from Eckman P: *In the footsteps of the Yellow Emperor: tracing the history of traditional acupuncture,* San Francisco, 1996, Cypress Book Co., pp. 2, 9.

Eckman[15]; the version presented here is described in greater detail in the more recent publication by Eckman.[4] This model is used in this chapter to help readers recognize the parallels between Western and Oriental medical thought. The model makes it easier for Westerners to understand OM and provides a convenient format for presenting the core concepts of OM.

The Circle model describes the structure of any complete, rational medical system. At position One is the paradigm (explanatory model, "theory"), a unified conceptualization that underlies and nourishes or informs all the other aspects of the given medical system. In OM, the concept of vital energy or *Qi* (a Chinese word pronounced "chee"; also often printed as *ch'i*) provides an emblem of this paradigm that is outside the realm of physics and chemistry. The concepts of OM cannot be reduced to biomedical or bioscientific categories; there is always something intangible at the root of OM, such as "vital energy," "spirit," or any other indication of OM's close connection with the philosophy called Daoism from and with which it evolved. OM has three primary philosophical roots: Daoism, Confucianism, and Naturalism. These correspond sequentially to the three realms of Heaven, Human, and Earth, which form a principle that extends

throughout all of OM. The realm of Heaven is the least tangible of the three, associating it with Daoist thought.[4] Biomedicine, which is built on a materialist paradigm, is similarly based on the belief in underlying intangible phenomena: the probability functions of quantum mechanics are accepted as an accurate description of the nature of subatomic reality, but they are by definition intangible.

Positions Two and Three on the Circle describe the makeup of a healthy living organism—a human being. In OM, function is more important than structure, so the twelve Officials or Organ systems are presented, later in this chapter, from a functional viewpoint before their Meridian or structural associations are discussed. This is opposite to the traditional Western approach where medical students learn the body parts (anatomy) before delving into their functions (physiology). All the positions on the Circle introduced so far relate to the normal healthy organism, and it is important to indicate that OM has a different concept of health and illness than does biomedicine. In the latter system, illnesses are defined states that, potentially at least, have unique names and causes, in addition to pathology. In OM, however, any deviation in positions Two or Three on the Circle (i.e., any abnormalities of function or structure) are by definition states of ill health or illness, even if they are totally devoid of "objective" somatic pathology.

Next are positions Four and Five on the Circle, the equator, which divides the top half (state of health or balance) from the bottom half (state of ill health or imbalance). Position Four includes all factors that can upset or create imbalances in the organism. Western medicine recognizes various categories of etiology: infectious, degenerative, hereditary, immunologic, traumatic, and so forth. OM organizes these "causal factors" into three categories: exogenous, endogenous, and miscellaneous. Whereas biomedicine posits the basic cause of most disease as being an invasion from without (e.g., germs, toxins, allergens), OM places more emphasis on the maintenance of health from within. Health is said to be maintained by the activity of Righteous Qi (*Zheng Qi* in Chinese, also known as Antipathogenic, Correct, or Normal Qi), which repels any incursion by pathogenic factors known as Evil Qi (*Xie Qi* in Chinese, also known as Pathogenic or Heteropathic Qi). Position Five shows the results of these pathogenic factors—the pathologies induced by them. In Western medicine, etiology and pathology are quite sharply differentiated, whereas in OM there is much less of a distinction between the two at this central horizontal axis of the Circle. Indeed, the same term, for example, *Wind* or *Dampness,* may be the name for both the cause and the kind of imbalance it induces in the organism. For example, Wind as an etiological agent is a form of Xie Qi, whereas Wind as a pathological state in addition to being a form of Xie Qi, is also a pattern of disharmony, or *Zheng,* which is discussed at Position Seven of the Circle. Thus both the etiological and pathological states called Wind are classified as type of Xie Qi. The etiological aspect may be emphasized by the use of the term *yin* (a homophone of the Yin in Yin/Yang, written with an entirely different character) meaning causal agent, while the pathological aspect may be emphasized by the use of the term *Zheng* (a homophone of the Zheng in Zheng Qi, also written with a different character), meaning pattern or syndrome.

Positions Six and Seven represent the realm of clinical practice, starting with the encounter of patient and physician in the examination at position Six (see Chapter 3). Whereas biomedicine has become increasingly reliant on technology to improve the collection of data (e.g., chemical and biochemical analysis of every bodily fluid, imaging using ultrasound, radio-

graphs, radioisotopes, and magnetic resonance), OM in each of its traditional styles relies only on the data gathered by the practitioner's senses: looking, listening, smelling, palpating, and questioning. The "four examinations" are strictly codified (listening and smelling are curiously treated together as one kind of examination*) and because they are both subjective (always gathered by the practitioner's sensory acuity), and interactive (practitioner and patient are in constant communication during treatment), researchers have found it necessary to develop alternate assessment approaches to replace the conventional double-blind and placebo designs used to verify clinical perception in biomedicine (see Chapters 11, 13, 15, and 18). The practitioner of OM is involved in an endless quest to develop awareness, sensitivity, and interpersonal rapport, all qualities that have contributed to the high level of Western interest in OM by patients (see Chapter 12) and practitioners alike, the latter of whom aspire to incorporate some form of spiritual growth into their experience of being in the healing profession (see Chapters 7, 8, and 10).

Position Seven takes the data from the examination and uses them to determine the diagnosis. Again, biomedicine places great emphasis on being able to name the disease, whereas in OM the pattern of imbalance underlying the symptomatology is given more weight. For example, two patients might have rheumatoid arthritis in Western medical terms, but their Oriental diagnoses could be as different as Deficiency of Kidney Qi in one case and Excess Liver Fire in the other. OM does have a concept of naming specific diseases,† but this is seen as secondary to identifying the Energetic imbalance that allows the disease to manifest. This distinction becomes even more important in the final position, treatment, where it is expressed as the difference between "roots and branches."

Position Eight is treatment. Just as biomedicine has many modalities of therapy (pharmaceutical medications, surgery, physical therapy, nutrition, psychotherapy, and so forth), so too has OM, including herbal medications, acupuncture, moxibustion, massage, therapeutic exercises, and diet, all discussed in later chapters (see Chapters 4 through 6). In this chapter, the discussion of treatment focuses on acupunc-

---

*The Chinese term *wen* refers to both acoustic and olfactory perception.
†Naming diseases is called *bian bing* in Chinese, while naming their underlying Energetic imbalance is called *bian zheng.*

ture, the most popular of these modalities in the Western world.

The purpose of acupuncture treatment, in addition to alleviating the patient's symptoms (i.e., the branch diagnosis), is to reestablish normal Energy (Qi) flow and balance so that patients can heal themselves, with nature's help, from whatever affliction has developed as a result of Energy imbalance or blockage (i.e., their root diagnosis). Just how acupuncture treatment is able to influence Energy flow and balance is as much of a mystery as is the nature of the Vital Energy itself. Thus position Eight harkens back to position One of the Circle, forming its vertical axis, and signifying its unitarian concept. If the Energy flow is balanced, the twelve Organs and their Meridians will perform normally, there will be sufficient Righteous Qi to repel or expel any Evil Qi, and so the patient will have nature's support in recuperation from previous ailments.

Bioscientists can study the epiphenomena that accompany acupuncture treatment—the neurological, neurohumoral, and endocrinological changes it may provoke—but will never be able to fully explain how acupuncture works because it is ultimately rooted in an intangible Vital Force that, by definition, is beyond the realm of physics and chemistry. Thus to understand traditional acupuncture, one must "suspend disbelief" in phenomena outside Western scientific categories, and judge this Oriental science by the consistency of its own internal logic (as outlined in the Circle) and by the results it provides in the hands of well-trained practitioners. That this practice is compelling is shown both by rapid increases in use of acupuncture in Western nations and by increasing amounts of research recently publicly assessed at a National Institutes of Health consensus conference. Their encouraging conclusions are listed in the Appendix.

BASIC ENERGETIC THEORY: QI, YIN, AND YANG

With this presentation of the framework and general outline of the components involved in the practice of traditional acupuncture in mind, let us study each in greater depth, the goal being a coherent exposition of the core teachings of OM. We start at position One with the concept of Qi, a Chinese word that can be variously translated as breath, energy, steam, or gas. As a technical term in OM, it is perhaps best translated as

Vital Force—the equivalent of the "vis medicatrix naturae" of homeopathy, and common in 19th century biomedical thinking as well. Qi can be both a generic term, indicating the ultimate principle behind all of nature, and a specific aspect of nature, for example, the Vital Energy that moves the Blood in the human body. In this latter context, the organism is viewed as an expression of the dynamic balance of two components, Energy and Substance, or Qi and Blood. The general theory for interpreting phenomena that express two complementary inseparable aspects is called the theory of Yin and Yang. These technical terms, which share a common etymology in Chinese with the word Qi,[4] can also be translated in various ways depending on the context. In essence they depict the difference between the shady and sunny sides of a hill, an image that provides the following associations: Yin is shady, therefore dark, cold, and inactive; Yang is sunny, therefore bright, hot, and active. Various laws describing the relationship of Yin and Yang can be understood from this image of the hill, which changes as the sun moves over it from dawn to dusk:

1. Yin and Yang always exist together. Everything consists of variable proportions of these two.
2. There is always some Yin within Yang and vice versa. The sunny side has bits of shade, and the shady side has its patches of light.
3. Yin and Yang are in opposition. The sunny side gets hot and dry, while the shady side gets cold and damp.
4. Yin and Yang are always waxing and waning. At dawn almost the whole hill is dark, while at noon it is almost all sunny.
5. Yin transforms into Yang and vice versa. The sunny side in the morning becomes the shady side in the afternoon.

In the human organism, these same five laws of Yin and Yang can be observed, whether in the relationship of Energy *(Qi)* and Blood *(Xue),* Nutrition *(Ying)* and Protection *(Wei),* or any other bipartite analysis. Yin and Yang theory is used for both classifying data (e.g., the findings on examination) and for guiding treatment (choice of Acupoints and methods of stimulation), because the goal is always to foster the natural harmony and balance of Yin and Yang. If Yin is excessive (causing the organism to become too cold), then Yang (which is necessarily relatively deficient in this situation) can be stimulated (causing the organism to become warmer). Nature usually takes care of adjusting this balance, but in a state of illness the natural mechanisms may malfunction, and it is just here where this elementary law of OM can be used to promote a return to health by a simple stimulation.

This introduction to Yin and Yang should be sufficient to understand its general application and to appreciate how fundamental it is in all of OM. It is the rationale underlying homeostasis, and many parallels can be found in Western medical thought (e.g., the sympathetic and parasympathetic nervous systems, the use of antipyretics in fevers). Two specific elaborations of the theory of Yin and Yang that are emphasized in different styles of acupuncture practice are mentioned next, because a knowledge of their terminology is essential for developing even a cursory understanding of how traditional acupuncture is used clinically by different practitioners and in different countries.

SIX STAGES AND EIGHT PRINCIPLES THEORY

The first special theory of Yin and Yang can be called either the "six stages" or the "six levels" theory. The former term is more common in herbal medicine, whereas the latter is more common in acupuncture, but both are based on the same idea: Yin and Yang can each be divided into three aspects or phases. Focusing on acupuncture theory, the levels of Yin and Yang are the origin of the theory of the twelve Meridians along which the acupuncture Points are located (Table 2-3).

The Yin Meridians flow (transport Qi) from below

to above and can be divided into Lesser Yin, Greater Yin, and Fading Yin levels. Each level is represented by a Great Meridian with one branch on the lower extremities and another branch on the upper extremities; thus there are six Yin Meridians made up of three Yin Great Meridians. In the same way, the Yang Meridians flow from above to below and can be divided into Lesser Yang, Greater Yang, and Bright Yang levels, each with its own Great Meridian composed of one upper extremity and one lower extremity branch. Thus there are six Yang Meridians made up of three Yang Great Meridians. In total there are twelve Meridians (each connected to a major internal Organ) made up of six Great Meridians. The Great Meridians relate to the specific levels of Yin and Yang, each of which has a characteristic description relative to technical parameters of the evolution of Energy in space and time. For example, the Yang Energy that is closest to the surface of the body is the Greater Yang; the Yin Energy that is quantitatively the least intense is the Fading Yin; and the Yin Energy that has just developed is the Lesser Yin. These technicalities are too advanced for an introductory book but are presented to explain one rationale for the effect of various Meridians and Points on the different Energy imbalances that lead to every form of illness. The unifying concept is that of "resonance." For example, an imbalance of Yang at the surface of the body resonates with the Greater Yang Meridians. Thus it is along these Meridians that specific Points are stimulated to encourage nature to restore balance or homeostasis.

The model of the Six Energetic Levels (SEL) of Yin and Yang is especially important in the style of practice characteristic of the French Medical Acupuncture Association's teachings. Because this style forms the core of its teachings, this model is also used by North American physician-acupuncturists trained in programs coordinated by the American Academy of Medical Acupuncture (AAMA). The AAMA is largely composed of graduates of the continuing education course in acupuncture sponsored by the University of California–Los Angeles School of Medicine. Its curriculum was principally developed by Helms,[16] whose own training in acupuncture occurred in France between 1974 and 1978 under several leaders of the French Medical Acupuncture Association (l'AFA).

The second special theory of Yin and Yang is called *ba gang bian zheng* in Chinese, which means "differentiating syndromes by the Eight Principles." There are various popular alternative English translations of this Chinese phrase including Eight Principal Syn-

TABLE 2-3

The Great Meridians

Yin-Yang character	Functional organ	Location
Greater Yin—	Lung	Arm
Taiyin	Spleen	Leg
Lesser Yin—	Heart	Arm
Shaoyin	Kidney	Leg
Fading Yin—	Pericardium	Arm
Jueyin	Liver	Leg
Bright Yang—	Large Intestine	Arm
Yangming	Stomach	Leg
Greater Yang—	Small Intestine	Arm
Taiyang	Urinary Bladder	Leg
Lesser Yang—	Triple Warmer—	Arm
Shaoyang	*San Jiao*	
	Gall Bladder	Leg

dromes, Eight Leading Principles, Eight Parameters, Eight Principal Patterns, and Eight Diagnostic Categories. All are acceptable choices. For citations of usage, see Eckman[4] (p. 181). This methodology is central to the style of acupuncture currently most widely known in the West; it is the one promoted by the Chinese government under the name TCM.

The Eight Principles are Yin, Yang, Cold, Hot, Deficient, Excess, Interior, and Exterior. These form two groups as follows: (1) Yin, Cold, Deficient, Interior, and (2) Yang, Hot, Excess, Exterior.

By using these sets of Yin and Yang descriptors, each patient's imbalances can be classified into various patterns that can then be addressed by the appropriate prescription of acupuncture Points and methods of stimulation. In practice, the diagnosis should be carried one step further—to either the Organ or Meridian or Great Meridian involved—to fully specify the pattern and correctly choose the treatment.

This Eight Principle approach was developed rather late in the historical evolution of acupuncture in China mainly as an adaptation of herbal prescription theory, and so it is not used, for example, by most acupuncturists in Japan. Japan acquired its knowledge of acupuncture from China long before the development of the Eight Principles theory, so Japanese tradi-tional acupuncturists are more likely to choose a different paradigm, most often either Five Element theory or Extra Meridians theory.

FIVE ELEMENTS THEORY

After Yin and Yang, the next most widely known and clinically used theory of Energetics is that of the Five Elements. The Five Elements is a translation of the Chinese term *Wu Xing*. Many authors have objected to this translation as being inaccurate, and insist on a more process-oriented translation, such as Five Movements or Five Phases. Both connotations are actually present in the Chinese use of the term *Wu Xing*. Its translation as Five Elements has a long history of prior usage and is retained here, but the reader is encouraged to always envision the other connotations whenever the term Five Elements is used. These Elements (also called Phases) are thought of as descriptive labels to name categories of phenomena that resonate with each other, and not as primordial substances (Table 2-4). The Five Elements are Wood, Fire, Earth, Metal, and Water. To illustrate the idea of resonance, it is commonly observed that patients who are irritable tend to shout, have a greenish complexion and a wiry quality

TABLE 2-4

Correlates of the Five Elements*

	Wood	Fire	Earth	Metal	Water
Direction	East	South	Center	West	North
Climate	Wind	Heat	Damp	Dry	Cold
Flavor	Sour	Bitter	Sweet	Pungent	Salty
Zang organ	Liver	Heart Pericardium	Spleen	Lung	Kidneys
Fu organ	Gall Bladder	Small Intestine, Three Heater	Stomach	Large Intestine	Urinary Bladder
Tissue	Tendons	Vessels	Flesh	Skin	Bones
Sense organ	Eyes	Tongue	Mouth	Nose	Ears
Emotion	Anger	Joy	Sympathy	Grief	Fear
Odor	Rancid	Scorched	Fragrant	Rotten	Putrid
Sound	Shouting	Laughing	Singing	Weeping	Groaning
Color	Green	Red	Yellow	White	Blue
Season	Spring	Summer	Late summer	Autumn	Winter
Stage	Birth	Growth	Transformation	Decline	Storage

From Eckman P: *In the footsteps of the Yellow Emperor: tracing the history of traditional acupuncture,* San Francisco, 1996, Cypress Book Co., p. 16.
*Not all compilations of the Five Element associations are in agreement. This list reflects the associations that are made in Leamington Acupuncture (LA). The most controversial entries are the colors for Wood (often stated to be Blue-Green) and Water (often stated to be Black), and the emotion for Earth (often stated to be pensiveness or "overthinking").

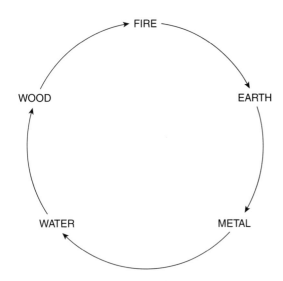

Figure 2-1 The Creative *(Sheng)* Cycle of the Five Elements. This cycle flows clockwise (the apparent direction of the sun through the Heavens) and illustrates how each Element engenders the succeeding Element, much as a parent creates (and nourishes) a child. Thus an alternate name for the relationships depicted in this cycle is the "Law of Mother-Son." From Eckman P: *In the footsteps of the Yellow Emperor: tracing the history of traditional acupuncture,* San Francisco, 1996, Cypress Book Co.

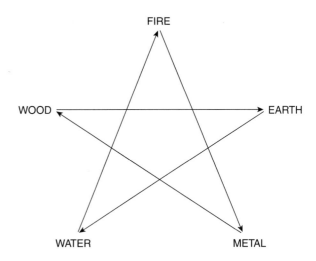

Figure 2-2 The Control *(Ke)* Cycle of the Five Elements. Each Element controls the one located two positions further along in a clockwise direction and is in turn controlled by the one located two positions prior in a counter-clockwise direction. For example, Fire controls Metal but is controlled by Water. From Eckman P: *In the footsteps of the Yellow Emperor: tracing the history of traditional acupuncture,* San Francisco, 1996, Cypress Book Co.

to their pulses, and tend to respond favorably to stimulation of Points on the Meridians of the Liver and Gall Bladder. This is because these emotions, voice qualities, facial colors, pulse types, and Organs are all associated with the Wood element, to which they resonate. This is one way in which nature indicates the quality of Energetic imbalance present, which in turn suggests an appropriate acupunctural response to the practitioner who perceives these resonant diagnostic signs. It does not matter whether the symptom or illness is (biomedically speaking) a migraine headache or a case of hepatitis; the underlying Energetic imbalance might be redressed by the identical treatment.

Like Yin and Yang theory, Five Element theory also can be described in terms of various laws. Of these, the following two have the widest clinical application:

1. Every Element is created by another Element (called its Mother) and creates in turn yet another Element (called its Son or Child). This is commonly known as the Mother-Son (Mother-Child) law, and is depicted as a creative cycle (Figure 2-1) that has neither beginning nor end.

2. Every Element is kept in check or controlled by another Element and in turn controls yet another Element. This is commonly depicted as a control cycle (Figure 2-2) that likewise has neither beginning nor end.

Clinically these two laws may be used by applying the following principles. To strengthen the Energy of a weak Element, the Meridians of the Element itself can be tonified (strengthened), the Meridians of the Element's Mother can be tonified, or the Meridians of the Element's Controller can be sedated (weakened). Conversely, to weaken the Energy of an overly strong Element, the Meridians of the Element itself can be sedated, the Meridians of the Element's Son can be sedated, or the Meridians of the Element's Controller can be tonified. These examples are more advanced than the general introductory level of this text but should serve to familiarize readers with the language and mode of thought used by many acupuncturists trained primarily in either Japanese or Korean traditions, both of which commonly emphasize Five Element theory, and both of which are practiced far from their homelands.

TABLE 2-5

Five Element Associations Emphasized in Leamington-Style Acupuncture

	Wood *(Hun)*	Fire *(Shen)*	Earth *(Yi)*	Metal *(Po)*	Water *(Zhi)*
Mental	Inspiration Creativity	Concentration Attention	Recollection Memory	Instinct Reaction	Determination Will
Emotional	Anger	Joy Excitement	Sympathy Anxiety Worry	Grief	Fear Fright
Spiritual	Benevolence	Propriety	Loyalty	Righteousness	Wisdom

Another Five Element style of acupuncture, sometimes called Worsley-style after its most famous teacher, but more appropriately labeled Leamington Acupuncture (LA) after the school in England where it was initially collated, is largely derived from Japanese teachings. It is widely practiced in both the United States and Europe. This style is distinctive for emphasizing the mental, emotional, and spiritual resonances that are part of Five Element theory (Table 2-5).

Contemporary Western medicine recognizes that psychosomatic mechanisms may be involved in many common ailments, but has no general approach to treatment in such cases. OM, on the other hand, specifically associates individual mental, emotional, and spiritual faculties with each of the Five Elements. When these faculties are malfunctioning at the same time that the other resonances of the associated Element (i.e., coloration, odor, and vocal quality) are also manifesting themselves, that Element is said to be out of balance Energetically. Acupuncture treatment to restore Elemental balance can not only alleviate psychosomatic complaints, but at the same time can lead to improvements in mood, cognition, and a general sense of well-being. The focus of LA on these areas is certainly one reason for its popularity in the West, where individuality and personal growth are socially valued more than in many Asian cultures, where fitting into the social group occupies a higher priority.

BASIC SUBSTANCES THEORY

Although the various styles of traditional acupuncture mentioned so far differ in their relative emphasis on either Yin/Yang or Five Element theory, it is im-

portant to note that both theories are recognized and used to some degree in each of these styles of practice. They are alternative ways of assessing the state of balance or imbalance in the Qi. Another method commonly used subdivides the unitary category Qi (in its generic sense) into its separate constituents, the building blocks or Basic Substances of the organism, as follows:

1. Qi or Vital Energy (in its more specific sense), which is responsible for movement, protection, transformation, and warmth
2. Blood (*Xue* in Chinese), which is responsible for nourishment
3. Essence (*Jing* in Chinese), which is responsible for reproduction and development
4. Body Fluids (*Jin Ye* in Chinese), which are responsible for lubrication and cooling
5. Spirit (*Shen* in Chinese), which is responsible for consciousness and personality

This differentiation of imbalances into patterns of the Basic Substances is the form in which TCM would usually interpret the same mental, emotional, and spiritual problems that are addressed by Five Element theory in LA. There are yet more ways of differentiating individual subcomponents of Qi,* each of which can serve as a focus for pattern discrimination, leading in turn to different strategies in acupuncture treatment, but the previous discussion has sufficiently explained basic Energetic theory. Position 2 on the Circle in Table 2-2 is the next topic.

---

*Porkert[12] lists 32 distinctions or types of Qi, but these do not form a commonly used clinical rubric for differentiating patterns of imbalance.

BOX 2-1

The Twelve Officials*

1. The **Heart** holds the office of lord and sovereign. The radiance of the spirit stems from it. It is called the Supreme Controller.
2. The **Lungs** hold the office of minister and chancellor. The regulation of the life-giving network stems from them. They are called the Receiver of the Pure Qi of Heaven.
3. The **Liver** holds the office of general of the armed forces. Assessment of circumstances and conception of plans stem from it. It is called the Controller of Planning.
4. The **Gall Bladder** is responsible for what is just and exact. Determination and decision stem from it. It is called the Decision-Maker and Judge.
5. The **Pericardium** has the charge of serving the Heart as resident [residing in the center] as well as envoy [carrying the Heart sovereign's messages]. Elation and joy stem from it. It is called the Protector of the Heart.
6. and 7. The **Spleen and Stomach** are responsible for the storehouses and granaries. The five tastes stem from them. The Stomach is called the Controller of Rottening and Ripening. The Spleen is called the Controller of Transport.
8. The **Large Intestine** is responsible for transit. The residue from transformation stems from it. It is called the Drainer of the Dregs.
9. The **Small Intestine** is responsible for receiving and making things thrive. Transformed substances stem from it. It is called the Transformer of Matter and Separator of the Pure from the Impure.
10. The **Kidneys** are responsible for the creation of power. Skill and ability stem from them. They are called the Controller of Water.
11. The **Triple Heater** is responsible for the opening up of passages and irrigation. The regulation of Fluids stems from it. It is called the Official of Balance and Harmony.
12. The **Urinary Bladder** is responsible for regions and cities. It stores the Body Fluids. The transformations of Qi then give out their power. It is called the Controller of the Storage of Water.

*My summary, based on translations of Su Wen Chapter 8, following the terminology of Claude Larre and Elisabeth Rochat de la Vallee.[17]

THE FUNCTIONAL ORGANS

The second position on the Circle concerns the 12 primary functions. These were specified as early as the *Yellow Emperor's Inner Classic,* in which they are compared with government officials with specific "charges" or areas of responsibility. Almost all of these primary functions are designated by the names of organs that likewise play a major role in the Western medical concept of physiological functioning, but it is imperative to recognize that these names are technical terms in OM and have significantly different meanings than their linguistically apparent Western counterparts.

The difference stems from the fact that Western terms primarily denote *structure* (e.g., liver, kidney, spleen), whereas the corresponding Oriental terms bearing the same names are both connotative and denotative labels for *functions* that are not bound by anatomic structure.

As an example, the Liver in OM connotes the functioning of a "general of the armed forces. Assessment of circumstances and conception of plans stem from it."[17] Thus all planning (including the ability to foresee the outcome of behavioral choices) and self-defense (including immunological reactions) evoke "Liver" functions in Oriental, but not Western medicine. One implication of this difference of perspective is that in OM the physical structure called the liver cannot be studied to determine whether a given illness is related to the Liver. In fact, cases of hepatitis are more likely to be diagnosed in OM as disorders of the Spleen than of the Liver, because the functional changes (e.g., anorexia, fatigue, yellow tinge to the skin) resonate to the Spleen and not the Liver. Box 2-1 lists the 12 functions with their charges from the *Yellow Emperor's Inner Classic.*[17] The understanding of Organ functioning based on this analogy to twelve "Officials" is typical of the style of practice designated in this book as LA. Box 2-2 presents the same 12 functions as they are conceptualized in TCM, which is obviously quite different.[18,19] Both of these traditional approaches, however, share the same method of defining the Organs functionally, and in a way that is independent of the physical structures of the same

BOX 2-2

The Twelve Zang-Fu Organs

1. The **Heart** dominates the Blood and Vessels, houses the Mind, opens into the tongue, and manifests on the face.
2. The **Lungs** dominate the Qi and control respiration, regulate the water passages by dominating the dispersing and descending of Fluids, dominate the skin and body hair and open into the nose.
3. The **Liver** stores the Blood, maintains the free flow of Qi, controls the tendons, opens into the eyes, and manifests in the nails.
4. The **Gall Bladder** stores the bile and assists the Liver in maintaining the free flow of Qi.
5. The **Pericardium** protects the Heart.
6. The **Stomach** receives the food, begins its decomposition and descends it.
7. The **Spleen** governs transportation and transformation leading to the production of Qi and Blood, and the elimination of Dampness; it ascends the Qi, controls the Blood (keeps it in the Vessels), domi-

nates the muscles and limbs, opens into the mouth, and manifests on the lips.
8. The **Large Intestine** receives the waste, transports, and excretes it.
9. The **Small Intestine** digests the food and separates the clear from the turbid.
10. The **Kidneys** store the Essence, dominate reproduction, growth and development, dominate water metabolism, help the Lungs receive the Qi, dominate bone and marrow to form the brain and spinal cord, dominate the anus and urethra, open into the ears and manifest in the head hair.
11. The **Triple Heater** *(San Jiao)* serves as the passage for Original Qi and Body Fluid. The Upper Heater dominates dispersion and distribution, the Middle Heater dominates digestion, and the Lower Heater dominates separation of clear from the turbid and the drainage of fluids and waste.
12. The **Urinary Bladder** stores and discharges the urine.

---

names. For this reason, these functions are spoken of as "delocalized."

MERIDIAN THEORY

Position Three on the Circle, or structures, introduces an even bigger discrepancy between Western medicine and OM. Although the anatomy of the internal organs was recognized early in OM, including descriptions of their size, shape, and location, this information was rarely used in clinical practice because of the absence of surgery as a therapeutic option, except in a limited number of anecdotal references that are mainly of historical interest (e.g., the alleged exchange transplant of human hearts by Bian Que [407-310 BCE] and the visceral operations attributed to Hua Tuo [110-207 CE] as described in Hume[20] and Chuang,[21] respectively).

In place of anatomy, OM developed a theory of human structure in terms of the pathways by which Qi (and its various constituents) is distributed to every part of the organism from embryonic to adult stages of development. These pathways are commonly known as acupuncture Meridians. Some translators

have argued that the term Channels would be a more accurate linguistic choice,* and certainly it is easier for a Western scientist to conceive of a somewhat ethereal substance, Qi, being conveyed in Channels where it might be subject to blockage (congestion, stagnation) or deficiency, leading to pathology, than the alternative conception of pathology in an intangible Meridian analagous to the earth's lines of latitude and longitude. In fact, however, the search for a material substrate corresponding to the Energy pathways has so far proven fruitless.† The two methodologies that have proven most promising for establishing the

---

*The Chinese term is *Jing,* using a different character than that for Essence. The first serious Western practitioner and translator of acupuncture texts was George Soulié de Morant (1878-1955), and his terminological choices of Meridian for Jing and Element for Xing, which have been retained in this chapter, are a tribute to his enormous contributions to the knowledge of acupuncture in the West. Each of these translational choices has led to scholarly debate. See the original text by Soulié de Morant[22] for the locus classicus of these terms.

†There was one well-publicized red herring, the research findings of Kim Bong-Han, which claimed to document the Channels histologically using radioisotopic techniques; however, according to my own observation of the literature, Kim's work was never successfully duplicated by other scientists and is generally discredited.

reality of Meridians are again functional rather than structural. From the earliest times, there have been reports of "sensitive" individuals who feel something happening along the classic Meridian pathways when certain Points along them are stimulated in a variety of ways. Research into this phenomenon in China has been done under the rubric of "propagated sensation of the Channels" or PSC.[23] The conduction velocity of these sensations is slower than would be predicted for a mechanism dependent on neural transmission, underscoring the importance of the fact that the Meridian pathways do not correspond to any known nerve, blood vessel, or lymphatic structures. The one area of Western science that has seemingly had the most success in providing plausible hypotheses for Meridians and acupuncture Points is electrophysiology, and a recent textbook on "medical acupuncture" deals with this model of how acupuncture might work in some detail. Helms' text[16] is the most accessible introduction to acupuncture for those with a strong attachment to the Western biomedical tradition, and is practically the only English language source of information on the SEL style of practice. For many years researchers have claimed that acupuncture Points are unique locations on the body surface at which the skin's electrical conductivity is maximal compared with neighboring spots. The initial research on the unique electrical properties of acupuncture Points was reported by Niboyet[24] in 1951 and later elaborated on by Niboyet[25] and others. This research was inspired by an observation of Cantoni and was carried out in collaboration with Borsarello (personal communication from Borsarello, 1998; see Niboyet, Borsarello, and Dumortier[26]). It is also claimed that the conductivity between two Points along the same Meridian or Great Meridian is greater than that between Points not sharing this relationship.[16] These findings have led to the theory that the Meridians are reflections of the pathways of least electrical resistance throughout the body. Structurally this may represent fascial cleavage planes where extracellular ionic fluids can spread electrical potentials over great distances without needing to overcome the resistances of cellular membranes. It is even conceivable that these low-resistance extracellular fluid pathways might have branches connecting them to the internal organs, thus providing some concrete, albeit hypothetical, basis for the traditional Organ-Meridian associations.

What is less amenable to explanation by the model under discussion is the specificity of the acupuncture Points. Although they share the low electrical resistance phenomenon of the Meridians, being located at sites of local minimal resistance, they classically have unique therapeutic properties that distinguish even different Points along the same Meridian, one from another (see examples in Chapter 4). In addition to their characteristic electrical profiles, acupuncture Points also frequently coincide in location with "motor points," the spots along the surface of muscles where the threshold for electrical excitation is lowest.[27] Finally, many acupuncture Point locations are commonly found to be the sites of "trigger points," sensitive spots at which pressure can elicit pain either locally or referred to distant locations.[9] These fundamental correlations of acupuncture Points are interesting and even provide the rationale for one Western style of nontraditional acupuncture, but offer no insight into the mechanisms of traditional acupuncture's efficacy in treating any of the other manifestations of imbalance in the body, mind, or spirit than the various pain syndromes. To comprehend this expanded scope of traditional acupuncture, it is necessary to examine its own teachings about Meridians and Points.

Traditionally there are descriptions of several different kinds of Meridians (Figure 2-3), *of which only the Principal Meridians that connect directly to the 12 major Organs are commonly discussed in elementary books about acupuncture. These 12 Principal* Meridians* do form the "skeleton" of the Meridian system in the adult, but are actually preceded in embryonic life by a system of eight Extraordinary Meridians† that develop sequentially and seem to provide a sort of grid or Energetic Field within which the Principal Meridians and Organs organize themselves and take on form. The Extraordinary Meridians transport all forms of Qi, with an emphasis on the inherited component called Essence, and are responsible for determining the primordial Yin/Yang distinctions of the developing embryo: front/back, top/bottom, left/right, center/periphery, interior/surface, and so on. Although these 8 continue to exist and function after the 12 Principal Meridians develop, only 2 of the Extraordinary Meri-

---

*Jing is the generic Chinese term for all the Meridians but is also used in a narrower sense when discussing the Principal Meridians, as referring to them specifically.
†Qi Jing Ba Mai in Chinese. Various alternatives to the English translation "Extraordinary" include Curious, Marvellous, Extra, Odd, and Irregular.

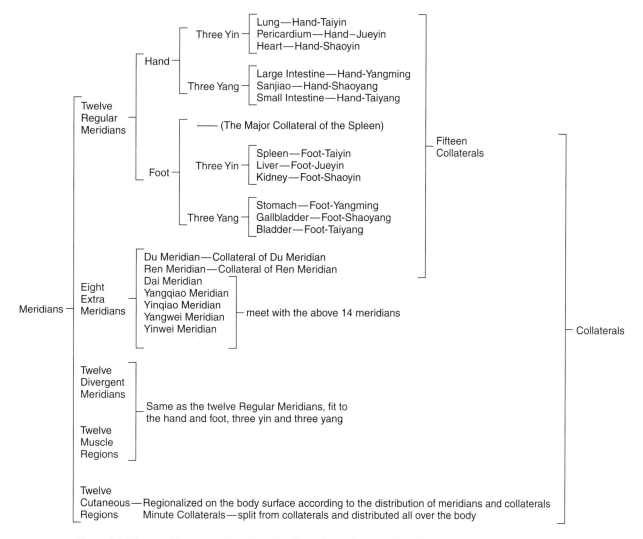

Figure 2-3 The Meridian Complex: classification of Meridians and Collaterals. (Modified from Cheng X (ed): *Chinese acupuncture and moxibustion,* Beijing, 1980, Foreign Languages Press.)

dians have acupuncture Points of their own. These are the Governing *(Du)* and Conception *(Ren)* Vessels marking the posterior and anterior midlines of the body. The other six Extraordinary Meridians are accessed by Points they share with the Principal Meridians.

The Principal Meridians, as noted, develop along with the organic functions they help coordinate. Thus each Principal Meridian has an internal branch that enters its pertaining Organ (however, there are no acupuncture Points along these internal branches). All the Points are located on the external branches of the Meridians, which are close enough to the body's surface to be reached safely by acupuncture needles. Each of the external branches of the 12 Principal Meridians is bilaterally symmetrical and either starts or ends at one of the extremities and connects to another Principal Meridian on either the trunk of the body or the head. There are many theories about how Qi flows in its various forms along the Meridians, but for simplicity, only three are described.

The most common image of Qi flow along the Principal Meridians is that of a closed loop in which each of the 12 pass their Qi on to the following Meridian, as in

Figure 2-4. This closed circulation of Qi is said to be governed by the Lungs, which traditionally play the initiating role that is analogous to the heart's role in blood circulation, a scientifically established function documented in the West only thousands of years after the Qi cycle was initially described. This cyclical flow of Qi, although continuous, has a wavelike character, so that each Meridian in sequence is said to be at the crest of its activity for a 2-hour period, and likewise has its lowest level of activity 12 hours later for a similar 2-hour period. This correlation of Meridians and their associated Organs with the diurnal cycle has important clinical applications, both in diagnosis and in therapy,* and although the details are beyond the scope of this introduction, it is pertinent to mention that Western medicine has taken a growing interest in the related field of chronobiology.

A second, and seemingly contradictory image of Qi flow, is along each of the Principal Meridians starting from the tips of the extremities and flowing toward the trunk of the body. In this image, or model, the Qi is said to appear at the tips of the fingers and toes like water collecting at a well, and as it flows centripetally it gathers strength, breadth, and depth as it transits Points likened to springs, streams, rivers, and finally seas. This model of Qi flow is known as that of the Five Transport Points (*Wu Shu Xue* in Chinese), and is used in many if not all of the variant styles of traditional acupuncture. Because the Five Transport Points coincide with the Five Element Points, this model is crucial to the application of Five Element theory to clinical practice. However, the same model is also the basis for choosing Points to access other (more minor) Meridian systems such as the Tendinomuscular (*Jing Jin* in Chinese, also translated as Channel Sinews and Muscle Conduits) and Divergent (*Jing Bie* in Chinese, also translated as Distinct Meridians, Branch Conduits, and Channel Divergences) Meridians to be described shortly. The common factor of these uses of the Five Transport Points is that the Qi from the periphery is constantly flowing toward the center of the body where the Organs can receive it. Thus it would seem that the image of Qi flow being evoked by the

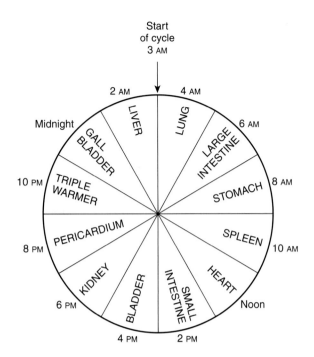

Figure 2-4 The Chinese clock: flow of Qi through the organs in the 24-hour day. (From Mann F: *Acupuncture, the ancient Chinese art of healing and how it works scientifically*, rev ed, New York, 1971, Vintage Books.)

Five Transport Points is the ultimate connection of the Meridian's external branch to its internal branch and Organ.

For example, in the Lung Meridian, the Qi is commonly said to flow from the first Point (L 1) on the chest down the arm to the last Point (L 11) on the thumb. However, the direction of Qi flow for the Five Transport Points along the Lung Meridian is from the thumb (L 11) up to the elbow (L 5). It would be simplistic to expect the movements of Vital Energy in living organisms to exactly follow any kind of linear model.

As if it were not difficult enough to conceptualize Qi moving simultaneously in opposite directions as in these two models, there is also a movement of Qi between Principal Meridians that seems to take place outside of any spatial context. Although the Connecting (*Luo Mai* in Chinese, also translated as Reticular Conduits and Junctional Meridians), Divergent, and Extraordinary Meridians all provide alternate

---

*The law of Midday-Midnight specifying the succession of 2-hour peaks forms the basis for biorhythmic applications in acupuncture. It is known as *Zi Wu Liu Zhu Fa* in Chinese. A more technically accurate translation would be Midnight-Midday, but once again Soulié de Morant[22] established the common usage of Midday-Midnight.

routes for Principal Meridians to exchange Qi, what is being alluded to is a delocalized movement of Qi that occurs presumably by the same sort of Energetic resonance that underlies the concepts of Yin and Yang, the Five Elements, and the Organ functions themselves. There are many examples of traditional acupuncture techniques that presumably operate by these delocalized mechanisms including those codified by the "laws" of Husband-Wife, Midday-Midnight, and Five Elements (i.e., Mother-Son and Grandparent-Grandchild, otherwise known as the creative and control cycles). As one example, using acupuncture at a Point on the Lung Meridian to strengthen Lung Qi (e.g., tonifying Lung 9) will also strengthen Heart Qi (Husband-Wife law), strengthen Kidney Qi (Mother-Son law), and disperse Bladder Qi (Midday-Midnight law), although none of these Principal Meridians is linearly connected. These delocalized interactions are not commonly discussed in TCM acupuncture but are part of the daily practice in various Japanese, Korean, Vietnamese, and European styles of acupuncture.

L 9 is an alphanumeric code name for the acupuncture point on the Lung Meridian at the wrist crease. Originally, acupoints were referred to by individual names only, but this led to some discrepancies and confusion as acupoints were given multiple names, so different alphanumeric systems have been proposed to standardize terminology. Most traditionally trained acupuncturists (i.e., by apprenticeship) still learn the names first, and perhaps the numbering system afterward, in order to pass licensure examinations. In contrast, most Western-trained acupuncturists learn the numbers first and may never proceed to learn the classic names of the hundreds of Points. See the next discussion of the grouping of acupoints for an explanation of the importance of learning the point names.

All the Meridians other than the Principal Meridians are grouped together as Secondary Meridians or Vessels. The Extraordinary Meridians have already been described, and many Japanese styles of acupuncture focus exclusive attention on treating through them. The recently deceased physician-acupuncturist Yoshio Manaka pioneered the integration of Eastern and Western thought in this context by experimenting with the use of semiconductors to "pump" electrical charges between the Points that control the Extraordinary Meridians.[28] Today his system of "ion-pumping" is widely taught and practiced as a hybrid form of acupuncture.

If the Extraordinary Meridians are conceptualized as the deepest level of Energetic organization in the body, then the Tendinomuscular Meridians represent the most superficial level. There are 12 Tendinomuscular Meridians, each one starting at the most distal Point of its associated Principal Meridian and extending proximally. But rather than connecting internally to its pertaining Organ, it traverses the exterior of the body in zones rather than lines, encompassing all the superficial structures located therein: skin, flesh, vessels, muscles, tendons, and connective tissue. Thus the Tendinomuscular Meridians are treated mainly when the complaint is of trauma or other acute problems of the body's surface that have not evolved from internal organic malfunctioning. The Tendinomuscular Meridians do not have unique Points, but borrow Command Points from the Principal Meridians and local tender or "Ah Shi" Points that have no fixed locations. Treatment of the Tendinomuscular Meridians is prominent in the teachings of the French Medical Acupuncture Association's style of practice.[16]

The term *Connecting Meridians* is sometimes used as a generic term for all the interconnections between and minute ramifications of the Principal Meridians. In this context, there is a hierarchy of three kinds of Connecting Meridians: 15 named Vessels, Superficial Vessels (*Fu Luo* in Chinese) and Lesser Vessels (*Sun Luo* in Chinese; also translated as Minute Connecting Vessels). Each of the Principal Meridians has a Connecting Point from which its named Connecting Vessel makes contact with its opposite polar-paired Principal Meridian (e.g., Connecting Point L7 connects the Lung Meridian to its partner, the Large Intestine Meridian). These 12 Connecting Meridians therefore serve to coordinate and balance the Qi flow in the 6 pairs of Yin and Yang coupled Meridians. Some acupuncture traditions also distinguish a Transverse Connecting Meridian that serves this coupling function and a Longitudinal Connecting Meridian that accounts for the therapeutic effects of stimulating the Connecting Points on a wider range of symptomatology.[29] In addition to these 12 Connecting Meridians, there is 1 each for the Governing and Conception Vessels and a Great Connecting Meridian of the Spleen that is said to tie together all the Connecting Meridians into a network of 15 Vessels.

The next category of Meridians, the Superficial Connecting Meridians, is associated with the blood vessels, and particularly the veins. When these Superficial Vessels are in an Excess state, they can be seen as blue (cold) or red (hot) structures (Meridians) that can be directly needled or bled to promote circulation. Certain Japanese schools of acupuncture focus extensively on this bleeding technique.

Finally, the Lesser Connecting Meridians appear to be a miscellaneous group accounting for the distribution of Qi down to the most minute components of the organism; these are of more theoretical than clinical interest.

Surveying the Meridian system from most superficial to sequentially deeper levels, are the Tendinomuscular Meridians, followed by the Connecting Meridians. Then before reaching the (deep) Principal Meridians, there is a level associated with what are called the 12 Divergent Meridians. These are best conceptualized as pathways of Qi flow that share properties of both the more superficial and the deeper Meridians. They branch off or diverge from the Principal Meridians and connect with their coupled Organs and their coupled Divergent Meridians to create another mechanism for Yin/Yang coordination. Also the Divergent Meridians all terminate on the head, and because the Yin Principal Meridians do not go to the head at all, the Divergent Meridians explain how Yin Meridians and Organs are able to exert their influences on the head. Treatment of the Divergent Meridians is emphasized in certain schools of both Japanese and European acupuncture.

QI TYPES CARRIED BY THE MERIDIANS

One way to summarize the Meridian system is to look at the kinds of Qi each preferentially transports. On the surface, outside any actual vessel, the Tendinomuscular Meridians mostly transport a kind of Yang Qi known as Defensive Energy (*Wei Qi* in Chinese) responsible for warming the tissues and protecting them from invading pathogenic factors. At the deepest level of the body, the Extraordinary Meridians mostly transport a more Yin kind of Qi known as Essential Energy* responsible for the genetic blueprints of the organism, including the

timing of its growth and development. These blueprints result in the formation of the Organs and their Principal Meridians, which mostly transport a relatively Yin form of Qi known as Nourishing Energy (*Ying Qi* in Chinese) to maintain the Organs' functions. The Connecting Meridians tie all these Energies and pathways together, and the major form of Qi they transport is the Blood, which is warm like the Defensive Qi, and nutritional like the Nourishing Qi, said to provide an abode for the Spirit like the Essential Qi, and is composed of all of these forms of Energy. Finally, the Divergent Meridians appear to act as a mechanism for carrying the Wei Qi from the exterior to the depths and simultaneously carrying the Essence and Nourishing Qi out to the surface, so that they play a major role in the integration of the human organism with its environment.

THE ACUPUNCTURE POINTS

There are more than 401 named acupuncture Points on the human body. In addition to the grouping that emerges from location on the Meridians, Points are also traditionally grouped in other ways. The Five Transport Points have already been mentioned; these are a subset of a larger group of Points known as Command Points.* The Command Points are all the Points that, as members of a group, have characteristic effects on the flow of Qi.

There is no universal agreement on a complete list of Command Points, but in addition to the Five Transport Points, they most often include the following:
1. Connecting Points (*Luo Xue* in Chinese; also known as Passage points, they activate the Connecting Meridians)
2. Source Points (*Yuan Xue* in Chinese; also known as Original Points, they infuse Original Energy into each Principal Meridian via the Triple Heater)
3. Cleft Points (*Xi Xue* in Chinese; they are mostly used for acute problems)
4. Posterior Associated (or Back Shu) Points (*Bei Shu Xue* in Chinese; they connect directly to their pertaining organs)

Jing Qi in Chinese. This term implies both Essence (Jing) and Original or Source Energy (Yuan Qi), which can be thought of as the material and Energetic bases of heredity.

Zong Xue in Chinese. The term Command Point was originally introduced by Soulié de Morant[22] to describe the effects of all Points that had a specifically identified impact on a patient's Qi. His use of the term was thus very broad in its connotation; however, subsequent Western authors, starting with Niboyet,[25] have used this term in a much narrower sense as indicated in the text.

5. Anterior Collecting (or Front Mu) Points (*Fu Mu Xue* in Chinese; often called Alarm Points in Western texts)

Other groups of Points that are considered to belong in the list of Command Points vary by the various traditions of acupuncture practice. They include the following:

1. Confluent Points (*Jiao Hui Xue* in Chinese) of the Eight Extra Meridians.
2. Entry and Exit Points (Chinese technical terms are not identified for these acupoints whose use derives from the biorhythmic tradition *[Zi Wu Liu Zhu Fa]*).
3. Influential Points (*Ba Hui Xue* in Chinese; also known as the Eight Meeting or Gathering Points).
4. Barrier Points (grouping developed by the French Medical Acupuncture Association, reflecting the SEL tradition, best described in the text by Kespi[30]).
5. Windows of the Sky Points (*Tian Chuang Xue* in Chinese; described as having a special influence on the Spirit in LA, but also commonly used in SEL and other styles of acupuncture).
6. Four Seas Points (*Si Hai* in Chinese; they are the Seas of Blood, Marrow, Nourishment, and Energy).
7. Group Connecting Points (Chinese technical terms are not identified for these acupoints, whose use was first described by Niboyet[24]).
8. Reunion Points (*Jiao Hui Xue* in Chinese; also known as Intersecting Points. These are Points where two or more Meridians cross. Treating them creates a similar effect on all the Meridians involved).

This listing is not exhaustive but is extensive enough to show that acupuncture Point theory is a complex subject.

A simpler way of classifying Points is into two categories: extremity or distal Points and body or local Points. Distal points are located between the fingertips and elbows, and between the toes and knees. All other acupoints are classified as body points. To a first approximation, this distinction separates the Command Points from the ordinary points, but there are many exceptions to this rule. In many traditions, the distal Points are believed to influence all the functions of the Meridians on which they are located, while the local Points are believed to have a more restricted influence on nearby structures and their associated functions. This classification scheme is a drastic simplification of traditional teachings, but it does allow for a clearer understanding of the various options in choice of treatment Points adopted by different traditions. The classic texts did not provide extensive dis-

cussions of Point functions, but contemporary practitioners have found such an approach useful and several such rubrics have been developed. For example, in TCM, Points are discussed in terms of their effects on the Basic Substances; in the French medical acupuncture tradition, Points are discussed in terms of the dialectics of the Six Levels of Yin and Yang; in LA (a tradition that attaches great significance to the ancient names chosen for each Point), Points are discussed in terms of their "spirits."

Historically, however, Points have most often been discussed in relationship to symptomatology for which they have been found useful.

CAUSES OF ILLNESS

Position Four on the Circle diagram represents the causes of illness. In OM, these are traditionally divided into three groups: endogenous, exogenous, and miscellaneous causes.

Endogenous means from within an individual, and it is curious that to a Western practitioner such a classification would most likely represent a genetic disorder, whereas in OM this category represents what might be called the "inner life" of an individual—their thoughts, feelings, and emotions. Traditionally there are seven emotions that have deleterious effects on the flow of Qi if they are experienced beyond an individual's tolerance. These emotions are joy, anger, melancholy, worry, grief, fear, and fright. Each of these emotions is an appropriate reaction to many of life's situations, and as such is a part of healthy functioning, but should such a reaction become fixed, habitual, exaggerated, or inappropriate in any other way, it would then disrupt the flow of Qi and thus imbalance the organic functions that depend on proper Qi flow, leading to a deterioration in the state of health. OM cedes pride of place to these psychoemotional factors, which is quite the opposite viewpoint to that of biomedicine. The classics of OM repeatedly claim that an individual whose Qi is not internally disrupted (i.e., one who is not subject to any endogenous disharmonies) will be immune to the invasion of exogenous pathogenic factors. For this reason, some styles of acupuncture (such as LA) place primary etiological emphasis on the emotions. In contrast, TCM in its evolution as a competitor to biomedicine has put its primary emphasis on the exogenous pathogenic factors that correspond to the etiological mechanisms characteristic of that medicine (i.e., infectious, toxic, and allergic).

There are six exogenous pathogenic influences known as Wind, Cold, Heat, Dampness, Dryness, and Fire. Undoubtedly the original conception was that climatic stresses can disrupt Qi flow in a manner analogous to that evoked by emotional stress. In other words, the Six Climatic Factors are normally handled in a healthy manner when they represent the natural fluxes of the seasons, to which we are biologically adapted. If, however, especially in a vulnerable individual already weakened by emotional imbalance, these climatic factors happen to be present with exaggerated intensity or duration, or occur outside their proper season, then they can overcome the individual's Defensive Qi, and penetrate the organism. In so doing, the climatic factors become Perverse or Evil Qi *(Xie Qi)*, which, by disrupting the flow of Normal Qi, leads to a pathological condition.

The miscellaneous (literally, neither endogenous nor exogenous) category of pathogenic factors is no less important than the endogenous and exogenous ones, only less systematized. It includes such diverse causes of ill health as trauma, poisoning, animal or insect bites and stings, parasites, epidemic pestilences, genetic and constitutional factors, spiritual possession, and improper lifestyle. The last three of these groupings merits further discussion.

Genetic and congenital factors were mentioned earlier as fitting a Western interpretation of what would be an endogenous cause of illness, and some acupuncture traditions have adopted an almost identical point of view. Others have adopted its antithesis. For example, LA uses the technical term "causative factor" as the crucial issue to be determined before any treatment plan can be formulated. The causative factor is one of the Five Elements, whose chronic state of imbalance cannot be completely corrected by nature itself. Thus the individual is likely to develop malfunctions in a somewhat predictable pattern guided by the causative factor. Because LA also includes a presumption that the causative factor is almost always determined before the end of childhood and then remains fixed for the remainder of life, the model tends to implicate a genetic or congenital mechanism. Another style of practice, Korean Constitutional Acupuncture (KCA), is even more explicit in teaching that each individual's energetic constitution and predisposition to disease is an inherited situation, the recognition of which must precede any treatment plan. KCA integrates both Five Element and Yin/Yang theories, with no presumptions about their relative importance in determining one's genetic constitution. Other Korean styles of practice do attempt to carry constitutional development one step further. Korean Hand Acupuncture (KHA) integrates several earlier theories of constitutional etiology, resulting in the assignment of a double constitution to each individual determined by the climatic (exogenous) factors predominant at the times of the individual's conception and birth. The concept of constitutional imbalances, although obviously amenable to differing interpretations, is firmly rooted in the classics, being present even in the seminal *Yellow Emperor's Inner Classic.*

Spiritual possession as an explanation for the cause of illness is the explanation least compatible with biomedicine. It was, however, probably the earliest etiological concept in OM, and it has persisted in traditional writings throughout China's entire dynastic history and into the 20th century.[2] The materialist beliefs of the political powers responsible for formalizing TCM in the People's Republic of China after the revolution precluded "demonic possession" from being listed as a cause of disease, but those styles of acupuncture that had emigrated overseas did not necessarily accept the Chinese decision. LA, for example, includes methods for the diagnosis and treatment of demonic possession, defined somewhat variably and quite inclusively. Sometimes it has been described as the literal usurpation of an individual by a discarnate spirit; commonly a more functional interpretation is offered in which possession merely denotes an individual's loss of control over his or her own life force (Qi), or spirit (Shen), with no further metaphysical imagery. Almost all traditional medical systems recognize this category of spiritual disease that they share with many religions, including those honored and respected by many, if not the majority, of proponents of biomedicine. The power of this position for traditional OM lies in the following: in avoiding the creation of a rigid distinction between science and religion, it allows for a more open approach to maladies that biomedicine has difficulty treating, but which are successfully treated by shamanic and other spiritual practitioners. An analogy that may help to develop an acceptable context for this pathological mechanism is to conceive of possession as an extreme case of psychoemotional (endogenous) disturbance requiring specific therapeutic strategies in the same way that epidemics (*Li Qi* in Chinese) are extreme cases of exogenous disturbance that also require unique therapeutic strategies. The concept of epidemic pestilential factors provides an interesting example of convergence between OM and biomedical thought.

Improper lifestyle is a conglomerate category that is open to multiple interpretations. Traditionally, the primary concerns were with a balanced approach to exercise and rest, nutrition, and sexual behavior. Anyone familiar with the practice of medicine is no doubt aware of the tremendous range of individual difference in both interest and tolerance of prescriptions for any of these behaviors. OM and biomedicine have their share of dogmatists who claim that a given diet, exercise program, or approach to sexuality will keep anyone in the best state of health, but there are so many conflicting theories in both Eastern and Western approaches that it would appear as if moderation in all is the best general advice, allowing that individuals may need to vary from moderation because of their unique needs. The fuzziness of standards for a proper lifestyle in no way diminishes its importance in Oriental medical theory and practice (see Chapter 6). A modern Japanese approach to health care known as macrobiotics is almost entirely focused on diet, and all other Oriental medical traditions incorporate dietary advice based on Yin/Yang and Five Element theories along with acupuncture treatment. Macrobiotics was the name chosen by Nyoitchi Sakurazawa, better known as George Ohsawa (1893-1966), for his unique interpretation of OM.[31] It is popular both in Japan and the West, although it has many idiosyncratic differences from other Oriental medical traditions.

There are many well-known Oriental systems of exercise including Tai Ji Quan, Dao Yin, Qi Gong, and the various martial arts, all of which combine exercise with mental concentration. There is actually a continuum between therapeutic exercise and therapeutic meditation, both of which are rooted in Daoist and Buddhist religious traditions. The same origin is also shared by the teachings about sexual behavior, which because it involves activity of the Essence, has always been thought to have enormous implications for both health and spiritual development in the Orient. The religious goal of "enlightenment" is seen as a result of the proper development of one's Essence, Energy, and Spirit, the basic constituents at the core of OM. Again, medicine and religion form a continuum, with strategies for spiritual development running the gamut from pure meditation to the ingestion of medicinal herbs and foods, to specific sexual practices taught

only to advanced initiates. Although popular books have been written on all of these methods, they are properly studied only under an accomplished teacher, just as is the study of acupuncture itself.

PATHOLOGY IN ORIENTAL MEDICINE

Position Five is allocated to the pathological results induced by the factors operating at Position Four. Although in general it may be acknowledged that disruptions in the normal flow of Qi will always be present in a state of ill health, how this is manifest and conceptualized is open to alternative points of view. One extreme position was adopted by a Japanese school originating in the late 17th century* that reduced all forms of pathology to a single phenomenon—the stagnation of Original Energy (*Yuan Qi* in Chinese), which was differentially treated depending on where it manifested on examination. The concept of stagnation led to extensive use of moxibustion, a type of heat therapy at acupuncture Points that counteracts stagnation by facilitating movement (kinetic energy).

Oriental theories of pathology, being metaphysical speculations, are not dependent on physical confirmation as are Western approaches to pathological conditions. In fact, Rudolph Virchow's introduction of the theory of cellular pathology in 19th-century Europe may have been the single most important point of divergence between allopathic medicine and OM. Because Oriental theories of pathology are not evidence-based, there must be other criteria for their acceptance or rejection. The primary criterion is whether or not any pathological theory is empirically useful in guiding the choice of an effective therapeutic intervention. Many theories fulfill this criterion in OM, only a sampling of which are mentioned.

LA, for example, attributes most disorders to an imbalance of the Qi, with the major pathological states being either Excess or Deficiency in one of the Five Elements or their associated Organs/Meridians. However, LA does acknowledge an ill-defined pathological category of "polluted Qi" including such conditions as Aggressive Energy and demonic possession. "Aggressive

---

*Gonzan Goto (1659-1733) was an early popularizer of the Koiho (Ancient Thought) school, which based its teachings on the *Treatise on Cold Induced Disorders,* an early Chinese medical classic.

Energy" is a phrase derived from the French teachings of Jacques Lavier, who was himself a teacher of the founder of LA, J. R. Worsley. It is almost certainly a translation of Perverse Energy or *Xie Qi*.[4]

The focus of LA on imbalanced Qi as the primary pathological entity reflects its largely Japanese derivation. Later developments in Japanese thinking led to an expanded theory in which pathology was differentiated into disorders of either Qi, Blood, or Fluids, and this model is still used by many Japanese practitioners, where it plays more of a role in herbal medicine than in acupuncture. This theory was developed by Nangai Yoshimasu (1750-1813).[4]

As another example, TCM often comingles discussions of etiology and pathology. These are not rigidly differentiated for the simple reason that the same Chinese term, *Wind* for example, is both an etiological factor and the name of the pathological state it provokes. Thus each of the six exogenous factors can lead to a pathological state of the same name, but this apparently simple schema is actually much more complex. On the one hand, these six pathological states may arise as a result of an invasion by their corresponding exogenous etiological factor. But they may also arise endogenously without any exogenous factor being involved. Staying with the example of Wind, Exogenous Wind is the pathological factor involved in many acute infectious diseases, whereas Endogenous Wind is the pathological factor implicated in many cases of stroke or cerebrovascular accident. Both OM and biomedicine share the notion that the former group of illnesses is associated with exogenous factors (germs or inclement weather), whereas the latter group of illnesses is associated with endogenous factors (be they diet, heredity, or psychoemotional stress). A second complexity in this TCM model is that these pathogenic factors are not static but undergo transformation as a result of their struggle with the organism's antipathogenic Qi. Thus an invasion of pathogenic Cold can transform into a state of Heat and vice versa (to help make sense of this, recall the discussion of Yin and Yang earlier in the chapter). In addition, the interaction between pathogenic and antipathogenic Qi can lead to the development of secondary pathogenic factors such as phlegm and stagnant Blood, which in turn are further damaging to the organism if not appropriately treated. Finally, TCM attaches great importance to the maintenance of the proper direction of Qi flow including ascending, descending, outward, and inward movements. Any variation of these movements from the norm is classified pathologically as Rebellious Qi (*Qi Ni* in Chinese).

There is very little information in English on the unique contributions of Korean medicine to the understanding of pathology, but the originator of KCA, Dowon Kuon, has been developing a hybrid model in which Western concepts, such as inflammation, infection, allergy, and neoplasia, play a role in determining the specific illness developed by an individual of a given constitution. Dr. Kuon has yet to publish anything more than an abstract of his work, even in Korean, but a textbook is said to be forthcoming.

EXAMINING THE PATIENT

Position Six on the Circle, examination, represents the initial interaction between patient and practitioner (see Chapters 3 and 7). As previously mentioned, the major difference between biomedicine and OM in this regard is in the absence of technologically based methods in the latter in contrast to their ever-increasing prominence in the former. This is not an absolute rule, as several essentially traditional styles of acupuncture have incorporated electrodiagnosis to a limited degree. For example, TCM practitioners often use electrical Point finders to locate reactive spots in the ears that provide useful information for both diagnosis and treatment. A similar situation exists in KHA where the hand rather than the ear is electrically scanned. These two exceptions might be said to prove the rule, because in both of these styles the other forms of direct sensorial examination of the patient easily account for more than 95% of the process of data gathering.

The traditional acupuncture examination consists of the four steps of seeing, hearing/smelling, questioning, and feeling. The order in which the steps are listed is not arbitrary, as it seems to follow a hierarchy of the senses, starting with the top of the body and proceeding inferiorly: the eyes for seeing, below which are the ears and nose for listening/smelling, below which is the mouth for questioning, below which are the hands for feeling. Hierarchies such as this are common attributes of spiritual or metaphysically based, as opposed to materialist systems such as biomedicine. However, in modern clinical practice these four steps are rarely carried out strictly in the traditional sequence.

Seeing implies anything that can be observed by looking at the patient. Each style of practice has its own point of view, however, so that, for example, the main focus of LA is on the subtle coloration of specific areas on the face (looking for correlations to the Five Elements), whereas the main focus of TCM is on observation of the tongue (looking for information about such Yin/Yang parameters as Hot/Cold and Excess/Deficiency, in addition to indicators of specific pathogenic factors and the Organ systems they might be affecting). KCA places more emphasis on overall body morphology, whereas KHA obviously focuses its attention on the hand, with particular interest in the five fingers, which are correlated to the Five Elements. There is a description by one Japanese author[31] of "diagnosis at a glance" that would appear to be based on a more spiritual type of seeing—seeing with the "mind's eye" perhaps. The majority of Japanese acupuncturists have historically been blind and have thus skipped this stage of the examination entirely. These accounts of various approaches to "seeing" are brief caricatures and in no way purport to describe the totality of this component of the traditional examination in any of these styles of practice. They are presented merely to provide a feeling for the differences that may be experienced in examination by acupuncture practitioners of differing backgrounds, which holds equally true for the other steps in the examination process.

Hearing/smelling is grouped together because the Chinese term for this type of examination does not distinguish between them. In LA, however, each of these procedures is given great emphasis because both vocal qualities and body odors are classified via the Five Element schema central to LA (see Table 2-4). The Japanese Five Element tradition known as Meridian Therapy (MT) was the major historical source for the LA teachings in this regard and uses a similar approach. TCM, on the other hand, tends to assign the least importance to this step of the examination, and the information it does gather is mainly related to indicators of the Yin/Yang dichotomies of Excess/Deficient and Hot/Cold.

Questioning is the part of a traditional examination that is the most similar to a biomedical examination, but even here there are significant differences and variations between styles. Almost all practitioners ask about the reason for seeking treatment, or the chief complaint, along with a description of how it developed and what has been done to address it so far. Other complaints are surveyed (review of systems) as is the past medical history and frequently both social and personal history and family medical history. Thus it is not so much the scope of questioning, but its

manner or point of view, that distinguishes OM and biomedical examinations. With regard to manner, LA places relatively less emphasis on the content of the patient's verbal communication and more on how the patient is using communication to elicit a response from the practitioner. This is the stage at which the emotional balance of the patient is investigated, again from a Five Element perspective. Most other styles of acupuncture, by contrast, are strongly focused on gathering information on the nature of the symptoms: what do they actually feel like, what makes them better or worse, when do they typically occur or subside, are they accompanied by complaints referable to any other part of the body? At this point, the patient's taste preferences, seasonal likes and dislikes, dietary, exercise and sexual behaviors might be discussed. Although there is an historically important codification of this step as the "Song of the Ten Questions," in clinical practice the variation in questions that might be asked is almost infinite, and depends ultimately on the kinds of information needed to make a diagnosis in Position Seven. Because each style of acupuncture has its corresponding diagnostic model, the questions needed to reach this stage vary from one style to another.

Perhaps the most well-known part of an Oriental medical examination is the feeling of the pulse (Figure 2-5). Quite naturally, a practice that has been in continuous use for thousands of years has developed regional and stylistic variations. Typically the pulse being examined is confined to the radial arteries of both wrists, but even this description has its exceptions. For example, KHA and some Japanese practitioners instead use a comparison of the pulses of the carotid and the radial arteries, a technique originally described in the *Yellow Emperor's Inner Classic*. The important role assigned to pulse diagnosis of any kind in the Oriental medical examination may be questioned. The answer is that the crux of OM is the life force or Qi, and the traditional teaching is that the pulse is an expression of the Qi moving the Blood. These two, Qi and Blood, stand as emblems of Yang and Yin, which must be in balance with each other for health to be maintained. Any abnormality of Qi or Blood thus shows up as an alteration of the pulse in some way. This global interpretation of the pulse has been refined in the differentiation of 28 variations of pulse quality, each indicating a specific abnormality of Yin/Yang balance.

Ascertaining the abnormal pulse qualities is of greatest importance to styles of acupuncture practice

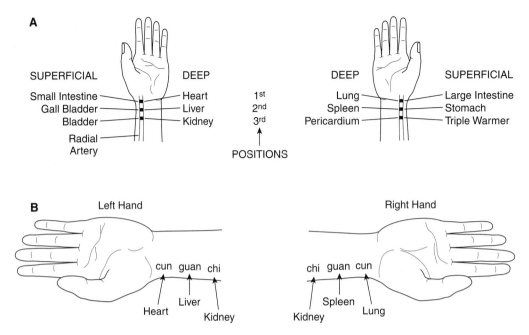

Figure 2-5 Two common models of pulse diagnosis. **A,** Model popular in Five Element style. **B,** Model used in TCM. (**A** from Mann F: *Acupuncture, the ancient Chinese art of healing and how it works scientifically,* rev ed, New York, 1971, Vintage Books; **B** from Xinnong C (ed): *Chinese acupuncture and moxibustion,* Beijing, 1980, Foreign Languages Press.)

that are primarily governed by the theory of Yin and Yang, such as TCM. Although there are many classic descriptions of associations between the Five Elements and various pulse qualities, clinically most acupuncture practitioners (at least of the Japanese and European styles) who base their practice on Five Element theory use an equally ancient but alternate paradigm for examining the radial pulse, called 12-position pulse determination. The theoretical explanation, or rationalization, of 12-position pulse determination is based on the fact that the rhythmic distribution of Qi in the body is traditionally governed by the Lungs. Therefore, any abnormalities in the distribution of Qi should manifest along the pathway or Meridian of the Lungs, and the acupuncture Point Lung 9 *(Tai Yuan),* adjacent to the radial artery at the wrist, is traditionally described as the "Influential Point" for all the Vessels in the body. Therefore the pulse at this Point most closely reflects the functioning of the Organs that cause the Vessels to pulsate: the Lungs and the Heart, each assigned by Yin/Yang theory to one side of the body. The Lungs—relatively Yin—are reflected in the right radial pulse, whereas the Heart—relatively Yang— is reflected in the left radial pulse. From this crucial

position at Lung 9 called the "inch" *(cun),* two further proximal positions on the radial artery are readily palpable, called the "barrier" *(guan)* and "foot" *(chi)* positions, respectively. Because they are proximal in terms of the flow of Blood and Qi, they are assigned sequentially to the "Mother" Organs by Five Element theory.* Finally, because each Element is associated with both a Solid (Yin) and Hollow (Yang) Organ, the superficial (Yang) aspect of the pulse is associated with the Hollow Organ, and the deep (Yin) aspect of the pulse is associated with the Solid Organ of each Element. This complex reasoning results in the schema in Figure 2-5, which was described in both the *Pulse Classic (Mai Jing* in Chinese) and the *Classic of Difficulties (Nan Jing* in Chinese), each written shortly after the *Inner Classic.* In this model, any abnormality in a given Organ's functioning is reflected in a change in the pulse wave at its corresponding location on the radial artery. It must be emphasized again that Oriental and Western ideas

---

*On the left wrist, the sequence of deep pulses from proximal to distal is Kidney (Water) to Liver (Wood) to Heart (Fire). On the right wrist, the sequence from proximal to distal is Pericardium (Fire) to Spleen (Earth) to Lung (Metal).

about the Organs are quite different, so that this type of pulse evaluation can neither confirm nor deny illnesses attributed to the organs in biomedicine.

Twelve-position pulse determination has been used clinically in its original form since its inception, but like every other facet of OM, it has been subject to variations and alternate interpretations. One of the most significant was the replacement of Five Element theory by a somatotopic correspondence system known as Three Heaters theory, to assign Organ correspondences to the 12 pulse positions, which was advocated in the Ming dynasty (1368-1644 CE) in China. This alternate 12-position system was the variant that remained dominant in China and was officially incorporated into TCM in the 20th century, the epoch when all the contemporary styles of "traditional acupuncture" achieved their present form.

There have been numerous modern systems of pulse diagnosis, reflecting the intuitive recognition by practitioners that the pulse more clearly reflects Energy flow than any other sign or finding on examination. KCA, for example, uses a segment of the radial artery even more proximal for its "genetic" diagnosis. Interestingly, this segment of the radial artery was identified by Soulié de Morant, the grandfather of Western acupuncture, as being associated with the central nervous system and its higher faculties.[22] In OM the cephalic central nervous system is described as the "Sea of Marrow," which is derived from the Essence or genetic endowment. There also have been attempts to measure pulses objectively, but the technological barrier this introduces between patient and practitioner has not found wide favor. Perhaps the most interesting observation about pulse diagnosis is a statement by the eminent British physician, Felix Mann,[32,33] who practices and teaches acupuncture from a completely Western scientific standpoint, rejecting all Oriental Energetic theories as unnecessary mystification. Quite simply, he has said, "I use pulse diagnosis because it works."

Although it may seem incomprehensible that neighboring sections of the same artery can pulsate differently, two plausible explanations come readily to mind and others may be awaiting discovery. The most obvious factor to consider is the autonomic innervation of the arterial walls, whose level of activity controls vasomotor tone. As the Organs themselves are under autonomic control, an interaction between Organ and pulse is certainly conceivable. A second mechanism to consider is the phenomenon of standing waves, which can occur in any closed system like the circulatory system. Standing waves typically display different pulsations at neighboring positions.

Although pulse palpation is the most frequently discussed part of the feeling examination, palpation of other parts of the body may also be emphasized in various traditions. The Japanese in particular have developed quite an elaborate system of abdominal examination known as Hara diagnosis. In this approach, the center of Energy in each individual is believed to be located in the abdomen, so changes in the tension, texture, warmth, or sensitivity in this area are thought to most clearly reflect Energetic imbalances. The abdomen happens to correspond to the location of the majority of Anterior Collecting Points, also known as Alarm Points in the West because of their usefulness in the palpatory examination. Similarly, changes in the Posterior Associated Points can be found on examination, and the palpation of the Points and Meridians throughout the body for sensitivity or other changes has always been a crucial part of the examination process. Finally, it is only through thorough palpation that the "Ah Shi" (ouch) points, which are of great therapeutic importance, can be identified.

DIFFERENTIATING PATTERNS OF DISHARMONY

Position Seven on the Circle diagram gathers all the information from the examination, analyses it in terms of the pathology it reflects and the causative factors that lead to such pathology, and determines what is occurring in the Organs, Meridians, and Basic Substances. Like biomedicine, OM has a tradition of naming individual diseases, but this approach to diagnosis is much less emphasized than that of differentiating diseases by their underlying Energetic patterns. Once again the two major guiding Energetic theories at play are those of Yin/Yang and the Five Elements.

The most well-known Yin/Yang diagnostic theory has been previously mentioned as the "Eight Principles," and TCM is often caricatured as a system based exclusively on Eight Principle acupuncture. Actually TCM encompasses many other diagnostic models including the "Six Levels of Yin and Yang," the "Four Divisions of Physical Resources," and the "Three Heaters," in addition to differentiating syndromes by the Organs or Meridians affected, and the Basic Substances involved. The reason for the characterization of TCM as Eight Principle acupuncture is that this dialectical system of applying Yin/Yang discriminations is not widely applied by practitioners of other styles of acupuncture, having been codified rather late in the historical development of acupuncture in China.[27,34] Because an Eight Principle diagnosis can frequently be determined simply from the examination of the pulse and tongue, this approach tends to be less dependent on the psychoemotional interaction of patient and practitioner, which plays such a predominant role in LA, for example.

The cardinal diagnostic rubric in LA has been described as the Causative Factor. Although the Causative Factor is one of the Five Elements that is identified by its corresponding color, sound, odor, and emotion, these findings are only reliably identified when they appear disproportionately in a patient who is experiencing a fluctuating level of stress on each Element in turn. It is precisely in the moment-to-moment encounter between patient and practitioner that situations arise that differentially stress each of the Elements. Thus practitioners of LA are trained in the use of interpersonal dynamics to gather the information needed for an Elemental diagnosis.

KHA uses a unique diagnostic model called "Three Constitutions" theory, which is based mainly on its own methods of pulse and abdominal examination. Although this model integrates aspects of Yin and Yang, Five Element, and Twelve Organ theories, the system as a whole bears a striking resemblance to the tripartite model of Ayurvedic medicine (a traditional Asian Indian medical system).[35]

KCA is almost wholly dependent on pulse determination; however, this system of acupuncture has never been given a full public presentation. However, there have been published research papers that purport to confirm that individuals of the same constitution have similar changes in blood chemistries when challenged with various types of diet,[36] so it is quite possible that a more objective method of constitutional diagnosis might be developed in the future.

There is no standard form of diagnosis in Japanese acupuncture because there are so many individual styles of practice. Many are focused on the symptomatic sites where local Energy blockages known as "Kori" are identified by palpation, and no further diagnosis is pursued. Other Japanese styles such as Meridian Therapy are highly dependent on pulse diagnosis, and some of the most interesting experiments in training practitioners to achieve a high degree of concordance in their findings, compared with those of other practitioners, have been done by this group, especially its blind members.

TREATMENT IN ORIENTAL MEDICINE

The Eighth or last Position on the Circle is devoted to treatment, which in this presentation refers to acupuncture, although it must be remembered that there are many other modes of therapy that are used by different practitioners. Acupuncture is actually called *zhen jiu* in Chinese, which strictly speaking means needles and cauterization, so moxibustion is implied by the term acupuncture. Both techniques are described in more detail in Chapter 4.

Many kinds of needles have been used throughout history, but presently only metallic needles are used. The most common type is called the filiform needle, composed of a handle and shaft, and typically measures from 0.5 to 3 in in length and from 0.12 to 0.34 mm in diameter. Because of concerns about transmission of infectious diseases, disposable stainless steel needles are typically used in Western nations; however, properly sterilized needles are as safe as dental or other surgical equipment. There are various schools of thought about the effects of using different metals to fabricate needles, and some practitioners routinely use gold needles to tonify and silver needles to sedate or disperse the Qi.* Obviously, treating such instruments as disposable would render the cost of treatment prohibitive.

In addition to filiform needles, specialized types are used for bleeding and semipermanent implantation. Bleeding needles usually have a triangular cutting point, whereas semipermanent needles are extremely short and are either inserted intracutaneously or into the cartilage of the ear (see Figure 4-9). They may be left in place from several hours to more than a week, but the longer a needle is left in situ, the greater is the chance of infection; therefore these needle sites require close observation and good patient hygiene.

Moxibustion is the collective name for any therapeutic process that applies heat to the body surface in an Oriental medical context. Most often the heat is applied to acupuncture Points, but there are many in-

---

*The differential effects of colored versus noncolored metallic needles are presumably related to their reduction potentials, which are highest for gold (colored) and lowest for aluminum (noncolored) of the common metals. The use of gold and silver needles, which is archaeologically at least as old as the Han Dynasty (202 BCE-220 CE) in China, was introduced to Europe by Soulié de Morant.[22] Using needles of different metals for tonification and sedation is common in certain Japanese and Korean (e.g., KHA) traditions, but is not espoused in TCM or LA.

stances where special Points for moxibustion only are used, whereas in other cases symptomatic areas of the body rather than specific Points are heated. Classically, the material used to provide the heat is composed of specially prepared leaves from the wormwood plant, *Artemesia vulgaris*. The word moxibustion is derived from moxa, an anglicized version of the Japanese term *moe kusa* (burning herb). There are three major styles of moxibustion in addition to numerous variants. These are known as scarring, direct nonscarring, and indirect.

Scarring moxibustion is rarely encountered in the West, although its results may be seen on clientele from Asia. In this procedure the moxa is applied directly to the skin spot to be treated, then ignited and allowed to burn all the way down. The same process may be repeated several times at the same spot. Such treatment is painful, producing a burn that blisters and eventually creates a scar. While this procedure may seem barbaric, it was formerly held in high repute because it was believed to produce the strongest response in the patient's Qi, particularly the Defensive Qi associated with the immune system. It was widely used to treat asthma, and contemporary research in China has confirmed its usefulness in treating both asthma and hypertension.[37]

Direct nonscarring moxibustion also involves burning cones of moxa on the skin itself, but these are snatched off as soon as the patient feels them as hot. Although a series of moxa cones is burned on each Point, because they are removed each time they are felt, no blister or scar results. Direct moxibustion is very commonly used in many Oriental traditions but is perhaps most widely used in Japan. One Japanese style, Structural Acupuncture* uses extensive direct moxibustion, a result of its evolution from the tradition of Sawada Ken (1877-1938), an influential practitioner who successfully treated the Japanese emperor with moxibustion. Reflecting its strong Japanese heritage, LA also uses direct nonscarring moxibustion, although not with the frequency used in Structural Acupuncture, where it is a mandatory part of every treatment.

Indirect moxibustion includes all methods that do not burn moxa directly on the skin. One method is to burn the moxa on a protective barrier applied to the skin. Examples of this technique include moxa on slices of ginger, garlic, beancake, aconite, clay, or a layer of salt. Another common technique is to use a "moxa roll," which is similar to a cigar made from moxa with or without the addition of other combustible herbs. The moxa roll is lit and held near the Point or zone to be heated and moved around sufficiently to produce warmth and erythema at the desired location. One advantage of the moxa roll is that in many cases patients can be safely taught to use moxa rolls for home treatment as an adjunct to the office session. All of these variations of indirect moxibustion are common components of TCM acupuncture treatment. Recently moxa tubes, which resemble small slices of moxa rolls suspended in a cardboard tube, have been developed. These can be affixed to the skin and allowed to burn all the way down, as the column of air between moxa and skin ensures indirect stimulation. Moxa tubes are now commonly used in various Chinese, Japanese, and Korean traditions.

Finally, it should be noted that needles and moxa are often used together, either sequentially or simultaneously. Sequential use at the same Point is common in LA and Structural Acupuncture. Simultaneous use can be accomplished by burning the moxa on the handle of the needle. Special moxa needles are available for this technique, but it is also possible to attach a special cup to the needle handle to hold the moxa, or even to have the handle transfix a slice of moxa roll, which is then ignited. In all of these simultaneous treatments, it is important to protect the underlying skin from dropping ashes.

A stronger variation of combined treatment is called "fire needling." In this technique a needle heated directly in a flame is rapidly inserted through the skin and immediately removed. Fire needling is said to be less painful than many other forms of acupuncture, but in spite of its description in the classic texts, it is rarely encountered in any of the contemporary traditions.

Both acupuncture and moxibustion are used to influence the patient's Qi. It is sometimes stated that needling is effective for moving or sedating the Qi, whereas moxibustion, by virtue of its introduction of warmth and other pharmacological properties, tonifies or reinforces the Qi.[38] Not all schools of thought in OM accept this dichotomy; some teach moxibustion techniques for sedation and acupuncture techniques for tonification. Styles of practice such as TCM that incorporate herbal treatments are more likely to use herbs for tonification and needles for dispersion

---

*Structural Acupuncture is the author's nomenclature for the style of acupuncture taught by Taiichi Sorimachi, which he calls Seitai Shinpo in Japanese. It is based on the work of Ken Sawada and Keizo Hashimoto, who emphasized palpation along with postural and mobility status in their examinations.

or sedation, but even this caricature is not entirely accurate.

The various styles of acupuncture use different methods of needle manipulation aimed at tonifying, dispersing, sedating, warming, cooling, guiding, or draining Qi. The parameters of needling vary widely in terms of the thickness of the needles, the depth of penetration, manipulation and intensity of stimulation, length of time the needles are left in place, and number of Points treated in a given session. Some styles of practice, such as LA, frequently use very few Points (ideally only one) with shallow penetration by very thin needles that are given a gentle manipulation that is often imperceptible to the patient, the needle then being withdrawn, in a matter of seconds. Most of the time in a typical LA treatment is involved in the examination process, previously described as involving the development of a very strong rapport between patient and practitioner, and many LA practitioners believe that their focused intention during the needling process is the most important part of treatment. This subtle approach to needling is characteristic of many Japanese styles of acupuncture that contributed to the development of LA.

By contrast, many Chinese styles of acupuncture including TCM profess a belief that for treatment to be effective, the patient must experience a strong feeling of *de Qi,* or needle sensation. De Qi can manifest as a soreness, aching, heaviness, distention, numbness, or other feeling, but not as the sharp pain associated with, for example, a pin prick. Typically more and thicker needles are used, manipulated at a deeper level, and then left in place for about 20 to 30 minutes. During this "retention" period they are periodically manipulated again.

Some Korean styles of practice use dozens of needles per session, but these are typically left in place for 20 to 30 minutes without manipulation. KCA uses a special type of needle inserter that allows a given sequence of Points to be stimulated rapidly a number of times, with the whole treatment taking only a minute or two to be accomplished. KHA uses tiny needles inserted at Points on the hands only, along with a number of other noninvasive methods of stimulation. Thus the process of acupuncture treatment is extremely heterogeneous.

Describing the physical characteristics and outcome of an acupuncture treatment without understanding the material discussed in Positions One through Seven would be akin to describing the color, size, shape, weight, and performance of an automobile to a medieval farmer—of course, to him it would seem like an exercise in delusion or magic. The reality is, however, that acupuncture is clinically effective, and automobiles do function in spite of the fact that drivers and patients alike may be wholly ignorant of the mechanisms involved.

The practitioner, however, does need to base his or her treatment on an understanding of the preceding information in this chapter. It is on this basis that suitable Points can be selected for treatment within a particular practice style. Points may be chosen according to the Organs or Officials found to be malfunctioning, the Meridians involved, the pathogenic factors or type of pathologic change detected, including any alterations of the Basic Substances. Any of the refinements of Yin/Yang or Five Element theory may be used to guide the choice of treatment Points, but usually treatment is conceptually divided into "root" and "branch" aspects. Root treatment is aimed at redressing the underlying Energetic causes, whereas branch treatment is aimed at relieving the presenting symptoms. Points for the former aspect typically have no special relationship to the location of the symptoms, whereas the latter are typically located mainly in the vicinity of the symptoms. The tremendous variety in possible treatment prescriptions for a given disease category in biomedical terms is one reason why it is so difficult to document the efficacy of acupuncture in the same way that Western pharmaceuticals are tested (i.e., with the standardized, double-blind, randomized clinical trial).

A growing body of literature addresses the issue of how acupuncture can be studied in a scientific fashion, both at the basic and clinical level.[39,40] The most difficult issues to be resolved include the need for treatment protocols to allow for individualized interventions for each patient with the same biomedical diagnosis (dependent only on the Oriental diagnosis), the need to address the tremendous variability in styles of acupuncture practice and skill of the individual practitioners, and finally the difficulty of devising suitable controls. To distinguish placebo from treatment effects, the control should be indistinguishable from the actual treatment, from the patient's point of view. This is easily accomplished with pharmaceuticals that can be swallowed or injected, but when it comes to inserting needles—either you use them or you don't—and, the patient knows which is which. There are also problems with "sham" acupuncture using needles at non-Points, because Point locations vary in different traditions, and some traditions believe the whole body is responsive to some degree to needle insertions, which are recognized as a stimulus by the body's own Qi. In any case, the range of possibly effective Points for a given individual can be quite large depending simply on the style of acupuncture practiced.

What then is a reasonable standard for both acupuncture research and for informed referral for acupuncture treatment by a Western practitioner? (See discussions in Part III.) At this time, the most useful clinical research in acupuncture would be comparisons of efficacy between acupuncture and standard biomedical treatment for as many conditions as possible. Because this type of study can only be single-blinded (i.e., the evaluator can remain ignorant of the therapy used), it does not discriminate against the possibility of an unusually strong placebo effect from acupuncture. However, if such an effect were to occur, it would in no way lessen the patient's benefit from the acupuncture treatment. In the present evaluation of acupuncture's role in health care, the establishment of safety and efficacy are far more important than is the discrimination of placebo from "real" effects.

Because of the enormous variety of acupuncture styles, some general guidelines are appropriate in referring patients for trials of acupuncture by interested physicians (see Chapter 21). The two most important issues are the qualifications of the practitioners and the expected outcomes of treatment. Historically, the majority of acupuncture practitioners in the Orient did not officially have credentials but practiced skills they had learned under family or apprenticeship to a Master willing to train them. In the late 20th century this mode of learning shifted to a school model, although apprenticeships are still an important mechanism of gaining intern and postgraduate skills. In the United States, acupuncture is regulated on a state by state basis, but there is a national organization that examines candidates for entry-level proficiency in acupuncture—the National Commission for the Certification of Acupuncture and OM (NCCAOM; see Chapter 20).* Some states accept NCCAOM diplomates for licensure, and others use their own examinations. Some make no provision for the practice of acupuncture, and still others

define acupuncturists as primary care practitioners (Table 20-2). This is an area of rapid change, and of course other Western countries have their own criteria for acupuncture practice.

In terms of the expectations of the outcome of acupuncture treatment, no absolute rule applies, but it is important to recognize that response to acupuncture treatment often takes time to become apparent. As with many medications that need an induction time of weeks to months (e.g., many psychiatric, antiinflammatory, and antihypertensive drugs), acupuncture may also not show its benefits for a few weeks to several months. Historically, in the Orient acupuncture treatment was often given on a daily basis, but in the West it is uncommon for treatment to be given more than once or twice a week. Although some patients may respond positively to even the first acupuncture treatment, this should not be expected, and there may even be an initial aggravation of symptoms that then subsides with further treatment. Most practitioners expect to see some improvement after 3 treatments, but generally a reliable trial consists of between 6 and 10 treatments. If the patient has experienced no benefit by that time, further treatment is unlikely to be helpful. It should be noted, however, that patients often experience benefits in areas unrelated to their chief complaints. For example, a patient with migraine headaches may experience improvements in sleep, digestion, or mood without achieving relief from headaches. These improvements are often harbingers of eventual success in pain relief, if treatment is continued.

The length of time that successful treatment should be continued is also extremely variable. Just as some medications need only be taken for a short time while others may need to be maintained throughout life, the same is true for acupuncture treatment. If the presenting problem resolves in a short time, no further treatment may be necessary, but if it recurs, ongoing treatment may be needed—an exact parallel to the situation with pharmaceuticals where diabetic patients, those with hypertension, patients with heart failure, hypothyroidism, or a host of other maladies must accept lifelong treatment. Thus, as long as a patient is experiencing ongoing benefit from acupuncture, it makes sense to continue treatment. The most significant difference with acupuncture is that the therapist's ultimate aim is to treat the roots of each patient's Energetic imbalance, so that the maladies or "branch manifestations" have the potential to resolve with ongoing treatment. For

*NCCAOM, PO Box 9072, Washington, DC 20090-7075.

some time, the World Health Organization has listed 40 conditions for which acupuncture has shown promise,[41] and this list is sure to grow in the future. It must be remembered, however, that as long as the causative factors responsible for each patient's imbalances are still operative, their symptoms are likely to recur. Thus the highest goal of the traditional acupuncturist is not to use needles at all, but to teach patients the right way to live. For some this is dietary advice; for others there are emotional lessons that need to be learned. The right way to live is like the Dao: it is unique from moment to moment and cannot be named or captured in any set of rules or norms. Only sensitive practitioners who are themselves ever learning from nature (the Western concept closest to the Dao) can effectively provide this highest level of healing.

References

1. Jiao S-f: *Head acupuncture* (translated by S Zhi-hong), Taiyuan, [1971], Shanxi Publishing House.
2. Unschuld PU: *Medicine in China, a history of ideas,* Berkeley, Calif, 1985, University of California Press.
3. Lu G-d, Needham J: *Celestial lancets; a history and rationale of acupuncture and moxa,* Cambridge, 1980, Cambridge University Press.
4. Eckman P: *In the footsteps of the Yellow Emperor: tracing the history of traditional acupuncture,* San Francisco, 1996, Cypress Book Co.
5. Lee JK, Bae SK: *Korean acupuncture,* Seoul, 1974, Ko Mun Sa.
6. Qiu M-L (ed): *Chinese acupuncture and moxibustion,* Edinburgh, Churchill Livingstone, 1993.
7. Nogier PFM: *From auriculotherapy to auriculomedicine* (translated by A Cousino and M Graff), Sainte-Ruffine, 1983, Maisonneuve.
8. Travell JG, Simons DG: *Myofascial pain and dysfunction: the trigger point manual,* Baltimore, 1983, Williams & Wilkins.
9. Baldry PE: *Acupuncture, trigger points and musculoskeletal pain,* 2nd ed, Edinburgh, 1993, Churchill Livingstone.
10. Chung C: *Ah-Shih point: the illustrated diagnostic guide to clinical acupuncture,* Taipei, 1982, Chen Kwan Book Co.
11. Needham J: *Science and civilization in China,* vol 2, Cambridge, 1956, Cambridge University Press.
12. Porkert M: *The theoretical foundations of Chinese medicine,* Cambridge, Mass, 1974, MIT Press.
13. Porkert M, Hempen C-H: *Classical acupuncture—the standard textbook,* Dinkelscherben, 1995, Phainon Editions.
14. Liu Y: *The essential book of traditional Chinese medicine,* New York, 1988, Columbia University Press.
15. Kutchins S, Eckman P: *Closing the circle: lectures on the unity of traditional Oriental medicine,* Fairfax, Va, 1983. (Reprints available from Peter Eckman, 4279 Army St, San Francisco, CA 94131.)
16. Helms JM: *Acupuncture energetics—a clinical approach for physicians,* Berkeley, Calif, 1995, Medical Acupuncture Publishers.
17. Larre C, Rochhat de la Vallee E: *The secret treatise of the spiritual orchid* (Su Wen chapter 8), Cambridge, 1985, Monkey Press.
18. Beijing, Shanghai, and Nanjing Colleges of Traditional Chinese Medicine: *Essentials of Chinese acupuncture,* Beijing, 1980, Foreign Languages Press.
19. Cheng X (ed): *Chinese acupuncture and moxibustion,* Beijing, 1980, Foreign Languages Press.
20. Hume EH: *The Chinese way in medicine,* Baltimore, 1980, Johns Hopkins Press.
21. Chuang Y-M: *The historical development of acupuncture,* Los Angeles: 1982, Oriental Healing Arts Institute.
22. Soulié de Morant G: *Chinese acupuncture,* Brookline, Mass, 1994, Paradigm Publications (original French version published in stages from 1939 through 1972).
23. *National Symposia of Acupuncture and Moxibustion and Acupuncture Anaesthesia,* Beijing, 1979.
24. Niboyet JEH: *Essai sur l'acupuncture Chinoise pratique,* Paris, 1951, Editions Dominique Wapler.
25. Niboyet JEH: *Complements d'acupuncture,* Paris, 1955, Editions Dominique Wapler.
26. Niboyet JEH, Borsarello J, Dumortier DO: Etude sur la moindre resistance cutanée a l'electricite de certains points de la peau dits "Points Chinois," *Bulletin de la Societe D'Acupuncture* 9:16-88, 1961.
27. Liu YK, et al: The correspondence between some motor points and acupuncture loci, *Am J Chin Med* 3:347-358, 1975.
28. Manaka Y, Itaya K, Birch S: *Chasing the dragon's tail,* Brookline, Mass, 1995, Paradigm Publications.
29. Van Nghi N, Recours-Nguyen C: *Medicine traditionelle Chinoise,* Marseilles, 1984, Editions N.V.N.
30. Kespi J-M: *Acupuncture,* Moulins les Metz, 1982, Maisonneuve.
31. Ohsawa GS: *L'Acupuncture et la medicine d'extreme Orient,* Paris, 1969, Vrin.
32. Mann F: *Acupuncture, the ancient Chinese art of healing and how it works scientifically,* rev ed, New York, 1971, Vintage Books.
33. Mann F: *The meridians of acupuncture,* London, 1964, William Heinemann.
34. Sivin N: *Traditional medicine in contemporary China,* Ann Arbor, Mich, 1987, Center for Chinese Studies, University of Michigan.
35. Eckman P: Ayurveda and Korean hand acupuncture, *Am J Acupunct* 2:153-158, 1995.

36. Kim SH, et al: A comparison of nutritional status among eight groups in relation to food preference on the viewpoint of constitutional medicine [English abstract], *Korean J Nutr Soc* 18:155, 1985.

37. Chen D, et al: *Proceedings of the National Symposia of Acupuncture, Moxibustion and Acupuncture Anaesthesia,* Beijing, 1979. p 57.

38. Turner RN, Low RH: *The principles and practice of moxibustion,* Wellingborough, 1981, Thorsons.

39. Birch S, Hammerschlag R: *Acupuncture efficacy: a summary of controlled clinical trials,* Tarrytown, NY, 1996, National Academy of Acupuncture and Oriental Medicine.

40. Bensoussan A: *The vital meridian,* Edinburgh, 1991, Churchill-Livingstone.

41. Mitchell ER: *Plain talk about acupuncture,* New York, 1987, Whalehall.

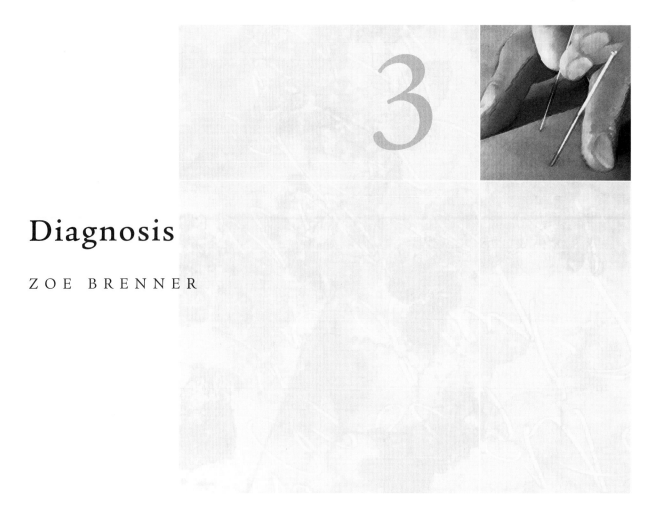

Diagnosis

ZOE BRENNER

The Chinese physician looks on the patient as a painter looks at a landscape—as a particular arrangement of signs in which the essence of the whole can be seen.

KAPTCHUK[1]

POINT OF VIEW

Diagnosis is at the heart of any medicine. It includes both gathering and combining information to identify a pattern of imbalance or disharmony, a syndrome, or a disease. In Oriental medicine, diagnosis surveys the surface of the body and explores the life of the individual to reach conclusions about the source of suffering. The practitioner's intent is to go beyond symptomatology to study the functioning of the whole person in the broadest context of his or her life.

In ancient Confucian China, it was essential to maintain the integrity of the body since the body ac-

tually belonged to one's ancestors. As a result, the Chinese were not inclined to anatomize or do surgery throughout most of their medical history. There are some exceptions, for example, the possibly legendary Hua T'o (second century CE) and some cataract surgery around the eighth century.[2] This began to change in the 19th century with contact with Western practices of medicine. Indeed, previous to the 19th century, the most "inside the body" practitioners could normally peer was at the tongue. In this context, very elegant, complex, and rich traditions of gathering information "from the surface" and via questioning developed. The goal was to know what was going on inside (physical) or within the depths (nonphysical) of the person. Early medical practitioners were fine observers and noted the correlations between such surface signs as colors and odors, and many others, with patterns of internal dysfunction. The information the practitioner gathers is quite broad and often can seem very subtle. These diagnostic procedures are still followed today.

Early Chinese philosophers were also keen observers of the interconnectedness and dynamism of the universe. They noticed that living beings acted differently in different seasons and that their survival depended on being congruent with the seasonal changes. They emphasized observing how change happens, noting that change is essential to life, stasis means death. All is in flux; beings are interacting, moving, changing, and responding. As a result, diagnosis is an assessment of how a person is functioning at a given moment. Diagnosis does not yield the name of a disease, which may have many states or possible manifestations, but a description of the process that is happening at that time in that person. Often the name given to that state implies movement or the lack thereof (e.g., Liver Qi stagnation; Rebellious Qi of the Stomach, moving the wrong way or in excess). For those who know Oriental medicine, the name also situates the patient on a continuum of progression from the subtle and mild early stages of imbalance to developed and serious degrees of disharmony. Very early Chinese medical texts often described the first signs of disorder and their extreme consequences if nothing intervened to help veer the patient off that course.*

In contrast, in biomedicine, patients are said to "have" a disease, sometimes permanently when it is defined as a "chronic" condition. Although biomedical conditions are understood to have many possible states or stages, only occasionally does the name locate the sufferer in that progression. Biomedicine focuses on the material and mechanical aspects of the life in the physical body and is generally far less interested in the being that inhabits that body and how that person lives in the world.

An important concept in Oriental medicine is that of "root and branch," in which the symptoms are considered the "branch," and the deeper level or not so obvious manifestation is the "root." The concept of "root" seems to approach the Western concept of "cause." However, it is not the same because in Oriental medicine, the pattern of imbalance is much more important than "cause" *per se,* and the "root" is really the underlying part of the pattern. In Oriental medicine, various styles focus on treating one or the other level more but generally paying attention to both is considered the most effective approach to treatment.

These patterns that are so important are not necessarily easy to apprehend. Single symptoms provide mere hints to what is occurring in the patient; to determine a diagnosis, the whole ensemble of symptoms and signs must be understood relative to one another. One way to explore this feature of relativity is through a review of the concepts of Yin and Yang. The original meaning of the Chinese characters were the shadyside (yin) and the sunnyside (yang) of the mountain. During the day, there cannot be a sunnyside without a shadyside, and where one finds sun and shade changes throughout the day and seasonally. Thus it is not possible to pick a place on the mountain and say it is Yin, because it can only be Yin in relationship to what is Yang at that time. This very basic point is pivotal to understanding Oriental medicine: observations are relative—as with *more* Yin or *less* Yang—nothing can be exclusively Yin or Yang. So it is with signs and symptoms: what in one context appears to be a sign of true excess heat, in another is heat coming from blockage caused by cold. One must know the whole context to understand the parts.

Besides the relativity of the signs, there is also relativity in the importance of the signs. For example, are the diagnostic signs in the tongue more important than those in the voice, or is the pattern seen in the medical history more important? Different styles of Oriental medicine emphasize different aspects of diagnostic observation, but what is always valued is the ability of the practitioner to have highly sensitive and discriminating perceptions. Practitioners thus must develop and hone their physical senses, and even more, must also develop an inner sensitivity. The latter demand reflects the influence of the culture of Taoism, which emphasizes the importance of the imperceptible. It is difficult to summarize this concept in a few words, but it is introduced in the first chapter of the *Dao De Jing* with the phrase "Names that can be named, but not the Eternal Name."

In other words, names can be assigned to things in our world, but the names are inadequate to express the

---

*The indications for acupoints in the *Chen Chui Jia Yi Jing* were written this way in the second century CE and later texts often followed this style.

underlying nature of reality. This same chapter goes on to say[3]:

So, as ever hidden, we should look at its inner essence:
As always manifest, we should look at its outer aspects.

LAO TZU

This is really the crux of diagnosis, perceiving the inner and using the outer signs as clues. This is the art of diagnosis in Oriental medicine. As summarized in the *Nan Jing (The Classic of Difficult Issues)*, compiled in the first or second century CE:

The sixty-first difficult issue: The scripture states: Anyone who looks and knows it is called a spirit [saint]; anybody who listens and knows it is called a sage; anybody who asks and knows it is to be called an artisan; anybody who feels the vessel [pulse] and knows it is to be called a skilled workman . . . That is what is meant when the scripture states: Those who know the (illness) from its external (manifestations) are called sages; those who know the (illness) from its internal (manifestations) are called spirits [saints].*

The skilled practitioner, then, must be capable of correlating context, perceptual data, and sensibility to diagnose what has been happening in each particular patient. Honing such abilities is emphasized in the education of the practitioner; it is now understandable why the development of technology to stand between patient and practitioner would not be encouraged in Oriental medicine.

THE FOUR EXAMINATIONS

Classic Oriental medicine names four parts in the examination of the patient. These are mentioned in the previous quotation from *Nan Jing*: looking, listening, asking, and touching. Listening includes smelling as the same word is used for both in Chinese. In the passage from the *Nan Jing*, the author seems to say that looking is more important and touching the least. I think this means the person who can assess the whole being with just a glance is of the highest ability. For an elegant description of this, see Kuriyama.[4] In practice, however, taking the pulse provides highly important clues to diagnosis.

Most practitioners of Oriental medicine complete all Four Examinations at the initial patient contact, us-

ing abbreviated versions as necessary at later visits. Some styles of practice stress some examinations over others, e.g., traditional Chinese medicine (TCM) emphasizes the condition of the tongue, whereas Leamington Acupuncture (LA) focuses more on the color, sound, and odor of the patient. Japanese Meridian therapy focuses on pulses and palpation of the abdomen.

Each category of the Four contains many assessments, and commonly some observations contradict others. Herein lies the art of the practitioner, for she must sort through data and impressions to reach a probable diagnosis. How soon will she know if her assessment is "right"—in the sense that her intervention is helpful? If she is using herbs, it may be some days, just as with pharmaceuticals. But if she is using moxibustion or needling acupuncture points, she may receive feedback so quickly that she can modify her treatment in the midst of a single session. I mention this feature to reemphasize the points made earlier about the dynamic and responsive quality of treating disharmonies of energy: the same markers—tone of voice, facial color, mood, pulse character—that signal disharmony and initiate treatment, can normalize rapidly, thus assuring the practitioner that she has made an accurate diagnosis. In short, diagnosis and treatment are temporally closely linked in Oriental medicine, particularly when acupuncture is used. Indeed, diagnosis is an ongoing process throughout treatment with acupuncture needles and moxibustion.

Box 3-1 summarizes the Examinations as discussed in this chapter. Note that the distinction made between symptom and sign in biomedicine is not emphasized in Oriental medicine. The oral responses of the patient are considered just as important as the signs gathered by the practitioner. The questions below need not be asked in a specific order, although there is some tendency to start "at the top" of the body and work down. In addition, the questions are so fundamental that they are discussed in all textbooks of Chinese medicine; thus specific references for further detail are not necessary.

Looking

This category comprises all that can be easily seen. It is usually what the practitioner first encounters (e.g., the appearance of the patient as he enters the office). *Looking* includes physical appearance, signs of vitality, quality of color on the face, and the condition of the tongue.

---

*Quote from Unschuld[2]; author translations in square brackets.

BOX 3-1.

The Four Examinations

Looking
Physical appearance and vitality
Color
Tongue

Listening and Smelling
Voice quality
Bodily Odor

Question Asking
Medical and psychosocial history
Heat and cold
Perspiration

Question Asking—cont'd
Headache and dizziness
Pain
Thirst, appetite, taste in mouth, dietary preferences
Excretion and secretion
Sleep
Gynecology

Touching
Pulse diagnosis
Abdominal diagnosis
Palpating acupoints

Physical Appearance, Vitality, Movement

When a practitioner first meets a patient, an early impression is of body type. In constitutional styles of Oriental practice, body type or shape is an important feature of diagnosis and prognosis. However, a general assessment rule is to expect excess conditions in those who appear strong, and deficiency conditions in those who appear frail.

Relative weight may also indicate a number of different things. In classic terms, overweight or underweight suggest the person is prone to deficient Qi. However, overweight people show a tendency to Dampness, whereas underweight people are more likely to display a deficiency of Yin or Blood.

Classically, certain body parts serve as indicators of the strength or weakness of individual Organ systems (see Table 2-4). The hair of the head reflects the strength of the Kidneys and the *jing* or Essence. The health of the body hair and skin signals the state of the Lung. The nails reflect the Liver, the flesh reflects the Spleen. The general state of the tongue is linked to the Heart; however, all the Organs express through the tongue (see text below). The condition of the Liver is reflected in the eyes. The nose corresponds to the Lung. The ears are the upper orifice connected to the Kidneys. Thus any unusual coloration, dryness, shape, or other unusual visible signs of any of these orifices or bodily parts can be noted to add to the information about how the whole system is functioning.

Another aspect of the appearance is what is called in Chinese *Shen*. Shen often is translated as spirit. A person with healthy Shen shows their aliveness; they are alert and thoroughly present, their eyes shine and their faces glow (Figure 3-1). Lack of Shen manifests as lusterless eyes and a veiled face. The Oriental practitioner looks to see if the person's spirit is intact. Whereas those with sight do this with their eyes, I have seen Japanese blind practitioners inspect for Shen with their hands. So perhaps Shen is a radiance that is not merely visual.

The practitioner also assesses the quality of the patient's movement. If it is quick and agitated, it is more Yang; if slow, passive, or sleepy, it is more Yin. Forceful exertions are more Yang and gentle and weak ones more Yin. Many other movement observations can be made, e.g., of shaking or trembling, of limping, of resistance to movement, or of protection of a body part.

Another component of movement is bodily and facial expression. The facies of anger may point to imbalance in the Wood Phase or the Liver, of sadness to the Metal Phase or the Lung, of fear to the Water Phase or Kidney, of pensiveness to the Earth Phase or Spleen, and of constant or inappropriate mirth to the Fire Phase or the Heart.

Color

A healthy skin has sheen, radiance, moisture, and both an overt pigmented color and a subtle shadow or tone

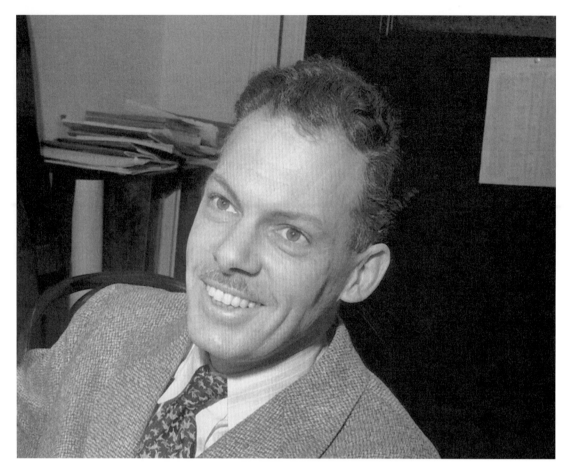

Figure 3-1 Shen shows as a radiance of the face, head, skin, eyes, and being. Shen is well illustrated in this 1949 photograph of a 42-year-old man who stayed healthy, kept working, and lived well for another 50 years.

to the skin. It is the latter tonality that is studied in Oriental medicine as a part of diagnosis. The tones can be seen on people of all pigment types and races. Color tone indications are sought on the face and on the inside of the forearm. On the face, one looks around the eyes, at the temples, and around the mouth; to catch sight of this subtle sign, it often helps to turn partly away, to view the face from the corners of one's eyes. Abnormal color or tones indicative of imbalance may be always present in a patient, or may appear during stress as in illness. Unhealthy colors may vanish quite suddenly with a good treatment, leaving the patient with both normal color and radiance.

Different styles of practice emphasize different color interpretations, but the following is a summary of the diagnostic use of color that most styles can accept.

- *White* is associated with the Metal Phase, which includes the Lung and Large Intestine; thus white may be pointing to an imbalance in these Organs. *Bright white* is a sign of Deficient Qi or of severe pain. *Dull gray-white* can be a sign of Deficient Blood or of disharmony in the Fire Phase.
- *Red:* A Fire Phase imbalance may also show up as *red,* a sign of heat. If the redness is everywhere and robust, it is Full Heat, but if it is confined mainly to the cheeks, it is a sign of Deficient Heat. Deficient Heat is a situation in which the person lacks the cooling aspects of Yin and thus shows spotty signs of Heat because of the

deficiency (rather than because of raging heat in the system). For example, one might expect to see a fully red face in a man who was infuriated and shouting, or suffering a sunstroke; however, red cheek spots in a woman in her mid-50s suggest the deficient heat response of Yin Deficiency, common in menopause.

- *Yellow* indicates Dampness. It can also show an imbalance in the Earth Phase, which includes the Spleen and Stomach. This is the yellow associated with jaundice, although true jaundice also often contains a tinge of red or green.
- *Azure* is a color that spans the range of blue to green and indicates imbalance in the Wood phase, which includes the Liver and Gall Bladder. In its presence the practitioner would suspect Stagnant Qi or Congealed Blood.
- *Black* is the color associated with the Water Phase, the Kidneys, and the Urinary Bladder. This tone on the face can indicate Congealed Blood (generally a painful syndrome) or serious chronic illness.

The study of color tones can be much further developed. Experienced practitioners can assess subtle tones and can use color change for prognosis; subtle differences in tone can indicate the seriousness of the imbalance.

Tongue

Tongue observation is a highly developed aspect of diagnosis, especially in styles that use Herbal medicine; for some practitioners, the information from the tongue is among the most reliable diagnostic signs; others barely look at it.[5] The tongue is also the only place that a classic practitioner of Oriental medicine looks "inside" the body.

In Oriental medicine, there is a distinction made between the *body* of the tongue and the *coat* or *moss*. A normal healthy tongue is defined as pale red and somewhat moist, with a slight or thin white coat.

Starting with the body of the tongue, if it is *redder* than normal, this indicates the presence of Heat. If it is *paler* than normal, there may be excess Cold or deficiency of Blood or Qi. If that pale tongue is *dry,* it is more likely deficient Blood, because the Blood has the function of moistening. If it is soggy *wet,* it points to Deficient Qi, because the Qi moves the fluids (implied: the fluids are not cycling through at an appropriate pace). An intensely red or *scarlet* tongue indi-

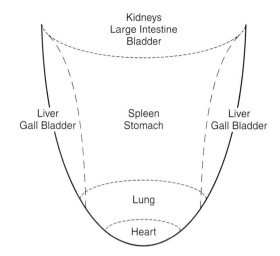

Figure 3-2 Map of the tongue.

cates extreme Heat, as in high fever. A *purple* tongue suggests either Stagnant Qi or Congealed Blood, but it also develops when Cold predominates because Cold also causes stagnation. *Red dots* on the tongue point to Heat or Congealed Blood.

The coat of the tongue is more quickly changeable and is important in more acute illnesses. According to Oriental medicine, a heathy moss is the product of a healthy digestive system. It is described as thin, evenly covering the tongue, white, moist, and "rooted not floating"—that is, it cannot be easily scraped off. A thick coat indicates Excess, and a thin (including absent) coat indicates Deficiency. If the coat is wet, there is excess Fluid; a greasy look like butter indicates Phlegm. A coat that looks like crumbly cottage cheese (as in thrush) is a sign of extreme Dampness with Heat. A tongue that looks peeled in places signifies Deficient Yin or Fluids or weak digestive Qi. If the color of the tongue coat is yellow, there is Heat; if the color is dark gray-black, it indicates extreme Heat or Cold. The normal coat color is white, but if the person is ill and the coat remains white, this points to excess Cold.

If they are not congenital, the pattern of *cracks* on the tongue is diagnostically important. The interpretation of cracks can become quite complicated because it depends on the color of the tongue, the configuration of the cracks, and their location. Figure 3-2 shows a simple map of the Organ-reflective regions of the tongue. The location of cracks suggests trouble in that area. For example, a crack down the center of tongue suggests digestive malfunction, whereas cracks near but not at the tip suggest Lung dysfunction.

The tongue map is also helpful in locating Organ linkages of some of the aforementioned indications. For example, a thick dark yellow coat at the root of the tongue suggests Damp Heat in the lower part of the body (e.g., a urinary tract infection). A thick yellow greasy area in the front of the tongue points to Hot Phlegm in the Lung (i.e., a severe upper respiratory tract infection such as bronchitis or pneumonia).

The shape and movement of the tongue are also important to diagnosis. A *thin* tongue points to Deficient Fluids, Blood, or Yin, whereas a *swollen* tongue suggests Dampness or Deficient Qi (because Qi is responsible for moving the fluids). A *contracted* tongue indicates excess Cold or blockage from Phlegm. A *weak trembly* tongue indicates that the Qi is too deficient to hold it still; it may be seen in extremely frail patients. But if the tongue is trembly and red, or red and hard, the cause is more likely Internal Wind, because Wind causes abnormal movement. Examples of Internal Wind syndromes include stroke and epilepsy. If someone moves his tongue abnormally in his mouth, or sticks it out without being asked, this suggests Disturbance of the Shen (mental illness, which in Oriental medicine is a problem of the Heart).

Listening and Smelling

As previously mentioned, the same Chinese character can be translated as both listening and smelling; both are used by some practitioners for diagnosis. The practitioner listens to the voice and breathing, smells the breath and the skin. Other sounds—joints creaking, flatulence—may also be noted.

Listening

In general, signs that are stronger and coarser are considered more Excess, and weaker, less forceful signs are more Deficient. This is generally the case for voice, coughs, and breathing patterns. Loss of voice as in laryngitis suggests invasion by External Pernicious Influence (e.g., Wind, Damp). A dry, hacking cough indicates either Heat or Dryness, whereas a really full wet cough and wheezing indicate Phlegm (recall that Phlegm in Oriental medicine is a Secondary Pathogenic Factor, not the same thing as mucus).

According to Five Phase theory, the character of the voice suggests specific types of imbalance. As with Color (see previous text), these voice qualities are subtle and the practitioner must develop considerable skill to use them in diagnosis. One kind of quality is called *shouting*—it is an intensity of voice use, a determined type of speaking that implies shouting even when the person whispers. *Shouting* correlates with Liver imbalance. *Laughing* tone, either a sound of constant amusement or actual frequent laughing at inappropriate moments, suggests a Heart imbalance. The quality called *singing* correlates to Spleen imbalance; this is a subtle lightness and dancing lilt to the voice that is neither accent-based nor language-based. A *weeping,* mournful voice tone points to the Lung. Finally, a *groaning* or slow, deep voice suggests Kidney imbalance.

Smelling

Some odors are overt and carried on the breath or skin—e.g., the odor of failing kidneys, of diabetic crisis, of an extreme sinus infection, or end-stage tuberculosis. The odors the practitioner of Oriental medicine seeks on every patient are, in contrast, subtle, something like the overtones that are left on the skin of a freshly washed person. These are qualities that can be difficult to detect, especially because in our society we train ourselves not to smell people. Practitioners who use smelling in diagnosis often sniff the mid-back, a locale where patients rarely apply scent and where they are unlikely to be anxious about being sniffed.

Again, Five Phase theory specifies which sorts of odors link to which Organ systems: *Rancid* (like rancid fat) is the odor of the Liver out of balance. *Scorched* (as from ironing) is a sign of Heart imbalance and can show up in the presence of a fever. A heavy, sickly *sweet* odor suggests problems of the Spleen. The odor of Lung/Large Intestine imbalance is *rotten,* like rotten meat or even stools. Kidney imbalance expresses as *putrid,* like old urine or an aquarium in need of cleaning. Interestingly, sometimes people report smelling these odors on themselves. One of my patients reported that she smelled like burning wood when she got overstressed, and another described herself as smelling like burning wet wood.

Asking

The classic texts of Chinese medicine specified 10 questions, or areas of concern, that the practitioner was to explore in reaching a diagnosis. These 10 were chills and fever, sweats, pain in head and body, state of urination and defecation, quality of diet, condition of chest, quality of hearing, character of thirst, history of previous disease, and perceived cause of disease. With some modification, these questions are still asked today.

Of course, today most Oriental medicine is offered in settings in which patients have also used other forms of medicine, particularly biomedicine. Thus modern patient record forms typically include questions that report the patient's biomedically defined laboratory results and conditions along with interpretations gleaned by a Oriental diagnosis (see Chapter 7).

Only during an intake interview is the full set of questions likely to be asked. And always, practitioners modify the basic set to follow a train of thought to name or confirm a diagnosis. This means that they may not ask the same questions of every patient, although they must be thorough enough in questioning to ensure that conflicting or complex signs are exposed. The practitioner's intention is to link the detail into a coherent whole, knowing that sometimes the pieces that do not fit an expected pattern are essential clues to an accurate diagnosis and subsequent treatment.

Interestingly, in this process realizing what the patient has *not* brought up is important. So also is the language in which the patient chooses to describe his distress. For example, a patient who states he is "drowning" in work may have an imbalance quite different from one who says he is "burnt out" by work. In the first case, the descriptive term suggests a Water (Kidney . . .) imbalance, whereas the second points toward a Fire (Heart . . .) imbalance. Sometimes what sounds irrelevant to the problem but is insisted on by the patient proves to be crucial to understanding how that particular person functions in the presence of the current illness. Finally, people often offer their Oriental practitioner bits of information that their biomedical physicians have said were not important; because Oriental medicine diagnosis is so different from that of biomedicine; such fragments can prove key in Oriental medical diagnosis.

The following text presents a brief examination of typical questions asked of Oriental medicine patients during the process of diagnosis. In each category, only the most classic questions and their associations are listed; in practice a practitioner might ask a far broader range of questions.

Medical and Psychosocial History

Usually the Asking part of the diagnosis begins with asking a patient to describe the problems that prompted seeking treatment. How the patient states what the problems are and how they are prioritized are valuable pieces of information. Sometimes, significantly, what appears to be the most serious issue is not what is bothering the patient most, and sometimes the patient only obliquely mentions the real issue. Attentive listening is vital to an Oriental medical diagnosis. Another aspect of this is to ask when these problems began and inquire about the whole context of the patient's life at both the time when the symptoms began and at the present time. Sometimes the clues to the diagnosis are in the context, not just in the actual medical condition.

Heat and Cold

This important category refers to the patient's subjective feeling of temperature, not what is measured on a thermometer. Heat corresponds with Yang and Cold with Yin. Cold is also experienced as the sensation of coldness and chills, or as aversion to cold, as in the patient who exclaims "I *hate* winter!" The opposite is true for Heat.

Fevers are extensively discussed in classic Chinese medicine because throughout human history febrile illness has been a major cause of death. In acute illness, fever with prominent chills often is classified as an Invasion of Wind-Cold Pernicious Influence, but when the fever is high without chills it is Invasion of Wind-Heat Pernicious Influence. The fever and/or chills are considered to be signs that the body is fighting the attack from the outside. There is considerable overlap between febrile conditions biomedicine has identified as being caused by microorganisms and conditions Chinese medicine defines as examples of Wind-Cold, Wind-Heat, or Wind-Damp-Heat Pernicious Influence.

Chinese medicine also recognizes patterns of lingering fevers, low-grade afternoon fevers, or alternating chills and fevers. Such fevers appear in biomedical conditions such as chronic fatigue immunodeficiency syndrome (CFIDS) and malaria. Chinese medicine states that the illness has penetrated deeper into the body, beyond the Defensive Qi (Exterior) level, but not yet into the Interior. It is stuck in a middle level called Lesser (Shao) Yang. In this situation, the patient is not strong enough to push the Pernicious Qi all the way out, but is strong enough to not allow further deterioration, so the illness lingers but not as an acute situation.

Finally, there is a category of chronic low-grade fevers that are said to be caused by a Deficiency of Yin.

This means that the Yin aspect of the body that cools and moistens is depleted. Yin Deficiency shows up as spotty patterns of heat, such as afternoon fevers, hot flashes, and hot hands and feet. This pattern is commonly seen in menopausal women, as well as in biomedical diseases such as tuberculosis and acquired immunodeficiency syndrome (AIDS).

Some people report being chronically cold. This is usually a sign of Deficiency of Yang or Qi (which warm the body and support movement). Often, however, the presence of cold or chilly sensations is not so straightforward. For example, there may be mixed signs of both heat and cold. A patient may report being cold, yet have a red tongue (a sign of heat). Or, a patient may have cold feet at the same time that her head is hot. The practitioner must sort all signs and symptoms to identify which predominate and how each interacts with the others.

Perspiration

Perspiration seems to be connected to Heat and Cold. However, in Chinese medicine, there is another factor: the ability of the body to control the opening and closing of the pores. The person who sweats frequently or with little exertion is believed to be weak, suffering one of the effects of Deficient Qi, because one of the functions of Qi is to control the pores. However, if excess sweating occurs in response to anxiety, it is interpreted as an imbalance of the Heart, because in Oriental medicine Mind is an aspect of Heart and the secretion associated with the Heart is perspiration. Night sweating is associated with Deficiency of Yin. The night is the most Yin time of day, a time when the body should remain cool as it sleeps. However, if there is not enough Yin, the heat of Yang bursts through, causing an inappropriate temperature rise relieved by sweating.

In the case of acute fevers, Oriental medicine views perspiration as a way for the body to eject the illness. In these acute situations, the Oriental clinician uses acupuncture and diaphoretic herbs to encourage sweating. However, when sweating is excessive, this is a sign of weakness of the body to retain its fluids. This can be countered by astringent acupuncture points and herbs.

Headache and Dizziness

Oriental medicine recognizes many patterns of imbalance that can manifest with headaches. The practitioner must ask many questions to reach an accurate diagnosis.
1. How do the headaches come on and when (e.g., with changes in the weather, particular activities, time of day)?
2. What is the character of the pain? Is it throbbing, sharp, one-sided, stuffy, boggy, and so forth?
3. What is the location? Is it stable or not, and with which meridian does it coincide?

Figure 3-3 illustrates meridians that pass through the head. When a headache coincides with the location of a meridian, the practitioner seeks other evidence for involvement of that meridian or Organ network; treatment includes that meridian and Organ. Particularly in treatment of chronic headaches, it is important to perform a complete pattern diagnosis of the patient. Chronic headache is a condition in which treating symptomatically is at best temporary and sometimes counterproductive.

The complaint of dizziness is, like headaches, nonspecific; it too requires a good general diagnosis to determine the pattern. Severe dizziness and vertigo is usually related to Wind, because Wind is often characterized by abnormalities in movement. Some patients do report dizziness after exposure to environmental wind, or when suffering from a simple Wind Invasion (a "cold" in biomedical terms). Internal patterns include those of slight dizziness or light-headedness associated with Deficiency of Blood (e.g., in low blood pressure), and a heavy, muddled dizziness that links to Phlegm.

Pain

Pain, in Oriental medicine, is caused by slow flow (stagnation) or blockage (stasis) of Qi and/or Blood. The first step in diagnosing pain is to determine if it is acute or chronic. Acute pain can often be treated locally, with rapid good results. For example, acupuncture can be used to relieve pain in strains and sprains, whereas cupping and moxibustion (see Chapter 4) can release congealed blood in bruises. Acupuncture or herbs can be used to relieve the pain of tension headache, achy muscles from overwork, acute diarrhea, and the like.

In chronic situations, the practitioner must perform a more complete diagnostic process to discover why Qi or Blood cannot move through the region of the pain. For example, the location of the pain is important because it may be on or near a particular meridian. Sometimes chronic dysfunction in an organ can show up along its meridian and the pain will not heal until the Organ dysfunction is addressed. An example is tennis elbow that does not heal. The patient may have a long weakness in the Large Intestine meridian that must be addressed to alleviate the pain in the elbow.

In addition, the practitioner must know what the pain feels like. Distending pain that moves about is as-

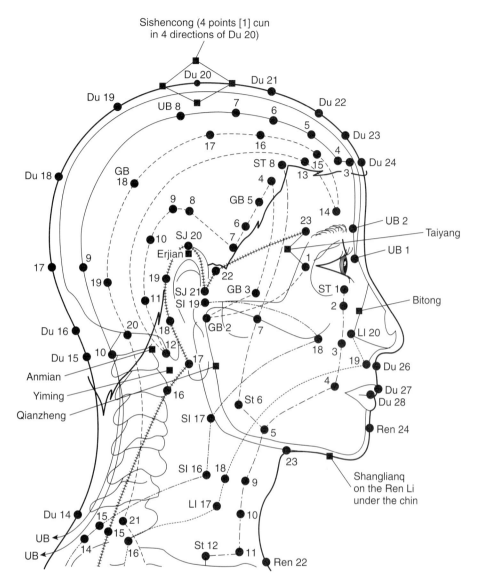

Figure 3-3. Lateral view of the head showing acupoints. In Chinese medicine the location and character of the headache are taken into account when selecting points for local stimulation. Points elsewhere on the body, particularly on the hands and feet, are added to complete a treatment prescription. (From Student manual on the fundamentals of traditional oriental medicine, ed 3, La Mesa, Calif, 1998, Living Earth Enterprises.)

sociated with Stagnant Qi, whereas pain that is stabbing and fixed is associated with Congealed Blood. If heat relieves pain, then part of the disharmony involves the presence of Cold and vice versa. If pressure relieves pain, it is associated with Deficiency, but if pressure increases the pain, it is an Excess condition. More questions of this nature are asked depending on the context.

In Oriental medicine, numbness is considered a kind of pain characterized by absence of sensation.

There are two major types. In one, Blood, which in Oriental medicine includes both the vascular and nervous circulatory systems, is Deficient. Because it is Deficient, Blood does not bring awareness and sensation to the area. In the second, numbness is related to the presence of Internal Wind, and secondarily, to the buildup of Phlegm. This combination results in symptoms such as hemiplegia (e.g., what biomedicine associates with stroke).

Thirst, Appetite, Taste in Mouth, Dietary Preference

Thirst for cold liquids is a sign of Heat, and thirst for warm liquids is a sign of Cold. Absence of thirst may be a sign of Cold, especially in the digestion. An unusually interesting sign is that of thirst without a desire to drink; this suggests Damp Heat. In this case, although Heat causes thirst, the simultaneous presence of internal Dampness means that there is no desire to drink.

Because Spleen Qi transforms the food consumed, lack of appetite often indicates a Deficiency of Spleen Qi. However, Dampness can also cause lack of appetite because Dampness makes the person feels distended and heavy, as if chronically overfilled. Excessive appetite is a key sign of Stomach Fire.

Each of the five Yin organs has a distinct taste associated with it, which, if constantly present, suggests abnormality in that network. Thus the Oriental practitioner asks patients if they have distinctive flavors in their mouths even when not eating. For example, the bitter flavor in food is said to nourish the Heart, but excess injures the Heart. A patient who reports a bitter taste in the mouth suggests Heat in the Heart or Liver Organ. Sweet is associated with the Spleen, but having this taste perpetually in the mouth may indicate Damp Heat of the Spleen. *Lack* of taste is also significant. It often indicates Spleen Qi Deficiency; sometimes it suggests a Heart imbalance because the Heart is responsible for making discriminations.

The five-flavor model is also applied to tending the patient's diet. Someone who overemphasizes (or underemphasizes) a particular flavor is pointing to an imbalance connected to that Organ system. Thus someone who overindulges in sweets or reports constantly craving a sweet would be suspected of having an imbalance in the Earth (Spleen/Stomach) network. This is equally true if a person insists that he cannot bear a particular type of food (e.g., "spicy" or "fatty"). The same model can be applied in making therapeutic dietary suggestions: not only would the patient who is hungry for sweets be treated to balance her Spleen, but she might also be encouraged to emphasize flavors such as sour and bitter, which might help to nourish and control the Spleen network (see Chapter 6).

Excretion and Secretion

In contrast to biomedicine, Oriental practitioners do not ask patients to provide samples of urine or stool for laboratory analysis. Instead, they seek the necessary information by asking questions. Excretions include urine, feces, and vomit; secretions include mucus, sweat, and milk.

There are many possible patterns for symptoms involving the stools, and the pattern can rarely be interpreted outside the context of the complete diagnostic picture. For example, constipation with dry, hard, and infrequent stools can be a sign of Heat (which dries the body), or a sign of dryness caused by Deficient Yin or Deficient Blood. Constipation that consists mainly of difficulty in moving a nonhard stool out of the body suggests Stagnation of the Liver Qi. Coldness or Deficient Yang can slow bowel movements or lead to watery, bland-smelling diarrhea. However, when diarrhea is urgent and smelly, it signifies the presence of Heat. Diarrhea from Deficient Spleen Qi or Yang is suggested by the presence of undigested food in the stool. Diarrhea that occurs primarily early in the morning is typical of Kidney Yang Deficiency. Alternation of constipation and diarrhea often indicates Stagnation of Liver Qi because the Liver is responsible for smooth and regular movement of the Qi.

In questioning the patient about urination, an important distinction is between Hot and Cold. In general, pale and copious urine is a sign of Cold, whereas dark yellow or reddish and scant urine is a sign of Heat. Incontinence and enuresis may occur in conjunction with several possibilities including Damp Heat of the Bladder, Kidney Deficiency, or Spleen Qi Deficiency. Difficulty in urination combined with pain can arise with blockage of Damp Heat in the Bladder, as well as with Stagnation of Liver Qi. What biomedicine identifies as a bacterial infection of the urinary bladder usually shows up as a Damp Heat Syndrome in Chinese medicine; sterile conditions such as interstitial cystitis can occur with Stagnation of Liver Qi.

The Qi of the Stomach normally moves down; vomiting is defined as Rebellious Qi of the Stomach, that is, it is moving in the wrong direction. When a patient reports vomiting, the practitioner asks additional questions similar to those concerning taste. Thus, sour vomit suggests the Liver is causing Stomach Heat, but bitter vomit indicates Heat in the Liver and Gallbladder. Thin, watery vomit can be a sign of Cold and Deficient Stomach Qi. Nausea, belching, and hiccuping without vomiting are also often signs of Rebellious Qi of the Stomach.

The assessment of mucus from the nose and throat follows the same pattern of analysis. Thin, clear phlegm is usually a sign of Cold, whereas thick, sticky, solid white, yellow, or green phlegm is a sign of Heat. Blood in the mucus is usually also a sign of Heat.

Sleep

In Chinese medicine there are many ways of not sleeping well. First, if a person has trouble falling asleep, this suggests difficulty in moving from Yang active time to Yin restful time; the patient may be Yin Deficient. However, because each meridian also has a particular time of day when it is primary (see Figure 2-4), the times at which a patient awakens also provide clues to the Organ network imbalance. For example, early waking can indicate disturbance in the Lung, Large Intestine, or Spleen. A general pattern of restless sleep during the night points to a Deficiency of Heart Blood. This is because the Shen (spirit) resides in the Blood and cannot rest calmly if its nourishment is insufficient. Dream-disturbed sleep (continuous dreaming) often indicates Heart or Liver Heat. Finally, excessive sleeping or the constant desire to sleep with lethargy can originate in a number of patterns of imbalance, especially Deficient Qi, Deficient Yang, and Dampness. Repetitious themes in dreams or nightmares also can provide information about the imbalance.

Gynecology

Whereas men are asked questions about their sexual and reproductive function when other symptomatology suggests the need, the classics proposed a set of gynecological questions and these are always asked of women. For example, the details of normal menstrual function help describe the characteristic functioning of an individual's Qi and Blood. Later, such data can help the practitioner interpret any changes the patient experiences. As already emphasized, to make sense of any one symptom, the whole pathological picture must be analyzed. This is well illustrated by the summary below, where a single sign may have several causes.

Periods that come earlier than normal suggest Heat, or Qi Deficiency. Late periods imply Stagnation of Blood, Deficiency of Blood, or Coldness. Irregularity of the cycle often points in the direction of Liver Stagnation because Liver regulates cycles. Menstrual blood that is intensely bright red indicates the presence of Heat, whereas pale or dark blood indicates Cold. Purplish blood means Stagnation of Blood, or Cold. Clots in the flow are often a sign of Congealed Blood, or Cold. Heavy bleeding or menorrhagia can come from several very different patterns: Heat in the Blood can cause intense bleeding, as can Qi Deficiency,

which can express itself as an inability to hold the Blood appropriately. Heavy bleeding also can be caused by Congealed Blood, as in what biomedicine calls fibroids. Finally, Cold also can cause excessive or inappropriate bleeding. Pain before periods often points to Liver disharmony, whereas pain during or after may point to problems with the Spleen.

The Oriental doctor also asks about vaginal discharges. As with most discharges, clear, thin copious discharges point to Cold, and thick, yellow ones suggest Heat. Itchiness, soreness, and specks of blood are also signs of Heat.

Infertility is a common reason for women to seek treatment in Oriental medicine. As in any kind of medicine, many possible causes are known, although in individual cases the cause may never be known. Oriental medicine can address some imbalances not recognized in biomedicine, thus furthering the chances of successful pregnancies. Some of the questions that lead to identifying contributing factors to infertility come from questions about menstruation. Thus, scant bleeding can be a sign of Deficient Blood, and dark blood and heavy clotting points to Congealed Blood; in Oriental medical theory, both of these can lead to infertility. Excessive Dampness, Heat, or Cold in the pelvic area (Lower Burner or *San Jiao*) can contribute to infertility. Kidney Essence *(Jing)* Deficiency can also be crucial.

Similar logic as that just presented is used to address women's issues linked to menopause. For detail on women's health issues, see Chapter 17.

Touching

This fourth part of the Four Examinations is considered by many to be the most important because it includes feeling the pulse. The other main parts of the examination are palpating the torso (especially the abdomen), and touching acupuncture points.

Pulse Diagnosis

The art of "taking the pulse" in Chinese medicine is subtle and complex, and provides remarkable feedback to the success of intervention. Pulse taking was already well described in the *Nei Jing Su Wen,* when pulses were taken on several arteries on the body. The later *Nan Jing* emphasized pulses at the radial artery, a locale that is normative today and is the focus of this section. Other locations are used by particular practitioners or under specific circumstances (e.g., carotid pulse or the pulse at the medial malleolus). For a wonderful history and explanation of the distinctions of feeling the pulse in Oriental and Western (Greek) medicine, see Kurigama.[4]

Taking the pulse in Oriental medicine yields information on the general quality of Qi and Blood flowing in the body, and additionally provides specific information about the character of the whole being. Reading the pulse demands sensitivity, skill, and experience, for there are many subtle variations that each practitioner must learn to identify by experience and continual practice.

Because taking the pulse depends on directly sensing, and has been practiced by a myriad of practitioners over much of the world for at least 2000 years, many different systems of correlation have developed. Commonly used schemas are summarized here; there are other, equally cogent, schemas that are not discussed here.[6]

Most schools of thought recognize three main positions on each wrist. Moving from distal (nearest wrist crease) to proximal (slightly closer to elbow) these are called *cun* or inch, *guan* or barrier, and *chi* or foot. In some popular traditions, each position has two depths, corresponding at the deeper level to the Yin Organs and at the superficial level to the Yang organs. In other styles, particularly some that emphasize herbal medicine, each position is thought to have three depths; these relate to the Yin Organs (deepest), the Blood (middle), and the Qi (most superficial).

Pulse positions given in Table 3-1 are based on the *Nan Jing;* these interpretations remain the most common even in modern textbooks. The set of positions that has been the most controversial is the right *chi* positions. Some styles interpret the deep level as reflecting the state of the Pericardium Organ, which translated from Chinese is actually "Heart Master," an aspect of the exterior function of the Heart. Other styles read this as reflecting the Yang aspect of the Kidney. The historical reasons for this conflict are complex; practically speaking, this position concerns the connection of Water and Fire.

In other styles practitioners have learned to "listen in" on other parts of the body through the pulses. For example, in the style of Leon Hammer (based on that of his teacher John Shen), there are pulse positions for the uterus, mitral valve, and diaphragm.[7,8] In short, in various traditions and over hundreds of years of observation, practitioners have discovered numerous correlations between various pulse positions and specific bodily functions and pathologies.

What does a practitioner feel for at these various positions? In a general sense, the pulse should be vibrant, soft but with a good strength and rhythm, filling the depths well, and repeating itself at an appropriate pace. The classics describe many possible pulse quali-

TABLE 3-1

Common Pulse Positions

	Left hand			Right hand		
	Superficial		Deep	Deep		Superficial
Model 1*						
cun	Small Intestine		Heart	Lung		Large Intestine
guan	Gall Bladder		Liver	Spleen		Stomach
chi	Urinary Bladder		Kidney	Pericardium/ Heart Master or Mingmen		Triple Warmer

	Superficial	Middle	Deep	Superficial	Middle	Deep
Model 2*						
cun		Heart			Lung	
guan		Liver			Spleen	
chi		Kidney			Kidney	

*Model 1 is used widely in Japanese and Five-Phase styles; Model 2 is used in TCM styles.

ties; these have been systematized as 28. The practitioner may find that all the pulses can have a particular quality, or some quality can occur in only one or two positions. Each position may combine several qualities. All of them are not reviewed here, but some examples will provide dimension to this discussion.

Some pulse qualities are paired in polarities, such as "superficial-deep," "fast-slow," "empty-full," and "long-short." A *slippery* pulse feels smooth and slides along under the finger "like a pearl in a white porcelain dish" (a classic description). Such a pulse is an indication of Dampness, Phlegm, or pregnancy. A *choppy* pulse is rough under the finger; it usually indicates Deficient Blood but can be a sign of Congealed Blood. The practitioner also distinguishes between *tight* and *wiry* qualities; these are close in sensation, but the latter is more extreme in its tautness and hardness. Both can indicate pain, but the tight pulse is more associated with Cold and the wiry pulse with Stagnation of Liver Qi. An interesting pulse quality is *hollow,* said to feel like the stalk of a spring onion where it is felt, lost and felt again as pressure is applied. This pulse indicates Deficient Blood, often from hemorrhage. The need to interpret pulses carefully is illustrated by the fact that if the hollow pulse is felt to be only slightly hollow, it may indicate impending hemorrhage. In this case, prompt intervention may prevent blood loss. Many pulse qualities suggest various types and causes of weakness, for example, *fine, minute, soft, weak,* and *scattered.* Because each implies a different source of malfunction, the practitioner is well served by developing discernment through practice in pulse reading.

An important feature of taking pulses is that they can provide the practitioner immediate feedback concerning the effectiveness of her treatment. With acupuncture and moxibustion treatment, pulse qualities can change literally within seconds. Sometimes a practitioner will check the appropriateness of a point selection by touching it and observing whether the appropriate change in the pulse occurs, before actually inserting the needle into the point.

The most common positions for the patient in pulse taking are sitting with the forearms on a small pillow or lying down with the practitioner holding the arm; usually the wrist is kept at about the same level as the heart. Generally the practitioner uses the index, middle, and ring fingers of the right hand for the distal, middle, and proximal positions respectively, of the patient's left hand, and those fingers of the left hand for the patient's right hand. In this way, one finger al-

ways feels the same pulse position. This allows that finger to specialize in the quality of Qi in those functions. In some systems of pulse taking, the practitioner moves the finger or rolls it in several ways to gather additional information.

Abdominal Diagnosis

Palpation of the abdomen is a common feature of diagnosis in Japanese and related styles of acupuncture. This technique was first described in the *Nan Jing,* a Chinese classic text that much influenced Japanese acupuncture practices. Figure 3-4 shows a basic map; as with most of Oriental medicine, this map has been elaborated over the years so other sources may show variants on this figure.

As in feeling the pulse, the practitioner doing abdominal diagnosis is trying to sense any deviation from a healthy quality. The healthy abdomen is resilient but not tight, soft but not flabby, and has Spirit or vibrancy. If an area is cold or hot, rough or too smooth, too soft or too hard, distended or sunken, dry or too moist, or if there is pain on palpation, it suggests a problem linking the symptom and its location. As with pulses, if diagnosis and treatment are correct, these indications often disappear immediately after treatment, thus providing the practitioner with a rapid feedback system on his intervention.

A similar diagnostic technique involves palpating the *San Jiao* or Triple Burner Organ. Recall that the Triple Burner is "the organ with a function but no body" and that it governs the flow of water in the body. Although it is an Organ identified primarily

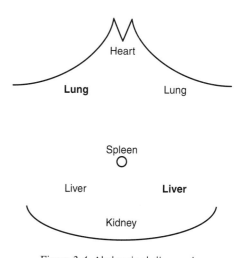

Figure 3-4 Abdominal diagnosis.

energetically, it has regions of effect within which are ordinary Organs. Thus the Upper Burner is in the chest (and contains the Lung, Pericardium, and Heart Organs); the Middle Burner is above the umbilicus but below the diaphragm; and the Lower Burner is in the lower abdomen. By comparing the temperature of the chest and the two regions of the abdomen, the practitioner learns about the relative activity of the various regular Organs, and about the general health of the *San Jiao* itself. For example, coldness in the Lower Burner might indicate Coldness or Deficiency of Qi of the Kidneys, Large Intestine, or the uterus, with many possible consequences including constipation, incontinence, edema, fatigue, and infertility.

Palpating the Points

Another possible means of gathering diagnostic data is from the palpation of acupuncture points. Generally sharp pain (Excess) or soreness (Deficiency) at a point is an indication that the point and its corresponding Organ network may not be balanced. Some styles of practice also consider other indications at the point to be significant (e.g., coolness, moistness, or lack of vitality suggest Deficiency, whereas an Excess may express as heat, swelling, or redness).

One often palpated set of points is the Front *Mu* or Alarm points, mostly found on the anterior trunk. Mu means a "call to arms." These points are particularly sensitive to imbalances, and each point relates directly to an Organ System. Another frequently palpated set is the Back *Shu* points; these parallel the spine and also correlate to each Organ System. Practitioners also palpate in regions indicated as painful by the patient; the most exquisitely painful spots, once accurately located, can be treated by insertion of needles and are called *ah shi* or "ouch" points. Practitioners may also palpate points to check their diagnostic hunches. For example, if the practitioner suspects a pattern of imbalance in the Extraordinary Meridians (see Chapter 2), the practitioner may check the sensitivity of the pairs of points that correspond to those Meridians.

MOVING FROM DETAIL TO PATTERN TO TREATMENT

Practitioners in all forms of medicine reach diagnostic conclusions by gathering detail, correlating it with theory, and constructing a "most probable" diagnosis. On this basis they treat with the expectation that follow-up of the patient will reveal the accuracy of the diagnosis and guide rediagnosis when necessary. In this sense, diagnosis in Oriental medicine is entirely typical. As shown, Oriental medicine recognizes numerous symptoms, assigns meaning to them, and follows a fairly standard theory-driven logic in constructing a diagnosis. Because the underlying theory is not biomedical, the conclusions reached are not biomedical ones. Nevertheless, biomedical readers will recognize many points of similarity of interpretation at a *clinical* level; the logic also "works" in the sense that patients of Oriental practitioners feel and function better (see Chapter 12).

As with all medicines, there is more than theory and logic to successful delivery—there is also art. Practitioners who treat a wider range of patients, who develop their skills in collecting and interpreting data, and who develop themselves so as to understand human beings deeply are most able to come to know why a person is suffering, most able to bring that person back into balance.

Each style of Oriental medicine offers somewhat distinct diagnostic and intervention procedures, and individual practitioners also have both preferences and strengths in practice. In sum, there is no single way to diagnose and treat a patient in Oriental medicine; there are many ways and all may be effective. Although mentioned previously, it is important to reemphasize that where one practitioner may see the signs of (for example) Stagnant Qi of the Liver leading to a condition expressing itself in the Lungs, another may choose to focus on the Deficiency of the Lung, which allows the Liver to overact upon it. Both interpretations are legitimate; both may be equally successful as they are translated into intervention protocols. Why? Because, as discussed at the beginning of this chapter, Oriental medicine works with the *flow* of energy through a *dynamic whole* organism. Thus, rather than being "right" or "wrong" in focusing on Liver or Lung, the practitioner has simply chosen to treat the imbalance from one side or the other.

Differences in diagnosis are to be expected with different styles of practice. Styles vary in how much emphasis is placed on understanding and treating the inherited constitution of the patient versus the symptoms reported by the patient. Most forms of practice agree that individuals have tendencies to certain types of imbalance. Some maintain that people have a constitutional type that does not change in their lifetime and that all or most symptoms show up through that constitution. That constitutional type determines strength as well as weakness. These discussions most often use the framework of the Five Phases. In some Korean and French styles, the practitioner identifies the basic constitution and thereafter always treats through that Phase (Element) guided by a logic that states that the symptoms arise from an imbalance within that constitution. If the basic Phase is working well, the person will be healthy. In contrast, other Five-Phase systems such as Japanese Meridian Therapy and Leamington (Worsley) styles identify central *tendencies*. These tendencies are not as unchanging as in the purely constitutional styles. Instead, there are general patterns that tend to last but do not necessarily do so—what is treated each time is what presents itself as needing attention. In the Japanese styles, the "root" treatment is often (but not always) on the same pattern, whereas the "branch" treatments address the particular symptoms and situations.

The largest group of Chinese and Western practitioners of Oriental Medicine practice TCM style. Codified in the 1950s in the People's Republic of China, this style is little interested in constitutional typing. Instead, practitioners analyze symptoms, using guides such as Yin and Yang and the other Eight Principles to identify dynamic states of malfunction. Practitioners then decide if they prefer to treat troublesome symptoms directly (a "branch" treatment), or indirectly and more deeply by addressing the affected Organ networks (a "root" treatment).

Many other interpretive models exist and are applied as necessary. For example, although the constitutional issue concerns mainly the major Organs, malfunction also may be focused in the meridians. Localized muscular pain may indicate a problem with a Regular or a Muscle Meridian; both can be treated directly. Other symptoms, such as those concerned with imbalance of the musculature between the limbs (including paralysis or developmental problems), can be treated by addressing the Eight Extraordinary Vessels.

A model applied in the treatment of Cold disease is called the Six Stages; another applied to the identification of Heat disorders is called the Four Levels. These models are often referred to in Oriental herbal medicine but also can be applied with acupuncture. This introduction does not further describe the application of these models (see Chapter 2). Both the Six Stages and Four Levels hold special interest for biomedical readers because they concern the barriers of protection of the body and the progression of dis-

ease. In both models, there are descriptions of what happens to the person who is experiencing an attack from on External Invasion as it progresses to deeper levels of the body. Survival is progressively more difficult the deeper the invasion. In a slightly different way, these models describe levels on which disease can occur, not just as a progression but where the person is suffering so that the practitioner can better direct the treatment to that level.

Treatment of Symptoms

Thus far the discussion has emphasized theory-driven intervention—diagnostic practices that lead to understanding the patterns that underlie symptoms, so that treatment may aim at the root. However, substantial literature in Oriental medicine concerns formulas, both herbal and of acupoints, for the direct treatment of symptoms. When properly applied, such formulas are appropriate and effective. For example, the acupoint P6 (Pericardium 6) is highly effective for stopping many types of nausea. This use has been popularized in the elastic cuffs worn over their wrists by people with a tendency to motion sickness. Each cuff has a small metal magnet; the user is instructed how to place the magnet, which is, of course, to place it over P6.

Formulaic approaches can be ineffective when they counter the pattern of an individual imbalance. In such cases, a treatment may work briefly but yield no sustained improvement. For this reason, most practitioners prefer to use symptomatic treatments as adjuncts and not as the main thrust of treatment.

The issue of the appropriateness of symptomatic formulas looms large in the design of "protocol-designed" controlled trial research. Because, as this chapter has shown, the use of symptomatic formulas does not represent the norm or the strength of Oriental diagnosis, it is not the best choice for research intended to test the effectiveness of Oriental medicine. A better design choice is that of "standard care"-controlled trials, in which standard care in one medical system is compared with standard care in another. In the latter design, participating practitioners perform a complete diagnosis and treat patients to the best of their ability. This means, of course, that people with the "same" symptoms from the point of view of biomedicine may prove to demand different interventions from the point of view of Oriental medicine. In designing research, or in assessing published research results, it is important to remember that the protocol design tests only the effectiveness of a particular formula, but not the effectiveness of Oriental medicine for that symptom or condition. These issues are discussed in more detail in Chapters 13, 15, and 19.

CONNECTING WITH BIOMEDICAL DIAGNOSES

Although the process used by biomedical and Oriental medical practitioners to reach diagnosis differs, the underlying goal is the same: to understand the character and source of a patient's distress. Accordingly, it is useful for both types of practitioners to know what diagnoses, and prognoses, the patient has received in the other practice of medicine.

A common difference between the two medicines concerns the ability to distinguish among expressions of a condition. For example, a biomedical diagnosis of "colitis" tells the Oriental practitioner that there is evidence of inflammation of the colon. The biomedical practitioner would be expected to focus intervention on the colon and possibly on the patient's emotional status (colitis is one of the disorders in which biomedicine recognizes an emotional component and categorizes as "psychosomatic"). In Oriental medicine, the label "colitis" does not necessarily guide the practitioner to treat the Large Intestine. While keeping open this possibility, this practitioner would also suspect malfunction at least in the Liver and Stomach networks, and would not be surprised to find a multi-network imbalance. Why? Because the human physiological system is integrated, Qi and Blood are moving, linking every part of the organism. Thus using a Five-Phase model of interpretation—while the Large Intestine (the Yang Organ of the Metal Phase, the "child" of the Earth Phase, Sheng cycle) may be signaling distress the loudest—the practitioner would automatically suspect weakness or blockage of its "mother" (Stomach, Earth Phase) and the controller of its mother (Ke cycle, Wood Phase, Liver Organ). The Oriental practitioner also would not be surprised to find Lung symptoms, because Lung is the Yin Organ of the Metal Phase, the partner in "taking in and letting go" of the Large Intestine. If the diagnosis is made again using a TCM interpretive process, the Colon is suffering from Internal Heat, a situation that can occur when the Liver is unable to keep the Qi and Blood moving smoothly. The Liver can malfunction this way both when the Stomach and Spleen fail to

provide Qi (from food) appropriately, and when the patient is suffering from excessive Emotion. To summarize this example, both medicines recognize symptoms focused on the Colon, both suspect an emotional component, but Oriental medicine may have reason to treat distant from the Colon. This issue of how the two medicines "divide up" a particular symptomatic set is developed in detail in Chapter 19 for the case of depression.

Biomedicine has diagnostic advantages over Oriental medicine in its ability to directly explore the interior of the body. Although the classic theory of Oriental medicine states that it is not necessary to have such information to make a diagnosis, in Oriental Medicine it can be helpful if the biomedical data can be translated into the physiological terms of Oriental Medicine.

This point also is valid if phrased the other way: the perceptions of the Oriental practitioner can serve the biomedical practitioner if he knows how to apply them. I and some of my colleagues have been able to help locate areas of infection and tumors, gallstones in a child, undiagnosed fractures, and other issues all of which were not clear to biomedical diagnosis. Our diagnostic procedures can also identify conditions such as cancer in nascent stages by, for example, reading oddities in the pulse—this should allow preventive care, allowing the patient to avoid development of an actual tumor.

A different issue concerns the situation in which patients seek Oriental medicine treatment when they have had limited success with biomedical intervention. Sometimes they arrive with biomedical diagnoses, sometimes not. Because Oriental medicine gathers different information and offers different diagnostic categories, it also offers novel possibilities for understanding what has gone awry. Although these may not directly serve biomedical practitioners, they may be helpful to the patient in offering new perspectives and treatment possibilities. Chapter 8 offers case histories with data on both biomedical and Oriental medical diagnoses, intervention efforts, and success levels from both practitioner and patient points of view.

SUMMARY

Diagnosis in Oriental medicine involves gathering a range of information and impressions, then applying theory and the sensitivity of experience to comprehending the patterns of disharmony that explain the patient's suffering. The emphasis is not laid on one symptom or aspect of the organism but on the interaction of all its parts. The best clues to overall pattern may seem unrelated to the overt symptomatology because the practitioner's goal is to expose an overall pattern of disharmony, and treat the "root" rather than the symptomatic "branch." To the extent that Oriental diagnosis differs from biomedical diagnosis, there arise new perceptions and thus novel possibilities for intervention.

References

1. Kaptchuk TJ: *The web that has no weaver: understanding Chinese medicine,* rev ed, Chicago, 2000, Contemporary Publishing.

2. Nan Jing: *The classic of difficult issues* (translated by PU Unshuld), Berkeley, Calif, 1986, University of California Press.

3. Lao T: *Tao Te Ching* (translated by JCH Wu), New York, 1961, St John's University Press.

4. Kuriyama S: *The expressiveness of the body and the divergence of Greek and Chinese medicine,* New York, 1999, Zone Books.

5. Maciocia G: *Tongue diagnosis in Chinese medicine,* rev ed, Seattle, 1995, Eastland Press.

6. Birch S: An historical study of radial pulse six position diagnosis: naming the unnameable, *J Acupuncture Soc NY* 1(3-4):19, 1994.

7. Hammer L: *Chinese pulse diagnosis: a contemporary approach,* Seattle, Wash, 2001, Eastland Press.

8. Shen JHF: *Chinese medicine,* New York, 1980, Educational Solutions.

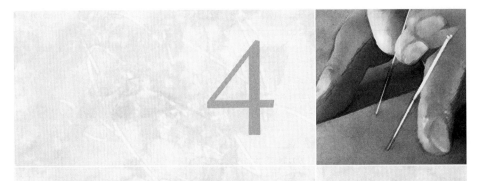

Acupuncture and Moxibustion

GRANT ZHANG

The marvel of the needle lies in its subtlety.

NAN JING #74

The word *acupuncture* is used both to define a medical technique and to refer to the entire theory and practice of one of the five major modalities of Chinese medicine.

As technique, acupuncture consists of appropriately inserting and manipulating special needles in selected points on the body. Use of acupuncture needles is often combined with *moxibustion* (burning the herb *Artemesia vulgaris* over acupoints) and with *cupping* (creating a local vacuum over acupoints). All these techniques are intended to draw Qi into or move Qi through the stimulated areas. Acupoints also can be stimulated by pressure alone, a procedure known as *acupressure;* a popular Japanese version is called *shiatsu.* Moxibustion,

cupping, and acupressure are discussed later in this chapter.

As a modality, the term *acupuncture* subsumes a large, ancient, and heterogeneous theory that guides technique—the main topic of this chapter. In China, acupuncture is generally viewed as secondary to herbal treatment, but outside China it is the most famous and most dispersed, as well as the most biomedically researched, of the modalities of Chinese medicine. This is so true that in many texts and in popular language, the term acupuncture is often used as a blanket term to imply the whole practice of Chinese medicine.

Acupuncture theory develops aspects of Chinese medical theory that emphasize locality and the relationship of parts (i.e., acupoints and meridians). Acupuncture is used to strengthen the body's defense system and open blocked energy circulation networks. This improves the production and circulation of vital materials such as Qi and Blood. Acupuncture's focus on enhancing homeostasis makes it suitable to treat a broad range of diseases.

WHAT ARE ACUPUNCTURE POINTS?

Defining Acupoints

An acupuncture point or *acupoint* is defined in Chinese medicine as a place on the body surface "where Qi and Blood gather." Because Qi* and Blood circulate throughout the entire body, virtually any surface area on the body can be stimulated as if it were an acupoint, particularly if it is aching or painful to touch. However, some locations are at all times responsive and can be mapped from person to person; these are termed *regular* acupoints, and it is these points that are discussed in medical theory and most often used in treatment.

Histologically, an acupoint is a three-dimensional structure composed of skin, submucosa, and muscle

*Qi, also spelled Ch'i or Chi, is pronounced chee.

fibers, sometimes tendons or ligaments, but so far no unique structures have been associated with acupoints. Although referred to as a "point," in fact both the diameter of responsive tissue, and its depth, clearly vary widely. This depends partly on the anatomical location (a point over a bone cannot have as great a depth as a point over soft tissue) and the size of the individual (point size is proportional to body size). More importantly, however, clinical observation and medical theory identify some points as unusually powerful, as having a wider sphere of effect, than other points. These issues matter both in the design of research (see Chapters 11, 13, 15, and 19) and in the appropriate selection of points and needling technique in delivering care. We recommend imagining the acupoint less as a point than as a region with both depth and width.

Acupoints fall into two main categories: those with fixed locations and those with changeable locations. Points with fixed locations are composed of Meridian acupoints (regular acupoints) and a growing list of "extraordinary" or new points that are gradually being added to the classic canon; there are more than 400 fixed acupoints. Each such acupoint carries a Chinese name, an alphanumeric name, and a precise anatomical location. Regular points occur along one of the 14 Meridians (12 regular bilateral Meridians and 2 midline extra Meridians). Regular points typically have several to many energetic features and physiological functions (Table 4-1).

TABLE 4-1

Comparison of Meridian, Extraordinary, and Ah-shi Points

Type of point	Example of type	Location	Related meridian	Special relation	Selected indications
Meridian point	Urinary Bladder 18 *Gan Shu*	On the back, below the spinous process of the ninth thoracic vertebra, 1.5 cun lateral to the posterior midline	Urinary bladder	Liver	Liver and Gall Bladder disorders, hypochondriac pain, mental problems, pain along the spinal cord
Extra point	EX-CA1 *Zigong* (Uterus point)	4 cun below the umbilicus and 3 cun lateral to the midline	None	None	Prolapse of uterus, infertility, premenstrual syndrome, lumbago
Ah-shi point	None	Unfixed	None	None	Local muscle or joint pain

The number of recognized Meridian acupoints has increased over time. In the classic *Nei Jing,* written in 475~200 BCE in China, there were only 160 points recorded; by 1817 in *Fu Yuan,* 361 points with their multiple functions were listed. This reflects a historical process of clinical trial and error, verification, and recognition of points. Currently most textbooks define 361 points as Meridian points.[1]

The extraordinary points have precise anatomical locations but may or may not be located along Meridians. For example, although *Yintang* (an extra point centered between the eyes at the top of the bridge of the nose) is on the midline in the same location as the Du or Governing Meridian, it is not considered a Du Meridian acupoint. *Erjian,* another extraordinary point, is located at the apex of the ear away from any Meridian. The group of extraordinary points claims an ever-growing list with mixed recognition. Some texts identify only dozens of these points; others name several hundreds.[2] Many extraordinary points have relatively simple and focused functions; they are usually used to enhance the effects of Meridian acupoints.

Points with changeable locations are called ah shi or "ouch" points. Found by palpation, these points become active and painful only in conjunction with a malfunction so are neither Meridional nor fixed in location. Ah-shi points are like trigger or tender points, and their number is virtually unlimited. They are often used in treating acute muscular pain.

In Europe and the United States, regular acupoints are given alphanumerical designations in addition to their Chinese name to facilitate point location. For example, ST 36 means Stomach Meridian, point 36 (the Stomach Meridian has 45 points; Figure 4-1). The Chinese names also have been translated into European languages, and some practitioners use these names as well as the numerical and Chinese designations. The English name for ST 36 is Leg Three Miles, a name that helps identify its location and remind one of its many functions (it is a point walkers can press to enhance their energy when fatigued).

The Meridian System

With more than 400 points known and in regular use, how do practitioners remember the distribution and distinguish among the functions? With only the points marked on a manikin, for example, the task simply of remembering the points becomes similar to remembering the stars in the night sky. Fortunately, acupoints are grouped by function in several different ways. The most familiar—and in terms of Chinese physiological theory, arguably the most important grouping—is called the Meridian (or Channel) system.

In this system, regular acupoints are organized into constellations with linear form, called *Meridians* or *Channels.* As with the points, there are regular channels as well as several additional groups of channels (see Table 2-3). Together these form a network that delivers Qi and Blood to every part of the body. The regular acupoints are distributed on the 2 midline Meridians and the 12 bilateral or regular Meridians distributed symmetrically on the body and extremities. Other Meridians can be accessed by using points on these 14 Meridians. Each major Meridian connects with an Organ system internally, as well as with acupoints externally.

Meridians are named by their corresponding Organ, distribution pattern on the extremities, and Yin-Yang property. For example, the full name of the Stomach Meridian is "Stomach Foot Yangming Meridian," because it connects with the stomach, moves from the head toward the foot, and is distributed on the lateral part of the leg, which belongs to the Yang category in Chinese medicine. Most important for understanding the logic of acupuncture treatment, all the points on (for example) the Stomach Meridian reflect, and can affect, the function of the Stomach, as well as its partner Organ, the Spleen. In addition, because of other connections, both of Channel pathway and of physiological influence, points on the Stomach Meridian can also affect the function of other Organs and Tissues. In short, by needling on the Stomach Meridian, the practitioner can directly affect the function of the Stomach and Spleen Meridians and Organs, and can also indirectly affect the function of the entire energy network of the body. This logic applies to all the Meridians and their acupoints.

An important feature of Meridians is that they help explain how remote points can have central effects. Thus each Meridian serves a specific Organ system, yet many of its component points are on the extremities well away from the Organ. It is probable that the Meridian system originated from clinical observations of the functions of individual points. For example, stimulation of the ST 36 point below the knee

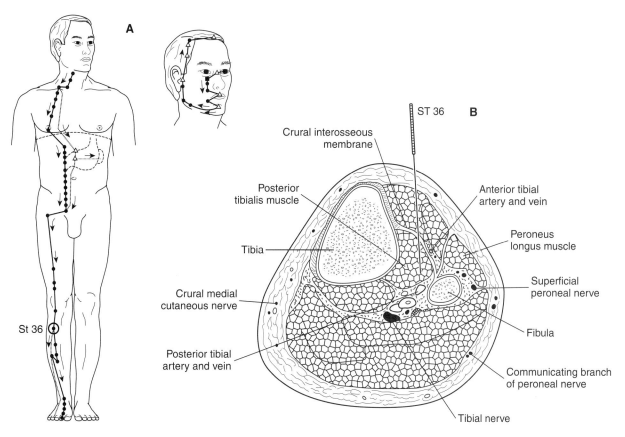

Figure 4-1 **A,** View of the Stomach channel. The first acupoint is located centrally below the eye. It runs over the face, neck, and down the front of the body, the front of the leg, and ends at the tip of the second toe. St 36 is highlighted. **B,** Cross-section of St 36 shows the anatomical structures traversed by the acupuncture needle. (**A** from Macioca G: *The foundations of Chinese medicine: a comprehensive text for acupuncturists and herbalists,* Edinburgh, 1989, Churchill Livingstone; **B** from Chen E: *Cross-sectional anatomy of acupoints,* Edinburgh, 1982, Churchill Livingstone.)

often results in changes in stomach activities. A connection between ST 36 and the Stomach Meridian could thus be established. It is a general rule that points on a given Meridian can treat the conditions caused by or associated with the dysfunction of that Organ.

However, equally important, many points have multiple functions, not all of which can be directly explained by their Meridian location. Thus ST 36 can also be used for treating asthma, insomnia, mania, and many other conditions besides gastrointestinal conditions. These uses were discovered by clinical experience; to date, scientific research has not been able to explain the specificity of acupoints.

Other Point Groupings

Independent of channel location, acupoints can be grouped by other features (see Chapter 2). For example, some points are especially effective for treating acute excess symptoms, others for reaching deep wells of Qi, others for affecting the spirit or emotion connections associated with an Organ, and yet others for connecting regularly with other Meridians so as to reach the superficial energy network rapidly. There are also points used in emergencies—to abort asthma attacks, revive the unconscious, alleviate shock, stop nausea, relieve urinary retention, arrest convulsions, and so forth.

Other Approaches to Acupuncture

In this chapter, we emphasize points on the whole body, especially along meridians. But there are other systems of points that are also often used by acupuncturists, including forms called Hand acupuncture, Foot acupuncture, Ear/Auricular acupuncture, and Scalp Acupuncture. The first three are based on the idea in Chinese medicine that the whole body is represented holographically in the parts. This idea also underlies the use of diagnosis of the tongue (or face) to diagnose for the whole body (see Chapter 3).

According to this understanding, the whole body can be reached by treating specific sites on the body part.

In this book, hand and foot acupuncture schema are not discussed. However, Chapters 9 and 14 discuss the use of auricular points in the treatment of substance abuse, and ear acupuncture is also frequently used in ordinary TCM acupuncture treatments. Scalp acupuncture points are based on bioscientific understandings of the basic function of the underlying brain structures. It too is becoming increasingly popular because it works well in treating central nervous system disorders including paralysis (see Chapter 19; also see Chapter 8, section 5).

These groups are discussed in Chinese medical textbooks and are not developed here. However, to illustrate the concept, we mention several important groupings.

Five Shu—or Command—Points

Five points on each bilateral Meridian located below the elbow and below the knees are therapeutically pivotal in most styles of acupuncture care. In traditional Chinese medicine (TCM) style, these points are metaphorized as Waterways, a model that was described in the *Ling Shu*.* Here the first point in the series, found on the tip of the digit, is the "well" point where Qi "starts to bubble" and the energy is deep and needs to be pumped out, as by pricking. The next four in the series are "spring," "stream," "river," and "sea" points, the names clarifying that the accessibility of Qi at these points progressively increases. Each type of point has special uses that correlate with its Qi proportionality. For example, well points are used in acute situations, such as syncope, when a degree of force ("pumping the well") is needed to restore the normal flow of Qi. In contrast, Qi is flourishing and stable at

sea points, and these are used to tonify the Qi of the whole body.

The logic for use of the same five points is rather different in Leamington style acupuncture practice, where the points are linked to the five Elements, as first described in the *Nan Jing*. Again starting with the tips of the digits, on the Yin Meridians the points correlate with Wood, Fire, Earth, Metal, and Water. On the Yang Meridians, the same sequence links to Metal, Water, Wood, Fire, and Earth. Each Element has particular characteristics, and the flow of energy through the elements, along with the expression of the elements, can be modified by appropriate needling of the Command points.

Source Points

Some of the Command points also have other special characteristics. For example, the third (Stream) point on any Yin Meridian is a powerful Source point through which the practitioner can access Original (Yuan) Qi of the associated Organ. Original Qi is the Qi that the individual receives at conception, hence the basis of the person's lifelong supply of Qi. (Additional Qi is gathered through life by eating, drinking, and breathing.) Source points are typically stimulated when the client has a deficiency condition such as a chronic disorder.

Source points frequently become sensitive or even painful when the associated Organ is malfunctioning, so practitioners can use palpation of Source points to guide diagnosis. For example, Lu 9 (Lung 9, palmar

---

*Centuries of oral tradition were compiled into the first classic of Chinese medicine, the *Huang-Di Nei Jing* or *Yellow Emperor's Classic,* in the Warring States, approximately 475 to 221 BCE. This text has two main parts, also referred to as texts: *Su Wen* or *Inner Classic of the Yellow Emperor, Simple Questions,* and the *Ling Shu* or *Classic of the Spiritual Axis* (or *Pivot*). The *Nan Jing* or *Classic of Difficulties* written in the second century CE contains interpretations and clarifications of material in the *Nei Jing*.

aspect, radial side of wrist, in transverse crease, lateral to radial artery) is often sensitive in asthmatic patients, whereas Sp 3 (Spleen 3, proximal and inferior to the head of the first metatarsal bone) may hurt in those with repetitive digestive complaints.

Influential Points

There are also eight special points with functions relating to the conditions of Qi, Blood, bone, tendon, and other Tissues. Scattered over the body, each of these points has multiple functions in addition to those covered by the term "influential point." For example, to tonify all the Qi of the body at once, the practitioner can needle at Ren 17 (midline of sternum, level with fourth intercostal space), and to strengthen bones and "soothe the sinews" one can needle UB 11 (level with the lower margin of the spinous process of the first thoracic vertebra).

THEORY OF THE ACUPOINT

It is easy to become focused on describing acupoints and easy to lose track of the reasons for studying them. In Chinese medicine, the reason for studying acupoints is that they serve as external signposts to the condition of the interior and provide gateways to the interior by which the practitioner can affect the movement of body energy and fluids and the functioning of the unseen internal organs. The classic terminology states that acupoints serve as sites to "access and regulate Qi and Blood." In bioscientific terminology, it may be stated that appropriate acupuncture needling improves bodily homeostasis, supporting efficient function of the organism.

Thus acupoints can be used both for diagnosing and treating an illness. Common pathological manifestations on acupoints include tenderness, redness, and hardness. These are interpreted as signals from the interior concerning malfunction in an Organ or in the flow of Qi through the Meridians. For example, it has been observed that respiratory disorders often show abnormality on LU 1 (upper anterior wall of chest), LU 7 (wrist), and UB 13 (upper posterior wall of chest), whereas disorders of the Liver and the Gall Bladder typically show tenderness at UB 18 and 19 (mid-posterior wall of abdomen), and at Liv 13 and 14 (lower edge of rib cage anteriorly), which are special points for these organs (Figure 4-2). In addition,

points in any location can be tender if the flow of Qi is blocked (which usually causes acute and painful symptoms) or flows too slowly and stagnates (causing dull aches and chronic symptoms such as a perpetually stuffy nose, abdominal distention, or emotional symptoms such as depression).

BIOSCIENTIFIC EFFORTS TO UNDERSTAND ACUPOINTS

The biophysiological properties of acupoints have been an intriguing research subject for the past 30 years among scientists worldwide. Studies with electrophysiology, cross-sectional anatomy, and histology have revealed that acupoints contain the following features: lower electrical resistance and higher current conductivity compared with the surrounding areas; a richness of free nerve endings, high concentration of sensory receptors (e.g., Meissner's corpuscle, Merkel's disk, and pacinian corpuscle) for touch and pressure, and a large number of small vessels and specialized cells, such as mast cells.[3] However, the hope of finding new, unique structures at the acupoint has not been realized. Indeed, it is important to understand that an acupoint is not just a gathering of anatomical structures. It is the combination of the functions of these structures that makes a point "microenvironmentally unique." For this reason, although it is important to accurately locate a point, it is more critical to reach to the right microenvironment below the skin surface. Thus the ancient practitioners developed a variety of needling techniques to reach and properly stimulate acupoints.

It has been proposed that an acupoint is a part of a communication network in the body that connects nervous, endocrine, and immune systems.[4] Many structures previously described are involved in this process. They synthesize, secrete, or bind small molecules, such as neurotransmitters and cytokines, to receive and transmit information. If this continuous, movable process is visualized as Qi, acupoints are the places where Qi is abundant and exchanged. It is thus understandable that the physiological status of an acupoint is changeable with change of environment, as well as during pathophysiological processes in the body. It is also important to emphasize that at the same acupoint, depending on the patient's symptoms and signs, the practitioner can sedate or tonify (Figure

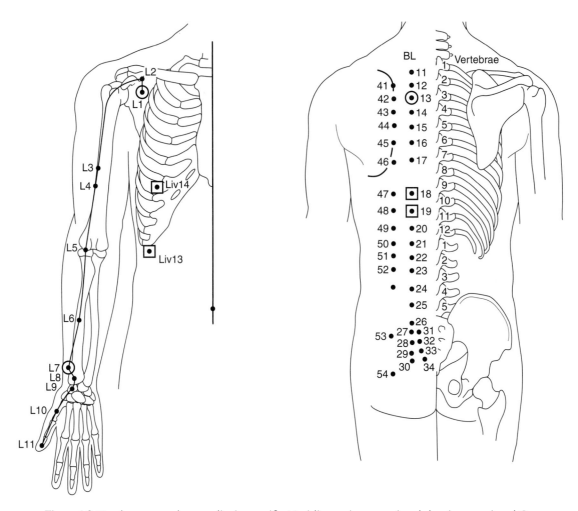

Figure 4-2 Tenderness or abnormality in specific Meridian points can signal that its associated Or-
gan is malfunctioning. For example, respiratory disorder may create pain at Lu 1 or Lu 7 or at UB 13.
Discomfort at UB 18 or 19, or Liv 13 or Liv 14, suggests malfunction of the Liver or Gall Bladder.
(*Right* adapted from Jacob J: *The acupuncturist's clinical handbook,* Santa Fe, 1996, Aesclipius Press.)

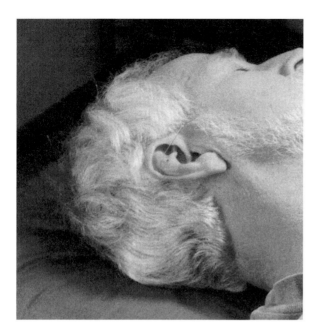

Figure 4-3 Note short needle inserted in the upper triangle region and the ear seed taped to the antihelix. The first location calms the body-person, whereas the second helps reduce pain in the lower back. (Courtesy C. Cassidy and D. Hutchinson.)

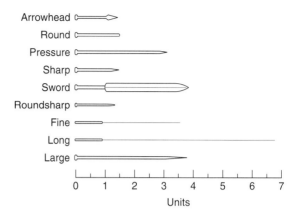

Figure 4-4 The Classic Nine Needles, as described in the *Nei Jing* over 2000 years ago. (From O'Connor J, Bensky D, editors/translators: *Acupuncture: a comprehensive text,* Seattle, Wash, 1981, Eastland Press.)

4-3).* This is discussed further in Chapter 11 as the phenomenon of "bidirectional effect."

USING ACUPUNCTURE NEEDLES

The practice of needling for therapy can be traced back to the Stone Age in ancient China, when people used pointed stone implements and pressure to alleviate illness. With the advance of technology, the stone-needle was replaced by bamboo, and later, metals. The *Nei Jing* described nine types of acupuncture needles with different shapes and functions, includ-

---

*Sedate (reduce) means to decrease the amount of Qi present at the point, in the Channel, or available to the Organ system; tonify (reinforce) is to increase the amount of Qi available. Because Qi flows, both sedation and tonification may occur in the same treatment at different locations, with the effect of "sending" Qi from some locations and "calling" Qi to other locations, thus smoothing the flow for the whole organism.

ing needles for puncturing, surgical incisions, and massage (Figure 4-4). By this date acupuncture medicine was already well developed, with 160 acupoints described. Much of the basic theory that guides needling today can be found in two classic texts, *Su Wen* and *Ling Shu,* as well as the later text, *Nan Jing.*

Acupuncture continued to evolve, changing in response to technology advancement and the interaction of various cultures as it spread to other countries. Today, acupuncture is so well known that the term is often used to encompass the entire system of Oriental or Chinese medicine. With its long history and worldwide extent, it is not surprising that acupuncture treatment is offered in several distinct styles, including Japanese styles, Korean hand acupuncture, Leamington Five-Elements acupuncture, French energetic acupuncture, and Chinese TCM style (see Chapter 2). There are also specialized formulations such as hand-foot acupuncture, auricular acupuncture, and scalp acupuncture. Although use of metal needles and moxibustion continues to be the most common technical approach, today both electricity and lasers are used to replace handheld needles in certain circumstances.

Modern Acupuncture Needles

One of the unique features of acupuncture is that the placement of needles does not usually cause pain. This

TABLE 4-2

Comparison of Gauges of Hypodermic and Filiform Needles*

	Hypodermic (hollow) needles				Filiform (solid acupuncture) needles				
Needle gauge†	16	22	25	30	32	34	36	38	40
Diameter (mm)	1.65	0.71	0.51	0.32	0.26	0.22	0.20	0.18	0.16

*Hypodermic needles, designed to carry fluids in or out of the body, are rigid and thicker than filiform needles, which are designed to be flexible and slip in with minimal tissue disturbance.

†Gauge diameters are approximate. Different gauges are used for different purposes, and only examples are shown here. The table could be continued in either direction. Gauge 16 syringe needle is used, for example, in fistulas for dialysis treatments; gauge 22 is the most common of three gauges used in Vacutainer blood sampling, and for injecting substances such as antibiotics. Gauge 25 is commonly used for subcutaneous injections, as for vaccinations. Gauge 30 is a fine-gauge needle often used by diabetic patients to deliver insulin; this gauge is also used by dentists. In acupuncture, the larger gauges are used to needle thicker and less sensitive regions such as the abdomen, hip, and buttocks; the smaller gauges are used in sensitive or thin-skinned areas (face, hands, feet).

is partly the result of using hair-thin needles, partly a measure of the practitioner's skill, and no doubt partly a feature of patient learning.[5] The most common modern needle is referred to as the filiform needle. It is a solid, stainless steel needle with an evenly pointed tip and highly polished smooth body. Above the body is a handle of steel, copper, or plastic that allows the practitioner to manipulate the needle body and tip.

Acupuncture needle diameter is always much less than those of hollow syringe needles. Commonly used gauges range from #32 to #38 (Table 4-2). Needle length (excluding handle) ranges from 0.5 in to 6 in; however, for most purposes, needles of 0.5, 1.0, and 1.5 in suffice. Good needles are fine, smooth, and straight, thus causing minimal discomfort on insertion. It is important that needles not be so dull as to cause pain on insertion nor be so sharp as to easily puncture vital structures such as organs, arteries, or nerves (Figure 4-5).

Needles are manufactured in China, France, Japan, and the United States. Traditionally, needles were made of gold or silver, but today most practitioners prefer stainless steel needles. Today's commercially available needles are presterilized and disposable (Figure 4-6), which helps control the risk of transmission of blood-borne pathogens and ensures the sharpness of needles.

In addition to the filiform needle, there are several other commonly used needle types. For example, the cutaneous needle, a noninvasive tool that does not have a sharp point, is used to apply pressure or friction on various areas of the body. The seven-star or plum blossom needles, which are composed of multi-

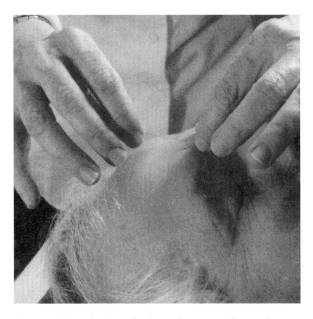

Figure 4-5 Technique for inserting a needle at Yintang (or wherever the flesh is loose) is to pinch up the loose flesh, then slip in the needle. (Courtesy C. Cassidy and D. Hutchinson.)

ple sharp needle tips, are used to stimulate a broad surface of skin. The triangular needle is used for bloodletting (a few drops of blood are often shed to release pathological Heat). These needles are variations on certain of the ancient Nine Needles. Newly invented needles include auricular dermal tacks for ear acupuncture and laser needles, which use a laser beam for stimulation. In 1996 the US Food and Drug

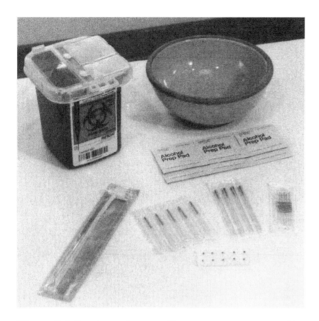

Figure 4-6 Basic equipment for acupuncture care. *Top from left,* Sharps box for used needles and bowl for waste, alcohol swabs. *Bottom from left,* Plum blossom needle; 1-inch disposable needles; 1½-inch disposable needles; ½-inch disposable ear needles; and block of ear seeds on individual adhesive tape squares. (Courtesy C. Cassidy and D. Hutchinson.)

Administration (FDA) reclassified acupuncture needles from an experimental device to medical instrument after a rigorous evaluation of the current usage of acupuncture. As a result of this reclassification, the standard of needle manufacturing and maintenance is now comparable to that of scalpels and syringe needles.

Locating Acupoints

Acupuncturists use several methods to locate regular acupoints, including finger measurement, proportional measurement, and anatomical landmarks. All demand relative measurement because each person's body proportions differ; however, descriptions of locations are precise and points are located similarly on all people.

Finger measurement uses the Chinese *cun* (pronounced *tsoun*) as a unit. One Chinese cun is equivalent to the patient's thumb width. Two cun is equivalent to the width of the patient's middle three fingers when these fingers are held together at the level of

the second phalangeal joint. Three cun is equal to two cun with the addition of the little finger. As an example, P6 (Pericardium 6, *Neiguan*), a popular point for treating nausea and vomiting, is found at 2 cun above the transverse crease of the wrist between the tendons of the palmaris longus and flexor radialis muscles.

Since early times, Chinese practitioners have also used a system referred to as proportional measurement that divides the body into proportional units. For instance, it is known that the total distance between the cubital crease of the elbow and the crease of the wrist measures 12 units and that P6 (Neiguan) is situated at 2 cun above the wrist crease. Based on proportional measurement, one can deduce that the location of P6 is ⅙ the total length of the forearm. Both finger measurement and proportional measurement are used to measure acupoints on limbs and the abdomen.

Anatomical landmarks also help to localize acupoints. There are fixed landmarks such as hairlines, shoulder blades, umbilicus, and the Achilles tendons, as well as movable landmarks that emerge only when the body is moved into a certain position. For example, GB 2 (Gall Bladder 2, *Tinghui*) appears as a depression behind the border of the condyloid process of the mandible only when the mouth is open.

Inserting and Manipulating Needles

It takes but a brief moment to properly insert and manipulate a needle, yet practitioners must spend many hours learning to do so effectively and painlessly (see Chapter 12). Before treatment, the patient is placed in a comfortable position that also allows the practitioner easy access to the selected acupoints. The various positions include sitting in extension or in flexion, or lying in a supine, lateral recumbent, or prone position. A general preparation of the patient's needling sites is done by using 75% alcohol swabs.

Needling occurs in three steps. First, the practitioner inserts the needle at the acupoint. Needles may be inserted perpendicularly (90 degrees), obliquely (30 to 60 degrees), or along the skin surface (10 to 20 degrees). One common method of insertion is the two-hand method in which the practitioner presses or pulls the skin taut with one hand while the other presses the needle through the skin, holding the needle by its handle. Some practitioners prefer to use a "guide tube" to assist the needle penetration process. In this case, a plastic needle tube is held at the point and the needle inside the tube is tapped into the skin with one quick motion of the index finger (Figure 4-7). An acupoint may be massaged or tapped briefly before insertion to relax the muscle around it.

After insertion the needle is often only about 1 mm below the skin surface. Rapid small-diameter alternate-direction twirling combined with downward pressure is used to push the needle deeper into the flesh. The needles are typically inserted 2 to 8 mm deep, depending on the particular region of the body. The depth of insertion also varies according to the season, nature of the ailment, and patient's constitution. It is said that shallow insertion is recommended in the summer, for an acute condition, for weak, thin-skinned, pediatric, or elderly patients. Deep insertion is necessary in colder climates, chronic conditions, or for people who are thick-skinned and a strong physical build. However, the depth of needle insertion can also be a characteristic of style of practice. For example, Japanese acupuncture typically practices shallow needle insertion. In this case, the needle is usually inserted less than 2 mm deep.

Although the appropriate therapeutic depth is defined for every point, in practice the practitioner seeks to feel a particular sensation called *de Qi* ("arrival of qi," "obtaining qi"). Obtaining this sensation means that the needle has reached the Meridian Qi; insertion is complete and therapy can begin. To the practitioner, de qi feels like a slight tug, a thickening, or tightening of the tissues around the needle tip; traditionally it is described as having caught a fish on the line. De qi (pronounced *day-chee*) can also be observed by the development of a red halo, or erythema, at the needle insertion site, which gradually dissipates during treatment as the Qi moves on.

Practitioners typically engage the patient in identifying if the point "feels right" and if they can feel the de qi.* To the patient, de qi is a sensation of mild aching, thickening, throbbing, soreness, or tingling. Sometimes the sensation moves from the point of insertion to another location, usually along a Meridian line. Most patients can distinguish this feeling from pain, which is not supposed to be a component of de qi sensation (however, occasional patients do experi-

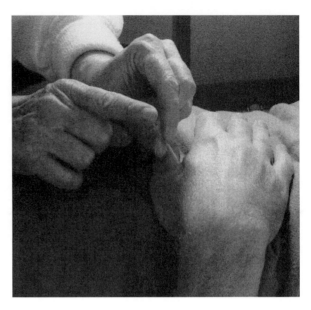

Figure 4-7 Acupuncturist tapping in needle, using a guide tube. Point selected is LI 4 *(hegu),* one of the body's most powerful points. (Courtesy C. Cassidy and D. Hutchinson.)

ence pain during the needling). The sensation of heaviness is usually a result of contraction or increased muscle tension, whereas soreness is felt when the needle tip touches periosteum, aponeurosis, tendon, or ligament. Direct stimulation of a nerve trunk or branch generates a fiery or numbing sensation. If a patient complains of pain, or if the de qi sensation does not arrive after appropriate stimulation, the needle is removed and reinserted nearby.

Therapy is achieved not only by the appropriate selection of acupoints but also by appropriate manipulation of the needle once inserted. The primary aim is to "regulate the flow of Qi" by guiding it in a certain direction. Practitioners may decide whether to slightly twist the needle for a light stimulation and then remove it immediately, or to leave needles in place for some time (15 to 45 minutes). Classic textbooks speak in detail about a number of manipulation techniques to achieve particular therapeutic effects. The basic three are the tonifying or reinforcing (to treat deficiency or chronic syndromes), sedating or reducing (to treat excess or acute syndromes), and even (for mixed conditions) styles. Manipulation consists of a complex of back-and-forth rotation, lifting, and thrusting of the needle, always within a small range of motion. Angle of the needle, speed of manipulation, the pattern of the patient's breathing, and other factors also modify the therapeutic effect.[1]

*The fact that the de qi sensation is shared between practitioner and patient means that traditional research design features such as double-blinding are difficult to use in acupuncture research. See Part III for discussion.

What Does Acupuncture Care Feel Like?

The practitioner's fingers palpate, tapping, measuring, locating the point ... "Oh! that's sore!" you say, surprised, as the point is pressed. A cool swab with alcohol, the tiny prick of the needle, and—suspense. Ahhh! the *de qi* sensation and maybe you jerk a little, or sigh, or simply affirm "you got it!" to the practitioner. De Qi, the arrival of Qi: Sometimes the point trembles and lets go, or it may sting mightily and elicit a brief painful gasp, but afterward there's nothing, no pain, no tenderness, no knotted tissue either, for the Qi has passed on through. Sometimes the needle goes in and sensation moves, lightning quick, from the point needled to a point somewhere else up or down the line. If you know your Meridians you can trace it, "yes, there it went, right down the Spleen Meridian!" "Good," says the practitioner.

At the beginning of the session, you notice the entrance of every needle but soon you relax, floating away as the tapping fingers of the acupuncturist trace the treatment through its effects on your pulse. If she leaves the needles in a while, and if she doesn't talk or leaves the room, you may well fall asleep. She will come back later, 10 or 15 or 20 minutes later, maybe laughing—"I could hear you snoring in the next room!" "Yes," you say sheepishly, "it sure felt good to sleep so deeply!" Then she takes out the needles, which by now you have almost forgotten.

Slowly you sit up, put on any clothes you have removed, pull on your shoes, and replace your jewelry. You move in slow motion. You sit again to write a check, make the next appointment. This is a slow time, relaxed time. The practitioner smiles, helps you name changes that have occurred—is pain diminishing or gone? Is breathing easier? Is nausea fading? Are knees less sore? Is sadness lifting? You listen and answer and try to feel your body and mind, the ceaseless circling of the Qi. She sees you out the door with a suggestion: "Notice what happens in the next couple of days. Call me if you have any questions or if you don't notice improvement." ∾

Manipulation may also be applied with a low-voltage electric device. Electric currents are introduced through conducting wires attached to the handle of the inserted needles (Figure 4-8). Light, heavy, continuous, or intermittent stimulation may be precisely adjusted.

Electrostimulation is efficient when manipulation must be maintained for a considerable length of time, for example, to prevent pain (acupuncture anesthesia) or to reduce severe pain.

The last therapeutic step in needling is needle removal. Because needles must be freed from subcutaneous tissues, including muscles that sometimes cling to needles, care is used to remove them slowly and with a light twisting motion. For superficially placed needles, quick withdrawal is recommended. If a drop of blood forms at an acupoint, it is simply wiped away with a dry cotton ball, which is also commonly used to "close" the acupoint. However, bleeding from head and face acupoints is prevented by pressing cotton balls for some time at the insertion openings immediately after needles are removed.

In chronic conditions, the most immediate effect of acupuncture experienced by the patient is, typically, relaxation; it is not uncommon for patients to fall asleep on the treatment table. Specific therapeutic ef-

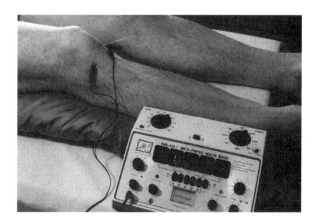

Figure 4-8 Electrodes are attached to needles inserted at *Xiyan,* the "eyes" below the patella. Battery-run electroacupuncture machine produces stimulation that the patient can control and is often used to treat musculoskeletal pain or weakness. (Courtesy C. Cassidy and D. Hutchinson.)

fects, in acute or chronic conditions, may be felt immediately or several hours or days later depending on patient responsiveness and the nature of the condition. Interestingly, some patients may feel their symptoms worsen after the initial treatment. These patients then gradually feel better. This response to acupuncture treatment occurs frequently enough that practitioners normally warn their new patients about this possibility.

The duration of the acupuncture effect also varies. It may last from several hours to several days. To the extent that acupuncture involves encouraging "balance" or homeostasis of bodily systems, it is also observed that the patient's ability to maintain comfort and ease of function increases from the initiation of acupuncture treatment. Thus in acute conditions or in active chronic conditions, twice a week treatment visits are common at the beginning. As the patient's distress calms, treatments become less frequent and may change focus from sickness treatment to health maintenance and prevention of future acute events. Practitioners and patients mutually establish effective treatment frequencies for chronic care that vary from monthly to seasonal visits.

Are There Unsafe Acupoints?

Acupoints are found all over the body and are safe to use when properly needled. However, there are a few acupoints that are absolutely contraindicated for acupuncture. Classic texts forbid needling of St 17 (Stomach 17, *Rhuzong*), located at the center of the nipples. This point is used solely as a landmark for locating other points in the chest area. Another point, Ren 8 (Shenque), located at the center of the umbilicus, is a point available for moxibustion therapy only.

A number of points are classified as high risk or dangerous. Points in this group carry adverse side effects if practitioners lack anatomical knowledge or neglect to observe the prescribed depth, angle, or stimulation pattern for the needles. For example, deep puncture is not advisable for points located below the occiput, such as Du 15 *(Yamen)* or Du 16 *(Fengfu),* to avoid harming the brainstem. UB 51 (Urinary Bladder 51, *Huangmen*), bilaterally located near the kidneys, is another example of a point that is vulnerable to deep needle insertion or vigorous manipulation. Points over the lungs, heart, liver, and other vital organs similarly must be needled with appropriate technique.

Finally, some acupoints are contraindicated in certain conditions. Many points are avoided during pregnancy either because they are local and may cause injury to the enlarged uterus (e.g., Ren 3, Zhongji, centerline abdomen below umbilicus) or because, although remote, they have been observed to produce strong stimuli including contraction of the uterus (e.g., LI 4, *Hegu,* on the web between thumb and index finger). Similarly, points that increase body temperature are avoided in fevers, those that increase blood pressure must be avoided in those with hypertension, and so forth.

Adverse Effects of Acupuncture

Compared with other surgical and pharmaceutical interventions and medical procedures, acupuncture has very few adverse effects. Although it is difficult to directly compare the primary biomedical interventions with acupuncture, estimates suggest that the rates of adverse effects with acupuncture are remarkably less. For example, estimates of serious harm from pharmaceuticals in hospitalized patients vary from a low of 1% to a high of 30% in different studies,[6] but major complications of acupuncture have been estimated as between 1:10,000 to 1:100,000.[7] Writing about Australia, Bensoussan and Myers[8] commented that even "if one presumes that only 1% of the actual Australian adverse events to [treatment with] traditional Chinese medicine are reported, then the number of cases currently on record over the past 20 years multiplied by 100 would not reach the number of adverse events due to pharmaceutical drugs in one year of medical practice." The relative safety of acupuncture was recognized by the report of the 1997 National Institutes of Health Consensus Conference,[9] which stated "one of the advantages of acupuncture is that the incidence of adverse effects is substantially lower than that of many drugs or other accepted procedures for the same conditions."

Nevertheless, needle insertion safety remains an issue for acupuncturists, who are trained to avoid adverse effects. The most potentially serious adverse events in acupuncture involve insertion of needles into vital organs, for example, causing pneumothorax, spinal cord injury, or cardiac tamponade. Such events are typically the result of improper practice.[10] Only one death has been reliably linked to acupuncture performed by a certified acupuncturist.[11] In this case, the acupuncturist inserted a needle at Ren 17, which is located over the heart on the sternum. Proper insertion is subcutaneous; unfortunately, in this case the patient had a hole in the sternum and the acupuncturist inserted the needle perpendicularly, accidentally puncturing the heart.

Not surprisingly, the rate of serious adverse events is lower among acupuncturists who have trained longer.

TABLE 4-3

Patients' Reports of Needle Experiences*

	No.	%
Type of Needle Used		
No needle used	5	0.9
Disposable filiform needle	488	85.3
Reusable filiform needle	48	8.4
Electric with filiform needle	31	5.4
Total	572	100.0
Adverse Experiences With Needles		
No adverse experiences	397	71.9
Drop of blood, small bruise	136	24.6
Fainting, sore after treatment	19	3.4

Representative Comments (each phrase from one respondent)
Bruise:
　"Once or twice in 10 years"
　"Twice in 7 years"
　"Occasional bruises—no big deal"
Blood:
　"My ear points bleed"
　"Occasionally and very minor"
　"Some points bleed—no problem"
　"1-2 drops blood stopped immediately"
Faint:
　"Fainted once years ago"
　"Fainted once"
　"Fainted—needle shock—first treatment"
Continued soreness:
　"Needles were painful years ago"
　"Severe sting on insertion"
　"Once hit a nerve in left hand"

*Previously unpublished data from a questionnaire study of 575 users of Chinese medicine, in five states and six clinics. For other details of this study, see Cassidy CM: *J Altern Complement Med* 4:17-27, 1998 and Cassidy CM: *J Altern Complement Med* 4:189-202, 1998.

In one study, those with less than 1 year of training averaged 2.07 adverse events per year, whereas those who trained 49 to 60 months averaged only 0.92 adverse events per year.[8] Previous biomedical training did not appear to minimize adverse events. In a Norwegian study comparing 201 professional acupuncturists with 202 biomedical doctors who used acupuncture, researchers found that 75% of 33 pneumothorax events occurred during acupuncture performed by physicians, along with the majority of skin infections reported.[12] Although this number of pneumothorax events appears significant, based on the frequency of treatments, the authors estimated that acupuncture care is likely to cause only 1 pneumothorax every 120 years.

Minor adverse effects are far more common than serious ones. The most common side effect, according to a recent survey, is transient hypotension, manifested during the acupuncture treatment as dizziness, discomfort, sweating, and sometimes syncope.[13] This problem usually disappears quickly after needles are removed and the patient lies down with the legs slightly raised. Transient hypotension is likely to appear in patients who are new to acupuncture (and anxious), constitutionally frail, hungry, or fatigued. Other minor adverse effects include local pain, minor bleeding externally, or internally (a small bruise), and local pruritus with or without redness (Table 4-3). All of these can be prevented or alleviated by using time-tested remedies detailed in many acupuncture books.

One of the most worrisome side effects of acupuncture, the potential transmission of infectious agents, is now well controlled by the use of presterilized and disposable needles.[14] A "Clean Needle Technique" training program is incorporated into accredited acupuncture school curricula in the United States. Acupuncturists are required to pass the "Clean Needle Technique" examination as a prerequisite for obtaining professional recognition by the National Certification Commission for Acupuncture and Oriental Medicine (NCCAOM).

DELIVERING ACUPUNCTURE THERAPY

Knowing the location of acupoints and how to insert and manipulate needles are necessary steps in delivering acupuncture therapy, but more important is the task of point selection. Point selection in turn is guided by diagnosis (see Chapter 3) and knowledge of the characteristics of the points, plus knowledge of how Qi moves within the body.

Characteristics of the Points: Close-up of a Single Acupoint

As noted, there are more than 400 predictably located acupoints. Each has the following characteristics:
- Precise location

- Predictable functions or spheres of influence, including the ability to affect physiology at locations remote from the point
- Multiple functions
- A homeostatic character so that either stimulation or sedation can be elicited, as needed, at the point.

To illustrate, we examine the characteristics of one point, Liver 3 (*Tai Chong*, Great Thoroughfare) located at the top of the foot between the tendons of the large and second toe. Box 4-1 summarizes the characteristics of Liver 3 in terms of its energetics and its indications. Like most acupuncture points, Liver 3 has a variety of indications assorted quite differently from what might be expected from familiarity with pharmaceuticals.

BOX 4-1

Description of a Single Acupoint: Liver 3 Tai Chong *Great Thoroughfare**

Type of Point
Shu-Stream Point, Earth Point, Source Point

Energetics
Promotes the smooth flow of Qi
Sedates Liver Yang
Clears heat, especially damp-heat
Expels interior wind
Calms Shen
Calms spasms
Tonifies Liver Yin and Blood
Expels cold in Liver Meridian and Organ

Indications
Qi Stagnation, dampness, fullness
Deviated mouth
Red eyes, burning, itching eyes; dry eye
Red face
Dizziness, vertigo
Insomnia
Headache, especially migraine type
Depression
Hyperthyroidism
Epilepsy
Menstrual problems; uterine bleeding
Hernia
Pain and fullness in hychondriac region

Technique
Insert needle perpendicularly 0.3 to 0.5 cun.
  Moxibustion OK.

*Characteristics listed are from just one text (Jacob, 1996); other texts may give a slightly different list or add more detail.

However, the indications derive logically from the energetics of the point. As discussed earlier, because acupoints are located along channels that course the entire body, passing through limbs as well as regions with internal organs, and because each point relates directly to two particular organs, and indirectly elsewhere, each is actually a semispecialized node in a body-wide communication network.

Given its location on the Liver Meridian, Liver 3 is expected to affect the function of the Liver Organ as well as its partner, the Gall Bladder Organ. The functions of the Liver are many and important: (1) it maintains the free flow of Qi, ensuring that the other Organs receive Qi when they should so that breathing, emotions, digestion, and elimination all can take place with ease; (2) it stores and regulates the flow of Blood, thereby helping to moisten the body parts; (3) it controls the sinews and tendons, helping to ensure ease of movement; (4) it houses the Ethereal Soul *(Hun),* which influences the ability to plan and make decisions, and supports the virtues of courage and resoluteness. The accessory organs associated with the Liver include the eyes, fingernails and toenails, sinews and tendons, tears, and the emotion anger. Every point on the Liver Meridian can aid any of these functions; however, some points are more efficient at effecting specific types of change.

Liver 3 is a powerful point that is frequently needled. It is a *shu-stream point* in the TCM method of naming points, meaning that it falls midway between the "well" (the first waterway point on the 12 Meridians) and the "sea" (the fifth waterway point on the 12 Meridians). It is an Earth point in Five-Element thinking, because Yin Meridians begin with the element Wood and move through Fire—Earth—Metal—Water. Finally, Liver 3 is also a Source point, that is, a point so powerful that it can source Original Qi for the entire Liver Meridian and strongly affect the associated Organs.

Using Box 4-1, we combine material from the energetics and indications columns to detail the logic of use of Liver 3. First, needling Liver 3 "promotes the smooth flow of Qi." Although needling any Liver point should achieve this end, using Liver 3 is particularly efficacious because it is a Source point. The practitioner may logically choose to needle Liver 3 any time that he detects factors that limit the free flow of Qi, such as dampness, stagnation, or sensations such as fullness or bloating (especially of the hypochondriac [liver and gallbladder] region). The presence of the emotion anger (or its variants such as irritability or complaining about unfilled desires), and often the mixed emotions connected with depression, also can be treated via Liver 3: malfunctioning emotions prevent the free flow of Qi and often cause stagnation.

Needling Liver 3 also "sedates Liver Yang." The Liver organ is highly active (= Yang, associated with heat or fire) and when its activity is not sufficiently controlled by other Organs, its energy tends to increase, metaphorically like the wind caused by a fire burning out of control, causing upper body disorders. Thus Liver symptoms are often seen in the face (red, distended), eyes (red, dry, sore . . .), or head (headache, dizziness, vertigo, insomnia). By treating so far from the head, energy can be pulled down, thus relieving congestive symptoms in the head.

Needling Liver 3 also "clears damp-heat," "expels interior wind," and "calms Shen." Hyperthyroidism is an example of an internal damp-heat condition, whereas epilepsy is an example of an interior wind condition. The *Shen,* commonly translated as the "spirit" of the person, is linked to the Heart, but strongly controlled by the Liver as well. Thus when there is malfunction of the Shen (e.g., depression, as well as insomnia and epilepsy) it makes sense to treat at Liver 3.

The Liver Meridian passes through the genital area, so points on the Meridian frequently are selected to treat conditions such as menstrual problems, uterine bleeding, and hernia. In addition, such problems often reflect deficient Blood or Yin, and because Liver is a storehouse for Blood, one might again select a powerful Liver point to treat Blood-related conditions. Hernia is considered a cold condition in Chinese medicine, hence the potential to use Liver 3 to expel cold in the Meridian as it passes through the genital region.

Finally, needling Liver 3 can help calm spasms, such as those that cause headache, menstrual cramps, or pain in the hypochondriac region.

Some points have synergistic effects when used in combination. For example, Liver 3 is commonly combined with Large Intestine 4 (the famous *Hegu* point on the web between the thumb and index finger). Although separately these points have different effects, used in combination, they are uniquely effective to ease tension and stress, and to treat facial paralysis. The combination is called Four Gates because both points are Source (Gate) points, and four needles are needed to treat both hands and both feet.

Selecting Acupoints

In most circumstances, Liver 3 would not be used alone. It would form part of a combination of points, each of which was selected to address the issues presented by the patient. Acupuncture practitioners learn not only the indications for each point, but also how to form appropriate combinations of points to serve the particular needs of the patient. Each style of acupuncture practice provides somewhat different guidelines for point selection. We develop an example for TCM style.

In this style, during diagnosis the patient is assessed for deficiency or excess, Yin/Yang and heat/cold imbalances, and the cause of the complaint, either external or internal. These so-called Eight Principles are further linked to an Organ or a system of Organs. Suppose a patient reported chronic asthma. The practitioner observed a person who was thin and fatigued, had a pale tongue, and a deep thready pulse. Wheezing was severe, with indrawing of the soft tissues of the neck and great difficulty exhaling. The patient stated that he sweated easily yet felt cold much of the time, and could not exercise without wheezing. In analyzing this situation, the practitioner would consider the several forms of "asthma" known to Chinese medicine, trying to determine if she was seeing an excess or deficient expression, an asthma primarily of the Lung or Kidney, and so forth. In this case, she would be likely to conclude that the patient had asthma linked to Kidney deficiency. As a major textbook explains, "Long-standing asthma affects the kidney which is the source of qi. The kidney . . . fails to receive qi, and therefore dyspnea on exertion, severe wheezing and short breath appear. When there is deficiency of the kidney qi in a chronic case, emaciation and lassitude happen. Exhausted kidney yang may lead to weakening of superficial defensive yang, hence sweating. If the yang qi fails to warm up the body surface, cold limbs appear. Pale tongue, deep and thready pulse are the signs of weakened kidney yang."[1]

To treat this situation, the practitioner would choose to needle points that influence Kidney, and probably Ren (Conception Vessel) as well, both on their Meridians and elsewhere. Because the main problem is that the Kidney cannot grasp the Qi arriving from the Lung, points would be chosen to enhance the Kidney's ability to grasp Qi, for example, the Source point K 3 (Kidney 3, *Taixi*), the Back Shu point UB 23 (*Shenshu,* over the anatomic kidneys), and/or Kidney points on the chest, which are often very sore in asthmatic patients; all tonify the Kidney and those in the chest serve the Lung as well. The practitioner also might choose to tonify the Qi of the whole body by needling on the Ren meridian, especially Ren 17 (*Tanzhong,* sternum at fourth intercostal space), and Ren 6 (*Qihai,* midline below umbilicus).

Having addressed the root or major imbalance, the practitioner would usually also choose to address "branch" issues, by using other acupoints to achieve specific purposes. For example, in this case the practitioner might wish to address the Lung to strengthen the body's defense capacity *(Wei Qi)*. She could do this by needling Lung points (e.g., Lu 1 on the chest or Lu 9 on the wrist). However, she also could choose to create a dual treatment effect by treating the Lung using local points that belong to the Kidney (on the chest) or its linked Organ, the Urinary Bladder (on the upper back).

If this practitioner were following a Five-Element theoretical model, the logic of point selection would change but the points selected might not, because the ways that the points influence physiological function are reasonably well known and perceptually do not vary much between styles. However, style would affect such features of needling as sequencing and depth of needling, and retention time for needles. It should be noted that many practitioners use a combination of stylistic logics to analyze patients; it is entirely possible to use the logic of (for example) Japanese, Five-Element, and TCM styles in one treatment session.

Points are selected to produce a synergistic effect for improving a condition. Indeed, it has long been observed clinically that appropriate combinations of acupoints yield superior results than needling singly. Over the centuries, this observation has led to knowledge of point combinations that are uniquely effective at achieving specified therapeutic goals. The application of such combinations without the necessity for a complete diagnostic workup is referred to as the use of "Formula theory." Numerous classics of Chinese medicine, many of them collections of experience from generations of practice, describe formulae for a myriad of conditions, including ways in which the features of points change when used in combination (the synergism feature). Formulae are still used today, and most textbooks will provide some examples (Table 4-4).

TABLE 4-4

*Selected Points for Common Symptoms**

Condition	Therapy	Location
Shock	Moxibustion	Du 20 (Bai hui, vortex of head)
		Ren 4 (Guan Yuan, below umbilicus)
	Needle	St 36 (Zusanli, laterally below knee)
Insomnia	Needle	Ht 7 (Shenmen, medial wrist)
		Sp 6 (Sanyinjiao, medial above ankle)
		Kid 3 (Taixi, posterior to medial malleolus)
Paralysis of hypoglossal muscle	Needle	Du 15 (Yamen, below spinous process C1)
		Ren 23 (Lianquan, upper border hyoid bone)
		LI 4 (Hegu, web thumb and index fingers)
Palpitations	Needle	P 6 (Neiguan, forearm 2 above wrist crease)
		P 4 (Ximen, forearm 5 above wrist crease)
Indigestion	Needle	St 36 (Zusanli, laterally below knee)
		Sp 4 (Gongsun, base first metatarsal)
Retention of urine	Needle	Sp 6 (Sanyinjiao, medially above ankle)
		Sp 9 (Yinlingquan, inferior border medial condyle of tibia)
Impotence	Needle	Ren 4 (Guanyuan, below umbilicus)
		Sp 6 (Sanyinjiao, medially above ankle)
Spasm of gastrocnemius	Needle	UB 57 (Chengshan, below belly gastrocnemius)
Pruritus	Needle	LI 11 (Quchi, lateral angle of elbow)
		Sp 10 (Xuehai, above patella)
		Sp 6 (Sanyinjiao, medially above ankle)
General weakness	Needle	Ren 4 (Guanyuan, below umbilicus)
		St 36 (Zusanli, laterally below knee)

*Modified and abbreviated from Bensky D, O'Connor J, editors/translators: *Acupuncture: a comprehensive text,* Seattle, Wash, 1987, Eastland Press, pp 556-557.

In summary, formula-based treatments can be very effective when conditions presented match those originally described because formulae represent results drawn directly from time-tested clinical trials.

For the same condition, some practitioners may routinely use as many as 20 acupoints, whereas others prefer to limit themselves to a few or sometimes 1 point. The difference results from the action of many factors. For example, because points have different functions and work synergistically, it usually makes sense to use several points, unless the complaint is distinctively linked to malfunction at one point, or unless the practitioner makes a clinical decision to address a single issue during an acupuncture session. When patients are frail, young, or highly sensitive to needles, it is appropriate to use fewer needles. Finally, as practitioners gain skill in point selection and manipulation, they can often reduce the number of points needled. Generally, in a chosen prescription of acupoints, one or two points serve as chief points, and other points function as supplemental points.

Indications for Acupuncture Treatment

Chinese medicine, like biomedicine and ayurvedic medicine, provides comprehensive care, that is, it views its task as that of addressing all forms of malfunction, as well as monitoring and maintaining normal function. As a major modality of Chinese medicine, acupuncture has been applied to improve and maintain health, and to treat numerous conditions over thousands of years.

In contrast to biomedicine, which defines many distinct "diseases," Chinese medicine concerns itself with the dynamic of health, the movement of Qi and Blood, and thus does not define disease as existing apart from the sufferer. For example, even though we named the condition in our previous example as asthma arising from Kidney deficiency, Chinese practitioners would understand that this is simply a physiological description of what is occurring right now in the patient, akin to stating that a biomedical patient "is acidotic." As soon as therapy has brought Kidney back into homestatic balance, the named condition no longer exists. And because that patient may never again experience that particular dynamic, it is not appropriate to say, "This patient is a Kidney patient" or some similar formulation. Instead, at every visit, the

practitioner listens again to the symptoms, again assesses the signs, and then decides, on the spot, what needs to be done to encourage homeostasis. Although it is true that some patients experience a similar form of imbalance time after time, still, in Chinese medicine, that patient would not be labelled as belonging long-term to a disease category.*

In the Western world, where the language and concepts of biomedicine have dominated for a century, the concept of distinct stand-alone "diseases" is normative. As a result, it is common to ask "what acupuncture can treat" and expect answers in terms of biomedically designated disease categories. The resulting lists are restricted compared with what classic texts report treating and what practitioners actually confront daily. Nevertheless, they do serve a useful cross-cultural communication purpose.

For example, in 1971, the World Health Organization of the United Nations issued a list of about 40 conditions suitable for acupuncture treatment (Box 4-2). This list is based on clinical experience in different parts of the world and does not reflect research data or the comprehensive intentions of Chinese medicine as a health care system. In an effort to assess the existing research findings, in 1997 the US National Institutes of Health sponsored a Consensus Conference.[9] The experts concluded that there is substantial scientific evidence to recommend 13 conditions for acupuncture treatment, among them chemotherapy-induced nausea and vomiting, postsurgical dental pain, osteoarthritis, asthma, and drug addiction (see Appendix). As public experience and research findings in the West both grow, it is probable that the comprehensive character of Chinese medicine will increasingly be recognized. In the future, patients and health care practitioners may more easily be able to select and recommend acupuncture when they wish to enhance homeostatic balance, regardless of the biomedical disease label and the symptoms.

The third section of this text offers a series of chapters on conditions and research results. The choice of chapters is partly guided by the frequency with which the named conditions are treated by profession acupuncturists, and partly by the availability of search data on the subjects. In summary, practiti

---

*On the other hand, some styles of practice do emphasize "c tutional types" to help explain why some individuals have dency to respond similarly each time they are stressed.

BOX 4-2

Conditions Appropriate for Acupuncture According to the World Health Organization, 1971

Infectious
Colds and flu
Bronchitis
Hepatitis

Musculoskeletal and Neurological
Arthritis
Neuralgia
Sciatica
Back pain
Bursitis
Tendinitis
Stiff neck
Bell's palsy
Trigeminal neuralgia
Headache
Stroke
Cerebral palsy
Polio
Sprains

Internal
Asthma
Hypertension
Ulcers
Colitis
Hemorrhoids
Diarrhea
Constipation
Diabetes
Hypoglycemia

Mental-Emotional
Anxiety
Depression
Stress
Insomnia

Dermatological
Eczema
Acne
Herpes

Eyes-Ears-Nose-Throat
Deafness
Ringing in the ears
Earaches
Poor eyesight
Dizziness
Sinus infection
Sore throat
Hay fever

Genitourinary/Reproductive
Impotence
Infertility
Premenstrual syndrome
Pelvic inflammatory disease
Vaginitis
Irregular period or cramps
Morning sickness

From chart in Beinfield H, Korngold E: *Between heaven and earth, a guide to Chinese medicine,* New York, 1991, Ballantine, p. 249.

expect good results in treating pain and pain-associated illnesses; problems originating from the digestive system, such as nausea, heartburn, and diarrhea; respiratory malfunction, including asthma and allergies; gynecological problems such as premenstrual syndrome, irregular menstruation, infertility, and symptoms common during menopause; emotional dysfunctions such as anxiety and depression; substance abuse issues including the misuse of prescription drugs; infectious conditions including human immunodefiency virus infection; and neurological conditions such as Bell's palsy, coma, and stroke.

MOXIBUSTION

Moxibustion is an ancient method of introducing heat into the body to correct Yin-Yang imbalances and to promote circulation of Qi and Blood. It is commonly used in conjunction with acupuncture; acupoint selection for moxa treatment follows the same principles as for acupuncture. Moxibustion involves burning moxa, an herbal substance made from *Artemisia vulgaris,* over an acupuncture point. This herb is unusual in that it produces an even, mild steady heat, making it ideal for warming a local region.

Animal Acupuncture: Susan Cushing

The old black mare stood shaking and pawing the ground, then she began to go down. For 2 hours she had suffered with colic, a serious and often fatal ailment horsemen fear. Standing by her side, I quickly inserted an acupuncture needle into Urinary Bladder 21 on her back and stimulated it with sedation technique. Before the next needle could be inserted, she lifted her head, walked over to a patch of grass, and began eating. A single needle seemed to do the trick; she recovered and never had a recurrence.

Happy was an ageing golden retriever who could barely walk because of arthritis and partial blindness. Each day, he was carried down the steps to go outside and rarely traveled far from the front doorstep. However, as weekly acupuncture treatments reduced his pain, Happy recovered the bounce in his stride and returned to taking long jaunts around the nearby park.

In barns, kennels, and veterinary clinics around the world, animals are benefiting from acupuncture for many of the same disorders for which people use it. Although the acupuncturist must have both a good working knowledge of animal physiology and clear understanding of Oriental medicine theory, animal acupuncture works much like human acupuncture; their meridians run in the equivalent locations and acupoints may be found by applying the same anatomical assessments proportioned to the animal's form. In addition, from cats to emus to horses, most animals have little or no objection to careful needling.

As an acupuncturist, I work in association with a veterinarian who makes an allopathic diagnosis before I offer Oriental medical diagnosis and treatment. This combined protocol provides a broad perspective on the problem and allows for the best treatments to be chosen. Acupuncture is often done in conjunction with either allopathic or other alternative therapies. As with human beings, it is a cost-effective therapy for chronic, degenerative conditions, and it strengthens the immune system and promotes the healing process in animals.

For more information, consult one of the many publications on animal acupuncture. The following are a good place to start: Schwartz C: *Four paws, five directions, a guide to Chinese medicine for cats and dogs,* Berkeley, Calif, 1996; Celestial Arts; and Schoen A: *Veterinary acupuncture,* ed 2, St Louis, 2001, Mosby.

To locate professional organizations, contact the American Academy of Veterinary Acupuncture (Box 419 Hygiene, CO 80533-0419; 303-772-6726, e-mail: AAVAoffice@aol.com) or the International Veterinary Acupuncture Society, which also publishes a directory (PO Box 271395, Fort Collins, CO 80527-1395; 970-266-0666, e-mail: ivasoffice@aol.com).

Moxibustion consists of burning the herb near or directly on the skin. The herb may be used in loose form, stick form, or in the form of small cylinders attached to sticky paper (Figure 4-9). The loose form is rolled into balls, tapped onto an acupuncture point, and lit with the tip of a thin moxa stick (Figure 4-10). It is removed when the patient says "hot," that is, the skin is not burned (Figure 4-11).* Slender moxa sticks or thick moxa cigars are used to warm points that cannot easily hold a moxa ball, such as the tip of a toe (Figure 4-12). Moxa attached to sticky paper is a new approach that provides indirect moxa and allows heat to be delivered to positions that cannot easily hold a moxa ball. Moxa also is formulated to rest on the handle of an acupuncture needle to be burned. This creates a warm needle that delivers heat comfortably into deep tissue.

Moxibustion is selected to treat conditions associated with cold, as well as chronic deficiency conditions such as asthma, diarrhea, hypothyroidism, or prolapse of organs. This unique modality also has been applied in some special conditions such as obstetrical and gynecological disorders. For example, UB 67 (Zhiyin, bilaterally at the outer corner of the small toe) is used classically to turn breech presentations. Recently, the *Journal of the American Medical Association* published a

---

*In Asia, burning for scarification is still sometimes practiced. This practice is rare in Western countries.

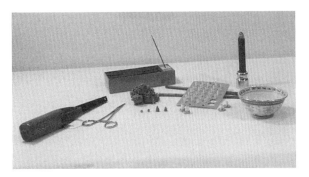

Figure 4-9 Set-up for moxibustion. A box of incense sticks *(back)*, which are used to light moxa rolls, next to a large moxa stick, which is lit with a steady flame, such as the flame of a barbecue lighter *(front left)*. A small bowl *(front right)* is filled with water to douse the moxa. Tweezers *(front left)* can be used to lift hot moxa cones. A loose pile of moxa *(center)* is shown with a selection of hand-rolled direct moxa cones *(front)* next to a plate of indirect moxa cones with adhesive backing. (Courtesy C. Cassidy and D. Hutchinson.)

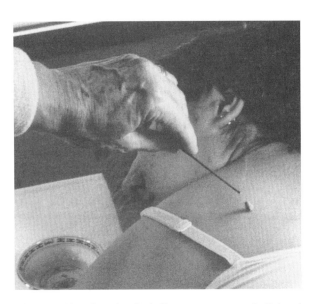

Figure 4-10 A hand-rolled direct moxa cone is lighted with a thin stick of incense. Moxa burns slowly and evenly and warms deeply without burning the skin. (Courtesy C. Cassidy and D. Hutchinson.)

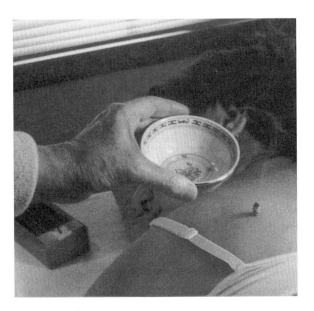

Figure 4-11 When it feels hot to the patient, the moxa cone is quickly removed and extinguished in a container of water. (Courtesy C. Cassidy and D. Hutchinson.)

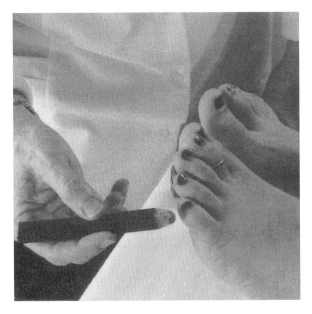

Figure 4-12 A moxa stick can be used to warm areas on which it would be difficult to burn moxa such as UB 67 at the tip of the small toe. Moxa stimulation at this point can turn breech babies and speed labor. (Courtesy C. Cassidy and D. Hutchinson.)

randomized clinical trial showing that use of moxibustion technique indeed increases fetal activities, which may prove favorable for the correction of breech presentations.[15]

Depending on the nature of the illness, moxibustion may be applied alone or with acupuncture in a treatment. The duration of a moxa therapy session ranges from 3 to 6 minutes per application, and 5 to 7 applications per treatment. Because the technique uses heat, caution is exercised when treating certain conditions such as high fever and hypertension.

The burning of the herb produces smoke and a distinctive odor, not unlike that of hemp. For this reason, most acupuncturists post signs in their offices explaining the odor, and some facilities, particularly hospitals, have forbidden the use of moxa. In fact, there is no biological relationship between hemp and *Artemesia,* and the overlap of odors is physiologically irrelevant. However, to address the issues of smoke and odor, new forms of moxa are now appearing. Some are "deodorized" herbs that are still burnable; some are in liquid form requiring the use of a heat lamp for activation.

CUPPING

Cupping is another ancient technique commonly used to supplement acupuncture (Figure 4-13). This technique helps the body expel pathogenic factors such as Cold, Dampness, and Wind, and treats conditions related to the stagnation of Qi and Blood such as bruises or sore muscles. It is particularly helpful for various types of pain in the lower back, shoulders, and legs. Cupping is also used to move stagnant blood out of deep bruises and to reduce swelling and pain in sprains.

Cupping consists of creating a vacuum by burning away the oxygen inside a cup, then clapping the cup over the affected area (Figure 4-14). Responding to the pull exerted by the vacuum, flesh pushes partway into the cup, and body fluids move into the area and may be extravasated (Figure 4-15). The cup is usually retained in position for 5 to 10 minutes. To remove it, one presses the skin around the rim of the cup to allow air into the cup so it can be easily lifted from the skin. The two most popular cups today are glass cups with large rounded openings, and cups that create a vacuum mechanically.

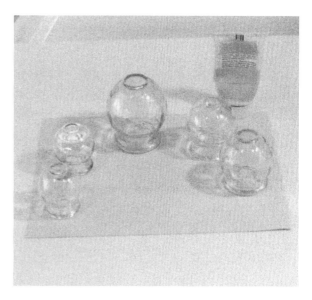

Figure 4-13 Three sizes of cups and cream used to enhance sealing. (Courtesy C. Cassidy and D. Hutchinson.)

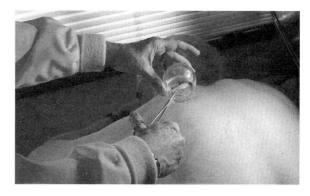

Figure 4-14 The acupuncturist creates a vacuum in the cup by burning an alcohol swab in the cup and quickly clapping it into the prepared region. (Courtesy C. Cassidy and D. Hutchinson.)

Cupping with acupuncture involves applying the cup over a retained needle; the goal is to enhance the effect of the acupuncture. Cupping also can be used to enhance the effects of bloodletting, for example, to move stagnant blood. In this case, the cup is applied immediately after an area has been pricked with a triangular needle. This technique is effective for blood stasis caused by trauma.

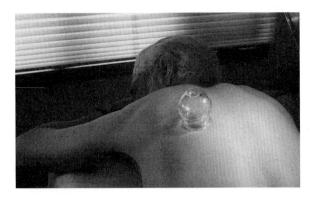

Figure 4-15 With the cup in place, the flesh of the back is drawn up into the cup by the vacuum. This process brings Blood and Qi to the surface and is not painful. (Courtesy C. Cassidy and D. Hutchinson.)

Cupping is generally avoided for the following situations: over the abdomen and lower back of pregnant patients; over large blood vessels; and over skin that is abnormal because of edema, allergic conditions, sores, or ulcers. Cupping is not recommended for patients with high fever or convulsions, or for those With Blood Dyscrasias.

ACUPRESSURE

Acupressure consists of exerting pressure on acupoints with the fingertips, rather than using needles. The effects of pressure are similar, although in some cases less intense, than the effects of needling. Selection of points follows the same guidelines as for acupuncture. Some practitioners specialize in acupressure and, indeed, may not be licensed to practice acupuncture. For example, the Japanese specialty of *shiatsu* can be practiced as a stand-alone health care specialty. It is taught in distinct facilities and has its own texts and its own theory of application. However, professional acupuncturists also often use acupressure. It is useful when patients are very young (children respond rapidly to acupoint stimulation and needles are rarely necessary before adolescence), when patients markedly fear needles, or when patients are pregnant, extremely weak, or have bleeding disorders. Because acupressure is safe and easy to learn, some practitioners teach stimulation of selected points to patients to allow them to perform self-care at home.

SUMMARY

Acupuncture is one of two major therapeutic modalities of Chinese medicine. It uses special needles and associated practices (moxibustion, cupping, acupressure) to stimulate unique bodily points called acupoints. The most common modern acupuncture needle is solid, hair-thin, stainless steel, sterile, and disposable; in 1996 in the United States, the acupuncture needle was classified as a medical instrument by the FDA.

Commonly used acupoints are distributed along Meridian pathways and have stable locations, names, and functions. Additional points have fixed locations but do not belong to meridian pathways, and yet others have unfixed locations. During therapy, points are selected and stimulated in accordance with the theories of Chinese medicine. Acupuncture produces few adverse effects and is extremely safe.

Although the mechanisms of acupuncture effectiveness are as yet not fully specified, it is clear that acupoints, with their associated Meridians, function as a communication system that links the organism to the outer environment, and also links the surface and the interior of the organism. Needling can achieve bidirectional effects—either stimulation or sedation—and the primary effect of acupuncture is to enhance bodily homeostasis. Accordingly, indications for acupuncture treatment are broad.

References

1. Cheng X, editor: *Chinese acupuncture and moxibustion,* Beijing, 1987, Foreign Language Press.
2. O'Connor J, Bensky D, editors/translators: *Acupuncture: a comprehensive text,* Seattle, Wash, 1987, Eastland Press.
3. Stux G, Pomeranz B: *Acupuncture textbook and atlas,* Berlin, 1987, Springer-Verlag, pp 20-24.
4. Pert C, Chopra D: *Molecules of emotion: why you feel the way you feel,* New York, 1997, Simon & Schuster.
5. Emad M: Does acupuncture hurt? Cultural shifts in experiences of pain. *Proceedings of the second Symposium of the Society for Acupuncture Research* 129-140, 1994.
6. Berkow R, editor: *Merck manual of diagnosis and therapy,* ed 16, Rahway, NJ, 1992, p 2642.
7. White A, Hayhoe S, Ernst E: Survey of adverse events following acupuncture, *Acupunct Med* 15:6770, 1997.
8. Benoussan A, Mysers SP: *Towards a safe choice. The practice of traditional Chinese medicine in Australia,* Sydney, Australia, 1996, Faculty of Health, University of Western Sydney Macarthur.

9. National Institutes of Health: *NIH consensus statement: Acupuncture,* vol 15, Bethesda, Md, 1997.

10. Yamashita H, Tsukayam H, Tanno Y, Nishijo K: Adverse events related to acupuncture [letter], *JAMA* 280:1563-1564, 1998.

11. MacPherson H: Fatal and adverse events from acupuncture: allegation, evidence, and the implications, *J Altern Complement Med* 5:47-56, 1999.

12. Norheim AJ, Fonnebo V: Acupuncture adverse effects are more than occasional case reports: results from questionnaires among 1135 randomly selected doctors and 197 acupuncturists, *Complement Ther Med* 4:8-13, 1996.

13. So TY: *Treatment of disease with acupuncture,* Brookline, Mass, 1987, Paradigm Publications.

14. Kaplin DC: *Acupuncture risk management: the essential practice standards and regulatory compliance reference,* Corvalis, Ore, 1997, CMS Press.

15. Cardini F, Weixin H: Moxibustion for correction of breech presentation, *JAMA* 280:1580-1584, 1998.

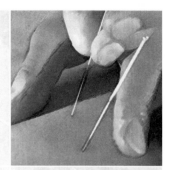

Chinese Herbal Medicine

TAO WANG

Chinese herbal medicine, like other modalities of Chinese medicine, has a history of more than 2000 years. It has been extensively used in Asia both as a form of dietary therapy to maintain good health, and as a major modality to treat disease. With the influx of East Asian immigrants and rising demand for Chinese medicine outside Asia, the use of Chinese herbs has spread to the United States and other Western countries and become part of the multibillion-dollar herbal industry.[1,2]

Increasing use of herbs is partially fueled by a perception among the general public that Chinese herbal medicine is natural and harmless. This perception is only partially correct: herbs are often efficacious in maintaining general health and are safe when they are prescribed by well-trained and experienced herbal practitioners. However, indiscriminate and unjustified use, especially for extended periods or for purposes other than maintaining well-being, can be harmful. The potential for misuse of herbs is higher than that for misuse of other Chinese medical modalities because herbs can be self-prescribed and obtained over the counter in many Chinese grocery stores in the United States and elsewhere.

With ever-increasing use of herbal medicine, biomedical practitioners can benefit from some understanding of how Chinese herbal medicine is practiced and from awareness of potential side effects and toxicity of herbs including interactions between herbs and pharmaceutical drugs. This chapter provides an introduction to the contemporary practice of Chinese herbal medicine by professional herbal practitioners. Readers who seek deeper understanding of this subject are encouraged to consult texts in the suggested

Current US Regulations on Chinese Herbal Medicine

Under the Dietary Supplement Health and Education Act of 1994, Chinese herbal patent medicines may be sold in the United States and bear "structure/function" claims—claims that the products affect the structure or function of the body—without prior review by the Food and Drug Administration (FDA). They may not, however, bear a claim that they can prevent, treat, cure, mitigate, or diagnose disease (i.e., a disease claim). The manufacturers or distributors of the Chinese herbal patent medicines must notify the FDA of the claims they are making within 30 days of marketing a given herbal product. They also are required to have in their files substantiation of any structure/function claims they make. Because raw herbs do not bear any claims, this regulation has little impact on herbalists who make up their own prescriptions; it does affect sales of patent preparations offered in public outlets. For a good summary of the Act and its impact on Chinese herbal medicine, refer to the review articles by Chang[2] and Upton.[3]

readings list at the end of this chapter. General information on herbal medicine (not limited to Chinese herbal medicine) can also be found at the US National Library of Medicine Web site (www.nlm.nih.gov/medlineplus/herbalmedicine.html). Note that the term "Chinese herbs" in this chapter and in many other texts includes more than botanical materials; the same umbrella term includes other natural products of both mineral and animal origin.

DESCRIPTION OF HERBAL PROPERTIES BY TRADITIONAL CHINESE MEDICINE

In Western society, people tend to select herbs based on images promoting singular health benefits. For example, people may select ginseng to increase overall energy or ginkgo biloba leaves to boost memory. They do so without concern for issues such as the herbs' inherent properties, or age or gender appropriateness for the user. In contrast, the selection of Chinese herbs by

herbal practitioners is guided by awareness of their health benefits and their properties based on theories of traditional Chinese medicine. A good understanding of properties of Chinese herbs enables Chinese herbal practitioners to select the most appropriate herbs among candidates with similar benefits to fit a patient's individual conditions and needs.

Properties of Chinese herbs can be described in one of three ways: *Qi, tastes,* and *channel tropism.*

There are four basic designations to describe *Qi:* hot, warm, cool, and cold. When used to describe the property of herbs, Qi is not a physical term and has no relationship to the measurable temperature of the product. Rather, it is a functional description of the herbs. An herb is said to be "hot" or "warm" when it has significant therapeutic effects on cold patterns (e.g., cold extremities, aversion to cold, preference for hot food or drinks, diarrhea with undigested food, pain without redness and swelling, pain relieved by warmth), or it results in certain unwanted reactions (e.g., dry mouth, thirst, sore throat, constipation, acne, or a sensation of warmness). In contrast, an herb is said to be "cold" or "cool" when it has a significant effects on heat patterns (e.g., fever, a sensation of warmth, thirst, dysenteric disorders, pain with significant redness and swelling, pain relieved by cold), or it results in certain unwanted reactions (e.g., lethargy, aversion to cold, tasteless sensation in the mouth, poor appetite, loose stools). A mild herb that does not result in noticeable cold or heat syndrome may be regarded as "neutral." It is important to note that the four Qi are not discrete descriptions of the herbal properties. Rather, they represent a continuum ranging from very hot to very cold.

The properties of Chinese herbs also can be described according to their "tastes." There are five designated tastes: acrid (pungent or astringent), sweet, bitter, sour, and salty. Herbs that have none of these tastes are said to be bland. Tastes in the Chinese herbal practice have two meanings: the true taste of the herb and the action of the herb. For example, when an herb has a significant diaphoretic effect, it is then said to have an acrid taste. The therapeutic actions associated with each Qi and taste are summarized in Table 5-1.

The properties of Chinese herbs can be further described by their channel tropism (i.e., their ability to enter specific Zang-Fu, or Organs, and their associated channels). For example, many herbs with the same warm property and sweet taste may have the same general tonifying effects. It is the channel tropism of the

TABLE 5-1

Typical Therapeutic Actions Associated with Each Qi and Taste

Properties	Examples
"Hot" and "warm"	To treat collapse syndrome
	To support Yang
	To dispense cold
	To warm up the interior
"Cold" and "cool"	To clear heat and purge fire
	To remove "toxins"
	To nourish Yin
Acrid taste	To act on the Lung (Fei)
	To cause sweating
	To expel external pathogenic factors
	To promote the normal flow of Qi and Blood to relieve stagnation
Sweet taste	To act on the Spleen (Pi)
	To tonify and replenish
	To coordinate between the Spleen and Stomach (Wei)
	To harmonize the action of different herbs
	To relieve tension and pain (particularly abdominal pain)
Bitter taste	To act on the Heart (Xin)
	To purge heat
	To dry
	To send down the adverse flow of Qi
Sour taste	To act on the Liver (Gan)
	To retain and arrest
Salty taste	To act on the Kidney (Shen)
	To purge
	To soften and resolve
Bland taste	To act on the small intestine (Xiao-chang)
	To promote diuresis

herbs that determines whether a particular herb in that grouping can best be used to tonify the Heart (mainly the central nervous and cardiovascular systems), the Lung (mainly the respiratory system), the Spleen (mainly the digestive and hemostatic systems) or the Kidney (mainly endocrine and reproductive systems). Full understanding of the channel tropism of herbs enables a Chinese herbal practitioner to treat complex conditions such as heat in the Lung with cold in the Spleen, or excess in the Stomach with deficiency in the Kidney. These two conditions frequently coexist in patients who have contracted infectious disease on top of a preexisting deficient condition. Proper use of herbs with opposite Qi and different tropism in these cases does not lead to reduced efficacy of each herb.

COMMONLY USED CHINESE HERBS

More than 1000 herbs are used in China; however, only a few hundred are exported to the other parts of the world. These exported herbs tend to be well documented in the Chinese herbal literature and are therefore frequently prescribed by herbal practitioners outside China.

Chinese herbs are typically categorized according to their most prominent action. The most commonly prescribed or purchased herbs in the United States are the tonifying herbs. These herbs may have one or more of the following actions: replenishing deficient fluids, increasing the body's vital energy, and enhancing certain Zang-Fu functions. Based on their specific func-

Commonly Used Tonifying Herbs

Category	Typical indications	Examples
Qi-tonifying herbs	Spleen-Qi deficiency (lethargy, weakness in the extremities, lack of appetite, abdominal distention or pain, loose stools or diarrhea); Lung-Qi deficiency (shortness of breath, shallow breathing, dyspnea on exertion, and spontaneous sweating)	Radix ginseng (Ren shen), Radix astragali membranacei (Huang qi), Radix dioscoreae oppositae (Shan yao or Chinese Yam), Rhizoma atractylodis macrocephalae (Bai zhu), Fructus zizyphi jujubae (Da zao or Chinese date), Radix glycyrrhizae uralensis (Gan cao or licorice root)
Blood-tonifying herbs	Blood deficiency (pallid face and lips, dizziness, vertigo, diminished vision, lethargy, insomnia, palpitations, dry skin, menstrual irregularities, pale tongue, and a fine pulse)	Radix rehmanniae glutinosae conquitae (Shu di huang), Radix polygoni multiflori (Shou wu), Radix angelicae sinensis (Dang gui), Radix paeoniae lactiflorae (Bai shao or peony root), Fructus lycii (Gou qi zi)
Yang-tonifying herbs	Kidney-Yang deficiency (systemic exhaustion, fear of cold, cold extremities, sore and weak lower back and lower extremities, impotence, spermatorrhea, watery vaginal discharge, infertility, enuresis, polyuria, and daybreak diarrhea)	Cornu cervi parvum (Lu rong or velvet of young deer antler), Cordyceps sinensis (Dong chong xia cao or Chinese caterpillar fungus), Semen juglandis regiae (Hu tao ren or walnut nut), Cortex eucommiae ulmoidis (Du zhong), Rhizoma cibotii barometz (Gou ji or chain fern rhizome)
Yin-tonifying herbs	Lung-Yin deficiency (dry cough, loss of voice, dry throat, dry skin); Stomach-Yin deficiency (lack of appetite, irritability, thirst, dry mouth, and constipation); Liver-Yin deficiency (diminished visual acuity; dry, dull eyes; night blindness; and tinnitus); Kidney-Yin deficiency (warm palms and soles, diminished sexual function, tinnitus, and so forth)	Radix adenophorae seu glehniae (Sha shen), Radix panacis quinquefolii (Xi yang shen or American ginseng), Tuber asparagi cochinchinensis (Tian men dong), Rhizoma polygonati Odorati (Yu zhu), Bulbus lilii (Bai he or lily bulb), Ramulus sangjisheng (Sang ji sheng), Plastrum testudinis (Gui ban or freshwater turtle shell), Fructus momordicae grosvenori (Luo han guo)

tion, these herbs can be further divided into one of the four subgroups shown in Table 5-2.

Qi-tonifying herbs typically are warm and sweet in nature and are used to treat patterns of Qi deficiency (reduced functions of one or more Zang-Fu). The typical indications for using these herbs are lethargy, lack of appetite, loose stool or diarrhea with undigested food, shortness of breath, shallow breathing, dyspnea on exertion, spontaneous sweating, pallid complexion, pale tongue color, and deficient pulse. Pharmacological studies of these herbs show that many can improve both stimulatory and inhibitory processes in the central nervous system, improve the function of the heart and peripheral vasculatures, enhance digestive functions, modulate endocrine functions, and increase immunities.[4-6] The most often used of all Qi-tonifying herbs is Radix ginseng (Ren shen), the pharmacological actions of which have been studied extensively by scientists around the world.[7-10] Other commonly used herbs are Radix astragali membranaceus (Huang qi) and Radix glycyrrhizae uralensis (Gan cao).

Properties of the *Blood-tonifying herbs* range from cool to warm in nature. Most of them have sweet taste. They are used to treat patterns of Blood deficiency. Some of the signs and symptoms of Blood deficiency are similar to those of anemia, heart failure, chronic hepatitis, or peripheral vascular disease. The best known herbs in this subgroup are Radix angelicae sinensis *(Dang gui)* and Fructus lycii *(Gou qi zi).*

Yang-tonifying herbs are primarily for patterns of Yang deficiency presented as systemic exhaustion, cold extremities, fear of cold, sore and weak lower back and lower extremities, impotence, spermatorrhea, infertility, enuresis, or polyuria. These herbs are found to increase functions of the endocrine system and improve overall energy metabolism. Many of these herbs are hot and very drying in nature and can consume Yin/fluids and assist the fire.

Yin-tonifying herbs are used to treat patterns of Yin deficiency in the Lung, Stomach, Liver, or Kidney. The indications for using this group of herbs are dry cough, dry throat, thirst, low-grade afternoon fever, night sweats, dull eyes, vertigo, tinnitus, insomnia, dark and scanty urine, or a red and dry tongue. These conditions may be the signs and symptoms of conditions such as chronic febrile diseases, hypertension, diabetes mellitus, or diabetes insipidus.[11]

The next category of commonly used herbs includes those that relieve stagnation of different sorts. Among them, herbs that regulate Qi movement, aid digestion, or improve blood circulation are well characterized in traditional Chinese medicine (Table 5-3). The indications for use of these herbs are not necessarily associated with deficiency. Rather they are the result of dysfunction of certain Zang-

TABLE 5-3

Commonly Used Herbs That Relieve Stagnation

Category	Typical indications	Examples
Qi-regulating herbs	Stagnant Spleen and Stomach Qi (epigastric and abdominal distention and pain, belching, acid regurgitation, etc); Constrained Liver Qi (stifling sensation in the chest, pain in the flanks, depression, hernial pain, etc.); Stagnant Lung Qi (coughing and wheezing, stifling sensation in the chest)	Pericarpium citri reticulatae *(Chen pi* or dried tangerine peel), Fructus immaturus citri aurantii *(Zhi shi* or immature fruit of the bitter orange), Rhizoma cyperi rotundi *(Xiang fu),* Radix aucklandiae lappae *(Mu xiang),* Radix linderae strychnifoliae *(Wu yao),* Lignum santali albi *(Tan xiang* or heartwood of sandalwood)
Digestion-aiding herbs	Food stagnation (severe bad breath; a feeling of distention in the abdomen; a yellow, greasy tongue coating; and a forceful, slippery pulse)	Fructus crataegi *(Shan zha* or hawthorn fruit), Fructus hordei vulgaris germinantus *(Mai ya* or barley sprout), Massa fermentata *(Shen qu* or rice sprout), Endothelium corneum gigeriae galli *(Ji nei jin* or chicken gizzard's internal lining)
Blood-invigorating herbs	Blood-stasis (localized, sharp pain, abscesses and ulcers, abdominal masses)	Radix ligustici chuanxiong *(Chuan xiong),* Radix salviae miltiorrhizae *(Dan shen),* Tuber curcumae *(Yu jin),* Herba leonuri heterophylli *(Yi mu cao),* Radix paeoniae rubrae *(Chi shao),* Semen persicae *(Tao ren),* Flos carthami tinctorii *(Hong hua),* Gummi olibanum *(Ru xiang),* Myrrha *(Mo yao),* Radix achyranthis bidentatae *(Niu xi)*

Fu, particularly the Heart, Lung, Liver, Spleen, and Stomach.

Qi-regulating herbs are frequently used to treat patterns related to stagnant Spleen and Stomach Qi (typically seen in patients with disorders of the digestive system), constrained Liver Qi (frequently seen in patients with hepatic disorders, stomach ulcers, or depression), or stagnant Lung Qi (may be part of presentation of depression or pulmonary dysfunction).

As suggested by the name, *digestion-aiding herbs* improve overall function of the digestive system (e.g., increasing appetite, helping relieve food stagnation, stopping diarrhea resulting from food poisoning). Some of these herbs contain enzymes that assist the digestion of specific type of food. For example, Fructus hordei vulgaris *(Mai ya)* contains amylase and is used to treat stagnation caused by the overeating of starch-containing food, whereas Endothelium corneum gigeriae galli *(Ji nei jin)* is used to treat all kinds of stagnation. Others may improve the food digestion through other mechanisms.

Blood-invigorating herbs are used to treat problems associated with Blood stasis that typically presents as localized and sharp pain, chronic and hard-to-heal abscesses and ulcers, or masses, particularly in the abdomen. Pharmacological studies have found that many herbs in this group have profound anticoagulant, vasodilatory, negative chronotropic and inotropic effects.[12,13] These pharmacological effects are often synergistically enhanced by herbs that regulate the Qi. Some of the Blood-invigorating herbs are also found to reduce plasma cholesterol concentrations.[13]

The third category of commonly used herbs includes those that address dampness-related patterns. Dampness-related patterns represent a very diverse group of medical conditions with symptoms such as nausea, vomiting, loose stool, cough with copious sputum, edema, and/or joint and muscle pain. According to their specific actions, this group of herbs can be further divided into the following subgroups: aromatic herbs that transform dampness, phlegm-transforming herbs, herbs that relieve coughing and wheezing, diuretic herbs, and herbs that dispel wind-dampness. Herbs from these subgroups are often used together to enhance their efficacy. Examples of herbs in each subgroup are listed in Table 5-4.

TABLE 5-4

Commonly Used Herbs That Eliminate Dampness

Category	Typical indications	Examples
Aromatic herbs	Dampness in the Spleen and Stomach (a feeling of distention and fullness in the abdomen, nausea, vomiting, diarrhea with some difficulty in defecation)	Herba agastaches seu pogostemi *(Huo xiang)*, Cortex magnoliae officinalis *(Hou po* or magnolia bark), Rhizoma atractylodis *(Cang zhu)*, Fructus amomi *(Sha ren* or grains of paradise fruit)
Phlegm-transforming herbs	Phlegm accumulation in the Lungs (coughing, wheezing, stifling sensations in the chest, and pain in the ribs), Phlegm accumulation in the Stomach (nausea, vomiting, loss of appetite, epigastric distention)	Radix peucedani *(Qian hu)*, Bulbus fritillariae cirrhosae *(Chuan bei mu)*, Caulis bambusae in taeniis *(Zhu ru* or bamboo shavings), Semen sterculiae scaphigerae *(Pang da hai)*, Rhizoma pinelliae ternatae *(Ban xia)*, Semen sinapis albae *(Bai jie zi)*, Radix platycodi grandiflori *(Jie geng)*
Herbs that relieve coughing and wheezing	Cold or heat in the Lungs (coughing, wheezing)	Semen pruni armeniacae *(Xing ren* or apricot seed), Fructus perillae frutescentis *(Su zi)*, Folium eriobotryae japonicae *(Pi pa ye* or loquat leaf), Cortex mori albae radicis *(Sang bai pi* or bark of mulberry root)

Continued

TABLE 5-4

Commonly Used Herbs That Eliminate Dampness—cont'd

Category	Typical indications	Examples
Diuretic herbs	Obstruction of normal fluid metabolism (acute edema, painful urinary dysfunction, damp sores, jaundice, and so forth)	Sclerotium poriae cocos *(Fu ling)*, Talcum *(Hua shi)*, Semen coicis lachryma-jobi *(Yi yi ren)*, Caulis mutong *(Mu tong)*, Medulla tetrapanacis papyriferi *(Tong cao)*, Semen plantaginis *(Che qian zi)*, Herba lysimachiae *(Jin qian cao)*, Herba artemisiae yinchenhao *(Yin chen hao)*
Herbs that dispel wind-dampness	Wind-dampness in the muscles, sinews, joints, and bones (pain, numbness in the joints and muscles, swelling of the extremities)	Radix angelicae pubescentis *(Du huo)*, Radix clematidis *(Wei ling xian)*, Ramulus mori albae *(Sang zhi* or mulberry twig), Cortex acanthopanacis gracilistyli radicis *(Wu jia pi)*, Fructus xanthii sibirici *(Cang er zi)*, Caulis piperis futokadsurae *(Hai feng teng)*

The last category of commonly used herbs includes those for treating patterns caused by external pathogenic factors. In biomedical terms, many herbs in this group have antimicrobial, anti-inflammatory, or antipyretic actions.[14,15] Some may also enhance the immune system to shorten the course of infection. In China, these herbs are frequently used in conjunction with antibiotics or antiviral agents to combat severe infectious disease. Depending on specific indications for use, this group of herbs can be further divided into the following subgroups: those that clear exterior wind-cold, those that clear exterior wind-heat, and finally, those that clear internalized heat (Table 5-5). Herbs that release the exterior are commonly used to treat the early phase of the infection, whereas herbs that clear internalized heat are used to treat infection with significant systemic presentation such as high fever, dysenteric disorder, and so forth.

PRACTICAL USE OF CHINESE HERBS

Herbs are commonly prescribed by Chinese herbal practitioners as formulas. In a typical formula, two or more herbs of the same group are used together to achieve additive or synergistic effects. This type of combination also reduces the risk of adverse events related to any one particular herb. In addition, herbs of different groups or categories are also used together in a formula. These herbs are combined based on their particular role in a formula as chief, deputy, assistant, or envoy. The roles of each component in a Chinese herbal formula are described in Table 5-6.

Such a hierarchy of ingredients can be exemplified using the *Regulate the Middle* Pill *(Li chong wan)*. This formula consists of the following four herbs: Rhizoma zingiberis officinalis *(Gan jiang)*, Radix ginseng *(Ren shen)*, Rhizoma atractylodis macrocephalae *(Bai zhu)*, and honey-fried Radix glycyrrhizae uralensis *(Zhi gan cao)*. The formula is indicated for a pattern of deficient cold of the Spleen and Stomach. Patients typically present with diarrhea with watery stool, nausea and vomiting, loss of appetite, abdominal pain, a pale tongue with a white coating, and a submerged, thin pulse. The principle in treating this particular pattern is to warm the interior and to strengthen the Spleen and Stomach. The chief herb, Rhizoma zingiberis officinalis *(Gan Jiang)*, warms the Spleen and Stomach and eliminates interior cold; it directly targets the principal pattern. Because the interior cold in this case usually results from Qi deficiency, Radix ginseng *(Ren shen)*, serving as a deputy, is used to tonify the Qi and to aid the chief to expel the interior cold. Rhizoma as-

TABLE 5-5

Commonly Used Herbs That Eliminate External Pathogenic Factors

Category	Typical indications	Examples
Herbs that clear exterior wind-cold	Exterior wind-cold (mild fever, severe chill, headache, body and neck pains, coughing, wheezing)	Herba ephedrae *(Ma huang)*, Ramulus cinnamomi cassiae *(Gui zhi* or cinnamon twig), Folium perillae frutescentis *(Zi su ye)*, Redix ledebouriellae divaricatae *(Fang feng)*, Radix angelicae dahuricae *(Bai zhi)*, Rhizoma zingiberis officinalis recens *(Sheng jiang)*, Flos magnoliae *(Xin yi hua* or magnolia flower)
Herbs that clear exterior wind-heat	Exterior wind-heat (severe fever, mild chill, sore throat, cough with yellow sputum)	Herba menthae haplocalycis *(Bo he* or mentha), Folium mori albae *(Sang ye* or white mulberry leaf), Flos chrysanthemi morifolii *(Ju hua* or yellow chrysanthemum flower), Radix puerariae *(Ge gen)*, Radix bupleuri *(Chai hu)*, Flos lonicerae japonicae *(Jin yin hua)*, Fructus forsythiae suspensae *(Lian qiao)*
Herbs that clear internalized heat	Excess heat in the Lungs and Stomach (high fever, irritability, thirst, delirium associated with febrile disease); Damp-heat pattern (dysenteric disorders, urinary difficulty or pain, jaundice, furuncles, and eczema, bitter taste in the mouth, a thick and yellow tongue coating); Heat in the Blood (rashes, nosebleed, vomiting, spitting or coughing of blood, blood in the urine)	Gypsum *(Shi gao)*, Rhizoma anemarrhenae asphodeloidis *(Zhi mu)*, Fructus gardeniae jasminoidis *(Zhi zi)*, Radix scutellariae baicalensis *(Huang qin)*, Rhizoma coptidis *(Huang lian)*, Radix gentianae longdancao *(Long dan cao)*, Radix isatidis seu baphicacanthi *(Ban lan gen)*, Radix sophorae tonkinensis *(Shan dou gen)*, Herba artemisiae annuae *(Qing hao)*, Radix rehmanniae glutinosae *(Sheng di huang)*, Cortex moutan radicis *(Mu dan pi)*, Cortex lycii radicis *(Di gu pi)*

TABLE 5-6

Roles of Each Component in a Chinese Herbal Formula

Component	Role
Chief	Is directed against the principal pattern or disorder
	Has the greatest effects on the principal pattern or disorder
Deputy	Aids the chief in treating the principal pattern or disorder
	Serves as the main ingredient against a coexisting pattern or disorder
Assistant	Reinforces the effects of the chief and deputy ingredients
	Treats a less important aspect of the pattern or disorder
	Minimizes or eliminates the toxicity or harshness of the other ingredients
Envoy	Directs the action of the formula to specific Zang-Fu, Channel, or area of the body
	Harmonizes and integrates the actions of the other ingredients

tractylodis macrocephalae *(Bai zhu)*, which tonifies the Spleen and dries dampness, serves as an assistant herb to reinforce the effects of Rhizoma zingiberis officinalis *(Gan Jiang)* and Radix gingseng *(Ren shen)*. Honey-fried Radix glycyrrhizae uralensis *(Zhi gan cao)* harmonizes the actions of other ingredients in the formula.

In practice, Chinese herbal practitioners may select one from hundreds of classic formulas that are well documented in textbooks or other technical sources. Practitioners frequently tailor the selected formula—remove some herbs from or add herbs to the existing formula—to fit the needs of the individual. For example, if a patient mentioned in the previous paragraph also has fever and chills (signs of exterior wind cold), an herbal practitioner may elect to use the *Regulate the Middle* Pill and add Ramulus cinnamomi cassiae *(Gui zhi)* to release the exterior wind cold. This new formula, called the *Cinnamon Twig and Ginseng Decoction (Gui zhi ren shen tang)* is also available in prepared form. If this same patient has no fever and chills but does complain of daybreak diarrhea and cold extremities, the herbalist may elect to use the *Regulate the Middle* Pill *(Li chong wan)* and add Radix lateralis aconiti carmichaeli praeparata *(Fu zi)* and Cortex cinnamomi csassiae *(Rou gui)* to warm the Kidney and to stop daybreak diarrhea. This new formula, called the *Prepared Aconite and Cinnamon Decoction to Regu-*

TABLE 5-7

Fundamental and Commonly Used Formulas That Treat Deficiency-Related Patterns

Formula	Main actions	Main indications
Four-Gentlemen Decoction (*Si jun zi tang*)	Tonifies the Qi and strengthens the Spleen	Pallid complexion, reduced appetite, loose stools, lethargy, pale tongue, weak pulses, and so forth
Tonify the Middle and Augment the Qi Decoction (*Bu zhong yi qi tang*)	Tonifies the Qi and raises sunken Yang	Intermittent fever, spontaneous sweating, preference for warm beverages, lethargy, chronic diarrhea, prolapse of the rectum or uterus, incontinence, chronic bleeding, and so forth
Generate the Pulse Powder (*Sheng mai san*)	Augments the Qi and generates fluids	Chronic cough with sparse sputum, shortness of breath, spontaneous sweating, a dry mouth and tongue, and so forth
Four-Substance Decoction (*Si wu tang*)	Tonifies the Blood and regulates the Liver	Dizziness, blurred vision, lusterless complexion, generalized muscle tension, irregular menstruation with little flow or amenorrhea, and so forth
Six-Ingredient Pill with Rehmannia (*Liu wei di huang wan*)	Enriches the Yin and nourishes the Kidney	Soreness and weakness in the lower back, vertigo, hot palms and soles, night sweats, nocturnal emissions, wasting and thirsting disorder
Sedate the Liver and Extinguish Wind Decoction (*Zhen gan xi feng tang*)	Nourishes the Yin, sedates the Liver and anchors the Yang	Dizziness, vertigo, tinnitus, headache, irritability, flushed face, progressive motor dysfunction of the body, or development of facial asymmetry, and so forth
Kidney Qi Pill from the Golden Cabinet (*Jin qui shen qi wan*)	Warms and tonifies the Kidney Yang	Lower back pain, a cold sensation in the lower half of the body, short of breath, urinary difficulty with edema or excessive urination, and so forth

late the Middle (Fu gui li zhong tang) can again be bought already made.*

Classic formulas, like *Regulate the Middle* Pill *(Li chong wan)* and their derivatives, not only provide an off-the-shelf selection of herbs for use but also pro-

vide an invaluable example in constructing a sensible and effective formula for a particular pattern or disorder. Well-trained Chinese herbal practitioners are all taught hundreds of classic formulas and the principles of constructing sensible formulas based on the theory of traditional Chinese medicine. Many practitioners also may elect to compose a formula of their own using different herbs. In this case, these new formulas also are built on well-documented principles. The most fundamental and commonly used formulas are listed in Tables 5-7 and 5-8. Many off-the-shelf formulas are derived from these fundamental formulas.

Other formulas such as *Ephedra Decoction (Ma huan tang), Cinnamon Twig Decoction (Gui zhi tang), Honeysuckle and Forsythia Powder (Yin quia san),* and *Ligusticum Chuanxiong Powder to be Taken with Green Tea (Chuan xiong cha tiao san)* are frequently used to clear exterior syndrome (i.e., conditions related to early stages of cold or influenza).

*Generally, Chinese herbal formulas are named in one of the following ways: (1) After the chief herb or herbs in the formula, e.g., *Ephedra Decoction* (Ma huang tang), *Honeysuckle and Forsythia Powder* (Yin quao san), *Tangerine Peel and Bamboo Shavings Decoction* (Ju pi shu run tang); (2) After the key action of the formula, e.g., *Tonify the Middle and Augment the Qi Decoction* (Bu zhong yi qi tang), *Sedate the Liver and Extinguish Wind Decoction* (Zhen gan zxi feng tang); (3) By a combination of the above, e.g., *Perrila Fruit Decoction for Directing Qi Downward* (Suzi jiang qi tang), *Honeysuckle Decoction to Relieve Toxicity* (Yi hua jie du tang). Occasionally the name of the formula is ancient and wrapped in mystery, e.g., *Drive Out Stasis in the Mansion of Blood Decoction* (Xue fu zhu yu tang), or *Four-Gentlemen Decoction* (Si jun zi tang). Because of difference in culture and language, accurate English translation of Chinese herbal formula names is often difficult, and names vary from translator to translator. The English names used herein are from Bensky and Barolet.[16]

TABLE 5-8

Fundamental and Commonly Used Formulas That Relieve Stagnation or Suppress the Reversed Yang or Qi

Formula	Main actions	Main indications
Drive Out Stasis in the Mansion of Blood Decoction (Xue fu zhu yu tang)	Invigorates the Blood and dispels Blood stasis	Pain in the chest and hypochondria, chronic headache with a fixed, piercing quality, depression or low spirits, a dark red tongue with dark spots on the sides of the tongue
Generation and Transformation Decoction (Sheng hua tang)	Invigorates the Blood, warms the menses, and alleviates pain	Retention of the lochia accompanied by cold and pain in the lower abdomen, a pale-purple tongue, and submerged pulse
Tonify the Yang to Restore Five Decoction (Bu yang huan wu tang)	Tonifies the Qi, invigorates the Blood, and unblocks the Channels	Sequelae of wind-stroke including hemiplegia, paralysis, atrophy of the lower limbs, facial paralysis, and so forth
Perrila Fruit Decoction for Directing Qi Downward (Su zi jiang qi tang)	Directs rebellious Lung Qi downward and stops coughing and wheezing	Coughing and wheezing with watery, copious sputum, shortness of breath marked by relatively labored inhalation and smooth exhalation, and so forth
Tangerine Peel and Bamboo Shavings Decoction (Ju pi zhu run tang)	Directs rebellious Stomach Qi downward and clears heat	Hiccup, nausea, or retching accompanied by pain, vomiting resulting from debility after a prolonged illness

FORMS OF CHINESE HERBAL MEDICATION

Patients obtain herbs either directly from their practitioners, or by taking an herbal prescription to a Chinese herbal pharmacy, which may be found in large cities worldwide; most Chinese medicine schools also have pharmacies on site. The herbal practitioner sees the patient and prescribes the herbs; the herbal pharmacist weighs and measures the raw herbs, then sends the patient home with directions for preparing the formula (Figures 5-1 and 5-2).

The most ancient way to take Chinese herbal medication is by decoction, commonly known as a "soup" or "tang"—the herbs are cooked, stored, and consumed according to specific directions (Figure 5-3). Other forms of Chinese herbal medicine such as powders, tablets, pills, capsules, tinctures, syrups, and medicinal wines are also used, and some of these are made up as patent medicines, obtainable at herbal pharmacies (or Asian grocery stores) with or without prescription.

Decoction remains the most popular individualized form among Chinese herbal practitioners because

Examples of Major US Manufacturers and Distributors of Chinese Herbs and Chinese Patent Medicine

In the United States, people can easily purchase Chinese patent medicine at Chinese herbal pharmacies or Chinese grocery stores, where supplies are either directly imported from China or obtained through US distributors. Some US companies have established manufacturing facilities in the United States. The following are some major US manufacturers and distributors of Chinese herbs (many in pill form) and Chinese patent medicines.

Bio Essence Corporation
5221 Central Avenue
Suite 105
Richmond, CA 94804
www.bioessence.com

Blue Light, Inc
111 South Cayuga Street
Ithaca, NY 14850
www.treasureofeast.com

Blue Poppy Enterprises
5441 Western Avenue
Suite 2
Boulder, CO 80301
www.bluepoppy.com

Crane Herb Company
745 Falmouth Road
Mashpee, MA 02649
www.CraneHerb.com

Golden Flower Chinese Herbs
4603 McLeod Road NE
Albuquerque, NM 87043

Jade Pharmacy
East Earth Herb, Inc
PO Box 2802
Eugene, OR 97402

Lotus Herbs
1124 North Hacienda Boulevard
La Puente, CA 91744

Kan Herb Company
6001 Butler Lane
Scotts Valley, CA 95066

Mayway USA
1338 Mandela Parkway
Oakland, CA 94607
800-262-9929
www.mayway.com

The Three Treasures, Classical Formulae
    for the Modern World
East West Herbs (USA) Ltd (Distributors)
1440 62nd Street
Emeryville, CA 94608

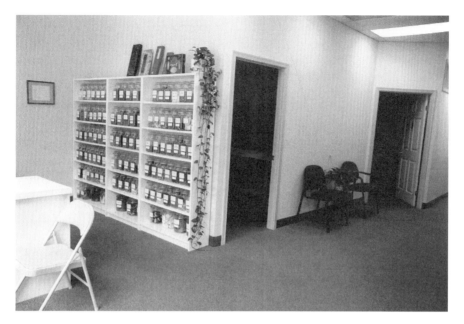

Figure 5-1 Raw herbs in airtight bottles line the walls at the on-site pharmacy in the front office of a practitioner in the District of Columbia. The patient waiting room is to the right and in the foreground. Pills and tinctures are stored elsewhere in the office suite. (Courtesy C. Cassidy and D. Hutchinson.)

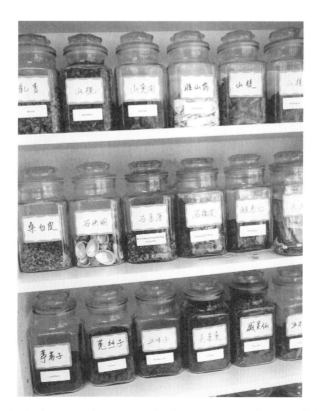

Figure 5-2 Raw herbs in the same pharmacy as in Figure 5-1. Note that not all the herbs are plant materials. For example, abalone shells show on the second shelf to the left.

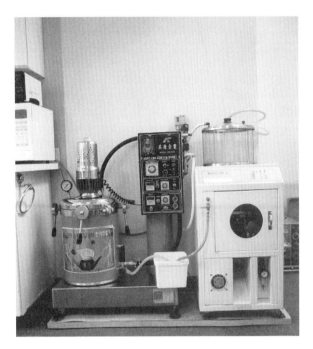

Figure 5-3 Raw herbs are mixed in an appropriate prescription and can be cooked and vacuum sealed into convenient individual servings in this machine in the acupuncturist's office shown in Figures 5-1 and 5-2. This technique is especially helpful when over-the-counter combinations will not serve the patient. (Courtesy C. Cassidy and D. Hutchinson.)

it offers superior flexibility for modification. Its two main drawbacks are the preparation time and the potential for an unpleasant smell or taste. Pills and capsules offer ease of ingestion but do not so easily lend themselves to creating individualized formulas.

RELATIONSHIP BETWEEN ACUPUNCTURE AND HERBS

Both acupuncture and herbs are major modalities whose use is guided by the same fundamental principles of traditional Chinese medicine. However, there are significant theoretical and practical differences in using these two forms. First, acupuncture tends to assert its therapeutic actions on the Zang-Fu Organs through channels and meridian points, whereas herbs tend to have direct effects on the Zang-Fu system. Herbs can also assert their therapeutic actions

through Zang-Fu to treat disorders related to the peripherals. Second, acupuncture is more effective in treating Zang-Fu dysfunction, whereas herbs are more effective in treating patterns caused by deficiency or external pathogenic factors in addition to Zang-Fu dysfunction. Third, acupuncture is more effective in reducing pain caused by obstruction of channels, whereas herbs are more effective in restoring the function of the Zang-Fu and maintaining the normal flow of Qi through the channels.

Sometimes herbs and acupuncture are used together to provide additive or synergistic effects. A typical example is the treatment of mild to moderate hemiplegia caused by wind-stroke (e.g., complications from but not limited to cerebrovascular accident). Herbs are selected to treat the underlying Zang-Fu dysfunction to improve overall wellness of the patients (e.g., by nourishing Liver-Yin, extinguishing Liver-fire, tonifying Yang-Qi, invigorating the Blood, or unblocking the channels, when appropriate; see Chapters 8 and 19). At the same time, points along the Du meridian and the Yang meridians of the affected side are needled to remove obstructions (e.g., by Blood, Phlegm) from the Meridians and collaterals. In the process, communication between Zang-Fu and collaterals can be restored in many stroke patients, that is, they can regain normal muscular function.

PRACTICE OF INTEGRATED TRADITIONAL CHINESE MEDICINE AND BIOMEDICINE IN CHINA

Since the mid-1950s, the Chinese government has established universities and colleges of traditional Chinese medicine throughout China. Hospitals of traditional Chinese medicine can now be found in every corner of the country down to the county level. Many doctors in these hospitals are trained and authorized to prescribe both herbal medicine and pharmaceutical drugs. They often use both for their patients. This practice is one aspect of the integration of Chinese medicine and biomedicine.

It is generally recognized by clinicians who practice both biomedicine and traditional Chinese medicine that pharmaceutical drugs are more specific and have faster action. In comparison, Chinese herbal medicines have broader actions. Herbal medicine also intends to return the body to homeostatic normalcy, in contrast to action aimed at specific malfunctions. Based on this understanding, severe and emergent conditions (e.g., heart failure, bacterial infection, cancer) are treated with pharmaceutical drugs for their specific actions, while at the same time patients are also given Chinese herbal medicines to relieve side effects of the pharmaceutical drugs and to improve their general condition. For example, chemotherapy or radiotherapy is used to destroy cancerous cells in cancer patients. Meanwhile, tonifying herbs are given to maintain a good digestive system, improve immune function, and increase the patient's general energy to combat cancer. Such combined use has been found to significantly reduce the side effects of chemotherapy or radiotherapy and increase the survival rate of the patients. For example, the 1-year survival rate of patients with lung squamous carcinoma was significantly higher in patients treated with chemotherapy plus herbal medicine than in patients who received chemotherapy only (67% vs 33%). Median survival time was 465 days for the former group and 204 days for the latter group.[17] In another clinical trial of 602 patients with gastric carcinoma (414 in experimental group; 255 in control group), the combination of chemotherapy and herbal medicine resulted in better tolerance of the chemotherapy, fewer digestive system side effects (reduced appetite, nausea, vomiting, and diarrhea), lower incidence of leukocytopenia and thrombocytopenia, and increased immune functions compared with chemotherapy only.[18] The same pattern of combined use is available outside China; however, most of the time success will depend on the ability of biomedical and herbal practitioners to work in tandem.

Another meaning of the concept of integrated Chinese and Western medicine is the use of contemporary biomedical theory and methods to study traditional Chinese herbs and formulas. Animal models and clinical trials have been used to study the efficacy of individual herbs and herbal preparations on clearly defined pathological conditions such as heart failure, hepatitis, neoplastic diseases, aging, and immune disorders.[6,19] Active ingredients in herbs are also isolated for research and therapeutic purposes. An important success story concerns the use of Qinghaosu (or artemisinin, a sesquiterpene lactone peroxide, prepared from the herb Qing hao, or Herba artemisiae annuae) to treat malaria. Qing hao was described in China in 168 BCE. It was specifically recommended for fevers in 341 CE. Thereafter Qing hao appears in many standard Chinese Materia Medica texts as a treatment for febrile diseases. The antimalarial activity of Qing hao was discovered in China in 1971 when a low-temperature ethyl ether extraction proved to have antimalarial activity against several microorganisms. A year later artemisinin was identified as one of the principal antimalarial compounds from Qing hao.[20-22] After extensive pharmacological, toxicological, and clinical studies, qinghaosu became the first herb-derived pharmaceutical drug approved by the Chinese health regulatory agency.

In addition to qinghaosu, many active ingredients from herbs have been isolated and proven to be efficacious in treating human diseases. For example, ginsenosides from Radix ginseng (Ren shen) and tanshinone from Radix salviae miltiorrhizae (Dan shen) have been found to provide profound myocardial protective action in patients with acute myocardial infarction and have been used extensively in China.[13,23]

As previously noted, single herbs are rarely used in Chinese herbal medicine. Herbs are generally combined in formulas. Although much of the research has been done using single herbs, research on formulas and their constituents is also being conducted extensively in China and increasingly elsewhere. One of the purposes of such research is to elucidate the mechanisms of action by combinational use of herbs and the role of each component in the formula. A good example is the in vitro and in vivo studies on the *Drive Out Stasis in the Mansion of Blood Decoction (Xue fu shu yu tang)*. This formula is primarily composed of two groups of herbs: one to invigorate the Blood and the other to regulate the Qi. The Blood-invigorating herbs in this formula are Semen persicae *(Tao ren)*, Flos carthami tinctorii *(Hong hua)*, Radix angelicae sinensis *(Dang gui)*, Radix ligustici chuanxiong *(Chuang xiong)*, Radix paeoniae rubrae *(Chi shao)*, and Radix Niuxi *(Niu xi)*. The Qi-regulating herbs are Radix bupleuri *(Chai hu)* and Fructus citri seu ponciri *(Zhi ke)*. The classic rationale for using these two groups together is that the effects of the former group of herbs can be reinforced by the latter group of herbs (i.e., promote the Qi movement to facilitate Blood circulation). In an in vitro test of this proposition, using a rat model of acute microcirculation failure induced by a rapid intravenous infusion of 10% high-molecular-weight D-dextran solution (mw 500,000 dalton), Blood-invigorating herbs dilated the constricted mesenteric arterioles. On the other hand, Qi-regulating herbs alone caused further constriction of the arterioles. When the two groups were used together, they produced profound effects in dilating the mesenteric arterioles more than the Blood-invigorating herbs alone, hence improving the microcirculation[24] (Table 5-9). Synergistic effects of the Blood-invigorating and Qi-regulating herbs on erythrocyte filterability and whole blood viscosity in rats were also observed (Table 5-10). Guided by these laboratory findings, the *Drive Out Stasis in the Mansion of Blood Decoction* has become extensively used in China to treat conditions such as coronary heart disease, acute diffuse intravascular clotting, headache caused by cerebral arteriosclerosis, and trauma.[24]

In China, medical professionals have established national or local associations and societies to encourage the use of biomedical knowledge and technology to study traditional herbs and formulas, and to guide the clinical practice of herbal medicine. Many peer-reviewed medical journals are also dedicated specifically to the topic of integrating Chinese and biomedical perceptions and practices. Unfortunately, most of these journals are published in Chinese and hardly accessible to the Western health care professionals. However, some English-language peer-reviewed journals do publish

TABLE 5-9

Effects of Drive Out Stasis in the Mansion of Blood Decoction (Xue fu zhu yu tang) *and Its Components on the Diameters of Mesenteric Arterioles during Acute Microcirculation Failure**

Group	Baseline diameter (μm)	Diameter change after 5 min (μm)	Diameter change after 30 min (μm)
Whole formula	26.6 ± 4.8	3.3 ± 2.2	4.7 ± 1.9
Blood-invigorating	25.8 ± 3.6	1.4 ± 0.6	1.8 ± 0.5
Qi-regulating	29.7 ± 5.7	−1.0 ± 0.4	−2.1 ± 0.8
Control	28.9 ± 6.4	−0.0 ± 0.3	−0.1 ± 0.4

Adapted from Zheng YW, Peng K: Laboratory study and clinical application of the Drive Out Stasis in the Mansion of Blood Decoction and analysis of its components. In Chou JH, Wang JH, editors: *Progress in pharmacological study and clinical application of Chinese herbal medicine*, vol 2, Beijing, 1993, China Science and Technology Press. (Printed in Chinese.)
*Acute microcirculation failure in rats was induced by a rapid intravenous infusion of 10% high-molecular-weight D-dextran solution (mw 500,000 dalton). Diameter of mesenteric arterioles was measured before and after injection of *Drive Out Stasis in the Mansion of Blood Decoction* or its components into the mesenteric artery bed.

TABLE 5-10

Effects of the Drive Out Stasis in the Mansion of Blood Decoction (Xue fu zhu yu tang) *and Its Components on Erythrocyte Filterability and Whole Blood Viscosity in Rats**

Group	Erythrocyte filterability index (% change)	Whole blood viscosity (mPa)
Whole formula	155 ± 10 (−25.85%)	4.39 ± 0.94
Blood-invigorating	187 ± 10 (−10.5%)	5.52 ± 0.79
Qi-regulating	183 ± 13 (−12.4%)	5.23 ± 0.47
Control	209 ± 13	7.31 ± 0.39

Adapted from Zheng YW, Peng K: Laboratory study and clinical application of the Drive Out Stasis in the Mansion of Blood Decoction and analysis of its components. In Chou JH, Wang JH, editors: *Progress in pharmacological study and clinical application of Chinese herbal medicine*, vol 2, Beijing, 1993, China Science and Technology Press. (Printed in Chinese.)
*Rats were fed with *Drive Out Stasis in the Mansion of Blood Decoction* or its components, twice a day for 3 days. Whole blood sample was collected 1 hour after the last dose and the erythrocyte filterability and whole blood viscosity were measured.

reports of herbal research, including the *American Journal of Chinese Medicine,* the *Journal of Alternative and Complementary Medicine, Botanical Medicine, HerbalGram,* and the *Chinese Journal of Integrated Traditional and Western Medicine.* Some are available in electronic form on the Internet (www.chinainfo.gov.cn/periodical/zgzxyjh-E/index.htm).

HERBAL SAFETY

Chinese herbal medicine is generally safe when used properly. However, many herbs and formulas have certain contraindications or precautions for use, and some are toxic if misused. Contraindications and toxicity information are not always available in books read by the general public, nor is it always stated in the labeling of patent medicine. Commonly used Chinese herbs with well-documented toxicity are listed in Table 5-11. Toxicity of some of these herbs may be eliminated or minimized by appropriate processing (e.g., by cooking with ginger for an extended time) or by appropriate combination with other herbs. To minimize the danger of toxicity in use, it is wisest to take herbal formulas under the guidance of a professional herbalist.

Toxicity or significant side effects of some Chinese herbs have recently been reported by Western observers.[25-27] As mentioned, only a small fraction of Chinese herbs are exported outside China. These exported herbs are typically well recognized by herbal practitioners as efficacious and safe when used properly. These herbs are also frequently used in combination to reduce the amount of individual herb in any formula, thereby reducing the potential for toxicity caused by one particular herb. Botanical herbs are usually used in doses between 3 and 12 g each; mineral products may be used in larger doses but generally not greater than 30 g. When these herbs are used in larger amounts in an attempt to achieve a rapid response, or when prescribed for prolonged use in efforts to achieve unphysiological outcomes (e.g., weight loss, increased sex drive), they may stress the body system, leading to adverse events.

In some cases, toxicity is not related to the herbs but to contamination with other substances, particularly heavy metals[28,29] or adulteration with pharmaceutical drugs in Chinese patent medicines sold over the counter.[30,31] The latter situation should be of concern to the general public outside China. As noted, an aspect of the integration of Chinese and biomedicine is the Chinese practice of combining pharmaceutical drugs with herbal formulas to achieve faster action. Most such combinations have been approved by the provincial (equivalent level of state in the United States) authorities in China, but when they are exported, information on the pharmaceutical drug content may not be included on labels.

The US Food and Drug Administration (FDA) maintains a database on imported Chinese herbal medicines that contain toxic substances or prescription drugs. This database (Import Alert, IA6610) can be searched at the FDA's site at www.fda.gov, using the keyword "IA6610." Published scientific literature on the safety of Chinese herbal medicines, albeit limited at the current time, can be searched at the National Library of Medicine's site (www.ncbi.nlm.nih.gov/

TABLE 5-11

Toxicity of Commonly Used Chinese Herbs

Commonly used herbs	Identified toxin	Toxic effects
Radix lateralis aconiti carmichaeli praeparata *(Fu zi)*	Aconitine	Neurological and cardiac suppression
Rhizoma pinelliae ternatae *(Ban xia)*	Conitine	Respiratory suppression
Semen pruni armeniacae *(Xing ren)*	Amygadalin	Respiratory suppression
Buthus martensi *(Quan xie)*	Katsutoxin	Respiratory suppression
Rhizoma arisaematis *(Tian nan xing)*	Triterpenoid saponins	Necrotic to mucus and nephrotoxic
Radix aristolochiae fangchi *(Guang fan ji)*	Aristolochic acids	Interstitial renal fibrosis

entrez/query.fcgi), using the keywords "Chinese herb" and "toxicity."

HERB-HERB AND HERB-DRUG INTERACTION

Through years of practice, adverse herb-herb interactions, particularly toxic combinations, have been identified by Chinese herbal practitioners. Examples of such pairs include Flos caryophylli *(Ding xiang)* and Tuber curcumae *(Yu jin);* Radix aconiti *(Wu tou)* and Cornu rhinoceri *(Xi jiao);* Radix ginseng *(Ren shen)* and Excrementum trogopterori seu pteromi *(Wu ling zhi);* and Cortex cinnamomi cassiae *(Rou gui)* and Halloysitum rubrum *(Chi shi zhi).* In addition, certain herbs are traditionally considered incompatible with many other herbs. For example, Radix glycyrrhizae uralensis *(Gan cao)* is considered incompatible with Radix euphorbiae kansui *(Gan sui),* Radix euphorbiae seu knoxiae *(Da ji),* Flos daphnes genkwa *(Yuan hua),* and Herba sargassii *(Hai zao).* Radix aconiti *(Wu tou)* is considered incompatible with Bulbus fritillariae *(Bei mu),* Fructus trichosanthis *(Gua lou),* Rhizoma pinelliae ternatae *(Ban xia),* Radix ampelopsis *(Bai lian),* and Rhizoma bletillae striatae *(Bai ji).* Rhizoma et radix veratri *(Li lu)* is considered incompatible with Radix ginseng *(Ren shen),* Radix adenophorae seu glehniae *(Sha shen),* Radix salviae miltiorrhizae *(Dan shen),* Radix sophorae flavescentis *(Ku shen),* Herba cum radice asari *(Xi xin),* and Radix paeoniae lactiflorae *(Bai shao).* Efforts are ongoing in China to verify the incompatibility of these herbs.

In comparison, herb-drug interaction is a newer issue. Although many combinations of herbs and prescription drugs are beneficial to patients, based on the Chinese experience of integrating the two medicines, certain combinations do result in adverse events. With many new pharmaceutical drugs being marketed each year, the potential for both beneficial and adverse effects of herb-drug interaction is enormous, yet difficult to assess. However, with some general knowledge of pharmacokinetics or pharmacodynamics, many potential adverse interactions may be avoided. Two recent articles provide excellent reviews of the subject.[32,33]

From a pharmacokinetic point of view, concomitant use of herbs and drugs may alter the absorption, distribution, metabolism, and elimination of the herbs or drugs or both, resulting in unexpectedly increased or decreased concentrations of biologically active compounds (either from herbs, from drugs, or from both). For example, Radix sanguisorbae officinalis *(Di yu),* which is typically used in charred form to treat bleeding, binds many drugs in the gastrointestinal tract and therefore prevents them from being absorbed into the body. Prescription drugs such as cholestyramine, colestipol, and sucralfate bind to certain herbs, forming insoluble complexes too large to pass through the intestinal walls, thus decreasing absorption of both substances. Radix glycyrrhizae uralensis *(Gan cao),* a common herb that can be found in more than half of the Chinese herbal formulas, has been found to decrease clearance of prednisolone and therefore raises its plasma concentration.[34] Some herbs affect the cytochrome P450 system mixed-function oxidase enzymes and therefore alter the normal metabolism of both herbs and pharmaceutical drugs.

Pharmacodynamic interaction occurs when herbs and drugs have the same pharmacological effects, either by the same or different mechanism. The risk of herb-drug adverse events is raised when the pharmaceutical has a narrow therapeutic index (e.g., warfarin, digoxin, phenobarbital, phenytoin, anesthetic agents). For example, warfarin (Coumadin) is a strong anticoagulant; enhancing its effectiveness promotes prolonged bleeding, while decreasing its effectiveness increases the risk of blood clots in the vessels. Most Chinese herbs that invigorate the Blood and dispel stasis have similar pharmacological actions; if used with warfarin, the risk of toxicity rises. Combining the two most commonly used Blood-invigorating herbs, Radix angelicae sinensis *(Dang gui,* which also contains coumarins, analogues of warfarin) or Radix salviae miltiorrhizae *(Dan shen),* with warfarin was found to increase international normalized ratio (INR), prolong prothrombin time (PT)/partial thromboplastin time (PTT), and cause widespread bruising (a sign of subcutaneous bleeding and potential internal bleeding).[18,35,36] On the other hand, the Qi-tonifying herb Radix ginseng *(Ren shen)* antagonizes the effects of the warfarin, decreasing INR.[37] Because ginseng has a reputation for enhancing energy and masculinity and is readily available, it is quite possible that practitioners might find this combination in use among their patients for whom they have recommended warfarin.

In addition to pharmacokinetic and pharmacological interaction between herbs and pharmaceutical drugs, herbs may interfere with the monitoring of certain drugs. For example, Radix eleutherococcus senticosus (Siberian ginseng) has been found to interfere with digoxin assay, resulting in falsely elevated digoxin concentrations. In this case, the patient did not have any adverse events despite "very high" serum digoxin levels.[38]

At present, only a few adverse herb-drug interactions have been confirmed, largely because the necessary research has not yet been done, thus some examples in this chapter are based on theoretical speculations or personal experience. Because of the difficulty in predicting adverse outcomes, health care professionals should warn their patients using pharmaceuticals with narrow therapeutic indices about the potential danger of concomitant use of herbal medicines. Again, cooperation between herbalist and biomedical practitioner is essential to maximize therapeutic success and minimize the danger of adverse events.

WORKING WITH AN HERBALIST

Practicing Chinese herbal medicine is both a science and an art. Peter Mere Latham (1789-1875) once said "poisons and medicines are oftentime the same substance given with different intents."[33] Like pharmaceutical drugs, Chinese herbs and herbal formulas have certain specificities, indications, and recommended durations of use. They can be of great benefit when prescribed by well-trained and experienced practitioners of Chinese herbal medicine. However, indiscriminant and unjustified use of herbs or herbal formulas—just as with pharmaceutical drugs—can be harmful.

Biomedical practitioners in Western countries should keep an open mind on the subject of Chinese herbal medicine, recognizing that many herbs and formulas have a long history of clinical efficacy in treating certain disorders. As the availability of Chinese herbs and over-the-counter formulas rises, it is increasingly important to know what patients are taking. Patients must be asked about their herb use in a nonjudgmental and relaxed manner to gain their cooperation and ensure full disclosure. In some cases, such use is self-selected, and in other cases a prescription has been given by an herbalist. In either case, the

biomedical practitioner is well advised to develop a collegial relationship with a well-trained and experienced herbalist. Such a professional can explain the uses of herbs and formulas, assess the appropriateness of herbal preparations being used by a patient, identify indications and contraindications for the use of particular herbs, and work with the biomedical practitioner to create an integrated drug-herb regimen when appropriate.[39] The utility of consulting is especially high when prescribing a pharmaceutical with a narrow therapeutic index. Understanding the properties of both prescribed drugs and the herbs will improve patient care and minimize the risk of adverse drug-herb interactions.

References

1. Tyler VE: What pharmacists should know about herbal remedies, *J Am Pharm Assoc* 36:29-37, 1996.
2. Chang J: Medicinal herbs: drugs or dietary supplement? *Biochem Pharmacol* 59:211-9, 2000.
3. Upton R: Traditional Chinese medicine and the dietary supplement health and educational act, *J Altern Complement Med* 5:115-118, 1999.
4. Wang J: Modern investigation on the nature of Pi (Spleen) in traditional Chinese medicine. In Zhou J, Liu G, Chen J, editors, *Recent advances in Chinese herbal drugs,* Beijing, 1991, Science Press, pp. 30-9.
5. Yang G: Immunologic effects of traditional Chinese drugs, *Chin Med J* (Engl) 109:59-60, 1996.
6. Wang Z: Licorice and immunoregulation. In Zhou J, Liu G, Chen J, editors, *Recent advances in Chinese herbal drugs,* Beijing, 1991, Science Press, pp. 141-8.
7. Nakajima S, Uchiyama Y, Yoshida Y, et al: The effects of ginseng radix rubra on human vascular endothelial cells, *Am J Chin Med* 1998;26:365-73, 1998.
8. Lee DC, Lee MO, Kim CY, et al: Effects of ether, ethanol and aqueous extracts of ginseng on cardiovascular function in dogs, *Can J Comp Med* 45:182-7, 1981.
9. Xiao PG, Xing ST, Wang LW: Immunological aspects of Chinese medicinal plants as antiaging drugs, *J Ethnopharmacol* 42:67-9, 1993.
10. Gillis CN: Panax ginseng pharmacology: a nitric oxide link? *Biochem Pharmacol* 54:1-8, 1997.
11. Zhang J: Clinical and experimental studies on Yin deficiency. In Zhou J, Liu G, Chen J, editors, *Recent advances in Chinese herbal drugs,* Beijing, 1991, Science Press, pp. 58-64.
12. Li L, Liu G, Sun H: Drugs for activating blood circulation to remove Blood stasis. In Zhou J, Liu G, Chen J, editors, *Recent advances in Chinese herbal drugs,* Beijing, 1991, Science Press, pp. 197-209.

13. Li R: Radix salviae miltiorrhizae (dan shen). In Wang B, Ma J, Deng W, Qi S, Li R, Li Y, editors, *Modern pharmacology of Chinese herbs,* Tianjing, China, 1997, Tianjing Science and Technology Press, pp. 880-9. (Written in Chinese.)

14. Ma J: Herbs that release the exterior. In Wang B, Ma J, Deng W, et al, editors, *Modern pharmacology of Chinese herbs,* Tianjing, China, 1997, Tianjing Science and Technology Press, pp. 29-32. (Written in Chinese.)

15. Deng W: Herbs that clear heat—introduction. In Wang B, Ma J, Deng W, et al, editors, *Modern pharmacology of Chinese herbs,* Tianjing, China, 1997, Tianjing Science and Technology Press, pp. 198-204.(Written in Chinese.)

16. Bensky D, Barolet R: Chinese herbal medicine—formulas and strategies, Seattle, Wash, 1990, Eastland Press.

17. Sun Y: Evaluation of Chinese drugs in the treatment of neoplastic diseases. In Zhou J, Liu G, Chen J, editors, *Recent advances in Chinese herbal drugs,* Beijing, 1991, Science Press, pp. 236-44.

18. Yu J, Sun G, Ren D: Treatment of late-stage gastric carcinoma using combination of chemotherapy and Tonifying the Spleen and Nourishing the Kidney Granules (Jian Pi Yi Shen Chong Ji)—experimental and clinical studies. In Zhou J, Wang J, editors, *Advances in pharmacological and clinical research of Chinese herbal medicine,* vol 2, Beijing, 1993, Chinese Science and Technology Press, pp. 286-97. (Written in Chinese.)

19. Zhou J: Twenty centuries of Chinese medicine: from traditional to integrative medicine. In Zhou J, Liu G, Chen J, editors, *Recent advances in Chinese herbal drugs,* Beijing, 1991, Science Press, pp. 3-18.

20. Klayman DL: Qinghaosu (artemisinin). An antimalarial drug from China, *Science* 228:1049-55, 1985.

21. Hien TT, White NJ: Qinghaosu, *Lancet* 341:603-8, 1993.

22. White NJ: Artemisinin: A current status, *Trans R Soc Trop Med Hyg* 88 (suppl 1): 53-4, 1994.

23. Chen X: Panax ginseng (Radix Ginseng) and ginsenosides. In Zhou J, Liu G, Chen J, editors, *Recent advances in Chinese herbal drugs,* Beijing, 1991, Science Press, pp. 91-9.

24. Zheng YW, Peng K: Laboratory study and clinical application of the Drive Out Stasis in the Mansion of Blood Decoction and analysis of its components. In Chou J, Wang J, editors, *Progress in pharmacological study and clinical application of Chinese herbal medicine,* vol 2, Beijing, 1993, Chinese Science and Technology Press, pp. 211-226. (Written in Chinese.)

25. Huxtable RJ: The myth of beneficent nature: the risks of herbal preparation, *Ann Intern Med* 117:165-6, 1992.

26. Angell M, Kassirer JP: Alternative medicine—the risks of untested and unregulated remedies, *N Engl J Med* 339: 839-41, 1998.

27. Ernst E: Harmless herbs? A review of the recent literature, *Am J Med* 104:170-8, 1998.

28. Espinoza EO, Mann M-J, Bleasdell B: Arsenic and mercury in traditional Chinese herbal balls, *N Engl J Med* 333:803-4, 1995.

29. Gertner E, Marshall PS, Filandrinos D, et al: Complications resulting from the use of Chinese herbal medications containing undeclared prescription drugs, *Arthritis Rheum* 38:614-7, 1995.

30. Huang WF, Wen SK, Hsiao ML: Adulteration by synthetic therapeutic substances of traditional Chinese medicine in Taiwan, *J Clin Pharmacol* 37:344-50, 1997.

31. Kang-Yum E, Oransky SH: Chinese patent medicine as a potential source of mercury poisoning, *Vet Hum Toxicol* 34:235-8, 1992.

32. Miller LG: Herbal medicinals—selected clinical considerations focusing on known or potential drug-herb interactions, *Arch Intern Med* 158:2200-11, 1998.

33. Fugh-Berman A: Herb-drug interaction, *Lancet* 355:134-8, 2000.

34. Chen MF, Shimada F, Kato H, et al: Effect of oral adminstration of glycyrrhizin on the pharmacokinetics of prednisolone, *Endocrinol Jpn* 38:167-75, 1991.

35. Izzat MB, Yim APC, El-Zufari MH: A taste of Chinese medicine, *Ann Thorac Surg* 66:941-2, 1998.

36. Page RL, Lawrence JD: Potentiation of warfarin by dong quai, *Pharmacotherapy* 19:870-6, 1999.

37. Janetzky K, Morreale AP: Probable interactions between warfarin and ginseng, *Am J Health Syst Pharm* 54:692-3, 1997.

38. McRae S: Elevated serum digoxin levels in a patient taking digoxin and Siberian ginseng, *Can Med Assoc J* 155:293-5, 1996.

39. Libster M: Guidelines for selecting a medical herbalist for consultation and referral: consulting a medical herbalist, *J Altern Complement Med* 5:457-62, 1999.

Additional Readings

Beinfield H, Korngold E: *Chinese modular solutions: handbook for health professionals,* San Francisco, Calif, 1997, Chinese Medicine Works.

Bensky D, Gamble A: *Chinese herbal medicine—Materia Medica,* Seattle, Wash, 1993, Eastland Press.

Duke JA: *CRC handbook of medicinal herbs,* Boca Raton, Fla, 1987, CRC Press.

Huang KC, editor: *The pharmacology of Chinese herbs,* 2nd ed, Bota Raton, Fla, 1999, CRC Press.

Kessler DA: Cancer and herbs, *N Engl J Med* 342:1742-3, 2000.

Naeser M: *Outline guide to Chinese herbal patent medicines in pill form,* Boston, 1990, Boston Chinese Medicine.

Nortier JL, Martinez MCM, Schmeiser HH, et al: Urothelial carcinoma association with the use of a Chinese herb (Aristolochia fangchi), *N Engl J Med* 342:1686-92, 2000.

The Pharmacopoeia Commission of People's Republic of China: *Pharmacopoeia of the People's Republic of China,* vol 1 (English version), Beijing, 1997, Chemical Industry Press.

Yu CM, Chan JCN, Sanderson JE: Chinese herbs and warfarin potentiation by "danshen," *J Intern Med* 241:337-9, 1997.

Zhou J, Liu G, Chen J, editors: *Recent advances in Chinese herbal drugs—actions and uses,* Beijing, 1991, Science Press.

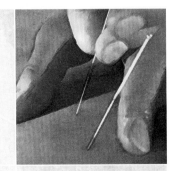

6

Other Treatment Modalities
Diet, Bodywork, and Qi Gong

PAULETTE MCMILLAN

BRYN CLARK

JEAN EDELEN

SECTION 1: CHINESE DIET THERAPY

PAULETTE MCMILLAN

*D*iet therapy in Chinese medicine, as in allo-pathic medicine, can be used to prevent dis-ease and promote longevity or it can be used to treat an already existing disease. The medicinal diet is usually an adjunct to acupuncture, herbal treatment, or both modalities. Diet can enhance or interfere with the action of the treatment. For example, a patient who needs a treatment plan "to clear the heat and soothe the Liver Qi" should avoid Liver-heating foods and bev-erages such as coffee, cola drinks, alcoholic beverages, and red meat; otherwise the diet will interfere with the corrective treatment. Therefore diet therapy means in-cluding as well as excluding specific foods based on their properties and the presentation of the disease.

Application of Chinese diet therapy is based on the traditional Chinese medicine (TCM) system of differ-entiation. Differentiation of the chief complaint is de-termined by the presenting signs and symptoms ob-tained through questioning, overall appearance of the patient and the tongue, pulse diagnosis, body smells, quality of voice, and breathing. For example, a chief complaint of migraine headache according to TCM can be differentiated into several syndromes such as Liver-Yang Raising, Liver-Fire, Dampness, Blood Defi-ciency, Stasis of Blood, and others. Accordingly, diet therapy for migraine headaches must vary in concert with the specific differentiation. This is an illustration of the case in which one disorder requires different treatments. In other situations, different disorders may respond to the same treatment, because their underlying energetic imbalance is the same. For example, both hypertension and migraine headache can present as Liver-Yang Rising. In this case, the practitioner might make the same dietary recommendations to patients who complain of different disorders. Thus the same disorder can receive different treatments, and different disorders can receive the same treatment. In short, diet therapy is prescribed according to the TCM differentiation and is not based solely on the chief complaint.

The Chinese recognize the importance of a healthy digestive system, and its role is considered privotal in treating and preventing disease. In TCM, the Zang-Fu Organ system referred to as the Spleen and Stomach most closely represents digestion and absorption in the biomedical system. (The Spleen in TCM should not be confused with the biomedical physiological understanding of the spleen). The Spleen and Stomach are important for taking in fluids and foods and transforming them into Qi and Blood and transporting them throughout the body. If there is an underlying Spleen/Stomach weakness accompanying a disorder, herbal medicine and diet must aim to strengthen the Spleen to better treat the chief complaint. The Chinese medical classics state that when the Spleen and Stomach are strong, then the Qi and Blood are abundant and the body is nourished.[1] As a result, patients recover faster and more easily. If the Spleen and Stomach are weak, dietary and herbal treatment may be hindered. According to TCM, irregular eating times, eating in haste, overeating or undereating, overeating greasy or sweet-tasting foods, or drinking iced beverages daily weaken the functions of Spleen/Stomach, ultimately leading to disease. The centrality of the Spleen-Stomach in Chinese medical thought contrasts with the situation in biomedicine, in which the state of the digestive system is given relatively little attention unless it is the patient's chief complaint.

Chinese diet therapy does not directly address current Western agricultural practices, the use of pesticides, herbicides, hormones, antibiotics, genetic engineering, food processing, and so forth. However, it does emphasize that only food of good quality and proper preparation are effective in the treatment of disease. Fresh food is said to contain Qi or Vitality. In the West, we might be tempted to think of these in terms of nutrients or phytochemicals, but Qi is more than these: Qi is the life force remaining in the food. Therefore it is

The Chinese Diet

The ancient Chinese advised people "to eat the five cereals to nourish the vital-Qi of the five Zang Organs, with the five fruits, the five meats, and the five vegetables as supplements" *(Su Wen)*. This seems to indicate that the center of the meal should be grains, and a variety of foods should be consumed. The five foods within each category represent each of the five tastes. For example, the five cereals include rice for sweet, sesame for sour, soybeans for salty, wheat for bitter, and broomcorn millet for acrid *(Ling shu)*. Traditionally, milk and milk products were not part of the daily diet in China. In fact, regular consumption is considered to weaken the Spleen's function causing Phlegm conditions such as asthma, nasal congestion, headaches, and fibroids. On the other hand, specially prepared milk can be used medicinally as a nourishing tonic when indicated. ∾

common sense that food from a local garden or a local farm is more likely to contain the Qi and nutrients needed for health than produce picked prematurely and consumed days later. It is also believed that fresh foods prepared at home contain more Qi than food bought from a local restaurant or fast food chain. Thus in general, Chinese medicine argues that processing and adulterating food alters its inherent properties. It is these inherent properties that are essential in the prevention and treatment of disease.

THE GENERAL PROPERTIES OF FOOD

The properties by which foods are sorted are the same as those used for herbs. There is a fine line between herbs and foods in Chinese medicine, and they are often used together in treatment. In general, herbal formulas are stronger and are meant to be used for shorter periods. However, some herbal tonification formulas can be taken for extended periods, although some foods such as coffee or frozen desserts should be permanently limited. The properties of food include the four natures, five flavors, channel propensity, and four directions.

Four Natures

The two most important properties are the four natures and the five flavors. The four natures of the food refers to the temperatures of cold, cool, warm, or hot. The nature of a food is determined by its effect on the body. For example, if it has antipyretic action, it is defined as cold, whereas if it promotes circulation and warms the body, it is considered warm or hot. Some foods are classified as neutral. The nature of the food helps balance the yin and yang of the body, and overconsumption of extremely hot or cold foods promotes disease. For example, ice cream or other frozen desserts, consumed habitually, weaken the function of the Spleen and Stomach (digestion). Poor digestion eventually leads to disease.

Five Flavors

The five flavors or tastes are sour, bitter, sweet, pungent, and salty. Different tastes have different actions on the body. *Sour* (includes astringent) "retains and arrests," meaning it can control such signs of loss or openness as diarrhea and excessive sweating. Sour can also generate fluids, which is helpful in promoting proper digestion. Foods that are sour include lemons and hawthorn berries. Some fruits are a blend of slightly sour and sweet such as grapefruit, apricots, and cherries. The *bitter* taste is drying and purging. Therapeutically these actions are good for treating constipation, moving perverse Qi downward as in acid regurgitation, and relieving some types of cough. Foods that are bitter include bitter melon and dandelion greens. *Sweet* can tonify or strengthen the body, help replenish fluid and blood, help harmonize the action of the Spleen and Stomach, and relieve spasms and pain. Sweet foods include many fruits, root vegetables, chicken, chicken eggs, and mutton. The *pungent* taste expels pathogens and helps promote the normal flow of Qi and Blood to relieve stagnation. Pungent foods include ginger, cayenne pepper, chilies, and Chinese spring onion. *Salty* taste softens and resolves masses. Salty foods include kelp and seaweed. Interestingly, these foods in ancient China were used to treat goiter. Today we know that some of these foods contain iodine, which treats simple goiter by providing this missing mineral.[2]

Each of the five tastes has an affinity for each of the five Zang Organs. Sour goes to the Liver, bitter to the Heart, sweet to the Spleen, pungent to the Lung, and salty to the Kidney. A balance of the five tastes promotes health. Too much of any one taste will create an imbalance and damage the corresponding Zang Organ. Overconsumption of salt weakens the bones because salt has an affinity for the Kidneys, which oversee the health of the bones according the TCM. This is interesting, as osteoporosis is most prevalent in industrialized nations where the salt intake from processed foods is very high. Research supports that a high intake of sodium promotes loss of calcium in the urine, possibly contributing to osteoporosis.[3]

Channel Propensity

Each food and herb has a propensity toward specific channels. Propensity is determined by the action of the food on different systems of the body. For example, many fruits such as lemons, tangerines, and pears can clear heat from the lungs to stop cough. Thus it is said that these fruits go to the Lung channel. Most foods go to at least two channels; for example, tangerines also treat nausea and loss of appetite, so they also go to the Stomach channel. By knowing the nature, taste, and channel propensity of a food, the food's action and clinical usefulness can be understood.

Four Directions

Once a food has been digested it can also have an impact on the direction of Qi. The four directions are ascending, descending, floating, and sinking. Therapeutically, foods with ascending action can treat diarrhea and prolapsed organs; foods with descending action can treat belching, hiccups, nausea, and vomiting; foods with floating or dispersing action can promote perspiration to treat the common cold; and foods with sinking action can relieve constipation or treat mania and hypertension related to upward movement of Yang Qi. The general law in TCM is that leaves and flowers are light and tend to move upward; roots, seeds, and fruits are heavy and tend to move downward.[4]

EXTERNAL AND INTERNAL ENVIRONMENTS

Diet is prescribed on the basis of TCM differentiation and the properties of foods. However, other factors are also considered including the patient's external environment and physiological status. The external environment refers to the seasons, indoor milieu, and geographical location.

Seasons

People naturally tend to consume different foods according to the seasons. For example, more sweet potatoes and soups are consumed in the fall and winter and watermelon and salads in the summer. The Chinese take this a step further and recognize that each season acts on the body differently, thereby guiding dietary preference and what is therapeutically best in different seasons. In the spring, the weather gets warmer and the Liver Qi is strong. "In spring man should eat more sweet food than sour food to nourish the Spleen Qi" *(Treatise on Health Preservation and Cultivation* by Qiu Chuji, the Yuan Dynasty). According to the Five Element theory, the Liver can invade or harm the Spleen. The above quote suggests that too much strengthening of the Liver may damage the Spleen; thus by nourishing the Spleen, a balance between the Liver and Spleen Qi is maintained. A common misunderstanding, using Five Element charts, is that because sour corresponds to Spring and Liver that sour foods should be consumed in the Spring. Actually sour has the action of retaining and drawing inward, which is the opposite of the desired action of dispelling and moving outward. This latter and desired action complements the natural Yang movement in the body during the spring.

In summer, the weather is hot and the gastrointestinal tract slows. The diet should be light and easy to digest. The diet principle for the summer is to clear heat and generate fluids. This is accomplished by consuming fruits and vegetables regularly while decreasing intake of foods that are difficult to digest such as animal meat and greasy foods.

In autumn, the Yang-Qi or the energy of the body is weakening while the Yin-Qi or the substance of the body is growing. The weather is cool and dry, so avoiding cold foods to protect the Spleen's function (digestion and absorption), and avoiding hot foods to prevent excessive drying is recommended. It is best to consume foods moderate in nature at this time of the year.

Generally in winter, the Yin Qi is in excess and the Yang Qi is deficient. After the Winter Soltice, the Yang Qi begins to rise again. This is the best time for people with weak or deficient constitutions to tonify and to rebalance the Yin and Yang. In general, it is the best

time to consume a nourishing and invigorating diet. Beef and mutton are often used because they are sweet and nourishing. Beef, in particular, can strengthen the Spleen. "To tonify the Spleen means to tonify all" *(Fundamentals in Compiling Medical Works* by Wang Fu, the Qing Dynasty).[1]

Indoor Environment

Today the indoor environment also plays a significant role in diet therapy. Many people live in air-conditioned environments for 2 months or more each year, and in heated ones much of the rest. In the first instance, although the summer temperature may be 95° F outdoors, the indoor environment is 70° F. Many people become easily chilled in air-conditioned environments. One dietary intervention combines a light summer diet of fruits and vegetables with some warming foods to protect the Spleen Qi and Wei Qi. Wei Qi is the Qi that protects the exterior layer of the body, preventing invasion of pathogenic external factors (i.e., Cold, Wind, Heat, or in biomedical terms, viruses or the common cold). In cool seasons, heated environments at home and at work tend to dry the body. To counter this, winter dietary tonification programs typically include moistening foods.

Geographical Location

The natural climate also affects the health of the body. For example, people living in unusually damp climates have a tendency to develop Damp syndromes, whereas those living in deserts tend toward Excess Dry Syndromes; the damp tendency may be exacerbated in late summer, while the dry worsens in autumn.

To complete the treatment plan, the patient's physical and emotional status must also be considered. Important physical characteristics include the patient's age, gender, and strength of constitution.

Age

Age is particularly important when addressing the young and the elderly. Children and infants have underdeveloped Spleen and Stomach Qi and as a result often have digestive difficulties. Weak Spleen Qi also allows fluids to accumulate, which leads to internal Damp syndromes that manifest as nasal congestion and runny nose, asthma, and ear infections. Good foods for children are root vegetables, well-cooked grains, and small amounts of animal protein. Cold and moist foods such as dairy products can aggravate Damp conditions.

The elderly also have a weak Spleen and Stomach function (weak digestive systems), in this case caused by wear. They should have small frequent meals that are warm, well-cooked, and easy to digest; soups and stews are particularly recommended in Chinese medicine.

Lifestyle and Gender

Women of child-bearing age have different physiological needs than men. Pregnant women, in particular, have special needs. During pregnancy, according to TCM theory, the fluids collect in the Ren and Chong meridians leaving the other meridians relatively dry, so drying foods must be avoided. Examples of drying foods are wine and hot spices.[5]

Workers who are sedentary have different nutritional needs than physical laborers. As in allopathic diet therapy, it is best to give more food during the day than at night because this is the time the greatest amount of energy is being expended. This is particularly important for the physically active patient.[6]

Patients with a deficiency syndrome need to use herbal treatments and make dietary alterations for extended periods to fully recover. Typically, those with deficiency conditions include people recovering from chronic illness, chemotherapy, radiation therapy, people with eating disorders, and the elderly.

Emotions

In addition to factoring in the external environment and the physical state of the patient, the practitioner making dietary recommendations must also consider the emotional state of the patient. Stress—whether physical, emotional, or from time pressure—hinders the proper function of the Spleen and Stomach (digestion). Patients with histories of chronic worry typically present with deficient Spleen function and need a diet that is easy to digest and tonifies the Spleen. In contrast, patients who are angry, are disappointed by life, or feel constantly pressured are likely to be prescribed a diet that soothes the Liver

Qi. In all cases of emotional distress, the patient must be encouraged to consume meals when the mind is calm, and to eat in a leisurely fashion so as to promote optimum digestion and absorption. Without proper Spleen function, the body cannot transform food into Qi and Blood, which are the essential elements of health.[7]

FOOD SELECTION AND PREPARATION

Chinese medicine acknowledges that the quality, freshness, and cleanliness of food is essential to maintaining its health-promoting properties. Foods are selected according to color intensity, freshness of flavor, and fragrance. Food preparation includes proper cleaning and preparing so that it is easy to digest and assimilate. Most importantly, attention is given to retaining the nutritional value of the food.

Medicinal food preparation includes cutting food into proper shapes and sizes, and using appropriate cooking methods and condiments. Steaming, braising, stir-frying, stewing, roasting, and quick boiling are among the common cooking methods. Condiments frequently added to foods include ginger, Chinese spring onion, mustard, salt, garlic, chilies, cilantro, and peppers. The medicinal diet can be dispensed in the form of teas, decoctions, fruit juices, medicated wines, gruels made of rice and millet, soups, pancakes, cooked dishes, candied fruits, and more.

Once food is properly selected and prepared, proper dietary habits are also important. Patients are encouraged to eat regularly, avoid overeating, to eat only when hungry, and to chew food well. Patients with weak constitutions are instructed to eat smaller meals more frequently.

As in allopathic diet therapy, some foods are contraindicated based on the patient's condition. For example, in biomedicine, it is not enough to consume more beans, fruits, and vegetables to lower serum cholesterol; it is considered equally important to decrease the intake of fats, especially saturated fats, to achieve the desired outcome. In the same way, the Chinese system instructs a patient with an Interior Cold syndrome not only to consume foods with warming properties, but also to avoid foods with cold properties to achieve the desired outcome.

SUMMARY

Chinese diet therapy can be used to prevent or treat disease. Generally, diet is used in conjunction with acupuncture, herbal therapy, or both modalities. The selection of diet is based on the traditional Chinese system of differentiation, not simply the presenting chief complaint. In addition, the patient's external environment is considered along with his or her physiological status. Most importantly, the health of the digestive system, known as the Spleen and Stomach, is considered fundamental to proper recovery from disease. A weak Spleen cannot transform food and beverage into Qi and Blood. Without adequate Qi and Blood, the patient cannot be expected to make a full recovery.

According to the Chinese medical system, food is able to promote health and longevity because of its inherent properties. The properties of food include the four natures, the five tastes, channel propensity, and the four directions. The four natures refer to the temperature that a food imparts on the body. They are cold, cool, warm, and hot. The five tastes are bitter, sour, sweet, pungent, and salty. Each taste is associated with specific actions. Channel propensity refers to the system on which the food will act. For example, if the food affects the Lung system, it is said to have an affinity for the Lung channel. In addition, many foods exert a directional movement and these movements are known as the four directions. The four directions are ascending, descending, floating, and sinking. All the properties of foods have clinical applications.

The properties of food are maintained or enhanced through proper preparation. Food preparation includes selection of fresh foods, proper cleaning, and retaining nutritional value. Food is cooked so that it is easy to digest and is appetizing. Patients are taught and encouraged to follow dietary habits that promote digestion and assimilation of food, and that take into account their reproductive status, age, and climatic environment. Thus Chinese dietary principles use the properties of food along with acupuncture and herbal therapy to achieve and maintain an ongoing state of health.[8]

Acknowledgments

Warm thanks to Dr. Jingiun Hou for her valuable selections in the completion of this chapter.

References

1. Jingiun H, editor: *Medicated diet of TCM,* Beijing, 1994, Beijing Science and Technology Press.
2. Robinson CH: *Normal and therapeutic nutrition,* ed 15, New York, 1977, Macmillan, pp. 115-6.
3. Nordin BE et al: Nutrition, osteoporosis, and aging, *Ann N Y Acad Sci* 854:336-51, 1998.
4. Li H: Class notes on Chinese dietary therapy, Bethesda, Md, 1997, Maryland Institute of Traditional Chinese Medicine.
5. Jilin L, Peck G, editors: *Chinese dietary therapy,* Edinburgh, NY, 1999, Churchill Livingstone.
6. Flaws B, Wolfe H: *Prince Wen Hui's cook,* Brookline, Mass, 1983, Paradigm Publications.
7. *Spiritual axis (Ling Shu Jing),* Beijing, 1981, People's Health Publishing House.
8. Ni M, translator: *The yellow emperor's classic of internal medicine (Neijing Su Wen),* Boston, 1995, Shambhala Press.

SECTION 2: ORIENTAL BODYWORKERS

BRYN CLARK

THE OLDEST FORM OF MEDICINE

Treating with our hands is a natural, instinctive human response to pain, injury, and sickness. For as long as we have been able to feel, human beings have been rubbing painful areas to make them feel better. In China, the theory and practice of medicine was developed by treating through touch, and the practices of acupuncture and herbology grew alongside bodywork treatment.*

Mastery of bodywork was required of traditional Chinese physicians. Viewed as integral to improving their sensitivity, it helped them learn the refined palpation skills necessary for competent diagnosis and practice of all aspects of Chinese medicine. Today in China, *Tuina-Anmo* is a doctoral discipline and requires 5 or 6 years of medical training depending on the particular specialization.

In the United States more than a dozen styles of Oriental bodywork base their practice on medical theory first written in the original medical texts of China. Although each is a full bodywork practice in its own right, two—*acupressure* and *shiatsu*—are so well known that practitioners of European massage use them to indicate that they have incorporated aspects of Oriental bodywork into their practices.

Although the origins of Chinese bodywork predate written records, written sources from the Qin Dynasty in the third century BCE call manual therapy *Moshou* (hand rubbing). (The phrase "manual therapy" is used to indicate treatment where the hands are used as the primary interventive tool.) A century later (Han Dynasty, 206 BCE-221 CE) it was called *Anmo* (press and rub), a term still used today. Palpatory techniques for diagnosis and manual techniques for treatment are described in the *Huang Di Nei Jing (The Yellow Emperor's Classic on Internal Medicine)*. Sadly, although we know that a considerable portion of the *Huang Di Nei Jing* consisted of the "ten classics of Qi Bo's massage,"† all of these books have been lost. Nevertheless, the fact that so much attention was given to this subject shows how important bodywork was at that early time in the practice of Chinese medicine.

By the fifth century of the Common Era, manual therapy had evolved into a discipline in its own right. A doctoral degree was created for it at the Imperial College of Medicine in Xian, the ancient capital of the Tang Dynasty.[1] During the Ming Dynasty (1368-1644) the term *Tuina* (push and pull) was added. Documents of the time reveal that one of the specialties of Tuina was in treating some illnesses of small children.

As China sent trade missions to open routes of commerce, Chinese medicine spread to the Korean peninsula and the Japanese archipelago. In each country these manual therapies were adapted and integrated into the local culture. In Japan this bodywork became known as *Anma* and in Korea it became known as *Amma*. There are today perhaps hundreds of forms of Oriental bodywork specialties in Asia.

Styles of Oriental bodywork recognized in the United States and Europe come primarily from China, Japan, Thailand, and Korea; the American Organization for Bodywork Therapies of Asia (AOBTA) recognizes a dozen forms. To simplify, these are described as six broad styles: *Tuina, Shiatsu, Jin Shin, Noad Bo Rom (Thai Massage), Amma,* and *Acupressure.* Although there is some overlap among these styles, they range from very specific treatment for common disorders to whole-body treatments that can profoundly shift the receiver's state of being. Self-treatment by the patient to support the body's healing process is also taught as part of Oriental bodywork practice.

Oriental bodywork developed within a number of different social environments. Some styles, such as *Noad Bo Rom,* evolved as part of monastic traditions to help the receiver practice sitting meditation. Other styles, such as aspects of *Tuina,* have come from the martial arts lineage. Here bodywork was used to heal traumatic injury and correct structural misalignments, as well as to keep the martial artist fit and healthy. Finally, practitionership was often learned through a family lineage of healers. Throughout Chinese history, nutritional support through diet and the art of bone setting also formed part of the bodyworker's set of skills.

THE THEORY OF ORIENTAL BODYWORK

Oriental bodywork is guided by much the same theory as other modalities in Oriental medicine. Because touch is primary to this modality, Oriental bodywork focuses on treating via the rivers of energy, the Meridians, that can be accessed at the surface of the body. Because the

*In his keynote address to the 1994 National Convention of the AOBTA, Professor Wang Jin-Huai spoke about the earliest known medical record in China. It is a prescription written by a practitioner for a woman of high social standing who was ill. The prescription describes rubbing down over the flanks to generate heat and flow in the lower abdomen. Then the patient was instructed to hold her hands there and breathe into the area until she could feel heat rising up to her shoulders. This remains an effective treatment even today, incorporating elements of both bodywork and Qi Gong. Professor Wang Jin-Huai was featured in Bill Moyers' documentary *Healing and the Mind.*

†Wang Jin-Huai in his key note address to the 1994 national convention of the AOBTA. Also in the *Han Shu Yi Wen Zhi* (Han's Book of Arts and Scholarship), it states that "during the reign of the Yellow Emperor, Qi Bo has written ten classics of An Mo ..." cited in *Chinese Qigong Massage: General Massage,* by Dr. Yang Jwing-Ming, 1992.

Meridians relate to Organs that in turn control the function of all the tissues, internal health is reflected in these pathways and can be affected by bodywork. In a very basic way, the goal of Oriental bodywork treatment is to help the body achieve and maintain balance between areas that are in excess and areas that are deficient.

The skilled practitioner's touch can both assess and treat at the same time. This is a kind of "loop" in which the practitioner is using his or her hands both to listen to (assess) the tissues being treated and to treat based on that assessment. Because Oriental bodywork is an energetic art, sensing Qi and its movement is an important aspect of knowing how to treat and to gauge the ongoing success of treatment.

DIAGNOSIS

Bodyworkers perform diagnosis using the same Four Examinations—asking, looking, listening/smelling, and palpation—used by other Oriental medicine practitioners (see Chapter 3). Tongue characteristics and quality of the pulse are also analyzed in the usual way, athough some Oriental bodywork traditions do not use these forms of diagnosis. And as in all of Oriental medicine, bodyworkers know that no one sign or symptom can establish a diagnosis. Instead, they seek a constellation of signs and symptoms that point to the pattern of disharmony and can guide treatment decisions.

An important component of diagnosis in many forms of Oriental bodywork, especially those that come from Japan, is *Hara diagnosis,* or *abdominal palpation.* First mentioned in the Han Dynasty text *Nan Jing,* this technique is based on the finding that reflex areas on the abdomen reflect the energetic state of the body. Numerous styles of Hara diagnosis exist, so depending on the map being used, reflex areas on the abdomen correspond to the Elements (in Five Element diagnosis), the twelve regular Meridians, the eight Extraordinary Meridians, and so forth. Each map is best used in concert with the style of treatment from which it is derived.

Practitioners also direct close attention to the signs and symptoms that present along the course of each Meridian because this provides clues to the pattern of imbalance. Important clues include pain or numbness, strained or twisted muscles, dysfunction, and the presence of energetically deficient or excess areas along the course of the Meridians. One of the most important abilities of an Oriental bodyworker is sensing the various manifestations of Qi as it flows in the body. This can be evidenced by, among other phenomena, the presence of heat or cold, the firmness or lack of tonicity of the tissues, the presence or absence of moisture, and the different qualities of pain.

With this information and the patient's report, a practitioner is able to estimate the etiology of the patient's condition and to formulate a course of treatment. To assess whether health is being restored, the practitioner seeks signs such as increased strength and pliability in the muscles near the Channels, reduction of pain, increase in functionality, a fuller flow of Qi where Qi was deficient, or a more appropriate flow of where Qi was excessive. In essence, better health reveals itself physically in improved energy, posture, skin, muscles, nails, hair, and membranes along the meridians affected, and in a brighter psychological outlook.

INTERVENTION TECHNIQUES

The main methods of treatment in Oriental bodywork involve influencing the Meridians throughout the body. Whereas a typical acupuncture chart emphasizes the acupoints and shows Meridians as slender lines that connect these points, the Oriental bodyworker experiences the Meridians as energetic rivers that run through and along the skin, muscles, tendons, bones, and joints. The bodyworker pays attention to the wider area influenced by these flows, and these areas are better represented by the *Tendinomuscular Meridians,* or the *Twelve Channel Sinews* (see Figure 2-8).

The primary goal of Oriental bodywork is to assist the body in creating balanced functioning within the Organs. When an energy imbalance is corrected, the body's own intrinsic healing power can produce remarkable cures. Treatment with Oriental bodywork can strengthen the Meridian system, clear blockages, and relieve pain. Clients report feeling energized with a calm sense of well-being.

A range of treatment styles characterizes the various forms of Oriental bodywork. As in acupuncture, a practitioner may work with a single point to effect a local response, or treat at a distal point to achieve a change along the Meridian or to address its Organ correlations. A set of points may be stimulated simultaneously or consecutively. A Meridian may be treated in its entirety from beginning to end. A practitioner may assist energetic movement between his or her hands along a Meridian. Stretches may be used to "open" the Meridian releasing heat or "evil" Qi, or to harmonize the Qi, facilitating flow within the Meridian. In another technique to open and encourage the energetic flow through the area, limbs and joints may be rotated to their full range of motion.

When doing bodywork, diagnosis and treatment become almost indistinguishable. For example, suppose a patient complains of a shoulder problem. Even when treating the local area, the practitioner continues to sense where the energy is full or empty around the shoulder, continues to correlate pain and dysfunction to Meridian and Organ theory, and remains responsive to ongoing changes as they occur in the patient. Then, to facilitate the balancing of excess and deficiency in the shoulder area, the practitioner may choose to work further down the Meridian, or use techniques to shift the flow of Qi and Blood and enhance healing (Figures 6-1 and 6-2).

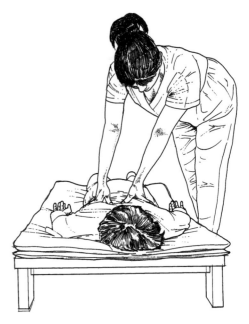

Figure 6-1 The practitioner manipulates small regions, particularly acupoints, with her fingertips, using her own body weight to control the depth of stimulation. (From Beresford-Cooke C: *Shiatsu theory and practice: a comprehensive text for the student and professional,* Edinburgh, 1996, Churchill Livingstone.)

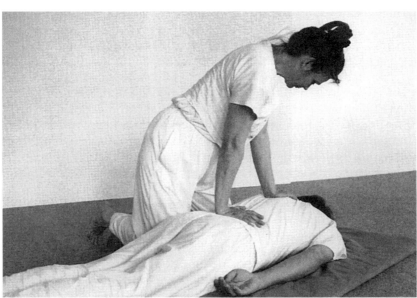

Figure 6-2 A variety of movements are used on different parts of the body to improve the flow of Qi and Blood. Here a practitioner kneels by a patient and uses her body weight judiciously to stretch and stimulate a patient's back. (From Beresford-Cooke C: *Shiatsu theory and practice: a comprehensive text for the student and professional,* Edinburgh, 1996, Churchill Livingstone.)

Adding Energy via Bodywork

An idea in Oriental medical theory that is often better developed in bodywork (and moving meditation practices) than in acupuncture and herbal care is that treatment can "add" energy to the system, thus offering another way of balancing those suffering from deficiency. This technique, called *Qi projection,* combines Qi gong and manual treatment techniques. After developing a personal abundance of Qi, a practitioner may focus Qi into points or an area of a patient's body.

Self-Care

Another important characteristic of bodywork is that some components can be performed by patients on themselves, outside the practitioner's office; it can be put to excellent use in daily life in the home. Practitioners often give homework to patients so that they can sustain or enhance their progress at home. Lessons may also be given in the treatment of family members. In fact, this is how many Asian practitioners first learn. Many of my Japanese clients say, "Oh yes, I learned shiatsu treating my Grandmother when I was young."

Finally, it is worth mentioning that in most, if not all styles of Oriental bodywork, the patient receives the treatment clothed. On the first visit, practitioners typically do an Intake Interview (patient's health history, living situation, diet, and so forth) and perform physical diagnosis. In subsequent visits, practitioners do follow-up interviews and assess the changing state of the body and health as described previously.

FIVE ORIENTAL BODYWORK PRACTICES

Tuina/Anmo/Amma

Tuina (push and pull) and *Anmo* (press and rub) are the most ancient and most Chinese of the bodywork systems, and their principles permeate all of the rest of the styles. Commonly combined under the single term Tuina, they provide a good example of the broad range of a practitioner's scope of practice. Indeed, a fully trained practitioner combines skills that in the West would usually be divided into massage, physical therapy, and chiropractic. A practitioner may also know and incorporate the use of Chinese herbs, plasters, bonesetting, and Qi projection. Originally, Tuina

was developed for the treatment of traumatic injury and for use in pediatric care, whereas Anmo was directed toward the treatment of internal disease. Amma is the same system coming to the United States from Korea, where Chinese medicine has been practiced since the sixth century CE.

Patients with orthopedic problems may benefit from Tuina and Amma. These modalities are specific for treating joint and injury problems, chronic conditions, and back problems. Because these modalities can affect the functioning of the body's internal organs, they are appropriate for internal medicine, gynecology, and trauma. They can affect the health of the five sense organs and help a person feel more alive. There are also specific applications for self-massage and massage for athletes.

Shiatsu

Literally meaning "finger pressure," shiatsu originated in Japan. Using the thumbs, palms, elbows, knees, and feet, the practitioner applies direct holding pressure sequentially to acupoints along meridians. Other techniques include stretching meridians to open and stimulate the circulation of Qi, and rotating joints to open the range of motion and move Qi blockages. Although there are many styles of practice, typically shiatsu practitioners treat whole Meridians as opposed to specific points. Diagnostic assessment focuses on identifying which Meridians are deficient *(kyo)* or in excess *(jitsu);* treatment aims to help the body achieve balance between the two.

Patients who can benefit from opening and facilitating flow of Blood and Qi within the body benefit from shiatsu because this treatment facilitates circulation in the body. One of the most influential shiatsu therapists in Japan, Shizuto Masunaga, was also a psychologist and outlined treatment based on psychological temperament in addition to physical conditions. The general ideas concerning psychological temperaments are first mentioned in Chapter 8 of the *Huang Di Nei Jing.*

Jin Shin

Jin Shin Jitsu is also from Japan and has numerous variations in America. For this text, the common body of these practices is called Jin Shin. This style of treatment uses gentle pressure on two or more acupressure points to facilitate the movement of energy. The point system is different from that of acupuncture, and the treatment is not directing, it is allowing. People who like active moving touch, or are hyperactive, may prefer one of the other therapies. The receiver is encouraged to go inward and participate in the release as fully as possible. This treatment has an affinity for facilitating movement at the levels of emotion and spirit, as well as at the physical level.

Noad Bo-Rom/Thai Massage

Noad Bo-Rom is the traditional name for the form of Thai massage that once flourished in the sequestered atmosphere of Buddhist monasteries. This form of Oriental bodywork is influenced by the ayurvedic tradition of India and the medicine of China; it also includes components that are purely Thai. Because it emphasizes stretching and extending the range of motion of the receiver's body, it looks somewhat like an assisted Yoga. However, it is a Yoga combined with the traditional techniques of Oriental bodywork that treats the Meridians and acupoints. Like shiatsu, this therapy is able to open the body and stimulate circulation. Another characteristic of *Noad Bo-Rom* is that it is practiced slowly—because the practitioner is seeking to induce a heightened or meditative state of consciousness in the receiver.

Acupressure

Acupressure employs stimulation of a single acupoint, or a combination of acupoints, to effect a specific therapeutic aim. Acupressure is a part of each previously mentioned Oriental bodywork practice, as well as a treatment modality in its own right. Stimulation of points is done primarily with the fingers and thumb, and the selection of points aims to create a specific shift in the body's physiology or condition.

OTHER BODYWORK IN AMERICAN PRACTICES

Many practitioners of Oriental medicine have learned other bodywork modalities that are not Oriental bodywork.[2] These might include Zero Balancing (ZB)[3] and Cranio-Sacral Therapy (CST), among other modalities. ZB was developed by an osteopath who learned acupuncture and began working where Merid-

ian Qi and bone Qi meet. ZB releases energy held in the body and helps the body to realign both pattern and function. CST is derived from osteopathic practice. Working the meningeal system of the central nervous system, CST can release the stresses held there and clear restrictions in the craniosacral system.

CONTRAINDICATIONS

Contraindications for treatment vary according to the hand techniques used. The fluid-mobilizing techniques of European massage and Meridian treatment are contraindicated in conditions such as thrombophlebitis; however, other techniques can be used if affected local areas are not directly stimulated. During pregnancy certain sites on the body must not be treated. In addition to predictable locations near the pregnant uterus, such sites include several points on inside of the lower leg, LI 4 (hand), and GB 21 (top of shoulder).

Oriental bodyworkers are also acutely conscious of conditions that cannot be appropriately treated by bodywork. Lists of such conditions (and how to identify them) are included in the curriculum of schools certified by the AOBTA. Most practitioners develop working relationships with biomedical doctors and seek advice when there are questions about appropriateness of treatment. For example, in work with cancer patients, some oncologists say to "do whatever makes the patient feel better," whereas others express concern about "moving cancer" via the lymphatic system. In the latter cases, treatment can be restricted to areas away from areas near the tumor.

CERTIFICATION AND CALLING A PRACTITIONER

The National Council for the Certification of Acupuncture and Oriental Medicine (NCCAOM) certifies practitioners of Oriental bodywork with the designation of Diplomate of Oriental Bodywork Therapy (Dipl. OBT). In addition, the AOBTA, founded in Kerhoset, New York, in August 1989, is part of an international network of practitioners, schools, and organizations that have developed international standards for the study and practice of Oriental manipulative healing arts.

The AOBTA has different levels of membership from Student to Associate to Certified; the highest level

Professional Oriental Bodywork Organizations

American Organization for Bodywork Therapies
    of Asia (AOBTA)
1010 Haddonfield-Berlin Road
Suite 408
Voorhees, NJ 08043
856-782-1616
Fax: 856-782-1653
E-mail: *AOBTA@prodigy.net*
Web site: *http://www.aobta.org*

Shiatsu Therapy Association of Canada
517 College Street
Suite 232
Toronto, Ontario M6G 4A2
Canada
416-923-7826
Toll-free in Canada and US: 877-923-7826
E-mail: *nmg.vanderpoorten@sympatico.ca*
Web site: *www.shiatsuassociation.com*

Shiatsu Therapy Association of British Columbia
PO Box 37005
6495 Victoria Drive
Victoria, British Columbia V5P 4W7
604-433-9495
E-mail: *www.shiatsutherapy.bc.ca*
Web site: *www.shiatsuatherapy.bc.ca*

The Shiatsu Society (UK)
Eastlands Court
St Peters Road
Rugby, England CV21 3QP
United Kingdom
01788 555051
E-mail: *admin@shiatsu.org*
Web site: *www.shiatsu.org*

Shiatsu Therapy Association of Australia
PO Box 598
Belgrave, Victoria 3160
Australia
039752 6711
Web site: *www.yogaplace.com.au/shiatsu*

of attainment is the Certified Instructor. Certified Practitioners have completed 500 hours of study including 160 hours of Oriental bodywork theory, discipline, technique, and practice; 100 hours of traditional Chinese medical theory; 100 hours of Western anatomy and physiology; 70 hours of observed clinical practice; and 70 hours of "red flags" concerning when referral is necessary, plus training in business, legal, and ethical considerations.

When calling a practitioner, patients should ask about the practitioner's experience and schooling. At the same time, it should be remembered that every practitioner has a gift that is unique to him or her. Patients should understand that practitioners will speak in different ways about the body and patients' health. An experienced practitioner will be able to speak to the patient's condition and ability to heal after the first or second treatment.

Ultimately, biomedical practitioners will understand Oriental bodywork better by experiencing it themselves. In my own practice, the physicians who have experienced my work are most proficient at referring patients who will benefit. Furthermore, those who experience Oriental bodywork will find that it helps their own practices of medicine by showing the power of hands-on care—its ability to improve sensitivity of palpatory skills, and its ability to facilitate the body's healing.

WHEN TO REFER

The great thing about bodywork is that patients do not need to be sick or injured to benefit from treatment; this modality can be beneficial or transformative when health is at its worst, and it can help maintain optimal function when health is at its best.

Oriental bodywork therapy can address health problems in each part of the life cycle. It can benefit people who have significant degenerative malfunctions, contagious diseases, or serious breakdown in the organs. When the body's ability to heal is permanently compromised, these therapies may still be used to assist and comfort. Those who are generally healthy but feel "not quite right"—sluggish, lacking appetite, tiring easily, poor facial color, frequent upset stomach or intestines—quickly benefit from Oriental bodywork treatment. For people who would like to better learn to promote their general health, these modalities are superlative.

Acknowledgments

Special thanks to Bill Helm, Jan St. Germaine, Cindy Banker, Barbara Clark, and Joseph Price, whose conversation helped to shape this chapter.

References

1. Changnan S, editor: *Chinese bodywork: a complete manual of Chinese therapeutic massage* (translated by Wang Qiliang), Berkeley, Calif, 1993, Pacific View Press.
2. Chaitow L: *Cranial manipulation, theory and practice,* London, 1999, Churchill-Livingstone.
3. Smith F: *Inner bridges: a guide to energy movement and body structure,* Atlanta, 1986, Humanics New Age.

Suggested Readings

Gach MR: *Acupressure's potent points: a guide to self-care for common ailments,* New York, 1990, Bantam Books.

Lee HM, Whincup G, translators: *Chinese Massage therapy: a handbook of therapeutic massage,* Boulder, Colo, 1983, Shambala Publications.

Masunaga S: *Zen shiatsu: how to harmonize yin and yang for better health,* New York, 1977, Japan Publications.

Mochizuki JS: *Anma, the art of Japanese massage,* St. Paul, Minn, 1995, Kotobuki Publications.

Serizawa K: *Tsubo: vital points for Oriental therapy,* New York, 1976, Japan Publications.

Sohn T: Amma: *The ancient art of Oriental healing,* Rochester, Vt, 1988, Healing Arts Press.

Teeguarden IM: *Acupressure way of health: jin shin do,* New York, 1978, Japan Publications.

Yang J-m: *Chinese qigong massage: general massage,* Jamaica Plain, Mass, 1992, YMAA Publication Center.

SECTION 3: MOVING MEDITATION

JEAN EDELEN

Qi gong (pronounced "chee gung") is the fifth major modality within Chinese medicine and may be the most comprehensive of all. Qi gong means the cultivation of Qi, the life force or human bioelectrical field. It has been called "acupuncture without needles" because, using only movement or meditation, it can open the energy gates and keep the Qi flowing smoothly, as well as balance the body as a whole. It is a broad term that encompasses virtually all of the Chinese movement arts. Most exercise systems that are slow or still and that focus on breathing are called Qi gong in China.[1]

Qi gong is the core of all self-care in the Chinese health care system.[1] The concept of self-care and health maintenance goes back many centuries in China. About 4000 years ago, the people of China were known to have danced to rid themselves of damp and arthritis. "Dancing made them hot, and the heat expelled the damp and poison from their veins and joints," remarks Michael Tse, in his book, *Qi gong for Health and Vitality*.[2] During the Three Kingdoms Period (280-220 BCE), a famous Chinese physician, Hwa Tou, created "Five Animal Play." He observed the movements of wild animals, noting how they maintained their balance. Thinking that people had lost this natural ability, he designed "Five Animal Play" to help them relearn this skill and strengthen their bodies. Adds Tse, "Hwa Tou explained that when you raised

your arms above your head, as if they were the horns of a deer, it stimulated the Qi circulation of the liver; when you stretched your arms out like a bird spreading its wings, it was good for the heart and relieving tension; rubbing and slapping yourself and moving like a monkey was good for the spleen . . . and bending forward like the bear was good for the back and kidneys."[2] Others also observed the natural movements and breathing of animals and used them as models for human exercise. These traditions came to be known as Qi gong and continued to be followed for hundreds of years. During the Cultural Revolution, most of China's traditional culture, including Qi gong, was prohibited. When the Cultural Revolution ended, people again began to practice Qi gong freely. Since then, enthusiasm for Qi gong has grown and it is again widely practiced.[2]

Indeed, self-care and health maintenance have long been central to Chinese medicine. "In China, illness is regarded as natural, a normal part of life, like a rainy day," states Mengda Shu, OMD. "Self-care is very important. Some people in America ignore illness, think it is terrible, think of it as the enemy. The Chinese believe that illness exercises the immune system. It makes you stronger."[3] After the Cultural Revolution, China experienced a severe shortage of biomedical personnel. Half had been killed, fled the country, or gone underground, while the general population doubled. In response, the government mandated a national program of Taijiquan, which incorporated many Qi gong principles. Before admittance to a hospital, nonemergency patients were required to first practice Taijiquan or Qi gong for 3 months. "The system worked," explains B. K. Frantzis. "Tai Chi and Chi Gung managed to keep health matters as stable as they could be kept given the poor sanitation and starvation diet most lived with. For the Chinese to get through this incredibly rough period, from the mid-1950s on, it is estimated that between 100 and 200 million people practiced Tai Chi or Chi Gung daily."[4]

There are literally hundreds of forms and traditions of Qi gong. Over the years old forms have evolved and new ones have been developed. Not all lineages of Qi gong are strictly concerned with physical health; many expand into systems of mental and spiritual development. Martial arts Qi gong develops the "warrior," using the Qi to enhance the practitioner's strength and endurance. Confucian Qi gong aims at self-cultivation, personal refinement, and ethical development. Some forms, such as the well-known Taijiquan (Tai Chi Chuan), are hybrids of the martial arts and healing traditions. Nor do all forms of Qi gong involve movement. Some forms, known as Jing Gong, or passive Qi gong, are done while lying or sitting very still. These use only breath, intention, and visualization to cultivate and enhance the Qi. Indeed, all forms of Qi gong have breath and intention in common, with the cultivation of the Qi as the primary focus. It could be argued that Qi gong is a form of meditation, whether a moving meditation, such as the familiar Taijiquan, or a still, strictly internal one. In his book, *The Most Profound Medicine,* Roger Jahnke, OMD, describes the range of Qi gong practice[1]:

There are many systems and traditions of Qi gong ranging from simple calisthenic type movements with breath coordination to complex auto regulatory type exercises where brain wave frequency, heart rate and other organ functions are altered intentionally by the practitioner. In extremely advanced levels of practice the Qi gong practitioner can transmit Qi or energy across distances and through substances. There are cases where the practitioner can manipulate the limbs of a subject from a distance and diagnose physiological disturbances without conversation or palpation.

The principles underlying Qi gong are the same as those of acupuncture. In Chinese medicine, disease is viewed as a disharmony of the body's energy system. The function of both acupuncture and Qi gong is to clear the energy blockage, allow the Qi to flow freely, and thus to reestablish a state of harmony and balance. Qi gong relies on breath, intention, visualization, and, in many cases, movement, to accomplish these aims.

The movement forms of Qi gong consist of slow, gentle, flowing movements, designed to cultivate and gather the invisible energy of nature and bring it to various acupuncture points, or "energy gates," where it can be taken in by the body. It is then circulated throughout the body, where it flows through the energy channels and nourishes all the organs and tissues. To the novice, virtually all of the movement forms of Qi gong look like Taijiquan; the practitioner is usually standing, raising and lowering the arms slowly, and occasionally bending backward or moving the legs. Unlike the aerobic exercise popular in the West, this is a slow, quiet, focused, moving meditation. Instead of listening to loud music or being mentally detached, the Qi gong practitioner is fully involved mentally. He or she visualizes the Qi, using intention and imagination, with the goal of bringing it to the various body organs to nourish and strengthen them. (See Figures 6, 7, and 8 on pp. 197-198.)

Visualization is thus central to both the movement and meditative forms of Qi gong; indeed, the meditative forms of Qi gong rely solely on breath, intention, and visualization. Whether standing, sitting, lying down, or perfectly still, the Qi gong practitioner visualizes the gathering and circulating of the Qi and the nourishing of the tissues. Jahnke[1] remarks:

The Qi circulates in the energy channels by virtue of the breathing, the movement and the visualization of Qi gong. There is an intricate network of bio-electrical circuits (71 named channels) and an endless number of minor channels that administer the Qi to every organ, tissue and cell of the body.

TAIJIQUAN

Taijiquan is a martial art, developed from and based on Qi gong.[4] Both use slow, flowing movements that relate to acupuncture points and serve to strengthen the internal organs. Both involve relaxation, visualization, and controlled breathing. Both build health through the cultivation of Qi. The distinction between

Sources for Further Learning

Recommended Books

Jahnke R: *The healer within*, New York, 1997, Harper-Collins. Explores Qi gong exercises and meditation from a Western perspective, with an emphasis on self-care.

Frantzis BK: *Opening the energy gates of your body*, Berkeley, Calif, 1993, North Atlantic Books. A fairly comprehensive introduction to Qi gong movement exercises.

Liang S-Y, Wu W-C, Breiter-Wu D: *Qi gong empowerment: a guide to medical, Taoist, Buddhist, and wushu energy cultivation*, East Providence, RI, 1997, The Way of the Dragon Publishing. A developmental survey of varieties of Qi gong exercises.

Huang CA, Lynch J: *Thinking body, dancing mind*, New York, 1992, Bantam Books. A Taoist approach to sports and other aspects of life. This book will be of interest to students of Eastern culture, but does not include any Qi gong exercises.

Classes and Seminars

The Chinese Healing Arts Center offers classes in Qi gong and Taijiquan, as well as training in Qi healing.

Call 203-748-8107 in Danbury, Connecticut; 914-338-6045 in Kingston, New York; or 212-579-5916 in New York City, or E-mail qihealer@aol.com for more information. They also offer acupuncture and Qi healing at these sites.

Master Shawn Liu conducts seminars on Qi gong worldwide, offers classes in Qi gong and Taijiquan, and performs Qi healing. Check his Web site at www.shaolin-world.com; E-mail at shawnliu@bellsouth.com, or call 334-343-6023.

The USA Wushu-Kung Fu Federation in Baltimore, Maryland, can also help prospective students find Qi gong or Taijiquan classes anywhere in the world. Call 410-444-6666, E-mail at usawkf@usawfk.com, or log onto www.usawkf.org.

B. K. Frantzis offers a variety of classes in North America and Europe, including 1 to 2 week retreats. He can be reached at 415-454-5243.

Roger Jahnke teaches throughout the United States; he can be reached at 805-682-3230. ∾

Qi gong and Taijiquan is a subtle one. Stuart Kenter, in his foreword to B. K. Frantzis' book, *Opening the Energy Gates of Your Body*, explains[4]:

Tai Chi . . . is an ancient Chinese system of movements based upon the development of the chi (life force) within the body. Cultivated chi can be used to rejuvenate the body, heal illness and injuries, maintain health, and enhance spiritual capacities. Tai Chi may also be used as a highly effective system of self-defense. . . . Chi gung . . . is the art and practice of internal energy development.

Taijiquan movements include some Qi gong; Qi gong is an integral part of Taijiquan. "Tai Chi Chuan without Chi Kung is no longer Tai Chi Chuan; it becomes a form of gentle exercise that may provide some benefits in terms of blood circulation and recreation but is unlikely to give the type of vitality and mental freshness commonly ascribed to Tai Chi Chuan training."[5]

Indeed, it is Qi gong that gives the Chinese martial arts their incredible strength and power. Through the cultivation and development of the Qi, Qi gong creates an inner strength, an internal power, that can neutralize an opponent's force and protect the practitioner against attack. Frantzis,[4] Qi gong master and teacher, states:

Chi Gung is the basis of the power of the Chinese martial arts, whether Kung Fu, or the more subtle internal forms, such as Tai Chi, Hsing I, and Ba Gua. It is almost impossible to determine from an external view how the seemingly gentle, smooth movements of the internal forms enable the advanced practitioner to defeat the most violent street fighter. This capability is basically derived from the practice of Chi Gung, which develops chi and internal power.

Jahnke agrees, "It is Qi gong in the martial arts that supplies the abundance of Qi that makes the practitioner seem to fly, absorb tremendous blows, and knock down opponents with what look like minor punches."[1] Without Qi gong, Taijiquan would be merely an engaging and graceful dance, without the power or strength needed for combat.

EXTERNAL QI GONG

External Qi gong, also known as "medical Qi gong" or "Qi healing," is the most challenging to Western notions of reality. Unlike the internal self-care forms of Qi gong, where the individual plays an active role in health maintenance, in external Qi gong an active practitioner treats a quiescent patient. The practitioner of external Qi gong does not measure pulses, observe the patient's tongue, or palpate reflexes. He seldom asks many questions. Instead, he or she relies on concentration, intuition, and his or her ability to "read" the patient's Qi, often through an off-the-body scanning technique, to find the energy blockages and enable the energy to flow freely again. Master X. (Shawn) Liu,[6] a Qi gong master and martial arts instructor, who also practices external Qi gong, says:

People have lots of blockages. The cells stick together and there aren't many white cells. These people are toxic; they will become malignant. I try to get the Qi circulating, to let the Qi flow and rechannel the blockage. You need to clean yourself, to give yourself oxygen, good nutrients, clean up the debris, and produce more white cells. Cells die every day; you need to clean up the debris.

Liu's patients may be seated or lying down. He tells them to relax and open their minds. Standing next to them and using his hands, he feels for an increase in body temperature and watches for a muscular response, such as a twitch, as the channels open up. "Sometimes they jump a little," Liu states. "Their skin may change color. The atmosphere is different. Blood circulation improves." Liu describes the external Qi gong practitioner as a satellite, which receives Qi and transmits Qi. "It depends on the Qi you're born with," he says. "Some people can project Qi; others can't." Communication also is important. Each patient has a code, similar to a computer password. "You have to break the code," Liu explains. "If the patient doesn't want to open up to you, it is much, much harder."[6]

Another Qi gong master and Qi healer, T. K. Shih, OMD, who founded the Chinese Healing Arts Center in Kingston, New York, teaches his students how to diagnose and correct energy blockages. Asked to describe how Qi healers do this, he explained, "We can see where there's a bad yin/yang balance, where the energy is too strong." He does not need to touch his patients, he says, because he "can feel the body's energy. You can't see it,

but we can feel it . . . Everybody has an aura. We can see it. From the aura we can see whether the body is healthy or unhealthy. We can see each organ's aura." When asked how, once diagnosed, the blockage is removed, he replied, "We just think about it."[7] (See p. 119.)

SAFETY

Most Qi gong is safe to practice, even for novices. However, some types of Qi gong are for specific health problems; others are more general. B. K. Frantzis notes that there are also a few extreme forms and advises against them, such as sexual Qi gong exercises and "Qi packing" techniques. He recommends weekly supervision with a competent and well-qualified instructor. But, he adds, "Most Chi gung systems are actually quite safe. Don't be afraid to practice Chi gung simply because some techniques may be dangerous."[4] Mengda Shu, OMD and Taijiquan instructor, prefers Taijiquan practice to Qi gong for many people. Some patients, because of age or temperament, do not have the patience to learn Qi gong, in her opinion. "Tai Chi is safer," she offers, "because it emphasizes body movement."[3] T. K. Shih, when asked about the safety of Qi gong and Taijiquan, replied, "You must choose the right Qi gong," but added, "correctly done, Tai Chi is OK for everyone."[7]

WHO CAN BENEFIT

Because Qi gong affects all body organs and tissues, it can treat a broad array of medical conditions. Certainly, all of the conditions generally ameliorated by acupuncture are good candidates for Qi gong. Qi gong or Taijiquan should be considered in the following cases:
- Those who might be helped by acupuncture, but who fear or dislike needles.[8]
- Patients with chronic pain, particularly when biomedicine offers little hope or when complex interventions are out of reach because of financial resources.
- Patients with acquired immunodeficiency syndrome (AIDS)/human immunodeficiency virus (HIV) who are not too sick to embark on a program of gentle movement or meditation. Indeed, any patient for whom biomedicine offers little or no hope.

- Patients restricted to wheelchairs or bed rest or those who are paralyzed (sitting or lying down or meditative Qi gong).
- Anyone who enjoys or could benefit from movement. The slow, gentle movements of Qi gong and Taijiquan are wonderful for seniors or for younger individuals for whom aerobic exercise would be too strenuous. Those who enjoy dance may also find the flowing movements appealing, particularly when set to music.
- Patients who prefer to play an active role in their health and healing.
- Virtually anyone who is receptive to new ideas and ready for lifestyle changes.[8]

Although the simpler Qi gong exercises are easily learned, many Qi gong instructors teach lengthy sequences of movements, which requires learning the name and location of many acupuncture points. This style of Qi gong requires a commitment of time and energy to learn and practice. Indeed, it takes time to learn either Taijiquan or Qi gong, whether a moving form or a strictly meditative one. Patients anxious for immediate improvement would be more inclined toward acupuncture, or acupuncture supplemented by a few simple Qi gong exercises. Some Westerners lack the confidence to "feel the Qi"; others find the culture

gap overwhelming, particularly as taught by Chinese instructors. Furthermore, Qi gong instructors and external Qi gong practitioners cannot be found in all geographical areas; in contrast, acupuncturists and Taijiquan classes are much easier to find.

Moving meditation is a safe and effective modality that offers tremendous healing potential for those patients open to a new paradigm. As Qi gong and Taijiquan become better known and more widely accepted, more patients, particularly those for whom biomedicine offers little promise, are likely to seek their benefits.

References

1. Jahnke R: *The most profound medicine,* Santa Barbara, Calif, 1991, Health Action Publishing.
2. Tse M: *Qi gong for health and vitality,* New York, 1995, St. Martin's Griffin.
3. Shu M: Telephone interview, April 3, 1998.
4. Frantzis BK: *Opening the energy gates of your body,* Berkeley, Calif, 1993, North Atlantic Books.
5. Kit WK: *The complete book of tai chi chuan: a comprehensive guide to the principles and practice,* Rockport, Ill, 1999, Element Books.
6. Liu X: Telephone interview, May 15, 1998.
7. Shih TK: Telephone interview, June 15, 1998.
8. Porvaznik M: Telephone interview, February 2, 1998.

II

DELIVERING CARE

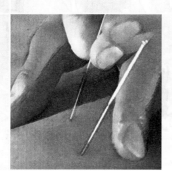

How does an Oriental medicine (OM) practitioner make patient care decisions? What kind of environment does he or she create to support the healing effort? Having examined the theory of OM and its major diagnostic and interventive techniques in the previous chapters, in Part II we consider how practitioners weave such information together into a deliverable whole.

Chapter 7 explores philosophical issues underlying OM care delivery in the West. Because in our setting delivery must take place in a cultural and historical environment different from that within which OM arose, the delivery task demands that the practitioner be unusually sensitive to expectation—his or her own and that of patients. The existence of this cultural and metaparadigmatic gap can also be clarified by offering some comparisons between the delivery assumptions that guide biomedicine and those that guide OM. To examine these issues, Dan Kenner draws on the literature

121

of medical anthropology and philosophy, as well as his own experience as practitioner and as designer of delivery systems for OM practitioners.

Chapter 8, "Grand Rounds," presents five case histories (all patient names have been changed). The first consists of the complete text of an editorial from an American medical journal, dated 1822, that describes "acupuncturation" and provides examples of successful musculoskeletal care. The second case history, by Carol Kari, concerns a subject not discussed elsewhere in the text, the care of skin and circulatory malfunctions. In this case a patient with chronic resistant ulcerations of the ankle responded to acupuncture care. As a result she was able to undergo reparative surgery to her toes. This is an example of Oriental medical care making it possible for the patient to benefit from biomedical care. Comparative costs of the patient's medical care are also reported.

The third case history, by Susan Cushing, deals with a common problem, chronic headaches. The case is particularly interesting because, although initially acupuncture and moxibustion reduced headaches, the client wanted to be free of them. The writer describes how she reconsidered her original diagnosis and initiated a second treatment plan. This involved team care—the acupuncturist, patient, and a massage therapist worked simultaneously to identify and address etiology—and after 20 years of frequent headaches the patient became, and remains, pain-free.

Lonny Jarrett, author of the fourth case history, emphasizes the "inner" tradition of Chinese medicine and has selected a case to illustrate a constitutional and psychospiritual approach to care. The author shares each step of his diagnostic process, helping the reader to develop deeper feeling for issues earlier discussed in Chapters 3 and 7. Chapter 8 ends with a report, from Haiyang Li, of treating stroke blindness with acupuncture. This case is included because, even though it is incomplete in the sense that a crucial test that might have shown if the acupuncture physically changed the status of the central nervous system lesion was not done, the patient reported marked functional improvement. This case history provides an example of a common situation encountered by medical doctors and acupuncturists—that of incomplete data. It also illustrates a little understood facet of acupuncture care—patients often experience functional improvement or "cure" even while "objective" tests show little change.

Chapter 9, drawing on the anthropological research of Martha Hare, describes the ideas and ideals behind the design of detoxification acupuncture clinics, group settings in which struggling individuals often find a second "home" and are empowered to give up drugs.

Finally, in Chapter 10, four acupuncturists and one publisher of Chinese medicine texts write autobiographical pieces. The resulting works describe typical days of work (Jane Grissmer, Jumbé Allen); the adventures involved in becoming both acupuncturist and teacher in China and the United States (Jingyun Gao); the struggle to integrate biomedicine and acupuncture especially in a hospital setting (Paulette Hill); and the long road to finding satisfaction through translating and publishing Chinese classics (Robert Felt).

Chapter 10 is followed by a Photo Essay that serves the whole book. ❧

Supplemental Readings

Case Histories

MacPherson H, KaptchukT, eds: *Acupuncture in practice: case history insights from the West,* New York, 1997, Churchill Livingstone.

History and Anthropology of Asian Medicine

Eckman P: *In the footsteps of the Yellow Emperor: tracing the history of traditional acupuncture,* San Francisco, 1996, Cypress Books.

Farquhar J: *Knowing practice: the clinical encounter of Chinese medicine,* Boulder, Colo, 1994, Westview Press.

Leslie C: *Asian medical systems: a comparative study,* Berkeley, Calif, 1976, University of California Press.

Leslie C, Young A, editors: *Paths to Asian medical knowledge,* Berkeley, Calif, 1992, University of California Press.

Lock MM: *East Asian medicine in urban Japan,* Berkeley, Calif, 1980, University of California Press.

Kleinman A: *Patients and healers in the context of culture: an exploration of the borderland between anthropology, medicine, and psychiatry,* Berkeley, Calif, 1980, University of California Press.

Kleinman A, Kunstadter P, Alexander ER, Gale JL, editors: *Medicine in Chinese cultures: comparative studies of health care in Chinese and other societies,* DHEW publication no. NIH 75-653, Washington, DC, John E. Fogarty International Center for Advanced Study in the Health Sciences, National Institutes of Health, 1975.

Porkert M: *The theoretical foundations of Chinese medicine,* Cambridge, Mass, 1974, Harvard University Press.

Unschuld P: *Medicine in China: a history of ideas,* Berkeley, Calif, 1985, University of California Press.

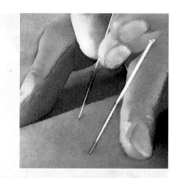

Putting It All Together
Practicing Oriental Medicine

DAN KENNER

Previous chapters in this book have examined characteristics of Oriental medicine (OM) that make it unique and distinguishable from other medical systems. This chapter serves as a bridge between the descriptive and theoretical material that has preceded it, and the task of actually delivering Oriental medical (OM) care, examined in this part.

In observing the delivery of OM, particularly in a large clinic or hospital setting, initially it might seem little different from the conventional biomedical approach apart from the use of needles, moxa, cupping, massage, or herbs to achieve change in symptomatology. For example, the questions asked and the issues covered during the clinical interview and patient examination are quite similar. However, a closer look reveals important differences. Some of these are apparent in the design of the physical delivery environment,

some in the details sought during interviews, and yet others in the underlying intentionality of the encounter. Beginning with a description of the characteristics of contact between patient and practitioner, this chapter examines a series of crucial, although often hidden and subtle, differences between the delivery characteristics of OM and those of biomedicine in Western nations.

THE MEDICAL ENCOUNTER: THE OFFICE VISIT

The patient who arrives at the office of an Oriental medical practitioner in private practice in North America or Europe might be greeted by a receptionist, but it is not unlikely that he or she would be greeted directly by the practitioner. It is possible that the office would have the feel of a conventional biomedical office with a glass enclosure for office personnel and a waiting room with rows of chairs and scattered magazines, but it is more likely that the waiting area gives the patient the feeling of being in someone's home. Soft lighting, soft music, artwork with an Oriental theme, furniture that invites lounging, and a display of plants and flowers are typical (see Photo Essay after Chapter 10). Patients, practitioners, and office personnel (if any) mingle and talk freely and there is laughter, although the environment nevertheless stays rather quiet and often contemplative.

At the beginning of the treatment session, even a return visit, the practitioner typically spends 15 to 30 minutes listening to the patient's story and discussing the patient's condition and needs. The discussion ranges from formal and direct questions about the patient's physiological functioning to informal discussion about work responsibilities, family, and the stress load of the patient. Time spent in this manner helps the practitioner create rapport, puts the patient at ease, and serves as the initial step in treatment. Through listening, the practitioner also develops a treatment strategy for the visit. Even if a long-term treatment plan already exists, each visit will introduce variations.

After the initial discussion, the patient lies on the treatment table, sometimes clothed and sometimes partly unclothed (but with flannel or paper sheet wrapped around himself or herself). Most acupuncturists use comfortable padded massage tables, and here the practitioner performs the physical examination. During this examination the practitioner often continues the discussion from the first part of the visit and may ask further questions or request clarifications based on the physical findings. Physical examination usually consists of visual examination of the face, the tongue, and the general skin tone, palpation of the pulse, palpation of the abdomen and potential treatment points on the arms and legs (see Chapter 3). Sometimes points are located on the limbs or ear with a rheostat point finder.

Treatment follows directly after physical examination. If the practitioner has decided to use acupuncture, needles are inserted using clean needle technique. Sometimes needles are removed immediately and sometimes they are left in place. Sometimes the original needle stimulus is augmented with heat from moxa or electrical stimulation ("electrostim"). Sometimes points are not needled but are heated with moxa alone, or sometimes with a special heat lamp called a TDP lamp. When needles are left in place, the practitioner checks frequently to ensure that the patient is comfortable, and to monitor the progress of the treatment by rechecking the pulse or function in areas related to the patient's complaint.

As an example, suppose a patient reports irregular menses. The practitioner uses interrogation, observation, and palpation to arrive at a diagnosis. If the time of menstrual flow is shortened with a scant flow, there is breast or subcostal pain, as well as nightsweats and irritability, the pulse is "wiry" (also called "bowstring"), and the tongue shows a thin yellow fur, then the practitioner would most likely diagnose a Pattern called Liver Congestion (Liver Qi Stagnation). The treatment might include use of an herbal formula such as "Powder of Leisure" (also called "Free Wanderer" and "Tang Kuei and Bupleurum Formula") or one of its variations. For acupuncture, points of the Liver or Gall Bladder Channel or points related to Liver function would be needled (e.g., Liver 2, Liver 3, Liver 14, or Gall Bladder 41). At subsequent visits the practitioner would question the patient about changes in her menstrual pattern or other health changes, would repeat the physical examination, and would adjust both diagnosis and treatment according to the ongoing findings.

Patient visits typically last from 45 minutes to 1 hour. Those who receive acupuncture with or without moxibustion often become quite relaxed and may fall asleep. At the end of the treatment, the practitioner withdraws the needles and disposes of them in a sharps container. The patient rouses, often being told to "take your time, do not hurry." The patient and the practitioner may discuss the immediate effects of the treatment. The practitioner makes comments about the patient's condition, the prognosis, and the progress thus far and may offer recommendations about steps to take in daily life to enhance (in this case) her menstrual health and health in general.

The patient is now nearly ready to leave. Quite often the patient writes a check and hands it directly to the practitioner, who enters the fee in the record book, makes the next appointment, and often also delivers any herb formulas the patient may need, along with instructions for use. In other cases, the practitioner directs the patient to a pharmacy that can make up Chinese herbal formulas. In a minority of cases, insurance billing is done. In larger offices a receptionist receives the payment and schedules follow-up appointments.

The tone of the visit is intentionally relaxed and low-key with ample time allowed to address the patient's concerns. Patients often perceive the practitioner as a friend or confidant, who, in turn, may share his or her own life experiences and information about family and personal background with the patient.

Although the occasional biomedical office, particularly in rural areas, may deliver patient care somewhat as described, the current urban norm contrasts significantly. The biomedical setting bustles with personnel—medical doctors, nurses, nutritionists, bookkeepers, receptionists, and records personnel—and quite often delivery personnel or others cleaning or moving equipment. The tone is one of urgency to stay on schedule and not to use the physician's time unnecessarily. The examination may be performed by the physician the patient came to see, but parts or all may equally be done by a nurse or physician's assistant, and the treatment itself may be relegated to yet other providers. The examination may further be distributed among personnel by deferring diagnosis pending the results of a laboratory examination of blood or urine with both collection and examination

being done by personnel other than the physician. The treatment is rarely hands-on; more commonly it is divorced from the health care setting by consisting of a prescription to be picked up on departure or ordered at a later time after laboratory test results. The patient makes a follow-up appointment and pays (or initiates payment by third-party payers) with personnel other than the physician. Currently total contact time with the physician averages less than 10 minutes in the United States[1]; rarely do patients think of their physicians as "friends," nor does the setting encourage this image of the practitioner. This delivery context is anonymous, busy, and technological, with industrial overtones both in the manner of personal care and the bureaucratic realm of third-party payment.

These differences in tone and timing of the office visit between biomedicine and OM (as delivered in the Western world) represent predictable expressions of differences in medical discourse and valuing, a point developed later in this chapter. At the moment it suffices to state that the typical Western practitioner of OM fulfills a different role from the biomedical practitioner by offering a high-relational medical experience. This is an experience that many patients enjoy (see Chapter 12) and relate to images of the old-fashioned "country doctor" who knows the patient and the patient's family, has a personal relationship with them, and understands their suffering. This "good doctor" offers personal counsel, advises about self-care, and provides nontoxic treatments.

The differences between the two care delivery styles reflect the differing histories and goals of the two medical systems and should not be interpreted simplistically as issues of "quality." The high-relational or "patient-centered" elements of alternative medicine practice do not so much usurp the biomedical practitioner's role as fill a humanistic and even metaphysical void left in the wake of technological development. That both options are available to patients is to everyone's advantage: the harmonious coexistence of the technological and humanistic can greatly benefit a society with complex health care needs. Indeed, there is considerable demand from American consumers for the chance to participate with the clinician in their own treatment strategy. A 1989 survey conducted at Harvard University identified 39% of medical consumers in the United States as "activist" health care consumers,[2] while a survey of American users of Chinese medicine showed that a major component of satisfaction was their sense that they were "partners" in guiding the medical encounter.[3,4]

Facilitative Relationships Preferred by Oriental Medicine Patients

In a large-scale (N = 575) survey of patient attitudes toward acupuncture and their OM practitioners, respondents reported high satisfaction with their practitioners and described their relationship to their practitioners in warmly relational terms.[3,4] For example, on a 5-point scale, 69.3% claimed to be "extremely" satisfied with their OM practitioner, and 21.9% stated that they were "very" satisfied. The comparative values for their biomedical practitioners were 15.3% and 28.5%, respectively. Requested to select one among nine vertical (authoritarian) or horizontal (facilitative) words to describe their sense of relationship to their OM practitioner, two thirds selected facilitative terms. The most popular horizontal term was "partner"; the second most popular term was "friend." Of the vertical terms, only "doctor" was selected with any frequency, and this only at sites where the practitioner used the title Doctor. ❧

THE MEDICAL ENCOUNTER: EXAMINING THE PATIENT

In both types of medicine, the format of the medical examination is similar and consists of the chief complaint, present illness, past history, family history, social history, systems review, physical examination, other investigations, diagnosis, and treatment plan.[5] However, there are differences in what is communicated between patient and practitioner in the two types of encounter (Table 7-1). As discussed in the last section of this chapter, many of these differences are the result of ideological or paradigmatic differences.

The first task of the medical encounter, to elicit the chief complaint, is as much a developed skill in OM as it is in biomedicine. In both cases, interrogation is biased to steer the dialogue to those details that most closely match diagnostic categories defined by the system and used by the practitioner. Thus, because the OM practitioner is looking for a Pattern instead of a disease, he or she does not emphasize the chief complaint as a stand-alone disease or condition, but fits it inside, and sees it as a component of, the second task, understanding the present illness. In recognizing a Pattern that leads to a diagnosis, the chief complaint may *not* be of central importance to the treatment strategy.

Taking the patient's medical, personal, and social history differs little between the two systems. The OM practitioner is interested in major illnesses, hospitalizations, surgery, prescription drugs used, and allergies and drug sensitivities, just as is the biomedical practitioner. However, the OM practitioner is more likely to seek information on sometimes minute details of lifestyle, diet, herbs and supplements used, type of exercise, quality of sleep, and cravings and preferences for food, drink, sex, and so forth.

The systems review is also painstaking. Like the biomedical physician, the OM practitioner is interested in the minutiae of urinary habits, bowel habits, how easily colds develop into respiratory infections, and other habitual pathological tendencies. Acupuncturists, especially, are interested in details of subjective pain sensations that patients are sometimes at a loss to describe, requiring the practitioner to prompt them with descriptions (e.g., "Is the pain aching, dull, heavy, burning, sharp, throbbing . . . ?").

TABLE 7-1

Medical Interview Emphases in Biomedicine Versus Oriental Medicine

Clinical encounter component	Biomedicine	Oriental medicine
Chief complaint and present illness	Central role in diagnosis; story-telling discouraged	Not always central to diagnosis; long stories tolerated or encouraged
Past history	Important, major medical events emphasized	Important, personal history and personal habits emphasized
Family history	History of diseases, causes of death in immediate family	History of relationships as important as history of diseases
Social history	Demographic data emphasized	Lifestyle issues, occupational hazards, past abuses emphasized
Systems review	Less detailed with experienced practitioner	More detailed with experienced practitioner, often lengthy
Physical examination	Seeks gross pathology compared with OM practitioner	Main source of data for diagnostic decisions
Other investigations	Considerable reliance on laboratory and other out-of-office tests	Little reliance on such data
Diagnosis	Seeking to name a disease	Naming a functional nosological unit that may vary as life moves
Plan	Pharmaceuticals, surgery, rest, exercise, counseling	Acupuncture, herbs, lifestyle suggestions on exercise, diet, meditation, relationship factors

Variations in the physical examination depend greatly on the background and training of the practitioner. The most common techniques include palpation of the cervical nodes (swelling), the abdomen (areas of tenderness, rigidity, temperature variations), the acupuncture Channels (sensitivity), and muscular and connective tissue (sensitivity, rigidity, atrophy), palpation of the pulse, and examination of the tongue (see Chapter 3). In most schools of thought in Oriental medicine, pulse and tongue signs are considered cardinal signs that are decisive in focusing the information from the patient interview into a diagnosis. Neither auscultation with a stethoscope nor percussion is common.

Other investigations are used considerably less extensively than in biomedicine. The historical context for this is Oriental medical theory: malfunctions of the Interior are expressed on the Exterior, thus the practitioner must develop skills in observation rather than a technology to "see within." A skilled practitioner is indeed very observant, and one of the pleasures of experience is in continuously developing finer clinical insight. Nevertheless, biomedical technological skills are increasingly being grafted into the practice of OM. Courses in using laboratory tests and diagnostic imaging are becoming part of the core curricula in OM schools. Continuing education programs in states where they are required usually have seminars in medical technology available. In California, licensed acupuncturists can qualify to become managing physicians in the state workers' compensation system, which requires considerable additional training in medical imaging, biomedical physical examination skills, and industrial injury evaluation.

Reaching a diagnosis in any system of medical thought is a cognitive process that requires sifting through data, assessing relevance and weight, and selecting what to include and exclude. The diagnostic categories of OM place strong emphasis on symptoms (i.e., the subjective experience of the patient). However, the evaluation of signs, based on the physical examination, is the OM practitioner's most important skill. To take the time to learn to make a sensitive and skillful physical examination is one of the most difficult and demanding hurdles of clinical practice. Development of these skills ultimately helps the clinician individualize patient care and observe changes during the course of treatment to make realistic prognoses.

The diagnosis, of course, is a function or subset of the system that the practitioner uses.[6] Disease names are not always helpful in reaching a diagnosis that determines a course of action for the clinician. Diagnostic methods and systems of phytotherapy and acupuncture offer divergent streams of thought. So-called traditional Chinese medicine (TCM) is historically the largest-scale organized attempt to create a unified system of acupuncture and phytotherapy. To do so, it espoused a concept of point specificity that endowed body points with characteristics that were traditionally associated with substances in the traditional pharmacopoeia. This system also created clinical algorithms for treatment of certain disease conditions, an approach to treatment that increases the rapidity of delivery but also creates rigidities and is thus sometimes derided as "cookbook acupuncture." Other styles of practice follow similar diagnostic methods, but emphasize the individuality of the patient and the complex layering of many, especially chronic, diseases. However, a *common* goal of Oriental diagnosis is to identify the "root" and focus care there rather than on the "branch" or "manifestation," that is, to treat the cause rather than the symptom.

The treatment plan is based on the practitioner's views on a wide variety of issues. In general, either acupuncture or phytotherapy will have ascendant importance. Acupuncture in general is associated with Qi problems, and phytotherapy and diet therapy are indicated for Xue (Blood) problems. Qi problems generically are functional problems in which pathological lesions have not developed. For example, Oriental medical diagnosis may find the Liver to be functionally impaired even though liver enzyme levels, as measured in a biomedical laboratory, are normal. Qi problems are also those that are related to stress and nervous system irritability (sympathicotonia, vagotonia). Blood problems are problems in which there are actual pathological lesions, tissue abnormalities, parenchymatous changes in organs, or blood circulation abnormalities.

Finally, the practitioner must make a decision as to which of the various Oriental medical modalities to use in treating the patient. For use outside the office, practitioners may try to enhance their treatments by encouraging patients to take up Qi gong or tai chi, and they may counsel them on diet and make lifestyle recommendations. Inside the office, they may offer some form of bodywork therapy, either as a substitute for needles or in addition to needles. Most often, practitioners offer phytotherapy or acupuncture care (hand needling, electrostimulation of needles, moxibustion, and other techniques).

Both phytotherapy and acupuncture are practiced in several forms, as noted elsewhere in this text (see Chapters 2, 4, and 5). A competent acupuncturist can use any of the forms, although most prefer or emphasize only some. Five main forms of acupuncture and their uses include the following[7]:

- Relief of acute and chronic pain (this usually requires the use of only a few needles, plus skilled manipulation; electroacupuncture is commonly used).
- Physical therapy to relax hypertonic conditions of muscle and connective tissue by releasing tension at trigger points and motor points. (This requires anatomical knowledge of muscle origins, insertions, and their dermatomes or cranial nerve innervations. Treatment of the tendinomuscular Meridians of classic acupuncture tradition belong to this category; needles are often used locally or at the site of the dysfunction.)
- Meridian acupuncture, a type of "polarity therapy" based on using the system of Channels and collaterals of classical acupuncture as a master physiological regulation apparatus, with the aim of restoring normal self-regulation to the whole system, especially the autonomic nervous system. (Treatment points are often physically remote from the area of the main complaint.)
- "Holographic" acupuncture, based on the idea that certain body structures are "fractals" that contain topographic representations of the entire body (e.g., ear acupuncture; points in the ear are used symptomatically, and may be provided with stay-in needles to maintain stimulation away from the acupuncturist's office).
- "Scalp" acupuncture, based on needling the scalp over brain functional areas to alleviate paralysis or other malfunction in those areas. (Treatment lines overlie brain regions mapped by bioscience; used increasingly in patients after strokes.)

As described in Chapter 4, traditional practitioners may want the patient to experience a strong sensation (*da qi*) but others, equally traditional, often use very fine needles (or spherical "seeds" and "beads" or magnets) to create stimulations that are not consciously detectable. Although it is not yet known exactly what happens when needles are inserted (see Chapter 11), practitioners and patients often speak of "changing the energy field" of the body or altering the skin currents.

Herbal prescription is a conspicuous part of practice for most acupuncturists, and as can be expected with a practice so ancient and widespread, phytotherapy theories are numerous (see Chapter 5). There is *Kampo* from Japan (originally from China during the *Han* Period) and several distinct Chinese schools of thought extant. However, at least in the United States, these have been largely overshadowed by the phytotherapeutic principles of TCM. As noted, the TCM approach often depends on algorithms, which emerge in phytotherapy in the form of prefabricated herbal formulas to be used for specific symptom-sign complexes. This is convenient both for the busy practitioner and for the patient, although the individualized prescription is lost in the process. Western research on phytotherapy is in its infancy, but the clinical effectiveness, accompanied by low side effects, of Oriental phytotherapy is widely attested.[8]

Although not everyone prefers the TCM approach, or uses it, adoption of the system by state bureaucracies in the United States has resulted in a standardized system used for curriculum design and testing for licensure (see Chapter 20), given the profession a common voice, and to a large extent done for the OM profession what the *Diagnosis and Statistical Manual of Mental Disorders III* classifications did for the psychiatric profession. It has established a set of principles for bureaucratic and legal consumption, and provided a common language for the profession.

PARADIGMATIC DIFFERENCES

As shown, the OM clinical encounter is similar to that in biomedicine (and other medicines) in seeking to know as much as possible about the patient and his or her complaint. At the same time, they differ in essential focus, timing, and tone. OM (at least in the West) has been termed "patient-centered" and "relational," in contrast to the heavy technological bias of biomedicine. This section examines these observations at a deeper level by brief discussion of the contrasting values and reality models that fuel the two medicines.[9-13]

In current biomedical school curricula, academic training examining the theoretical structure of scientific and medical thought is seldom emphasized. Students are told that biomedicine is a "scientific medicine" (which is defined as a "good thing") yet receive little exposure to the issues, commonly discussed in medical anthropology, that could shed light on the systems of thought and logical structures that comprise the alternative practices available in the marketplace, including the values of science or their own medical system. This lack of teaching reflects the fact that conventional bioscience, and biomedicine, rarely are regarded as philosophical systems. Indeed, their cultural normalcy—their "truth power"—is so taken for granted that as late as the 1970s, even the field of medical anthropology tended to "test the validity" of the health care practices of other cultures by measuring them against a biomedical standard.[14] Nevertheless, "normal science" contains many propositions that are not universally shared. One is a belief that facts are "uncovered" by scientific method, and that science is (or can be) above ideology, objective, and neutral in values. From a paradigmatic point of view, however, *facts and other data are the products of the methods of investigation used.*

Underlying root assumptions and intrinsic biases can be grouped as *metaparadigms,* and the specialized assumptions of a particular profession or practice derived from the metaparadigm belong to the *paradigm* or explanatory model. The importance of assumptions that belong to a metaparadigm is that they are invisible to us. They are the conceptual water in which our mental activity swims. Conceptual features of the metaparadigm and their logic are defined as normal, obvious, and even as reality itself. Because of its unconscious influence, it is often difficult to perceive how one's own metaparadigm influences cognition. Reasoning derived from a different metaparadigm can also evoke suspicion or even derision caused by a disparity in different modes of cognition.

The metaparadigmatic underpinnings of biomedicine and OM are different, and these differences can help explain the differences in the delivery characteristics described previously, as well as others to be discussed in the following text (Table 7-2). Specifically, biomedicine proceeds from the assumptions of the *reductionistic* metaparadigm, whereas OM is guided by the assumptions of the *relational* metaparadigm. Biomedicine belongs to the tradition of science that began 400 years ago. This bias focuses on analysis, objectivity, and delving into the microworld to develop understanding. This vision of the world has created the dazzling technology that pervades all aspects of modern life. The emphasis on dividing the world from

ever-narrower segments into intricate detail has created a great variety of specializations.

Adherents of the relational metaparadigm, in contrast, emphasize understanding the connections between disparate elements of a system. For this reason they are drawn to pre-Enlightenment philosophies (i.e., Chinese philosophy) and cognitive structures, or to cutting-edge science based on the belief that the next wave of scientific progress will result in a new synthesis of scientific specializations and the humanities. The emphasis is on the macroworld of whole systems and on the "postmodernist" idea that science can never be completely objective or value-free.

The bioscience and biomedical proposition that science is a method that can be neutral or objective—that is, free from assumption or metaparadigm—is one important idea characteristic of reductionism as applied to science and medicine. Another belief of this metaparadigm is expressed in the view that scientific method is progressively and incrementally discovering the secrets of nature, which, when fully realized, will give science the ultimate resolving power, intellectually and technologically, to all problems confronting humanity. There is a theological aspect to this sometimes conscious quest for the ultimate truth, commonly known as "scientific progress." Herbert Hensel, MD, comments, "I find it noteworthy that the belief in scientific method is strongest among those who use it second hand, and among these there is hardly anyone who accepts the belief more unquestioningly than people in the field of medicine."[15]

Treating this apotheosis of scientific progress as a pathway to ultimate power and knowledge elucidates a basic difference in how theories and hypotheses are perceived within the framework of an Oriental medical system. This *relational* system is much less likely to perceive differing cosmologies as competing, is not interested in ultimates such as "truth," and does not seek a "theory of everything."[16] There are often overlays of Taoist and Buddhist philosophy; in the medical field these traditional concepts have been source material for the development of *overlapping systems for clinical problem solving.*

Thus Yin and Yang, the Five Phases, the Eight Entities, and so forth are flexible conceptual tools that have been repermuted and recombined in innumerable ways by individual clinicians over generations and over a vast range of geographical area to adapt medical practice to varying climatic and cultural environments.

TABLE 7-2

Contrasting Assumptions That Guide Biomedicine and Oriental Medicine*

Item	Biomedical approach	Oriental medicine approach
Metaparadigm	Hierarchic, reductionistic, ontological	Egalitarian, holistic, individualized
Characteristic assumptions concerning science and "truth"	Scientific method can be objective, data can be value-neutral	Scientific method and data reflect the values of the cultural setting and historical periods that produced them
	Science is making incremental steps toward distinguishing "fact" from "falsehood"; science progresses and is the ultimate arbiter of Truth; heresies exist	Science seeks evidence, since all things are interrelated and complex; all contain some "truth" or utility; there is no heresy but differing perceptions and opinions
Effect of the "truth" issue on medical practice	Low diversity of practice; standardization sought	High diversity of practice accepted
Locus of power in the clinical encounter	Clinician	Patient
	Practitioner delegates diagnosis and treatment, has legal power to diagnose and to prescribe controlled drugs, uses technical terminology	Practitioner counsels patient on lifestyle, offers health care to support the body-person's own regenerative capacity
Locus of responsibility in the clinical encounter	Clinician	Patient
Intervention tonality	Active, forceful, heroic; "fix it"	Minimalist, cooperative, "regulate it," "bias toward recovery"
Image of the body	Machine analogies common; body breaks down, requires correction; treatment aimed at correction and repair	Nature analogies common, body self-regulating and self-correcting, treatment aimed at enhancing self-regulation
Malfunction	Specific disease entities, external malefic forces that must be conquered	Dynamic states of internal discord, internal imbalances to be harmonized

*The distinctions made in the table are for pedagogical purposes more intense than are found in daily life.

How such conceptual schemes have been used to design different theoretical constructs is like writing a "software" for the purpose of developing a system of correspondences to use for clinical practice. It is intended to be a tool for correlating data and phenomena, rather than a model of reality.

In short, for the East Asian practitioner, theoretical principles of practice are an instrument rather than the quest for an ultimate system of knowledge.[17] Contradictions in the vast OM literature are regarded as differences in interpretation and not the polemic of truth versus error. For this reason, the practice of OM is as diverse as the number of its practitioners. This is especially true in modern times among populations less subject to intellectual and social controls, such as Japan or the United States.

Another fundamental difference is the way in which symptoms and signs are organized. OM uses different nosologies from conventional medicine.[18] In conventional medicine patterns of symptoms and signs are reified into "diseases," specific entities with powers to "victimize" their hosts. This nosology is ontological and localized, described as a pathological lesion afflicting a specific anatomical structure or system. The idea is conveyed that a disease is an entity, with a specific name and characteristics, and in this sense disease is "external," an invader to be conquered. The more serious the illness, the greater necessity for force in "fighting" it.

In contrast, the nosology used in most of OM is functional and individualistic. Disorder is viewed as primarily "internal" in the sense of a physiological discord to be harmonized, and both practitioner and patient strive to reenact an elusive "balance" (homeostasis). As in the conventional nosology, here there are also nosological units with specific features, but in this case each nosological unit is a disorder of the *whole system*. Thus a "Spleen-Damp" condition could manifest as a gastric ulcer, Crohn's disease, epileptic seizures, or chronic joint disease, to name only a few possibilities. The history taking and physical examination would lead to evaluating this "symptom-sign complex," but the paradigm of evaluation uses a whole-system explanatory model that is more physiological than anatomical.

Additionally, assigning an interpretive label to a condition does not imply that the condition will remain unchanged. In OM, labels are temporary and dynamic, reflecting the fact that living bodies change. One practical result of this point is that different practitioners may reach different, yet equally valid, conclusions about the movement of malfunction within a patient, and that practitioners reexamine and reinterpret—at every patient visit—the patient's health status and thus may select a different label to reflect the changed condition. Another implication is that treatment is not usually forceful. Instead, the body-person is "led" or "encouraged" to function smoothly and remain in physiological balance.

The contention of an underlying ideology implies that there are messages conveyed by the context of the medical encounter that reflect a deeper communication based on the traditional cultural roles of physician and patient and the expectations created by the framework of the conventional Western metaparadigm.[19] There are other differences between the conventional biomedical and the Oriental medical occupational paradigms in addition to the ones previously noted. For example, the issue of responsibility for the patient's illness or condition is often perceived by the American Oriental–style practitioner as belonging to the patient. The practitioner views his or her role as that of a consultant to the patient. The patient then must take responsibility for his or her health with the tutelage and assistance of the practitioner. This provider of OM attempts to help, commonly phrased as "educate," the patient to take responsibility for his or her health by means of talk (the long clinical encounter fosters specificity of educational efforts), diet change, Qi gong exercises, or other lifestyle modifications in combination with the interventions such as acupuncture, manipulation, and herbal prescription. This approach to the patient is relatively horizontal and patient-centered.

Biomedicine, in contrast, is hierarchic and interventionist; responsibility belongs to the clinician. There is an inherent social structure of domination wherein the clinician has the power to diagnose the problem in the context of the law and for third-party payment. Diagnoses are often couched in a Latin- and Greek-based nomenclature that sometimes obscures their meaning to patients. The clinician has the power to prescribe controlled (prescription) drugs. There are many cases, of course, where this hierarchic structure is appropriate. Crisis management situations require a physician or an emergency medical technician to take charge of the situation. This is also true when patients feel unable to cope with their problems or feel themselves to be a threat to others. But in the ordinary clinical contact situation, the hierarchical structure reflects more of ideology than the practical demands of the situation.

The conventional scientific metaparadigm reveres "objectivity" and often is unwilling to diagnose without measurable data. As this bias acts in biomedicine, subjective complaints become peripheral, even stigmatized, and placebo (clinical suggestion, expectation) factors are distrusted and trivialized. In the OM context, however, subjective complaints are of central importance, and the practitioner is aware of the potentially healing or harming power of his or her words and attitudes. The patient's actual experiences, sometimes described in rich detail, are of obvious importance to the clinician. What may appear to be minutiae ("do you prefer hot liquids to cold?" "do you have more difficulty breathing in or out when you wheeze?") provides important details to the clinician. In a physiology-based nosology, disease is always systemic. Thus if a patient complains of asthma, the practitioner bases the treatment plan on attempting to determine its origin—if, for example, it is related to the Liver (allergic), Spleen (digestive tract, immune system), or a weak Lung or Kidney (lack of Essence) system.

The OM practitioner's intention is generally to maximize the placebo factor, thus tapping into "inner healing" resources. Some strategies, apart from simply being patient-centered, are to provide a quiet environment with soft music, lead the patient in guided visualization, teach "energy" exercises, or simply to offer hope, encouragement, and a positive outlook. The social context of the OM practitioner allows this because the practitioner does not have a legal obligation to alert the patient to all potential worst-case scenarios.

A belief conveyed in the conventional paradigm is that the body makes mistakes and requires correction in the form of scientific expertise. The belief conveyed in the natural medicine context is that the body is self-regulating and self-correcting, and the practitioner assists what the body is trying to do to restore harmonious self-regulation. In the conventional context, symptoms are undesirable. In the OM context, symptoms are not always undesirable because they may be caused by a self-regulating process or possibly a detoxification process. Symptoms can function as "friends" that alert the patient to the early signs of failure of homeostasis.

This belief that the body is self-correcting is based on belief that the body manifests an innate higher intelligence. This intelligence is responsible for the self-manifesting and self-regenerating vital processes. This view is the launching point from which spring many of the metaphysical and religious overtones found in healing systems, with OM as no exception to the rule. For the OM practitioner, clinical science is a type of human science rather than the efficient application of a powerful scientific technology. This humanistic approach is without doubt partly responsible for its considerable growth in the health care marketplace.

SUMMARY

The OM practitioner strives to create an environment in which the patient can relax and feel nurtured, takes careful note of subjective complaints, and factors the patient's biological and social individuality into the health care plan. This approach to the patient contrasts with characteristics of biomedical service delivery, which is divided into several components involving different personnel and multiple sites, which displays marked technological presence, and which offers less detailed attention to the subjective experience of the patient. These differences can clearly be traced to differences in underlying metaparadigmatic value structures.

Today in the rapidly changing metaparadigmatic environment of the West, the distinctive health care emphases of OM are part of a cultural countertrend toward a new humanism in health care delivery. The OM practitioner belongs to a new class of "alternative" medical practitioner that meets needs of health care consumers that are commonly unaddressed and unfulfilled in the conventional biomedical system. It remains to be seen if and how consumer needs currently being addressed in alternative contexts will be integrated into national-level health care systems.

References

1. Waitzken H: A critical theory of medical discourse: ideology, social control, and the processing of social context in medical encounters, *J Health Soc Behav* 30:220-39, 1989.
2. American Board of Family Practice: *Rights and responsibilities,* Lexington, Ky, 1987, American Board of Family Practice, p. 38.
3. Cassidy CM: Chinese medicine users in the United States. I. Utilization, satisfaction, medical plurality, *J Altern Complement Med* 4:17-28, 1998.
4. Cassidy CM: Chinese medicine users in the United States. II. Preferred aspects of care, *J Altern Complement Med* 4:189-202, 1998.
5. Waitzkin H, Stoeckle JD: The communication of information about illness: clinical, sociological and methodological considerations, *Adv Psychosom Med* 8:180-215, 1972.
6. Kenner D, Requena Y: *Botanical medicine: a European professional perspective,* Brookline, Mass, 1996, Paradigm Publications.
7. Kenner D: A taxonomy of acupuncture. In *Proceedings of the First Symposium of the Society for Acupuncture Research.* Bethesda, Md, 1993, Society for Acupuncture Research.*
8. Tsutani K: The evaluation of herbal medicines: an East Asian perspective. In Lewith G, Aldridge D, editors: *Clinical research methodology for complementary therapies,* London, 1993, Hodder & Stoughton.
9. Cassidy CM: Cultural context of complementary and alternative medicine systems. In Micozzi M, editor: *Fundamentals of complementary and alternative medicine,* New York, 1996, Churchill Livingstone, pp. 9-34.
10. Cohen J, Stewart I: *The collapse of chaos,* New York, 1994, Viking.

*Available from SAR, PMB 106-241, 4200 Wisconsin Avenue NW, Washington, DC 20016-2143, www.acupunctureresearch.org.

11. Lock M, Gordon D, eds: *Biomedicine examined,* Dordrecht, The Netherlands, 1988, Kluwer Academic.

12. Stein HF: The *psychodynamics of medical practice, unconscious factors in patient care,* Berkeley, Calif, 1985, University of California Press.

13. Stein HF: *American medicine as culture,* Boulder, Colo, 1990, Westview Press.

14. Kleinman A: Social, cultural and historical themes in the study of medicine in Chinese societies: problems and prospects for the comparative study of medicine and psychiatry. In *Medicine in Chinese cultures,* Washington, DC, 1975, John E. Fogarty International Center for Advanced Study in the Health Sciences, National Institutes of Health.

15. Hensel H: *Toward a man-centered medical science,* Armonk, NY, 1977, Futura.

16. Unschuld PU: *Medicine in china: a history of ideas,* Berkeley, Calif, 1992, University of California Press.

17. Unshuld PU: Epistemological issues and changing legitimation: traditional Chinese medicine in the twentieth century. In Leslie C, Young A (editors): *Paths to Asian medical knowledge,* Berkeley, 1985, University of California Press.

18. Unschuld PU: Traditional Chinese medicine: some historical and epistemological reflections, *Soc Sci Med* 24:1023-29, 1987.

19. Habermas J: Technology and science as ideology." In *Toward a rational society,* Boston, 1970, Beacon, pp. 81-122.

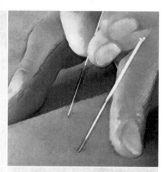

Grand Rounds

ANONYMOUS (1822)

CAROL KARI

SUSAN CUSHING

LONNY S. JARRETT

HAIYANG LI

SECTION 1: EDITOR'S COMMENTS FROM *THE NEW YORK MEDICAL AND PHYSICAL JOURNAL**

FOREIGN

Acupuncturation

This is a surgical operation, and implies puncturing by means of a needle. The operation is of Asiatic origin, and is employed for the removal of local pain. But, notwithstanding the boasted efficacy of the measure among the Asiatics, it has only recently attracted general attention in Europe, where some favourable reports have been made on it in the public journals. It is considered as peculiarly adapted to diseases of a rheumatic character, unattended by inflammation or excitement of the vascular system. According to Berloiz of Paris, acupuncture dissipates instantly that state of distress which sometimes attends rheumatism of the external muscles subservient to respiration. "In the space of one or two minutes, a patient whose suffering drew from him tears, exclaims he is quite well."

In favor of this operation, we have likewise the experience of Dr. Haime of Tours, who has lately published an interesting memoir on the subject, in the 13th volume of the "Journal Universel des Sciences

*From *The New York Medical and Physical Journal* 1:242-45, 1822.

Medicales," from which we shall extract the following case:

A woman had suffered for several days with wandering rheumatic pains, which continued daily to increase in violence; there were, however, at all times, fixed pains in the shoulder and in the right arm, which required such a degree of intensity by intervals, that the patient could not refrain from crying out. She was in this state when she came to consult me: finding, however, neither alteration in the pulse, nor increase of heat, nor redness of the skin, nor tension, nor swelling in the part affected, I considered the case to be simple rheumatalgia, and passed the needle in the middle of the arm, between the fibres of the triceps brachialis muscle: the place designated by the patient as the seat of the pain. The pain was driven into the fore arm, and the second puncture caused it to descend into the hand, and a third being made in this part, caused it totally to disappear, and the patient said, with delight and astonishment, she was cured; and was so satisfied with this treatment, that she spoke of it to everybody.

A treatise on acupuncturation has also been published in England by Mr. Churchill, Member of the Royal College of Surgeons, in London. The author of this work does not attempt to give any theory respecting the rationale of the remedy, but he speaks very decidedly in favour of its efficacy in "local diseases of the muscular and fibrous structure of the body," to which he has hitherto confined its use. He considers the operation as inapplicable in diseases of an inflammatory character. We will give the details of one or two cases from Mr. C.'s book, which will convey a more correct notion of the nature and effects of the operation, than any general description.

The first case is that of a bricklayer, aged 30 years, who came to Mr. C.'s house, supporting himself by a stick in one hand, and resting the other against the wall as he proceeded.

The body was bent at nearly right angles with the thighs, and his countenance indicated acute suffering. He had been attacked, he said, three days before, with darting excruciating pains in the loins and hips; every motion of the body produced an acute spasmodic pain, resembling an electric shock; and the attempt to raise the body to an upright position was attended by such insupportable agony, as obliged him to continue in this state of flexion rather than encounter it by altering his position. There was no more constitutional disturbance than was to be expected from three days and nights of constant pain; the pulse was a little quickened, and the tongue white, but I attributed this derangement to the irritation set up by the pain and

loss of rest. I directed him to place himself across a chair for support during the operation, and I immediately introduced a needle of an inch and a half in length into the lumbar mass on the right side of the spine; in two minutes time, I observed that he seemed to rest the weight of his body more on his limbs, and in the next instant, without any inquiry being made, he observed, that he felt his limbs stronger from the 'pain having left his hips.' He next plainly indicated that the disease was lessened, by raising his body; from which he only desisted, by being desired to remain at rest, through fear of the needle being broken. The instrument having remained in its place about six minutes, the patient declared he felt no pain, and could, if he were permitted, raise himself upright; it was then withdrawn; the man arose, adjusted his dress, expressed his astonishment and delight at the sudden removal of his disease, and having made the most grateful acknowledgements, left the house with a facility as though he had never been afflicted. (p. 49)

A young man, employed in a timber yard, whilst in the act of lifting a heavy piece of mahogany, was attacked suddenly with a violent pain in the loins. The weight fell from his hands, and he was unable to raise himself. He was immediately cupped and blistered on the part; but two days passed without much relief.

On the third day the operation of acupuncture was performed upon the part of the loins pointed out as the seat of the injury, which, as in its former case, dissipated the pains in five or six minutes, and restored the motions of the back. He returned, however, the next day, with the same symptoms as at first, but in a mitigated degree. A needle was now passed to the depth of an inch on each side of the spine, which, as I expected terminated the disease in a few minutes, and it was with pleasure that I understood the next morning, that the man had gone to his usual employment. (p. 51)

The instrument employed by Mr. C. is a common sewing needle, adapted to a small ivory handle. The mode of introducing the instrument he thus describes:

The handle of the needle being held between the thumb and fore finger, and its point brought into contact with the skin, it is pressed gently, whilst a rotatory motion is given it by the finger and thumb, which gradually insinuates it into the part, and by continuing this rolling, the needle penetrates to any depth with facility and ease. The operator should now and then stop to ask if the patient be relieved; and the needle should always be allowed to remain five or six minutes before it is withdrawn. This mode of introducing the needle, neither produces pain (or at least very little) to the patient, nor is productive of hemorrhage, which Dr. Haime says arises from the fibres being separated, rather than divided, by the passing of the needle; the former of which (the absence of pain) is a point in its favour, which few surgical operations possess. (p. 81)

We have now presented to our professional brethren sufficient matter to direct their own attention to the operation of acupuncturation—and here our duty ends. We have had no experience of the remedy, and will therefore refrain from offering any opinion concerning its efficacy.

SECTION 2: AN EXCRUCIATING LESION: A CASE OF NONHEALING ULCERATIONS

CAROL KARI

Karen was referred to me by another acupuncturist in my region because of her complex medical problems. When we first met, she was a 53-year-old part-time administrative assistant. She hobbled into my office and in a slow, somewhat disconnected way began to tell me about her main concerns.

Like many of my patients, Karen had spent the year before consulting me and running the full gamut of allopathic medical care for her problem with no success. She had complained of pain during this entire year. According to her account, some of her health care providers even doubted that she was in pain. When her condition worsened, and she developed more physical manifestations, she tried all offered allopathic options, although costly, but at best achieved only brief relief. At her initial visit with me she was angry and frustrated by her experiences. Her decision to try acupuncture was based on the fact that it had helped her in the past during an emotional crisis.

Later, when I sought her permission to tell her story in this case report, Karen wrote, "I regret not being aware of the wide range of health conditions which might readily respond to acupuncture treatment. . . . I would have been spared the many months of pain and discomfort before any diagnosis was made, the many different trial drugs administered and their side effects, the many office visits to a well-known medical center where my cries of pain were discounted and not believed, and the expenditure of precious time and money."

KAREN DESCRIBES HERSELF

Karen's Main Concern

Karen's main concern was the pain in both of her ankles related to nonhealing skin ulcerations, which she described as excruciating. She had been in pain for more than 1 year when we met for her initial 2-hour assessment. The problem had begun with edema at the inner ankles and pain at the soles of her feet. When ulcerations appeared, however, they erupted bilaterally at the lateral malleolus. These were preceded by waves of dizziness and blurred vision. Her pain became excruciating, her ankles felt very tight, and at times she needed a wheelchair because she could not bear to walk. Any kind of pressure, extremes of temperature, and anger intensified the pain. The pain also was aggravated by cold, so that even air conditioning was unbearable. She could not exercise, all activity was limited, and she had a minimal social life.

During the year of allopathic care, Karen actively sought help from her internist, her hematologist, a rheumatologist, a dermatologist, and a plastic surgeon. She tried topical medications, hyperbaric oxygen treatments, surgical skin grafting, and medications to promote blood circulation by decreasing blood viscosity. The ulcers did not heal. Another skin grafting procedure was being considered when we met. Karen was very frustrated by the lack of success in treating her problem, even though she had tried all options suggested to her. In addition, the skin ulcers were preventing corrective foot surgery for bilateral bunions and other deformities in her toes.

Her Other Concerns

Karen hoped that the acupuncture could help her skin ulcers to heal and thus decrease her pain level. But she was also concerned that she was "having no energy" and "I'm tired all the time." In addition, she "felt out of balance," had "no enthusiasm," "no fun" in her life, and had a "hot temper."

Karen reported psychological problems in her past. She had a "nervous breakdown" after a divorce in her late 20s. She also had started psychotherapy in her 40s because of episodes of unexplained crying. She stated that there were no feelings for her to connect to these episodes—she would just be in tears. She described herself as being "disconnected." In her psychotherapy sessions, she got in touch with anger and the hurt underneath her tears. Then she developed "real highs and lows" with a temper that was "hot and destructive." After an event of several days of crying for which she did not seek help, she "spun out of control." At that time a diagnosis of manic-depression was made.

In her own words, "I used to be superwoman, now I'm boring." Karen wondered if the medication that she took for her manic-depression and her other medical conditions could be contributing to her fatigue and mood. I felt that her constant pain must also be a factor.

THE ALLOPATHIC VIEWPOINT

Her biomedical practitioners' working evaluation of the leg ulcers was that Karen had microvascular clogging associated with her diagnosis of essential thrombocytosis. This rare disease had been diagnosed in 1991 after a hysterectomy. Postoperatively she had developed thrombophlebitis, received heparin, and was on bedrest. The diagnosis was made at that time.

Essential thrombocytosis is characterized by excessive amounts of platelet formation in the bone marrow. This can result in active bleeding or thrombosis. The cause is unknown, but in some cases it may be inherited as an autosomal dominant trait. It affects males and females in equal numbers, usually by the fifth to sixth decade of life. Treatment is usually geared to sup-

pressing the number of blood cells in the bone marrow with myelosuppressive agents. There is a high incidence of certain types of leukemia in this population.[1]

Karen stated that the only symptoms she ever connected specifically to her diagnosis of essential thrombocytosis were dizziness and blurred vision. These would worsen when her platelet count increased. She had never experienced unusual bleeding as part of her illness, but she believed she was at risk for thrombi because of her postoperative experience of thrombophlebitis. She understood that the excessive numbers of platelets circulating in her bloodstream could be disrupting blood flow in the tiny vessels in her legs.

Karen's platelet count was in the range of 700,000/mL when she was seeking biomedical help in the spring of 1994. A normal range for platelet count is 150,000 to 450,000/mL.[2] When we met in the spring of 1995 the platelet count was in the 500,000/mL range. She was taking hydroxyurea (Hydrea), a myelosuppressive agent, which resulted in anemia (hematocrit 31.4). The average hematocrit (volume of red blood cells in whole blood) for a woman is 35 to 45.[3] Other blood tests had been done to rule out rheumatoid and autoimmune conditions; results of these tests were negative.

As noted, Karen had been seen by five biomedical specialists for care of her ankle pain and had tried a variety of interventions. When Karen started acupuncture, she was taking pentoxifylline (Trental) to decrease blood viscosity. She was also seeing her plastic surgeon for cleaning and measuring of her ulcers once a week. Silvadene cream and dressings were applied to the ulcers twice a day. Elastic bandages covered her ankles to keep cold away from her skin and to prevent accidental bumps to the ulcers. Her plastic surgeon was recommending another skin graft procedure, even though the ulcers had recurred after the previous grafting. Karen was also taking lithium and sertraline (Zoloft) for bipolar disorder. She was not in therapy when we met, but had periodic visits with her psychiatrist if she felt the need to talk to him or to have prescriptions renewed. Blood studies were regularly done to monitor lithium levels, anemia, and platelet counts.

Causes of Leg Ulcers

Among the many causes of leg ulcers are arterial and venous diseases, diabetes, infections, vasculitis, vascular abnormalities, lymphatic diseases, cancers, trauma, drugs, and hematological abnormalities. Arteriovenous diseases and diabetes are primary causes. Treatments aim to enhance blood circulation, decrease edema and varicosities, and provide a moist environment to support healing of the lesion. Various compression bandages, compression stockings, and compression pumps are used. In addition, wound care with moist dressings and wound cleaning/inspection is performed. Modes of treatment for nonhealing ulcers include skin grafts, hyperbaric oxygen, electrical stimulation, whirlpool baths, surgical debridement, and other forms of compression therapy.[4]

Ulcers heal slowly, and even with intensive therapy, some do not heal. The cost of biomedical ulcer care is considerable. In 1991, Gilliland and Wolfe estimated that in Great Britain alone £50,000,000 was spent each year on treatment of leg ulcers, and 500,000 working days were lost by the patients; the average time to heal a leg ulcer was 6 months.[5] These authors estimated that the number of cases would double yearly to the year 2000 as the proportion of aged in the population increases. High cost was partly accounted for by the need for ample dressing supplies and to pay for a health care professional to perform wound care. The authors further estimated that if the healing time of only 100 ulcers could be reduced by 2 months (current average of 6 months), and the total number of ulcers reduced by 50 after 1 year, the savings would be £22,000 in dressings and £10,000 in nursing time.

To illustrate the high cost, Karen provided a partial cost list for 1 year of care of her leg ulcers:

- 1 hospitalization of 8 days: $33,000
- Surgical debridement of ulcers while in hospital: $1,059
- 23 hyberbaric oxygen treatments at $300 each: $6,900
- Rebandaging after each hyperbaric procedure: $1,500
- 1 or 2 visits per week for 1 year to the plastic surgeon for assessment and rebandaging of ulcers: $70 to $90 per visit
- 1 to 2 blood samplings and blood tests per week for 1 year at $50 to $150 per sampling.

Karen's insurance company paid more than $100,000 in costs for her feet in 1 calendar year; she also paid out-of-pocket fees for items not covered by her medical plan.

When Karen started acupuncture treatment, her blood test results were being monitored and she was still seeing the plastic surgeon once a week to assess and dress her ankle ulcers.

THE CHINESE MEDICINE VIEWPOINT

As a practitioner of Five Element style acupuncture, I am as interested in the patient's emotional/mental/spiritual well-being as physical concerns. I always look at and assess the entire person, body-mind-spirit. In this style of acupuncture, the body-mind interaction in an individual is described by the energy of the Five Elements: Water, Wood, Fire, Earth, and Metal. Each element has many correspondences that include color, sound, odor, emotion, season of the year, body organs, climate, acupuncture meridians, musical notes, food substances, and times of the day. The Elements interact in various ways to balance the entire system; they both create each other and control/balance each other. An imbalance in one of the Elements can therefore trigger problems in other areas of the energy system (see Chapter 2). Table 8-1 summarizes some of the more basic correspondences (see Figures 2-1 and 2-2, Tables 2-4 and 2-5, and Box 2-1).

In my initial and subsequent meetings with a patient, it is important to gather diagnostic information about the state of the patient's energetic system by asking questions, as well as by using my senses and the usual Chinese medicine diagnostic techniques (see Chapter 3). I assess the tone as well as the content of the patient's spoken words. I observe the colors on the skin, become aware of patient odors, and use touch to provide further information. I notice many details that are significant in Chinese medicine—such as yawning—that often do not form part of the diagnostic process in allopathic medicine.

My Observations of Karen

In the first 2 hours we spent together, Karen presented her story in a slow, somewhat disconnected manner. She was yawning and did not seem completely present. She related her concerns but was in obvious physical and emotional pain, at times becoming tearful and trying to restrain her emotions. My overall impression of her emotional state was a combination of frustration/anger and either sadness or grief. Table 8-2

TABLE 8-1

Review of Five Element Correspondences

Element	Organs and meridians	Emotions	Tissues	Climatic factors
Fire	Heart, Small Intestine, Pericardium, Triple Warmer	Joy and sadness	Blood vessels	Heat
Earth	Spleen, Stomach	Empathy	Flesh/muscles	Dampness
Metal	Lung, Large Intestine	Grief	Skin	Dryness
Water	Kidney, Urinary Bladder	Fear and lack of fear	Bones	Cold
Wood	Liver, Gall Bladder	Anger and lack of anger	Tendons, ligaments	Wind

TABLE 8-2

Karen's History at Initiation of Acupuncture Treatment

History	Details
Past medical	• Childhood through teens: allergies/eczema/asthma with frequent bronchitis and pneumonia starting in teens, missing much school, frequently entertained herself • Grew up in environment of abuse related to her father • Smoker for many years; quit early 1990s • Migraine headaches 1 week before menses • Late 20s: "nervous breakdown" after divorce; infant daughter to care for alone, sought psychiatric help • Many upper respiratory infections in 30s • Bipolar disorder diagnosed in 40s; taking lithium and Zoloft • Uterine fibroids in 40s cause pain/bleeding, has hysterectomy, develops post-operative thrombophlebitis, diagnosis of essential thrombocytosis • Motor vehicle accident leads to splenectomy • Bilateral ankle edema and foot pain 1993-1994; ulcers appear on both lateral malleoli with severe pain • Bilateral bunions and deformity begin with onset of ankle edema • Very dry skin since use of lithium began • Dizziness and blurred vision with increase in platelet count
Current bodily functions	• Sleep: normal, 7 to 8 hours nightly • Appetite: weight gain of 30 lb in 2 years attributed to pain in feet, reduced activity • Bowels: constipated, no regularity, uses laxatives • Bladder: no problems • Temperature: feels cold but denies cold hands or feet • Menses: no clots in flow; history migraines 1 week before flow since teens; later in life also migraines midway in period; hysterectomy for bleeding fibroids

summarizes her medical history and the status of her bodily functions when we met. Her main concerns were listed previously.

Examination of Karen's legs and feet revealed the following:

- Skin extremely dry and flaky
- Nails rough and ridged on her toes
- Feet warm with strong pedal pulses, no obvious edema, bilateral bunions with malformation of first toes
- Lateral malleoli: bilateral ulcers. Each ulcer was shallow, about 1 cm in diameter, with deep pink-purple margins approximately 0.5 cm around each ulcer, yellow coating over the ulcers, no odor, small amounts of yellow serous drainage on the dressings, no signs of acute infection.
- Ankles: no edema, many broken capillaries and distended veins, skin discolored brown-purple, right ankle more sensitive to palpation, patient very nervous about my being near the ulcers.

Application of Chinese diagnostic methods showed the following:

- Palpation of the abdomen revealed pain at the reflex site for the Liver (see Figure 3-3)
- Chou diagnosis: upper—chest cooler than the rest of the torso; middle—abdomen warm; lower—pelvis warm
- Akabane test* (to see if the same amount of Qi is present in each side of the bilateral meridians): Urinary Bladder meridian deficient on the right side, 9/15; Gall Bladder meridian deficient on the left side, 21/11; Lung meridian deficient on the right side, 9/16
- Tongue diagnosis: red-pink color with tinge of purple, no abnormal coating, narrow shape, dry, lateral cracks scattered over central region of her tongue
- Pulses: overall not excessively deficient, but notably tight in quality on the Wood (Liver/Gall Bladder)

and Water (Kidney/Bladder) pulses. Pulse rate normal.

- Color: overall pale complexion, with some white near her eyes
- Odor: none discernible
- Emotion: angry/frustrated; sadness or grief

My Diagnostic Assessment of Karen

Karen had multiple issues occurring simultaneously, but I believed those most crucial to address were the imbalance in her Wood energy and the presence of Congealed Blood. These problems had to resolve before additional progress could be made, but Congealed Blood can be one of the most difficult problems to move. In view of this, and what I also considered to be a history of imbalance going back to her youth, I honestly told Karen that I could make no promises, but that we should work together for 3 months and see what happened. (I usually expect to see progress with acupuncture within 10 to 12 treatment sessions, or within about 3 months.)

In terms of Five Element diagnosis, the major dynamic to address was one between Wood and Fire. The priority was the Wood imbalance, the energy of the Liver and Gall Bladder.

The Liver plays an important role in the body. It is responsible for the smooth movement in the entire system on all levels of the person. It relates to the smooth flow of joints (tendons/ligaments), the smooth flow of Blood and Qi, the smooth movement of the digestive tract and colon, and the smooth flow of the emotions. Anger and frustration especially affect the Liver. The Liver opens into the eyes and affects vision, both physical seeing and the psychic component of vision. It allows for the ability to plan and to see the future. Deficiencies in Liver Blood can manifest as brittle nails, dry eyes, tight muscles, numbness, spasm, and menstrual problems. The Liver's partner, the Gall Bladder, not only stores bile and secretes it, but also rules decision making, and can present as timidity/indecision when out of balance.

I chose to focus on Karen's Wood imbalance at the start of treatment for several reasons. Her Wood pulses were very constrained and tight, and she had numerous physical indications of lack of movement and flow in her lower extremities, her body functions, and her moods/emotions. Other signs pointed to

---

*The Akabane test is from Japanese style practice. A lighted incense stick is held near the toe and fingertip points bilaterally, while the practitioner counts at an even pace. The patient says when the heat of the stick becomes uncomfortable. If Qi is flowing evenly on both sides of the body or limb, the count should be the same (or very close) on both sides; that is, sensitivity to temperature should be equal on both sides. Uneven sensitivity signals pathology in the Meridian. In the first example above, the Urinary Bladder Meridian, which ends at the lateral edge of the small toe, had a count of 9 on the left side and 15 on the right, indicating reduced sensitivity (reduced Qi flow) on the right.

deficient Liver Blood in both her history and her physical examination. These imbalances in her Wood created the imbalance in her Fire, and created the pathology of Congealed Blood Pain.

Congealed Blood Pain is a sign of severe stuckness/obstruction. It can manifest as a very focal, usually severe stabbing pain. It can also manifest as a hard lump or swelling (swelling to the point of coagulation of Blood and Qi, as with a painful fibroid or tumor). A Liver imbalance is frequently part of the problem behind this condition, but it can occur in conjunction with other problems such as heat, cold, Blood deficiency, Qi deficiency, trauma from bruising, and scar tissue. Congealed Blood also occurs on the emotional level with wounds or traumas that act as psychic scars or long-term emotional pains. Abuse, traumatic incidents, a history of suspicious behavior, dissociative behavior, and hallucinations can be psychic manifestations of Congealed Blood. A rough pulse, a purplish tongue or tongue with red spots, a dark complexion, or purplish skin hues are also indicators of this condition. I knew that I needed to address Congealed Blood issues with Karen because of the severity of her pain in a fixed location, the purple color in her tongue/ulcers/ankles, her history of uterine fibroids with severe pain, and her history of being "disconnected emotionally" from her hurt and anger. In addition, this problem *was very stuck,* for no treatments she had tried previously were resolving her problems.

I hoped that correcting the constraint/stagnation in her Wood would reduce Karen's pain, relieve the ulcers, and feed her Fire, thus naturally assisting with other issues such as her circulation, the effect of cold on her pain, her "lack of enthusiasm," and her unsettled heart spirit (Table 8-3).

Acupuncture Treatment

Karen's acupuncture treatment was fairly straightforward. We met once a week for a 1-hour treatment session. Because of her complicated problems, I wanted treatment to be simple with clear feedback. I started by simply sedating/relaxing the constrained Qi of her Wood, the Liver, and Gall Bladder Channels with points on her lower legs. I focused mainly on treating the source points, sedation points, and Wood points. My needling technique for sedation involves retaining the needles for 15 to 20 minutes. I also corrected the akabane imbalances in her acupuncture Meridians that

TABLE 8-3

Chinese Medicine Diagnosis

Priority issues	Additional issues
Constrained/ Stagnant Liver Qi Congealed Blood Pain	Lack of Fire Blood Deficiency Wind-Cold Pain Issues Akabane imbalance

caused her to have uneven Qi flow, left to right, in the bilateral Meridians. After each of the first three sessions, Karen experienced temporary worsening of her pain. This is something that I had explained might occur, as some patients have a temporary worsening of their symptoms before improvement is noted. This usually occurs within the first 48 hours after an acupuncture treatment and does not last longer than 48 hours. In Karen's case the worsening decreased in duration from several days to only 20 minutes after the third session. She was feeling calmer and her energy level was increasing. By the fourth treatment, she had less yellow coating on her ulcers and the surrounding tissue was not red/purple, just a dark pink. At this point, 4 weeks into acupuncture treatment, Karen explained that her surgeon believed she ". . . was doing much better . . . has put off the surgery . . . and now will see me in two weeks instead of one. . . . " Her pain level, on a scale of 0 to 10, had dropped from a 6 to a 4 level. There were temporary spikes of stronger pain.

I began to treat several other pathways because I was certain that treating her Wood Element was making a positive shift for her. I moved Qi from her Wood Meridians to the Fire Meridians, using tonification points. The Fire Element controls blood circulation, calmness of the spirit, warmth, and so forth. I also treated her Earth Element, the Stomach and Spleen Meridians on her leg, for their effect on her Blood and to help control/balance the constrained Wood. One unexpected finding was that using a particular point on her Gall Bladder Meridian, near her lateral malleolus, always resulted in a temporary worsening of her pain. I subsequently avoided using that particular point (Table 8-4).

By the tenth treatment, the ulcer on the left ankle had healed sufficiently to no longer require a dressing, and the ulcer on the right ankle continued to decrease in size. Her pain level fluctuated to a level of 5 or 6 but

TABLE 8-4

Acupuncture Points Used in the Care of Karen's Leg Ulcers*

Meridian acupoints	Therapeutic goal of needling
Liver 1, 2, 3	Sedation
Gall Bladder 38, 41	Sedation
Spleen 1,3	Tonification
Stomach 36, 42	Tonification
Pericardium 7, 9	Tonification
Triple Heater 3,4	Tonification
Heart 7, 9	Tonification
Small Intestine 3, 4	Tonification

*At each treatment a selection of points is made to serve the needs both of the long-term treatment plan and the immediate needs of the patient. Only a few of these points are used at any one treatment session.

overall was still better than before treatment and was now mainly on the right side. The ulcer on the right ankle was healed by the nineteenth treatment session.

All treatments focused on sedation of her Wood, with some tonification of her Fire and Earth pathways. My needling technique for tonification involves inserting the needle into a point and then immediately removing it after a clockwise turn. No herbal remedies were used. The ulcers shrank and healed, and even before resolution became less painful. She had better range of motion in her ankles. She was more relaxed, even while dealing with her mother's critical illness and the impending loss of her own job.

With regard to her biomedical care while receiving acupuncture care, the plastic surgeon canceled the skin grafting procedure, recommended that she decrease the frequency of her visits, and allowed Karen to stop taking Trental. At the end of her acupuncture treatment for ankle ulcers, Karen had also ended her visits to the plastic surgeon.

Karen was thrilled and grateful for her progress. She went to religious services for the first time in 2 years and was able to start planning surgery for her bunions, something she had not dared to do previously because of her concerns about surgical wounds healing and possible postoperative blood clots.

In summary, 19 treatments assisted in resolving her ulcer condition over a period of 5 months, with obvious changes within the first few weeks. (In the last 2 months, I saw her only every other week.) The cost of this treatment was $1,260 ($120 for an initial 2-hour consultation, and $60 per each subsequent 1-hour acupuncture treatment session).

The only shadow in Karen's experience of healing occurred when she told her biomedical doctors about her acupuncture intervention. She remarked, "Much to my chagrin, when the ulcers began to respond to acupuncture treatment, and again when they were declared 'healed,' no credit was given to the obvious success of acupuncture treatment—the medical doctors only grinned and said, 'only God knows.'"

Long-term Acupuncture Treatment

Karen has now been under my care for a total of 3 years. She continues biweekly treatment. This is not the usual treatment interval for someone whom I have treated for this long, but considering her health problems and past emotional state, this seems to be an appropriate treatment interval for her current condition. At this point with other patients who have decided to continue to use acupuncture, treatments at 6-week intervals or seasonal treatments might be used.

On a physical level, Karen has used acupuncture over the last 3 years to help her healing process after 5 surgical procedures on her feet. She has had corrective bunion surgery bilaterally with no complications of thrombi. One surgical procedure resulted in a poorly approximated suture line. We both were concerned about this problem, but the area healed nicely.

Karen still uses acupuncture to deal with stiffness in her feet and ankles. The severe pain that she constantly experienced in the past is gone, and she finds her current discomfort manageable. There are temporary spikes of more intense pain, but she manages these better and they are usually of short duration.

Karen has had two episodes of small abrasion-like lesions on her left lateral malleolus that have been painful. They have healed, were not as severe as the previous ulcers, and were treated with acupuncture and topical herbs. I instructed Karen to revisit her plastic surgeon to assess the first abrasion-like lesion for any type of pathology; there was none.

Karen has been using acupuncture for a variety of other problems over the last few years: a neck injury after a car accident, bowel problems, shoulder pain, and headaches. In addition, she has used the acupuncture to help her deal with numerous emotionally traumatic events such as the loss of her job, the death of her mother, and the stress of caring for her father who has Alzheimer's disease.

Over the 3-year period I have also introduced herbs into Karen's treatment plan, with the focus on herbs that move blood stasis/congealed blood. Herbs are also used to moisten the sinews, decrease pain, moisten the stool and skin, and improve her mood. She has been using various formulas during this time depending on her needs. They have been administered mainly in capsule or tincture formulations.

Karen is the type of patient that I really enjoy working with. The complications of her medical history and the ongoing issues in her personal life make her treatments a challenge. There is a great benefit for me when I work with someone on a long-term basis. I have the opportunity to see their lives change and to support them with that process. Karen still has issues to work on. I have been unable to convince her to return to a regular type of exercise program, which would benefit her circulation and her emotional state. And yet, she is doing things that she had not done in years, such as take a vacation and be interested in social relationships. I am very grateful to be doing work that I can still find to be amazing and full of wonder, and yet so simple and low-tech. Karen's case is a great example of that for me.

A NOTE ON REFERRAL

A research assessment of acupuncture care for chronic foot pain, conducted at Kaiser Permanente Hospital in California, recommends that acupuncture be considered as a first line of treatment for foot pain of more than 3 months' duration and that surgery for foot pain should not be undertaken without a prior trial of acupuncture.[6] This recommendation was based on a study of 67 patients with medically unresponsive foot pain. These patients had used orthotics, nonsteroidal antiinflammatory medications, analgesics, physical therapy, exercise, local injections of steroids and analgesics, and surgery. Acupuncture provided complete relief of symptoms in 31 of the patients and better than 75% relief in 19.

Acupuncture care should be considered when allopathic physicians cannot find a cause for the problem or a specific diagnosis. Frequently the patient's symptoms will make sense when considered within a different paradigm or perspective. Acupuncture also can be considered when a patient cannot tolerate the recommended allopathic treatment or when that treatment is not providing complete relief.

References

1. Rare Disease Database, #577: *Thrombocythemia: essential,* New Fairfield, Conn, National Organization for Rare Disorders.
2. Tierney LM, McPhee SJ, Papadakis MA, editors: *Current medical diagnosis and treatment,* ed 37, New York, 1998, McGraw-Hill, p. 1535.
3. Tierney LM, McPhee SJ, Papadakis MA, editors: *Current medical diagnosis and treatment,* ed 37, New York, 1998, McGraw-Hill, p. 1533.
4. Margolis DJ: Management of venous ulcerations, *Hosp Pract (Off Ed)* 27:32-44, 1992.
5. Gilliland EL, Wolfe JHN: Leg ulcers, *BMJ* 303:776-9, 1991.
6. Erickson RJ, Edwards B: Medically unresponsive foot pain treated successfully with acupuncture, *Acupunct Med* 14:71-4, 1996.

SECTION 3: A CASE OF CHRONIC HEADACHE

SUSAN CUSHING

Sara looked tired, and was. Twenty years of daily headaches were wearing her down. At 40 years of age, she looked youthful and healthy except for the puffy circles under her eyes and a tired expression. She had a quiet manner and described her problem in a matter-of-fact way tinged with resignation.

Sara came to my clinic because her fiancé encouraged her to try acupuncture for her headaches. She had decided long ago there was nothing to do but live with the constant pain and was paying for her stoic attitude with fatigue and what seemed to me to be a lack of sparkle in life.

HISTORY

Daily headaches began for Sara when she became pregnant at age 20. For 9 days after the birth her bladder did not function; she was given medication and gradually recovered. During the years after her first pregnancy, Sara was dealing with marriage difficulties, going to college, a second child, and dependence on Medical Assistance. Stress and fatigue became constant aspects of her life, and the "always present" headache never went away. It continued through her second pregnancy several years later; by then it seemed a permanent part of her life.

Over the years she went to several different biomedical doctors and was given a number of medications; none improved her headaches. Six years after the headaches began she went to a neurologist who diagnosed "chronic muscle contraction headaches" but found only "tenderness over the posterior cervical muscles" on palpation. He noted that other examiners believed she might have temporomandibular joint syndrome apparently because of some malocclusion, but he found the temporomandibular joint "not tender on either side." The treatment plan stated "under usual circumstances she would be a good candidate for biofeedback relaxation training but Medical Assistance would not pay for it," so Sara refused the therapy. He prescribed maprotiline (Ludiomil) 25 to 50 mg at bedtime.[1] She did not return for a 2-month follow-up appointment because the medication "wasn't doing anything for me." She believed that the neurologist "was the headache expert; if he couldn't fix it, there was no point in going elsewhere."

Sara also sought chiropractic treatments from several practitioners. She would get a treatment "whenever the pain got too bad" and found relief for up to 2 weeks. In 1996 she began going to a chiropractor whose initial examination found "dramatic rotation to the left in the upper cervical area at C2" and "visible posterior of the seventh cervical on the first dorsal," as well as some reduced range of motion. It was noted that no physical therapy was used at the time, and treatment goals were to "eliminate pain and restore subluxation complexes so the problem does not return." After a few visits he noted "the patient's progress has been slow; however, positive changes are noted following spinal adjustments."[2] Believing there was no better solution, Sara "just took aspirin or ibuprofen (Advil) to manage the pain" and missed work once every 2 or 3 weeks because of pain.

I noted no other illness or injury when I explored her history except for two "minor" car accidents when she was a teenager that left her with bruises. She claimed a lifetime of good health, apart from headaches, in answer to all questioning.

PRESENTING SYMPTOMS

During Sara's first appointment in March 1997, she described pain that began at the base of the skull and spread toward the temples with a dull, achy, tight feeling. Throbbing accompanied strong headaches. Pain was "never less than a 2 or 3" with intense spells of "at least an 8" on a pain scale of 0 to 10 (0 indicating no pain, 10 unbearable pain). She took six to eight aspirin or Advil per day, every day, to reduce the intensity of her pain. The headaches were present at all times and worsened with fatigue, excessive stress, or before her period.

Her only other complaints were lower backache, neck and shoulder tension, cramps before her period, and mild fatigue. Sara's tongue was a pale pink-red with a thin coating but had a red tip and sides. Her pulse was thin and wiry and showed weakness in the Liver and Kidney positions. Her abdomen had even muscle tone and was soft and unremarkable. Tension in her shoulder area expressed as tenderness on deep palpation. Appetite, digestion, sleep, and all other areas of questioning elicited satisfactory answers.

Sara felt both her job as a laboratory technician and being a single parent for two teenage children caused much stress that continually exacerbated the headaches. She felt healthy in general but could not seem to stop reacting to the stresses of her daily life with a headache.

ETIOLOGY AND PATHOLOGY

I assessed Sara as suffering from Deficiency of Blood, Kidney Deficiency, Liver Qi Stagnation, and Liver Yang Rising.*

Pregnancy and childbirth deplete a woman's body of Qi and Blood and weaken the Liver, Kidneys, and

---

*A Chinese medical term such as Blood Deficiency does not mean a lack of the substance we call blood. All of these terms embody concepts of function quite different from the biomedical usage. See details in Chapter 2.

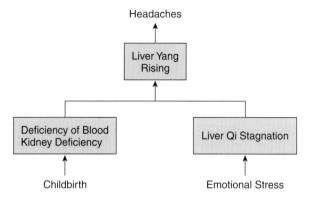

Figure 8-1 Etiology chart in a case of chronic headache.

BOX 8-1

Patterns of Disharmony in a Case of Chronic Headache

Blood Deficiency
Thin pulse
Pale tongue
Fatigue
Occipital achy pain

Liver Qi Stagnation
Wiry pulse
Menstrual cramps
Symptoms worse before period
Symptoms worse with stress

Kidney Deficiency
Weak Kidney pulse
Occipital achy pain
Fatigue
Low backache
Puffiness under eyes

Liver Yang Rising
Wiry pulse
Pain at temples
Red tongue tip and sides
Throbbing pain

Chong Mai. Normally these losses are rapidly repleted, but if not, they may prevent Kidney Essence from reaching the head or may allow Liver Yang to rise, either of which can cause headaches.[3]

Pregnancy and childbirth often lead to chronic health problems minor enough to be endured rather than treated. Over time, such minor problems become a major drain on the body's Qi as the wear and tear of life add to the original weakness. This seemed a likely scenario in Sara's case, as her headaches began during pregnancy and then a demanding and busy life seemed to prevent a normal recovery.

Occipital pain, low backache, puffiness under the eyes, a deficient pulse in the Kidney position, mild fatigue, and the chronic nature of the problem can all be attributed to Kidney Deficiency. Blood Deficiency symptoms were thin pulse quality, fatigue, and pale tongue. (Some symptoms, especially fatigue, may have several causes.) Liver Qi Stagnation is almost synonymous with chronic stress, especially unrelieved emotional distress. The smooth flow of Liver Qi ensures the harmony of all other Organ functions. When the Liver is affected by emotions of frustration, anger, or irritability, Liver Qi may surge upward because it cannot flow in normal patterns, becoming Liver Yang Rising, which in turn can cause headaches. Premenstrual tension, wiry pulse, menstrual cramps, and fatigue may be caused by Liver Qi Stagnation. Liver Yang Rising causes similar symptoms with the addition of pain in the temples, throbbing pain, and a red tongue tip and sides. Both Liver Qi Stagnation and Kidney Deficiency may cause Liver Yang Rising (Figure 8-1 and Box 8-1).

TREATMENT PROCESS

The treatment principles were to treat the Branch (stop pain) and the Root (rebuild the Qi and Blood) by sedating Liver Yang, Regulating the Liver, and Nourishing the Kidneys and Blood. Because several aspects of Sara's life were very stressful for her and thus continued to aggravate her Liver imbalance, I chose to focus the first treatments on this part of the Pattern of Disharmony.

The first treatment consisted of acupuncture points to regulate the Liver and open Meridians to allow correct movement of Qi, especially through the Shao Yang (Gall Bladder and Triple Heater) and Tai Yang (Urinary Bladder, Small Intestine) Meridians that flow through the temple and occipital regions of the head, respectively (see Figure 3-3). My first treatment goal was to stop pain and regulate energy. Points used were Gallbladder 20 and 41, Triple

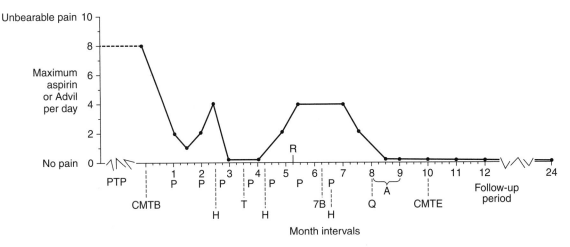

Figure 8-2 Change in use of aspirin and Advil during Chinese medical treatment of chronic headache. At initiation of treatment the patient had been taking eight painkillers daily for many years. Need and use rapidly decreased, and although variable over the first 7 months of treatment, never regained the initial level. After 8½ months of treatment, daily use had decreased to zero. It remained at this level until cessation of treatment at 10 months. In two follow-up reports at 12 and 24 months, the patient reported no daily use of painkillers. *PTP,* Pretreatment period (20 years of chronic headaches); *CMTB,* weekly Chinese medicine treatment begins; *P,* patient's menstrual period; *H,* patient's holiday; *T,* Tui Na therapy begins; *R,* practitioner reassesses treatment plan; *ZB,* Zero Balancing therapy begins; *Q,* Qigong therapy begins; *A,* patient has accident with damage to neck; *CMTE,* Chinese medicine treatment ends.

BOX 8-2

Acupuncture Point Functions in a Case of Chronic Headache

Liver 3: Top of foot between metatarsals 1 and 2. A Source Point (where Qi is easily accessed); subdues Liver Yang, regulates Qi.

Pericardium 6: Inner arm between ligaments 3 cun above wrist. Connecting Point with Triple Warmer, opens chest area, is effective for occipital neck ache.

Gall Bladder 20: Rear of head on occiput. Subdues Liver Yang.

Urinary Bladder 10: Rear of head on occiput. Removes obstruction from Tai Yang meridian

Stomach 28: Parallel to midline 2 cun below umbilicus. Regulates Qi of lower abdomen.

Lung 7: Near styloid process of radius on wrist. Regulates Qi of chest area.

Conception Vessel 4: Midline 3 cun below umbilicus. Tonifies Kidney, nourishes Blood.

Spleen 4: Inner edge of arch of foot. Opens Chong Mai, regulates menstruation.

Spleen 6: Located inner calf 3 cun above medial malleolus. Meeting point of Spleen, Liver, and Kidney meridians, regulates all three meridians.

Spleen 10: Just below knee, inner aspect of leg. Removes Blood Stasis from lower body.

Extra Point Tai Yang: Located on the temple 1 cun from outer canthus. Regulates Qi locally on side of head.

Small Intestine 3 with Urinary Bladder 62: Located lateral to fifth metacarpal or metatarsal, respectively. This combination opens the Yang Heel and Governing Vessels, affecting the spine and back.

Warmer 5, Liver 3, and Pericardium 6 (Box 8-2 and Figures 8-2 and 8-3).

After the first treatment Sara's headache was gone for most of the remainder of the day. The rest of the week headaches occurred as usual, but she took ½ less

aspirin tablet per day. Initially, Sara came for acupuncture once a week. After four treatments she had reduced her aspirin use to one tablet two times a day. Headaches were about three or four days apart and less severe.

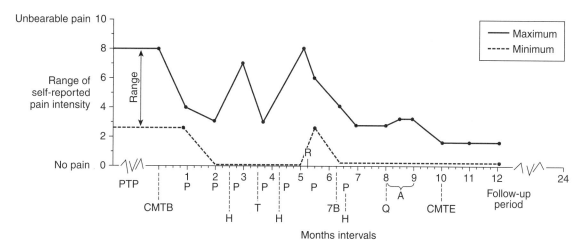

Figure 8-3 Change in frequency and intensity of headache using Chinese medical treatment of chronic headache. At initiation of treatment patient reported a 20-year history of continual headaches with intensities that varied from a low of 2.5 to a high of 8 (severe pain). With periodic exacerbations linked to menstrual periods and an accident that involved the neck, both intensity and frequency decreased gradually in the first 5 months of treatment. In the fifth month, changes in care resulted in rapid decrease in both frequency and intensity. By the tenth month when treatment was discontinued, the patient reported that she experienced only occasional mild headaches. *PTP,* Pretreatment period (20 years of chronic headaches); *CMTB,* weekly Chinese medicine treatment begins; *P,* patient's menstrual period; *H,* patient's holiday; *T,* Tui Na therapy begins; *R,* practitioner reassesses treatment plan; *ZB,* Zero Balancing therapy begins; *Q,* Qigong therapy begins; *A,* patient has accident with damage to neck; *CMTE,* Chinese medicine treatment ends.

In the fifth week she reported taking only one aspirin per day and was feeling quite well. Both of us were happy with the progress made, but for the next several weeks Sara had one or two headaches a week and took about one aspirin a day. Although this was a major improvement over the original situation, we agreed to continue working toward eliminating the headaches. The arrival of Sara's menstrual period and extra stress at work or with her children briefly but consistently increased the headaches, and with them, her aspirin use also increased.

Other acupuncture points used varied depending on the menstrual cycle and would include two or three of the following points: Spleen 4, 6, or 10, Ren 4, and Stomach 28, as well as burning moxa over points in the lumbar and sacral areas of the spine. I also used Back Shu points along the spine to strengthen the involved Organ systems. Gall Bladder and Liver points, and local points on the head and neck such as Bladder 10 or Extra Point Tai Yang, were used to affect Qi flow in the head and neck area. Points varied from one treatment to the next. Some points were used on a regular basis, whereas others were added or deleted to respond to the symptoms

and pulse presented by the patient on a particular day. By the third menstrual cycle after starting treatment, Sara had a period with no cramps and no headaches the week before. After this she went on vacation for 2 weeks, took no aspirin, and had no headaches. On her return she still had tension in her neck and a mild occasional headache, so I suggested she try Tui Na treatments from a massage therapist in my clinic (Tui Na is described in Chapter 6). Points that day consisted of Small Intestine 3 and Urinary Bladder 62 to open the Meridians along the spine and neck, facilitating response to the massage that was added to the treatment.

Sara canceled her next appointment because she had felt good all week, but soon after her period began and with it came a headache. Tui Na and acupuncture relieved the pain, but with the next premenstrual phase it again returned. At the same time, however, her headaches were much reduced in intensity. They now occurred mostly before her period or when stressed. During another vacation no headaches occurred, but her job or home life regularly caused upsets severe enough to cause pain and Sara would return for acupuncture and sometimes massage treatment.

Puzzled by the combination of initial rapid reduction in frequency and severity combined with stubborn recurrence, I decided to revisit her medical history. I wondered if the car accidents Sara experienced as a teenager had left Stagnation in the Meridians of the head and neck that was being overlooked.* Stagnation of Qi or Blood from an injury to the head may not cause headaches immediately, but years later a new health problem may intervene and the combination of factors triggers headaches.[3] Because Sara claimed chronic but minor neck tension and was unaware of any injury other than bruises from the accidents, I had not focused on the accidents in my original assessment. And although Sara did not have classical Blood Stagnation signs such as stabbing fixed pain or purple spots on her tongue, I believed it was possible that the small, recalcitrant imbalances in Sara's neck for which she sought chiropractic care, were mostly Qi Stagnation and a key factor in the headaches. I also considered that even though I had addressed energy blockage in the occipital area through acupuncture, this intervention must be insufficient because the problem had not resolved completely. Accordingly, I decided to try a more comprehensive and intensive approach to identifying and resolving Sara's continuing headaches.

By this time, the first massage therapist had moved away, so we began working with another therapist in my office who combined several body work techniques from Cranio-Sacral and Zero Balancing therapies.† Our goal was to discover the cause of the pattern of stress response. While the massage therapist worked with Sara, she encouraged Sara's growing awareness of the small changes in position, breathing, and muscle tension that were the early stages of a developing headache. By checking Sara's pulse while various body work techniques were done, we all learned how what happened in Sara's physical body was closely connected to what she felt emotionally. We now initiated acupuncture and body work in the same session. As the three of us worked together we discovered that Sara was holding her breath whenever she felt anxious; this directly caused tension in her neck and triggered a headache. My needling at Ren 17, which affects the diaphragm, while the massage therapist gently worked on the areas around T12 and C3, caused sensations of anxiety for Sara. She immediately held her breath and in a few moments felt a headache begin. The tension from feeling anxious began in her diaphragm and quickly spread upward to the neck and base of her skull. I promptly added Urinary Bladder 16 and Lung 7 acupoints to encourage diaphragm expansion and a free flow of Qi through the area between diaphragm and head. At the same time the massage therapist began hold-and-release techniques on the cervical vertebrae, T12, and at various locations on the ribs to relax the muscles and fascia and simultaneously release any possible impingement on the phrenic nerve, which affects the diaphragm. When the treatment was done, Sara was deeply relaxed and felt a new sense of openness and release in her upper body.

For several subsequent treatments the massage therapist and I worked together, focusing on the association between the diaphragm, the phrenic nerve connection to the cervical vertebra that were chronically misaligned, and the patterns of stress response that caused tension through these areas. I taught Sara to do two simple Qi Gong exercises to move energy in the chest area and we practiced correct breathing, which meant relaxation of ribs, scapula, and diaphragm with each breath.[4] Sara also learned new ways to adjust her posture from the massage therapist and began using these techniques at home to break through the tension-pain cycle.

This combination treatment, plus self-care exercises, seemed to move Sara past a barrier. Over the next few months Sara had only very mild and infrequent headaches, almost always just before her period (see Figures 8-2 and 8-3).

To treat these headaches, she often did not need to do anything other than relax and check her posture and breathing, or rarely, take one aspirin. We reduced the frequency of treatments to less than once a month. Acupuncture focused on Tonifying Kidneys and Nourishing Blood (treating the Root), with less emphasis on releasing blockage. Sara changed to a less stressful job and was preparing for her wedding a few months away when we decided the headaches were so rare that

---

*Stagnation is the blockage of normal flow of Qi or Blood in the Meridians. In Chinese medicine Stagnation may cause pain and conversely, there will be no pain if there is free, normal movement of Qi and Blood.

†Zero Balancing is a body work system that aligns the energy in the body with its physical structure through gentle manipulative techniques. For information, contact the Zero Balancing Association, PO Box 1727, Capitola, CA 95010. Cranio-Sacral is a gentle noninvasive technique developed to affect imbalances in the body by manipulating the membranes and tissues around the spinal cord and brain. For information, contact the Upledger Institute, Inc., 11211 Prosperity Farms Road, Palm Beach Gardens, FL 33410. (See also Chapter 6, Section 2.)

we could stop regular treatments. At this time her pulse was moderate and the weakness in the Kidney position was slight; some wiriness showed just before her periods. Sara rarely felt tired and usually had no complaints. The Blood and Kidney Deficiencies were essentially resolved, Liver Yang was Subdued, and Liver Qi Stagnation was mild and manageable.

A few months later Sara told me "I never thought it could change." Summarizing her experience she said, "I am forever grateful to my fiancé for urging me to try acupuncture. The first few months of acupuncture I would again just get temporary relief, but I continued to go every week. I started feeling better, then went every 2 weeks. Susan suggested adding body work—that was the ticket! The two combined was like heaven on earth—no more headaches! Occasionally, once a month around menstruation I have a relapse, so I come back for a treatment and am OK again. I would encourage more people to use Chinese medicine for their medical problems."

COST OF TREATMENT

Sara had 35 acupuncture treatments over 10 months. She paid $30 for each session, for a total cost of $1085. The massage therapy began in July 1997 and she had nine massage appointments at a cost of $35 each, an additional $315. Sara viewed the cost as reasonable and was pleased with treatment that caused no negative side effects.

SUMMARY

This case is presented because it exemplifies common clinical problems. What seems straightforward to each practitioner is not necessarily so. As with the tale of the blind men and the elephant, we each see a true part of the picture, but it is not always enough. In Sara's case, each practitioner over the years addressed one part of the problem but was unaware of or unable to deal with other aspects of Sara's health. Several therapies helped to varying degrees, but none alone resolved the problem.

Taking time to get to know a patient well is critical to good care because behaviors and habits that aggravate or even induce symptoms are often so ingrained that neither the patient or the practitioner easily notices them. For example, Sara's tendency to

hold her breath when stressed is something many people do. Yet when in my office she was not stressed, breathed normally, and so my attention was not drawn to her respiration. Further, I assumed that Sara's chiropractic sessions dealt effectively with her structural problems, and that the original car accidents were not very important because the headaches began years later and during pregnancy. From an acupuncturist's perspective there were several obvious systemic imbalances requiring treatment in a person who was reasonably young and healthy. Addressing them directly helped but did not provide a complete resolution to her pain, leading me to reassess her case. The changes made then led to resolution of Sara's headaches.

The treatments were successful from a clinical point of view not only because the patient was free of chronic pain, but also because she learned about ways she unconsciously dealt with stress and also how to choose different responses that gave her more control over her health. Meanwhile, all of us benefited from sharing the process of learning and change that led to Sara's healing. Sara's experience of the treatment results as "heaven on earth" eloquently describes how much the relief of pain meant to her.

Chronic pain problems require extra care and time to resolve. In the end, Sara, the massage therapist, and I concluded that the use of acupuncture to regulate, strengthen, and rebalance the body's energy combined with body work techniques that gently addressed somatic responses induced by stress, and Sara's willingness to make changes in her lifestyle and behavior, were all essential parts of our success.

In summary, adding or changing a therapy when treatment progress slows may be an effective option when faced with a chronic and recalcitrant problem; doing so cooperatively may enhance the outcome for everyone involved in the process.

FOLLOW-UP

I saw Sara more than a year after we had ceased regular care for an experimental treatment session with the massage therapist and a harpist. The experimental treatment focused on a general balancing of her energetic system. Sara continues to see the massage therapist approximately every 6 to 8 weeks. She takes no medication, uses no other therapies, and remains pain-free.

References

1. Hutter RD: Treatment notes, March 30, 1984, Gunderson Lutheran Hospital, LaCrosse, Wisconsin.
2. Erlandson M: Treatment notes, January 1, 1996, to November 20, 1998, Erlandson Clinic of Chiropractic, Westby, Wisconsin.
3. Maciocia G: Headaches. In *The practice of Chinese medicine*, New York, 1994, Churchill Livingstone, p. 4.
4. Xiangcai X, Ping YW: Various Qi Gong exercises. In *The English Chinese encyclopedia of practical TCM-medical Qi-Gong*, vol 8, Beijing, 1989, Higher Education Press, p. 56-7, 71-3.

SECTION 4: RECOVERY FROM CHRONIC FATIGUE: THE TRANSFORMATION OF INGRATIATION INTO INTEGRITY

LONNY S. JARRETT

In my writing I have referred to an "inner tradition" of Chinese medicine that emphasizes the use of medicine as a tool to assist in the fulfillment of individual destiny.[1] Notably, a patient's progress in treatment is assessed primarily according to indicators of balanced emotional and spiritual functioning and the degree to which he or she is consciously aware of his or her motivation for acting in life. In this paradigm, habitual unconscious functioning is seen as illness, and spontaneous, open, creative awareness is viewed as health.

Who an individual is at each moment is the sum total of all inherited (constitutional) and acquired influences. Chinese medicine offers unique tools for assessing the relative contributions of these variables to an individual's balance of health and illness at any moment.

The patient's constitutional endowment may be likened to a diamond that burns brightly in the depths. Five Element diagnosis provides a window through which the practitioner may gaze past the accretions of acquired conditioning back toward the patient's true inner nature. The Five Element model allows the practitioner to understand the qualitative nature of the patient's destiny and to strengthen the foundational influences that support its manifestation. On the other hand, the Eight Principle model may allow the practitioner to understand how acquired conditioning has become physiologically embodied as illness, obscuring the manifestation of original nature. Using both models, the practitioner can simultaneously access the potential of the inborn constitution and remove the acquired impediments that prevent one from evolving in life.

The case of Sheila, a woman with severe chronic fatigue, is presented. When she entered treatment Sheila had dropped out of school and could barely function on a daily basis. Several clinical signs including her pulse and tongue conditions indicated a high degree of vulnerability to serious disease. My discussion of her case highlights the diagnostic process and emphasizes the interpretation of clinical data that show how her physical symptomatology is the embodiment of her belief systems and behavior.

While receiving my treatments, Sheila also consulted a holistic physician, Steven J. Bock, MD. His description of his assessment and treatment follows mine. Sheila reports her own experience of Chinese medicine in the box on p. 153.

THE NATURE OF THE DIAGNOSTIC PROCESS*

The goal of my diagnostic process is threefold. First, it offers an opportunity to assess an individual's Five Element constitutional type, as well as important deficiencies, excesses, and stagnations, all of which may be harmonized with acupuncture and herbal medicines. Second, the diagnostic process involves the collection of a detailed patient history, which may be used as a reference point for assessing the patient's progress as treatment proceeds. Finally, the diagnostic session helps establish rapport between the practitioner and patient, initiating the patient's process of healing.

*For a detailed account of the diagnostic process, see reference 2.

Sheila's Experience in Her Own Words

I first came to acupuncture when I was very ill. My symptoms included severe fatigue, dizziness, weight loss on my already slight frame, headaches, diarrhea, night sweats, and insomnia. I felt as if I was dying. Prior to this, I lived a fast-paced life. I wanted to do well in everything I did. I was going to school full-time, working at making money in my spare time, and I was also recently divorced. To me, it seemed normal to be busy all the time. I seldom relaxed and was very unaware of what leading a balanced life meant. My symptoms seemed to hit me all at once, but I think I was ill long before I was forced to take notice. I was feeling rather desperate because allopathic medicine could not offer relief of my symptoms. I had no experience with Chinese medicine and did not know what to expect.

My first visit to the acupuncturist consisted of tongue and pulse diagnosis. He told me that I had Liver Blood deficiency. My tongue was very white on the side, which I had been unaware of until he showed me. I did not feel much improvement until after my eighth visit; then, I noticed a slight increase in my energy. If I had more energy, I used it. My acupuncturist explained to me how I had very little energy reserve, and that I must save my energy to invest in my recovery. The other symptoms took longer to go away but now, after 2 years, I am back in school finishing my degree in physical therapy. My tongue is looking pinker and healthier and so am I. I'm back to my normal weight and often feel better than I did, even before I became ill.

Through acupuncture, I've learned to live a more balanced life. I feel more accepting of life and better able to gracefully live within my limitations. I still get fatigued if I don't pace myself but have learned to accept this as an indication of needing rest rather than constantly trying to push beyond my reserves. ❧

One of the most powerful approaches I have incorporated into my practice is that of assisting the patient in acknowledging the connection between his or her specific symptoms and beliefs, thoughts, and actions. The verbal aspect of the diagnostic process may be divided into outer and inner components. On an outer level, the questions asked by the practitioner are necessary to collect specific information. Every interaction also offers an opportunity to establish trust and rapport. Therefore, on an inner level, the practitioner must have clear intention regarding the manner in which each question is asked, being absolutely clear about the nature of the messages he or she is sending and receiving. The context for the communication that the practitioner consciously creates is just as important as the specific meanings of the spoken words.

A patient's responses to the practitioner's questions also consist of outer and inner components. Superficially, the content of the patient's answers is informational. During the course of the interview each answer contributes to an elaborate story. As in a book, the story changes with every sentence as the interview progresses. However, the main concern of the practitioner is not with the unfolding story, but rather, with its theme. For the practitioner, of utmost import in forming a constitutional diagnosis is the way in which the patient relates to the events described during the telling of his or her story. Once the patient's quality of destiny and constitutional dynamics are determined, then secondary diagnostic measures such as pulse and tongue may be considered to provide a view of how the underlying constitutional imbalance manifests physiologically.

Diagnosis

Initial Impression

Box 8-3 and Table 8-5 summarize my diagnostic impressions of Sheila. The following text reports each step that led to this diagnosis. My twin tasks were to identify Sheila's constitutional type (using Five Element logic) and the functional imbalances that expressed through her symptomatology (using both Five Element and Eight Principle logic).

1. *First telephone communication.* The message left by Sheila on my answering machine was short, yet her voice clearly had the "singing" tone associated with the Earth element.
2. *First meeting.* On entering my office Sheila greeted me with a warm smile. I immediately

BOX 8-3

Diagnostic Assessment of Sheila

Sex/age: Female, age 36
Height: 5 foot 2 inches Weight: 95 lb

Reasons for Seeking Treatment
Severe fatigue
Poor memory
Dizziness
Hemorrhoids
Depression

Five Element Diagnostic Markers
Color: Yellow
Sound: Singing*
Odor: Fragrant†
Emotion: Excess sympathy‡
Constitutional type: Primary: Earth (Spleen); secondary: Wood (Liver)
Eight Principle pattern: Deficient Spleen Qi and Blood, Deficient Liver Blood

*"Singing" may be heard in the voice as a modulation of tone that occurs regularly between high and low frequencies.
†Patients are advised not to wear perfume or cologne to their sessions to facilitate diagnosis by odor. The physiological basis of the various odors is summarized in Table 8-5; also see Table 2-4.
‡The Five Element association of color, sound, odor, and emotion are summarized in Tables 2-4 and 2-5.

TABLE 8-5

Physiological Basis of Odors

Element	Odor	Physiological basis
Water	Putrid	Uric acid in the Bladder
Wood	Rancid	Bile in the Gall Bladder
Fire	Scored	Heat in the circulatory system
Earth	Fragrant	Yeast and fermentation in the digestive system
Metal	Rotten	Fecal material in the Large Intestine

noticed how thin and undernourished she looked and noted her yellow color and fragrant smell. Further, her smile revealed that her gums and tongue were extremely pale, a finding that initially suggests a fair amount of Blood deficiency. On shaking hands with me she looked around the office nervously. Noticing the waiting room she asked if she should wait there as she began walking toward it. I said that would be fine and that I would be with her in one minute. When I did let her know that I was ready, she again asked for permission to use the bathroom before we began. In both these instances I had a strong sense of her wanting very much to please me by doing the right thing. Although she had come to me for treatment, it appeared as though she was trying to take care of me by behaving correctly to avoid being an imposition. This is typical of the unbalanced Earth constitution's tendency to be ingratiating and habitually take care of the needs of others rather then attending to the needs of self. Also evident was her inability to stand up for and assert herself, which is often related to an inability of the Liver to promote healthy self-esteem. Her general jumpiness and too-thin build further suggested that Blood deficiency could be a clinical issue for her.*†

My initial impression, which was later borne out, was that Sheila is an Earth constitutional type,

*A function of Blood is to empower one to feel comfortable "inside" one's self.
†Throughout diagnosis, I freely associate the names and functions of the acupuncture points that match the patient's momentary expression. In this instance, the names of St-20 (Receiving Fullness) and Lv-3 (Happy Calm) came to mind.

specifically Spleen. This assessment was made based on my observation of her color, sound, odor, and emotion, which was yellow, singing, fragrant, and sympathy, respectively.

Intake Interview

Background

Parents. Sheila's parents were divorced when she was 9 and she was raised by her mother, seeing her father on weekends. Her father died of a heart attack at the age of 52 when she was 11 years old. While relating this information Sheila's voice grew weak and she began crying. I commented to her that it must have been difficult to have lost her father, and she laughed while drying her eyes and apologizing to me for crying.

Sheila described her mother as "75 years old and in 'good health' though she smokes cigarettes. I'm close to my mother but there are some 'difficulties.' I don't get what I need from her. She's not the type who hugs or who says 'I love you'; she's not emotional."

When I asked, "How did their divorce affect you?" Sheila sat up straight in her chair and raised her voice. "I felt that I was to blame that I wasn't good enough. If I had been they wouldn't have fought so much. I tried so hard to bring them together." At this point Sheila began crying and again apologized and asked if she could please have another tissue.

MY IMPRESSION. Her parents' divorce and the death of her father were major turning points in Sheila's life. That such strong emotion immediately surfaces relative to these two events suggests that she still carries unresolved feelings that currently limit her from full self-expression. Her two apologies for crying are further examples of her trying to take care of me during the therapeutic process, rather than being present to her own needs. This tendency to be "ingratiating" is a strong indicator of the Earth constitutional type.[1,3]

Observation of this nature, essential to constitutional diagnosis, emphasizes the importance of discerning the differences between what the patient says (his or her story) and the functional dynamics underlying the story (the theme). When I offered Sheila sympathy in an attempt to console her, she brushed it aside with a nervous laugh. Her inability to be present with and "take in" sympathy, the emotion associated with Earth, is a habitual tendency of the Earth constitution. In this context, sympathy may be thought of

as emotional nurturance and here, although she craves being cared for by another, Sheila demonstrates a habitual inability to be in the presence of that emotion.

The Earth element is comprised of the Stomach and Spleen "officials" who, in large part, are functionally responsible for abstracting nourishment from life and incorporating it into the individual in the form of Blood. Sheila's belief that she is "not enough" is perfectly embodied in her overly thin body. The dynamic is exemplified in her relationship with her mother. The Earth element may be thought of as governing one's relationship to mother through one's central connection (Earth rules the Center) through the umbilicus. After the umbilicus is cut, one must establish a new connection to the universal sources of nourishment both internally and externally. One's ability to do this is often modeled by the unconditional love of the mother. In Sheila's case, believing that her mother does not fulfill her needs suggests that she still unconsciously projects her need for fulfillment on her mother. The image of not being embraced by a mother whom she perceives as unaffectionate suggests the imagery contained in the functional relationship between acupuncture points Sp-21 (Great Enveloping) and Ht-1 (Utmost Source).

When asked about her parents' divorce, Sheila sat up in her chair and her voice increased in volume. This rise in volume is typical of the "shouting" sound associated with the Liver official. Trapped between her warring parents, Sheila absorbed their hostilities while trying in vain to make everything all right. Her ingratiating behavior may be explained as a compensatory mechanism that arose to help her avoid conflict.

It was at this point in the interview that the importance of the functional relationship between her Liver and Spleen officials began to assert itself. Both organs are located in the middle jiao.* The Liver (whose emotion is anger) tends to "overcontrol" the Spleen across the *ke* (control) cycle of the Five Element cycle (see Figure 2-2). At a young age Sheila determined that anger, which she perceived as having led to her parents' divorce, was not a safe emotion. Over time she developed the habit of trying to take care of others as a way of compensating and making the world "right." Predictably, her own healthy expression of the emotion anger became stifled as she struggled in vain

---

*The Triple Heater or *San Jiao* is represented by the division of the trunk into three regions, upper, middle, and lower *jiaos*.

to take care of everyone but herself. In time her Liver, whose function it is to empower directed movement and growth in life, ceased to function in a way that empowered Sheila to stand up for herself. Further, the function of her Spleen suffered as she grew increasingly exhausted from habitually catering to the needs of others.

Sexual relationship. "I've lived with Peter for 4½ years—it's a good relationship. I'd like to be married and have a child but he's wavering. I'm in therapy."

MY IMPRESSION. Sheila discussed her relationship with a heartfelt sadness. She simultaneously evidenced a strong desire to be married to her mate, and resignation about her felt helplessness to change her circumstances. The theme of Sheila's dependence on the actions of others for nurturance and fulfillment, present in her relationship with her mother, is also apparent in her intimate relationship.

Children. "I would like children but Peter isn't sure about either marriage or having kids. I don't know if I'm healthy or strong enough to have children now anyway."

MY IMPRESSION. Sheila's assessment that she may not be strong enough to bear children at the moment suggests that she has a fair appraisal of her health and a degree of consciousness about her condition which, from the standpoint of the inner tradition, supports a positive prognosis. In truth, Sheila has barely enough resources to keep herself going, let alone to carry and nurture a fetus. The theme of "mothering" is central to the Earth element as Earth is the mother of all beings.

A general principle in diagnosis is that when a patient makes statements about another, she is actually describing herself. Hence, when Sheila is describing her mother's inability to nurture her, she is actually discussing the emphasis that she places on nurturance as a virtue in life. Having been unfulfilled as a daughter she seeks to heal that wound by becoming a mother. The theme of unfulfillment in relation to nurturance runs from her mother who represents the past, to her longing for a child, which represents the future. Her demeanor is identical when discussing both her mother's lack of nurturance and her desire to have a child. In both instances, she appears unfulfilled (Earth) and grieving (the emotion associated with the Metal element, the "child" of Earth on the sheng (creative) cycle; see Figure 2-1).

Career. "I'm in school studying physical therapy, but I've had to go on academic leave for a year because of my illness. They were so nice to let me take time to get better—it's the first time they have ever done that for someone. Previously I had spent 12 years as a graphic artist but lost interest when the move to computers meant it was no longer a hands-on field. Now my garden is my palette."

MY IMPRESSION. Sheila's choice of a "hands-on" career in healing suggests her desire to nourish and care for others. When a person of a given constitution possesses a weakness in one area of life it is usually a strength elsewhere. Hence, Sheila's inability to nourish herself and meet her own needs is developed externally as a deep caring and sympathy for others. The Earth element is paired with late summer and the harvest when the fields are full with the fruits of one's labor. Sheila's statement about her garden being her palette is evocative again of her relationship to nourishment being directed externally. She is nourished by cultivating her garden yet ironically seems unable to be nourished by that which she cultivates.

Sheila expressed deep appreciation that the school board let her take a year's leave to recover her health. Clearly, this decision on the part of the school was humane and compassionate. However, I got the sense from Sheila that she was almost overwhelmed by the caring it exemplified. In a sense this decision on the part of the school board was merely the right thing to do, and Sheila's appreciation seemed to be almost too extreme, as if she were not used to such consideration. I also had the impression that she could not have stood up to the board had they denied her request. Again, she appears to view her care and nourishment as being entirely in the hands of another party.

Reasons for Seeking Treatment

"I used to get too much done. I was always working so hard pushing in school and not taking care of myself. I was under constant stress and really out of balance. I just want my health back. In May of 1995 I had the flu and started losing weight. I was really lightheaded and nauseous. Things have gotten slowly better and I have few headaches now. My appetite has come back, but I weigh 95 pounds down from 103. My memory is poor and I have trouble focusing. Often I feel disoriented when I'm driving and feel like I'm lost. I often feel dizzy and this can lead to fainting, particularly under stress."

MY IMPRESSION. The Earth constitutional type is inclined to two extremes regarding work. One extreme is characterized by momentum. When moving in a given direction the Earth constitution finds it difficult to stop or change his or her course. This may be likened to the movement of earth during a landslide or earthquake. At the other extreme, Earth tends toward inertia and all movement is slow and seems to occur in a geological time frame. Sheila exemplifies both these tendencies. Initially Sheila overworked, driven by some unconscious motivation (which became explicit during the pulse diagnosis). Eventually Sheila reached the point of exhaustion where she now barely possessed the energy to make it through the day. The issue of failing to take care of herself while striving to produce in the world is archtypical for the Spleen constitutional type.

Sheila had overworked to the point that her immune system had become compromised. The flu to which Sheila attributes her illness was merely a final event for which her weakened energy was unable to compensate. The symptoms of nausea, lack of appetite, and loss of weight suggest that, under stress, her digestive system is affected; this, too, is typical of the Earth constitutional type. One function of Blood is to house the spirit *(Shen)* so that conscious awareness may be brought to all aspects of self. Her trouble focusing is consistent with a systemic Blood deficiency that leaves her dizzy and disoriented. Her feeling lost while driving also suggests the involvement of Liver Blood, which has the function of empowering perspective both internally and externally. Liver Blood empowers vision externally in the form of orientation to one's surroundings and internally in the form of self-esteem, which springs from a clear vision of self.

Patterns of Function

Sheila's responses to questions about her patterns of function are summarized in Box 8-4. My interpretations of selected features are discussed in the following text.

The time that Sheila wakes up each night corresponds precisely to the high point of Liver function on the Chinese clock (see Figure 2-4). When an individual rests the Blood is said to return to the Liver, which both detoxifies and stores it. Insomnia that involves waking up, rather than difficulty falling asleep, is related to Blood Deficiency.

On the subject of her bowel habits, I made a note to advise Sheila to eliminate dairy foods (cheese and milk) from her diet and to decrease her intake of raw food. Bowel movements that fluctuate between being

BOX 8-4

Sheila's Systems Review Responses during the Intake Interview

Sleep: "Very poor, I wake up between 1 and 3 AM with my mind racing and cannot turn it off."
Exercise: "None, energy won't support it."
Energy: "Exhausted all the time."
Appetite: "Improving."
Cravings: "Salty food and bread."
Bowels: "Fluctuate between loose and constipated. I often have hemorrhoids."
Urination: "Up twice each night."
Surgeries: "One laparoscopy in 1986 relative to gynecological pain. They found I had endometriosis."
Menstrual period: "Regular and very light. I feel wiped out as soon as I get it and often have debilitating headaches."
Circulation: "I'm cold all the time."
Substance use:
Coffee: No
Alcohol: None
Tobacco: "Smoked from 17 to 20 years old."
Recreational drugs: "Before I was 20 I smoked pot daily for a couple of years."
Medications: None
Preferences:
Favorite color: Blue
Least favorite color: Yellow
Favorite season: Fall
Least favorite season: Winter

loose or constipated often indicate a functional problem with the digestive system as a whole. In the process of digesting food and abstracting nourishment from it, the digestive system has to effectively break down the food by "cooking" it (see Chapter 6, Section 1). The more the body has to work to digest foods, as it does with complex fats and raw (cold) vegetables, the more stress is placed on the digestive system. As it hyperfunctions, Qi, Yin, Yang, and ultimately *Jing* (Essence) are consumed, leading to a multitude of imbalances. Another function of Spleen Qi is to "hold the 'center.'" The presence of hemorrhoids may be interpreted as a sign suggesting that one's Spleen Qi is inadequate to the task of holding one's "center" in place.

Regarding urination, a central function of the Bladder official is its ability to store resources without dissipating them. Waking up twice each night to urinate suggests that Sheila's Bladder Qi is insufficient to support its function. From a Five Element standpoint this may be viewed as insubstantial Earth failing to control water across the *ke* cycle.

Scanty bleeding during menses confirms the finding of a generalized Blood deficiency. Because her functional Blood is already weak, it is to be expected that Sheila would feel particularly exhausted when she loses physical blood during her period.

The fact that Sheila feels cold all the time confirms Blood deficiency.

Sheila's lack of use of addictive substances enhances my impression that she has a fair awareness of her condition. Clearly she is trying to take care of herself by living a clean lifestyle, a fact that offers support for a positive prognosis.

A patient's preferences are of secondary value after color, sound, odor, emotion, pulse, and tongue, providing supportive evidence about constitutional or physiological diagnosis. In this case, it is interesting to note that Sheila's favorite color (blue) and least favorite season (winter) are both associated with the Water element. The Kidney is the residence of *jing* (Essence) and forms the foundation of one's inherited endowment. It is also the storehouse of human Will *(zhi)*.[4] Because Sheila has excessively drawn on her Will by pushing herself, her Kidney energy has been depleted as inherited resources are used to support the functioning of her other Organs, specifically the Spleen. Hence, her Kidney Yang has been depleted in an effort to support her Spleen Yang. This partly explains why she is continually cold (the other reason being Blood deficiency). Her internal state of Cold is exacerbated by the cold of winter and thus she does not like the season. On the other hand, the blue color subtly strengthens her Kidney function and so she is attracted to it.

The fall season is associated with the Metal element. It is important to note, however, that although in the West we speak of four seasons, the Five Element system refers to five seasons. The fifth season is the transition from summer to fall (Indian summer), which in the Berkshires runs from about August 15 through October 15. Thus Sheila's favorite season is late summer, which corresponds to Earth, her constitutional element. Yellow is the color associated with Earth and is her least favorite as it does not compliment her sallow complexion.

Physical Findings at Intake

Box 8-5 summarizes the physical findings, discussed in the next section.

Analysis of Data and Diagnostic Logic

Constitutional Analysis: Destiny and Virtue

My initial assessment of Sheila's color, sound, odor, and emotion was substantiated throughout the interview confirming her as being Earth constitutionally. Other findings consistent with the manifestations of this assessment include (1) a life theme of taking care of others needs while disregarding her own, (2) poor digestion and fluctuating bowels indicating deficient Spleen Qi and a weak digestive system, (3) the presence of hemorrhoids indicating deficient Spleen Qi, (4) nausea, poor appetite, and weight loss when under stress suggesting that her nervous system undermines the function of her digestive system (confirmed during pulse diagnosis), and (5) the tendency to favor the season (late summer) and dislike the color (yellow) associated with the Earth element.

Sheila's unbalanced relationship to nurturance and sympathy was apparent in the dynamic that emerged during the interview. Each time I offered concern and

---

BOX 8-5

Physical Findings on Initial Examination of Sheila

Blood pressure: Currently 100/70 mm Hg
Was 120/80 mm Hg before becoming ill
Tongue: Entire tongue pale, particularly the sides
Overall shape swollen with teeth marks on the sides of the tongue
Front third of tongue enlarged
Entire tongue has a wet coating
Pulses: Blood depth of the entire pulse *Thin*
Fine *Vibration* at the top of the entire pulse
Presence of a heart murmur detected in the left distal position
Tightness in the Heart Protector pulse
Both positions corresponding to the Heart and Lungs *Inflated*
Diaphragm pulse present bilaterally

support (e.g., while commenting how difficult her father's death must have been for her), she would laugh through her tears and immediately downplay her current need for the care offered. The theme of caring for others while ignoring her own needs was present throughout her life and extended to the way she interacted with me from the moment she entered the office.*

Sheila's tears were accompanied by a heartfelt sorrow that suggested that her Heart had never known fulfillment in life. It is as if she knew that she had sources of nourishment available to her throughout her life, yet somehow had never managed to be nourished by them. These qualities immediately called to mind several acupuncture points. Her quality of neediness, combined with her Heart sorrow, suggests the functional dynamic contained in the exit/entry combination of Sp-21 (Great Enveloping) and Ht-1 (Utmost Source), as well as the point Sp-14 (Abdomen Sorrow).[1,5] Her inability to access sources of nourishment in her life suggests the points St-20 (Receiving Fullness") and St-40 (Abundant Splendor).

The destiny of the Earth constitutional type is to transform ingratiating behavior (evidence of a distortion of the virtue "sincerity") into the virtues of "sincerity" *(xin)* and "reciprocity" *(shu),* which manifest as the balanced relationship between fulfilling one's own needs and the needs of others.† Sheila is habitually driven by the need to produce in life. She appears to be like a farmer who exhausts herself growing her crop yet never pauses to be nourished by the fruits of her labor. A key therapeutic issue for Sheila is that she must learn to nourish herself and to stop habitually reacting to her feelings of "not being enough" in the world by working excessively hard.

Diagnostic Analysis of Physical Findings

Tongue. The pink color of a healthy tongue is evidence of an ample supply and quality of blood. The

overall pale color of Sheila's tongue (Figure 8-4) suggests that systemic Blood deficiency is a critical issue in contributing to her poor health. The teeth marks on the tongue edges indicate that it is swollen, which suggests Spleen Qi deficiency. Combined with her complaint of always being cold, the tongue's pale color, swollen condition, and wetness suggest that Spleen Yang also is deficient. Therefore the Spleen is failing to produce Blood, and its deficiency of Qi and Yang is failing to transform Fluids; this causes the tongue to swell. The thick white area on the sides of Sheila's tongue suggests that the Liver is particularly affected by her Blood-deficient condition. The enlarged front third of the tongue suggests that there is Stagnation of Qi and possibly Damp affecting the Lungs. This is an example of the "mother" element, in this case Earth (Spleen), affecting the "child," in this case Metal (Lungs).

The degree of Blood deficiency found on Sheila's tongue suggests that the depth of her illness is manifesting strongly on a physical level. Even a small white spot this pale on a tongue can be indicative of a pathological state in an Organ proceeding toward a critical illness. That her entire tongue was this pale indicated the need for a strong treament approach. To achieve the desired results and avoid critical pathology, it

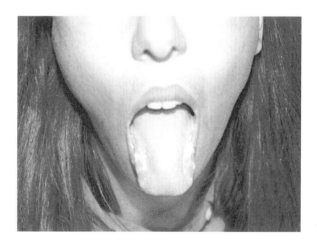

Figure 8-4 This photograph was taken during Sheila's second acupuncture session. Note that the entire tongue appears pale, indicating systemic Blood and Yang deficiency. The sides of the tongue are particularly pale, indicating the increased degree to which Blood Deficiency affects the Liver. The sides are also swollen as evidenced by teeth marks, which indicate Spleen Qi and Yang Deficiency.

---

*A hallmark of constitutional type is the form of emotional expression to which one habitually returns. During the interview the practitioner may interact with the patient to bring out each of the emotions present. This allows the practitioner to assess the ease with which the patient is able to transition through each form of elemental expression. During this interview, Sheila moved fairly easily through the expression of the other four elements. However, she continually returned to the theme of exhibiting an excessive need to give and receive sympathy.

†The virtues associated with the five constitutional types are discussed at length in references 3 and 6.

would be necessary for Sheila to be compliant in taking herbs, in making lifestyle changes, and in receiving acupuncture treatments fairly frequently.*

Pulses and pulse diagnosis. Five Element constitutional diagnosis by color, sound, odor, and emotion allows the practitioner to perceive the most subtle waveforms that spontaneously and continuously emanate from a patient. The pulse, in contrast, is the most subtle waveform that can be detected by physical touch. Incorporating considerations of the pulse allows for a fully integrated diagnosis, which permits the practitioner to discern precisely how the patient's constitutional and acquired dynamics manifest physiologically in the Organ systems.

My analysis of the pulse represents my own synthesis of 18 years of experience in the Leamington/Worsley Five Element system of *Nan Jing* pulse diagnosis, and 10 years of study with Leon Hammer, MD, author of *Dragon Rises, Red Bird Flies, Psychology and Chinese Medicine*.[7] Although much of my pulse nomenclature is taken from Dr. Hammer's work, my specific interpretation of pulse qualities often occurs within the context of constitutional diagnosis and does not necessarily correspond to his associations of these qualities.

I begin by taking the pulse on all six positions simultaneously. This allows me to quietly orient myself to the larger picture on the pulse while creating an atmosphere of stillness in the room. The impression of the pulse gleaned from all positions orients me to the largest therapeutic issues in the patient's life. The interpretation of the individual positions always occurs in the context of the bigger picture. When I see a new patient I always conduct a 40-minute pulse diagnosis. (Here I present only the major findings as they pertain to this case. The names of the pulse qualities are all capitalized at first usage.)

Major pulse findings. When Blood depth of the entire pulse is Thin, it indicates the presence of systemic Blood deficiency. This corroborates the tongue and interview findings.

The fine Vibration at the top of the entire pulse indicates that Sheila's Heart spirit *(Shen),* as it manifests through the function of the nervous system, was playing a crucial role in perpetuating her illness. The fact that this vibration was stronger on the right side, corresponding to the digestive system, suggested that Sheila suffered from excessive worry, an emotion associated with the Spleen official.

The presence of a heart murmur was detected in the left distal position, indicating, in this case, a functional problem with the mitral valve predicated on a deficiency of Heart Qi.*

Tightness in the Heart Protector pulse suggested that the function of this Organ had been compromised, most likely by pain or perceived betrayal in a past relationship.

Both distal positions corresponding to the Heart and Lungs were Inflated, which suggests that Stagnant Qi and Heat are trapped in the upper *jiao*. The finding of stagnation corroborates the swollen tip of the tongue (which also represents the Heart and Lung officials). Stagnation in the upper *jiao* can correspond with the inability to clearly communicate one's needs and a suppression of self in an effort to care for others. Physically it may be experienced as pressure in the chest or tightness in the throat, both of which Sheila felt on occasion. The sensation known as "plum pit in the throat" is well treated by acupuncture point St-9 (People Welcome), a point I subsequently used with Sheila.

The Diaphragm pulse was present bilaterally, suggesting that Sheila had possibly been divorced and that a painful conclusion of her previous relationship was still negatively affecting her.† This finding also indicated that separation may still be an issue in her present relationship. Here the entry/exit combinations of Lv-14 and Lu-1, and Sp-21 and Ht-1 offered an ideal way to move the stagnant Qi through the chest.‡

It is important that Sheila had not mentioned her previous marriage during the intake interview. When asked, she confirmed with amazement that, in fact,

---

*Sheila had one acupuncture session each week for 6 months and then "graduated" to treatments every other week. After 2 years she still comes for a treatment once every 3 weeks.

---

*Sheila's biomedical doctor independently identified a "mid-systolic click" and diagnosed mitral valve prolapse; see last section.

†An Inflated pulse in the diaphragm position (between the medial and distal position pulses, bilaterally) indicates Stagnation of either Qi, Heat, or both in the diaphragm. The bilateral presence of this pulse most often indicates the repression of tender feelings. The emotional basis of the Stagnation suggested by the diaphragm pulse results precisely from situations such as divorce. This concept was introduced to me by Dr. Leon Hammer; see references 2, 8, and 9.

‡Qi moves through the Meridians in specific sequence. An entry/exit treatment involves needling the last point (exit) on one Meridian and the first point (entry) on the subsequent Meridian.[5]

she had been married before. Being able to discern details of a patient's life from the pulse that have not been mentioned may help to instill a sense of confidence and makes the patient more likely to comply with the practitioner's therapeutic suggestions.

I therefore took this opportunity to ask how she felt when she looked back on her previous marriage. She answered, "God, I just can't think of anything good about it. He had a physical disability and I just could not bring myself to leave him for the longest time. I felt so bad for him—he depended on me. When I did leave I worked so hard to prove I could be something on my own, I had such low self-esteem. That's how I made myself ill, I just worked so hard."

As Sheila heard this admission pour out, her countenance changed subtly and she began to relax. It was clear that, on some level, she heard herself say that she had made herself ill rather than merely being the victim of a flu. She glimpsed that she had been driven by some unconscious motivation. This statement contains a major theme for Sheila that has played out often throughout her life: caretaking of another to her own detriment and exhausting herself trying to be "enough." At this point in the intake interview, a major part in Sheila's healing had been initiated, although she was not explicitly aware of that at the time. A major piece of her path to health would involve learning, at increasingly deep levels, to have awareness of how and when her motivations spring from an habitual tendency to push herself as a reaction to her sense that she cannot be enough.

Prognosis

The degree to which a patient is consciously aware of the reality of his or her condition is the degree to which a positive prognosis can be made. Sheila appears to realize that she is in need of a rest and that her health is seriously impaired. This is demonstrated by the measures she is now taking to care for herself. Further, she appears to have some insight into how she wore herself down, as well as her motivations for doing so. All of this points to her illness as serving as a possible turning point for the better in her life and thus suggests a positive prognosis. My expectation at beginning treatment with Sheila was that she had the potential to become substantially better. However, I assumed that recovery from this illness would be a slow process with ups and downs yet characterized by gradual and steady improvement.

THERAPY AND RESULTS

Therapeutic Strategy

The emerging clinical picture of Sheila suggested that the Spleen was not fulfilling its task of nourishing and creating a strong physical and emotional center. In turn, the weak Earth was not supporting the function of the other Organs, especially the Liver, whose Blood, Qi, and Yang deficiency failed to empower self-esteem. Thus Sheila found it difficult to stand up for herself in life both literally and figuratively.

In light of this assessment, I chose as my primary therapeutic strategy to help restore balanced function to Sheila by focusing treatment on her weakened constitutional Organ, the Spleen. I selected herbal prescriptions and acupuncture points to reestablish the functional relationships between the Spleen and the other involved Organs, particularly the Liver. The herbal formulas would nourish Qi, Blood, and Yang. Acupuncture points would be chosen to empower spiritual and emotional virtues associated with the balanced function of the Spleen and Liver officials.

I would gauge my success by observing whether, in the course of treatment, Sheila would exhibit more of a balance in her ability to stand up for (Liver Qi and Blood) and fulfill her own needs (Spleen Qi and Blood), and be better able to set limits when catering to the needs of others. I also hoped she would manifest a more dependable reserve of physical energy and strength. For example, increased weight would suggest that Sheila was embodying new balance and developing the capacity to assimilate nourishment in life.

Therapy

Perceptual Retraining

Suggestions and imagery. A risk in treating Sheila was that, if she were merely strengthened but not educated, she would soon deplete her newly filled reserves of energy by continuing her old habits of perception and action. I was concerned, in fact, that treatment could possibly make her sicker if she failed to gain awareness regarding the appropriate uses of her energy and thus drained even further her remaining reserves. Therefore, suspecting she would soon begin to feel an increase of energy from her treatments, at the end of the first several sessions I reiterated to her the importance, should she begin to feel better, to retain most of her new energy for herself so that it could contribute to her healing. I told her that she could "spend" 60% of her new energy but that 40% had to be "invested" in her recovery. The impression made by this message is shown in her own story of her healing (see p. 153).

Self-esteem and "not being enough." Clearly Sheila travelled through life collecting data for her thesis that she wasn't enough—enough to keep her parents together, care for her first husband, finish her degree, or succeed in having her current partner marry her. Eventually, Sheila also embodied this thesis in the form of weight loss and exhaustion predicated on Blood and Qi deficiency. Sheila's healing at the deepest level required her to become increasingly aware of her motivations. It was imperative that she learn about the beliefs that prevented her from being fulfilled in life.

For example, during one session Sheila began crying over her unfulfilled desire to marry her mate, Peter. Although she had been with him for many years he still seemed hesitant to commit to marriage. It was clear to me that she was projecting past patterns onto her present relationship, another instance in which Sheila's feelings of "not being enough" were preventing her from contacting available sources of nourishment. I mentioned the reality that, even though she was not married to Peter, he had stayed with her and cared for her through her entire illness, even supporting her and paying for her treatments while she could not work. That, in fact, he demonstrated a very high degree of devotion to her, and perhaps she was failing to be nourished by that which he offered her. I also noted that perhaps her conceptual attachment to the specific form of Peter's commitment was keeping her from being nurtured by a relationship of true value. She returned after that session and stated that she felt like a new woman.

This illustrates a point vital to the inner tradition of Chinese medicine. When, in response to pain in life, an individual suppresses an aspect of his or her true nature, Heaven (the highest aspect of Nature, that which instills innate nature and destiny) begins to try to reawaken that which has been lost. Internally, symptomatology is generated according to the dictates of that person's constitution. Thus symptoms are seen as warnings that, at a deeper level, some aspect of self has been lost. Externally, Heaven will send one life situation which, if heeded, will provide the lessons one needs to learn to repair the consequences

of lost self-expression. By looking at the momentary picture of "what is" in a patient's life, we gain immediate access to how he or she is generating reality. Hence, the nature of one's symptoms and life situation at any given moment always points to a deeper truth—the aspect of self that has been lost. When an individual masters a life lesson and reestablishes contact with that lost aspect of self, then, simultaneously, the signs of that imbalance resolve in that person's life both internally and externally as life becomes more simple.

This was true for Sheila, who was finally able to contact and accept sources of nourishment in life on the terms they were offered (as the virtues associated with Earth, integrity, and reciprocity emerged) and began to thrive both physically and spiritually. At last Sheila felt like an equal rather than merely at the mercy of another waiting for her needs to be met. Now she was able to accept and be nourished by her relationship as it stood, now she was able to meet her own needs. This in turn gave Peter more freedom to share himself with her, not out of reaction to her neediness, but rather from his own desire.

Herbs

Five herbal formulas (Box 8-6) were prescribed over the 2-year period covered by this case history.

For the first 6 weeks of treatment I prescribed Dang Gui Decoction to tonify the Blood in the form of raw herbs. This formula consists of two herbs, Astragalus *(Astragalus membranaceus)* and Danggui *(Angelica sinensis),* in a 30:6 ratio. Astragalus greatly tonifies *zheng Qi,* the "upright" Qi, that forms the core of immunity in human beings. *Danggui* tonifies Blood, which empowers one to be nourished by the fruits of one's actions. This is a strong formula for nourishing both Qi and Blood; I prescribed it early in treatment because of the severe deficiency evident on Sheila's pulses. It was my hope that by helping ro replenish Sheila on a deep level she would feel encouraged and hopeful about her progression of healing.

After seeing initial improvement I prescribed Ginseng *(Panax* spp.) and Astragalus, a strong Qi tonic, in combination with *Danggui* Four formula, a strong Blood tonic. Ginseng and Astragalus strengthen the Qi of the center and could therefore help improve Sheila's energy as well as empower her to "stand up" for herself. *Danggui Four* addresses Sheila's Blood deficiency and may also serve to help balance the Qi tonifying properties of Ginseng and Astragalus, which

BOX 8-6

Herbal Formulas Prescribed for Sheila over a 2-Year Period

1. Danggui Decoction (Dang Gui Bu Xue Tang)
Action: Strong Tonification of Blood and Qi

2a. Ginseng and Astragalus formula
Action: Spleen Qi and Liver Yang tonic

2b. Dang Gui Four combination
Action: Liver Blood tonic

3. Wu Chi Paifeng Wan (Black Chicken Pills)
Action: A gynecological formula that tonifies Blood and Yin Deficiency in the lower jiao and moves Blood stagnation resulting from deficiency

4. Tianma Shouwu
Action: An excellent formula for treating deficient Liver Blood and the associated signs of dizziness, fatigue, headache, and poor memory

5. Placenta Restorative Compound
Action: Tonifies Kidney, Heart, and Liver Yin, nourishes Blood, and tonifies Qi

can make some people feel nervous or "edgy." By tonifying Blood and Yin, *Dang Gui Four* can help to soften this edge. Herbs similar to these two formulas were prescribed regularly for more than 1 year and varied slightly according to Sheila's signs and symptoms. The dosage was 3 g in pill form of each, 3 times daily.

Wu Chi Paifeng Wan was prescribed concurrently with the previous two formulas to address Sheila's scanty menstrual bleeding, and because of the deeply nourishing nature of this formula. The presence of Ginseng and Astragalus in this formula make it an excellent Qi tonic in women who are also deficient in Kidney and Liver Yin and Blood. Although primarily used as a gynecological formula, I consider this prescription to be deeply nourishing in nature and not much different from giving a bowl of chicken soup in concentrated form. This formula was prescribed for 3 months and then occasionally afterward as needed. The dosage was 6 pills, two times daily.

I prescribed *Tianma Shouwu* intermittently for several months to address Sheila's Liver Blood deficiency. This formula helps to calm the mind by dispelling internal wind that rises to the head and presents as dizziness, fatigue, headache, and poor memory and focus. It is an excellent formula for clearing internal vision and empowering perspective. The dosage was 3 pills, two times daily.

Placenta Restorative Compound was prescribed to help reestablish Sheila's connection to universal sources of nourishment and to help heal the wound caused by initial separation from her mother. This formula is similar in intention to burning moxa on acupuncture point CV-8 (Spirit Deficiency) located in the center of the navel, a point that figured prominently in early stages of Sheila's treatment. This formula was prescribed for 3 weeks after about 3 months of treatment. Dosage was 6 pills, 3 times daily.

Acupuncture

The inner nature of acupuncture points lies in their ability to restore one's experience of original nature. Each point has the capability to evoke some aspect of functioning that has been lost, buried under the accretions of life's habituating influence. The process of point selection may be informed by input from many sources that are meaningful in the life of each practitioner. The practitioner must be able to hold his or her long-term vision of the patient's path of healing while simultaneously responding to the unique circumstances of the therapeutic moment. The process of point selection often recedes into the realm of intuition when the practitioner is doing his or her best work.

The central focus of Sheila's treatments lay in empowering her to contact sources of nourishment in life and embody them as Blood. Toward this end many points were treated that empower the production and enhance the quality of Blood. During the initial treatments moxa was also burned on many of the points for its virtue of deep nourishment and to add warmth to the Meridians. Box 8-7 summarizes the inner

BOX 8-7

Inner Nature of Three Acupuncture Points Used to Treat Sheila

Sp-21, Dabao (Great Enveloping)
Midaxillary line 6 cun below axilla
in seventh intercostal space
The ideograph *bao* reveals in its etymology the image of a fetus surrounded by the womb.[10] Sp-21 is the Great Luo point, which sends collaterals branching around the entire torso and effectively surrounds each person with an enfolding, motherly embrace. The term *baoyi* in Daoism means to "embrace the one."[11] This evokes the image of the Daoist making the spiritual journey of restoring original nature *(de)* and returning back to the womb by patterning himself on the primal *dao*. The sage who is "for the belly" receives the unconditional nourishment of the mother. The inner nature of Sp-21 is to empower one to feel surrounded by unconditional nourishment in life as though still in the womb.

St-9, Renying (People Welcome)
Anterior border of sternocleidomastoid muscle,
on the path of the carotid artery
Most of the Meridians contain a point or points known as "Windows to Heaven." These points are potent in empowering the virtues associated with the Element. It is interesting to notice that these points are all located on, or around, the neck, which may be thought of as being the region that physically separates the heart (body) from the mind (brain). A central virtue of the Earth element is reciprocity, which may be defined as emerging in the healthy balance between taking care of others and self.

St-9 is a main point for "people pleasing" and treating resentment that one has built up by being ingratiating. St-9 is ideal for the person who takes care of everybody else in an attempt to avoid conflict and eventually comes to resent others. This resentment is often evidenced as a constricted feeling in the throat at the level of this point. Often patients point at St-9 when they say, "I've had it up to here." This point may also empower a person who is unable to ask for his or her needs to be met to welcome others into his or her process.

Lv-14, Qimen (Gate of Hope)
Exit point directly below the nipple
in the sixth intercostal space
Lv-14 is anatomically the highest point on the Liver meridian and empowers the quality of aspiration. Here, at the top of the tree (Liver is the Wood Element) the branches reach up to touch Heaven, which is represented by its connection to the Lung meridian at Lu-1 (1 cun below lateral end clavicle in first intercostal space). Symptomatic of this Exit/Entry block is a loss of both aspiration (Liver) and inspiration (Lungs). The Qi in leaving the Liver meridian through the "Gate of Hope" helps one to keep one's eyes turned toward the future with optimism. Lv-14 may be useful for treating the person who can't see the light at the end of the tunnel. This point was used during several sessions when Sheila would become frustrated at her progress and lose hope of ever regaining her strength.

nature of just three of the many acupuncture points that were important in Sheila's process of healing.

RESULTS AND SUMMARY

Sheila's path to healing was steady and gradual. At the time of this writing, her tongue and gums have become a healthy pink, reflecting the improvement in her quantity and quality of Blood (Figure 8-5). She has regained her weight of 104 lb, signifying her increased ability to derive nourishment from life. Her blood pressure has increased to 124/72 mm Hg, which is in

her preillness range. Her energy now is significantly better, and she has not reported feeling dizzy or having headaches in several months. Further, she is generally joyful and has not reported feeling depressed for some time. Most importantly, Sheila has gained an awareness of what motivates her in life. Now when she feels the need to take care of another, or to strive excessively, she is able to take a step back and gain perspective. Rather than being a prisoner of habitual reaction to her feelings of "not being enough," she has the freedom to choose her actions based upon her own commitments. Within 1 month of Sheila reporting her major breakthrough and feeling like a "new woman,"

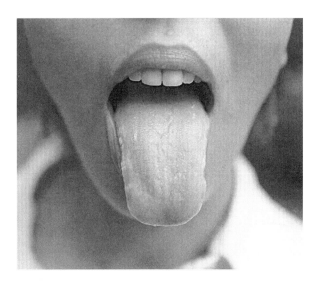

Figure 8-5 This photograph was taken 2 years later. Now the pale color can be seen only at the very edges of the tongue, which is otherwise generally pink, indicating increased quantity and quality of Blood. The teeth marks are greatly reduced, indicating less swelling of the tongue and therefore increased Spleen Qi and Yang.

Peter asked her to marry him, a proposal that she joyfully accepted.

BIOMEDICAL ASSESSMENT AND TREATMENT

Concurrent with her Chinese medical care, Sheila received biomedical care from Steven J. Bock, MD. The text below and the material in Box 8-8 are used with his permission.

This patient was first seen . . . for complaints of loss of weight, dizziness, nauseousness, increased fatigue, frontal headaches, decreased memory, falling asleep in her 1:45 to 3:30 class, drinking increase in coffee, had some palpitations.

[Sheila] was treated by myself and simultaneously by Lonny S. Jarrett, Acupuncturist, who treated her with acupuncture and Chinese herbs. She had a nutritional program including dietary management, nutritional supplementation, which included Coenzyme-Q10, Branched Chain Amino Acids, Desiccated Adrenal, Calcium Pantothenate, B_6, Vitamin C, Acidophilus, Phosphatidyl Serine, Licorice. On this combined treatment, she gradually

improved greatly. Dizziness went away. A low dose of DHEA was added to her regimen. She also had intravenous nutrients, specifically Vitamin C and B vitamins.

The patient started some psychospiritual counseling which complemented her medical and acupuncture treatment. She started having increasing return of her former weight, fatigue was better, headaches disappeared, sleep was better, she started noticing increased stamina and muscle strength. . . . She is feeling much improved. She is married. She is finishing up physical therapy school. Her physical findings are much improved. Her tongue picture improved with treatment.

In summary, we have a patient who was treated jointly from Chinese medical aspects and from a complementary medical aspect with symptoms of chronic fatigue, hypoadrenia, and a Chinese diagnosis of Liver/Blood deficiency.

References

1. Jarrett LS: *Nourishing destiny: the inner tradition of Chinese medicine,* Stockbridge, Mass, 1999, Spirit Path Press.
2. Jarrett LS: Chinese medicine and the betrayal of intimacy: The theory and treatment of abuse, incest, rape and divorce with acupuncture and herbs. III. Case study, *Am J Acupunct* 23:241-267, 1995.
3. Jarrett LS: Constitutional type and the internal tradition of Chinese medicine. I. The ever present cause, *Am J Acupunct* 21:19-32, 1993.
4. Jarrett LS: The role of human will (zhi), and the spirit of Bladder-52, *Am J Acupunct* 20:349-358, 1992.
5. Jarrett LS: The use of entry and exit points in traditional acupuncture, *J Natl Acad Acupunct Oriental Med* 1:19-30, 1994.
6. Jarrett LS: Constitutional type and the internal tradition of Chinese medicine. II. The ontogeny of life, *Am J Acupunct* 21:141-158, 1993.
7. Hammer L: *Dragon rises, red bird flies: psychology and Chinese medicine,* Barrytown, NY, 1990, Station Hill Press.
8. Jarrett LS: Chinese medicine and the betrayal of intimacy. I. The theory and treatment of abuse, incest, rape and divorce with acupuncture and herbs, *Am J Acupunct* 23:35-51, 1995.
9. Jarrett LS: Chinese medicine and the betrayal of intimacy. II. The theory and treatment of abuse, incest, rape and divorce with acupuncture and herb, *Am J Acupunct* 23:123-151, 1995.
10. Weiger L: *Chinese characters,* New York, 1965, Paragon Books.
11. Girardot NJ: Myth and meaning in early Taoism, Berkeley, 1983, University of California Press.
12. Kaptchuk T: Personal communication, 1989.

BOX 8-8

Summary of Findings by Steven J. Bock, MD

Past History
- Treatment includes treatment of endometriosis with laser.
- Allergies as a child consisting of sore throat, headaches, increased adenopathy.
- Positive streptococcal throat infections.
- Treated for allergy with shots at age 16.

Social History
Attends physical therapy school.

Review of Systems
- HEENT: She had dark circles under her eyes, lids felt droopy, some lid puffiness.
- Nasal: Increased sneezing in the morning.
- Mouth: Bad taste, postnasal drip, lips cracked.
- Gastrointestinal: Loose stools, anal itching, alternating constipation, diarrhea.
- Genitourinary: She had frequent urination after intercourse, especially at night, decreased libido.
- Gynecological: She had cramps the first day, slightly teary. Sleep was interrupted, awaking at 1-2 AM. Wheat caused bloating.
- Cigarette smoke would give her headaches and nausea; gasoline bothered her.

Physical Examination
Eyes: Pupils equal and reactive to light. Conjunctiva—within normal limits. UM is intact. She had puffy lids with dark circles.
- Nose: Clear
- Ears: Clear
- Throat: Clear
- Tongue: Showed white discoloration on the lateral surfaces where there is some scalloping. Some of the tongue was coated and the tip was red.

Physical Examination—cont'd
- Neck: Supple.
- Chest: Clear to percussion and auscultation.
- Core: Regular sinus rhythm with a midsystolic click.

Impression (at this time)
- Medically fatigued
- Weight loss
- Rule out malabsorption for parasites
- Rule out Lyme disease
- Rule out hypoadrenia
- History of endometriosis
- History of allergies to dust, mold, and foods
- Rule out food allergies
- Mitral valve prolapse
- Rule out chemical sensitivities
- History of hypoglycemia

Laboratory Testing
- Ova and parasites: Negative
- Stool analysis: Showed some imbalance flora *Anthrobacter cloacae*: 3+ and some pathogenic bacteria, *Citrobacter* and *Pseudomonas*.
- She had salivary adrenal testing, which showed on temporal salivary cortisols that she had a depressed morning cortisol suggestive of marginal adrenal performance. She had an elevation in the midnight value, suggesting a lack of sensitivity to suppression at the pituitary-hypothalamic axis.
- She had DHEAs done, which showed a DHEA of 245 and a DHEA sulfate of 95.

SECTION 5: A CASE OF STROKE BLINDNESS

HAIYANG LI with CLAIRE M. CASSIDY

ACUPUNCTURE PRACTITIONER'S CASE REPORT

A new patient, Harry, came to my office and offered the following explanation of why he was seeking Chinese medicine care.

Harry was a draftsman at a gas and electric company in Baltimore, Maryland, and reported being reasonably healthy at age 71, although he had been suffering from hypertension for 10 years (controlled to about 135/90 mm Hg with medication) and had a blood cholesterol level more than 300 for which he was not taking medication. One day, 3 months previously, he had had a severe right-sided headache all day. He went home after work and dozed off when reading the newspaper. When he woke up, he could not see. His wife drove him to the hospital emergency department. On the way, vision in his left eye returned. At the emergency department a stroke was diagnosed, and Harry was given a blood thinner. A few days later, he could see with both eyes. However, he had difficulty driving because he was experiencing blind spots. After a neurological examination, a diagnosis of bilateral upper left visual field defects was made.

He came to see me because the defect in the left visual field in both eyes had remained for 3 months and he still could not drive. Harry also reported occasional headaches, described as affecting his whole head. He said reading easily caused eye strain and worsened the headache.

On examination I found tenderness and tightness in the nape of the neck and in the upper back. The upper left visual field was missing in both eyes. The pulse was wiry. The tongue body was deep red, pointed, and covered with many fine wrinkles and purple spots. The tongue coat showed patches of yellow in the back and mid sections. There was no motor or sensory loss noted. He had normal tendon reflexes with no pathological reflex detected.

I diagnosed Blood Stagnation Blocking the Visual Orifice.

In the next month, I performed four acupuncture treatments, using both scalp points and regular body points. After four treatments Harry reported that he

had no missing visual fields and stated that he was free of headaches and eye strain after reading.

His treatment plan proceeded as follows:
- November 26, first visit. Needling of scalp vision points in occipital region, both sides. Needling of body points Du 16 *(Feng Fu)*, G 20 *(Feng Chi)*, G 21 *(Jian Jing)*, both sides. Electrical stimulation was applied to selected points using intermittent wave pattern for 20 minutes.
- December 2, second visit. No significant improvement noted. Acupuncture treatment same as the first.
- December 16, third visit. I examined Harry and found that he could see in all directions. He stated that he still sometimes had mild headaches. Acupuncture treatment: same as the first.
- December 30, fourth and last visit. Harry reported that he had had no headaches, even after reading. He is able to drive with no difficulty. He told me that an examination this morning by the neurologist showed total recovery of the visual fields.
- Acupuncture treatment: Needling of body points G 20, G 21, SJ 5 *(Wai Guan)*, LI 4 *(He Gu)*, Sp 9 *(Yin Ling Quan)*, Liv 3 *(Tai Chong)*, Kid 3 *(Tai Xi)*, both sides. I charged $140 for the initial visit and $40 for each subsequent visit, for a total cost to Harry of $300.

PATIENT INTERVIEW

The following is based on a telephone interview with Harry performed by Claire M. Cassidy, 10 months after he ended his acupuncture care.

Can you tell me what happened to you?

I had a "minor stroke" on my right side. It affected my eyesight—I lost my sight in the upper left corner of both eyes, like a pie wedge. I went to the emergency room and a series of doctors examined me; they agreed it was a minor stroke. I had an MRI [magnetic resonance imaging] and MRA [magnetic resonance angiography], blood tests, a CT [computed tomography] scan—the whole thing. The neurologist read all the information and established what it was, and put me on a blood thinner called Persantine [dipyridamole], and baby aspirin. After a few days my sight came back a little bit, but I couldn't drive the car because I was lacking peripheral vision.

I'm a draftsman. My eyesight is very important. With the stroke, I couldn't see—I had to move my eyes around a lot, computer, desk, people talking, point to point, and it was difficult. I couldn't read, I couldn't watch TV.

My wife had been seeing the acupuncture doctor, and suggested I go see him. I had nothing to lose—the medical doctors had said there was nothing they could do about it. My age, 71, was a factor. On my first visit, Dr. Li explained the procedures to me. Then he put needles in my ears and back of my head and all around—I couldn't tell you exactly where, because there was no pain. That lasted about one-half hour.

On my second visit I was lying on my stomach and couldn't see where he put the needles. I could feel them, but there was no pain. It lasted about 20 minutes. I got these treatments in the afternoon so when I left for home it was already dark so I couldn't gauge if the treatments had made a difference. But in the morning I could tell there was a slight change in the viewing area. My left eye had been worse, but vision was coming back.

On my third visit things got much much better. When I went to work the next day I didn't even know—wouldn't have known I had a problem, everything was so good! I use my work as a gauge. I could look down and read a brochure, look up and read the computer—my eyes adjusted just like I was 18 years old. I could go from close up, like 2 feet away, to looking up at people far away.

The fourth time, that was it. There had been quite a bit of improvement, and it's been like that since. What Dr. Li did really helped me. It happens that just at this time, in late December, I was scheduled to renew my driver's license. I had to take an eye test and I was worried that without my peripheral vision I would not be able to pass the test. But I passed the test! I'm glad that I went to see Dr. Li. All I can say, it did me good. I'm retired from my field of drafting, but I was back at work as a contractor. The stroke was a setback. Dr. Li's treatment helped me along—if I didn't go, I wouldn't have been able to work as a contrac-

tor; I couldn't drive! The treatment wasn't miraculous—I still have some loss—but my peripheral vision is back, I can drive, do work, read, do my job.

Now it's 13 months since your stroke, and 10 months since you saw Dr. Li. How is your sight now?

My sight now is not 100%, but I can live with this. I got at least 50% back, even in my left eye.

Why did you stop seeing Dr. Li if you weren't at 100%?

I felt like it was better. I hate to go to doctors! I got back into my normal way of life, and, I guess I just let things slide. But I'll go see him again if the ophthalmologist says my eyes aren't right.

Dr. Li also mentioned that you had headaches.

Yes, I did, but they were gone and they've stayed gone.

REMARKS FROM JOHN SORROW, MD, OPHTHALMOLOGIST

The following is a transcript from a telephone interview with Dr. Sorrow performed by Claire M. Cassidy, 10 months after Harry ended his acupuncture care.

I did not know, until he told me on this recent visit, that Harry had been to see an acupuncturist for care of his visual field defect. At this time Harry continues to have a left visual field defect in both eyes. My simple tests—finding the beginning of a sentence, and pointing his finger left—show this to be so. However, we did not repeat the visual field test to ascertain if there has been any change in the size of the defect since the first test in November 1999. It might be worth doing, though I'm not sure Medicare would pay for it. (Biomedically) I cannot explain why he feels he can see better; according to our theory, the kind of stroke damage he incurred cannot be reversed.

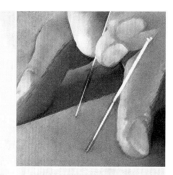

9

Inside an Acupuncture Detoxification Clinic

M A R T H A   H A R E

I figure if a needle got me into this fix, maybe a needle can get me out.*

For the past two decades, even though there has been controversy about the efficacy of acupuncture in general and for substance abuse in particular, detoxification acupuncture has enjoyed increasing acceptance both within and outside medical circles. In 1989, *The Lancet* published results of a controlled trial of acupuncture treatment for patients with severe recidivist alcoholism.[1] The investigators showed that 53% of patients in the treatment group completed treatment compared with only 2.5% of the control group. This study was groundbreaking not only because it suggested the utility of acupuncture in detoxification care, but also because it was the first substance abuse efficacy study of acupuncture treatment that fully conformed to standards of clinical research. Subsequent research, both quantitative and qualitative,[2,3] plus the day-to-day experience of providers, has continued to support the use of acupuncture for detoxification.†

Data concerning acupuncture research in the care of substance abusers is further developed in Chapter 14. This chapter describes delivery of acupuncture care in public detoxification clinics designed to wean patients from illegal drugs and alcohol. This is a complex subject because the task of detoxification commonly goes well beyond the usual conceptual boundaries of

---

*Remark of a jailed Baltimore detoxification patient.
†This chapter focuses on detoxification from such drugs as heroin, cocaine, crack, and alcohol. Acupuncture may also be used to reduce dependence on other substances such as caffeine, nicotine, and antidepressants.

169

what is medicine and what is not. In the care of addicted patients, not only chronic illness must be considered, but also legal and social issues, because many patients are referred to treatment from courts and some are concerned about qualifying for custody of their children. Thus a detoxification clinic must meet many patient needs and work with a variety of authorities. Two of the clinics discussed in this chapter are located in large publicly funded hospitals where most services are defrayed by Medicaid payments. The third, established later, relies on small grants, volunteerism, and donations.

The data for this chapter come from in-depth observations made at three acupuncture detoxification clinics, two located in New York City and one in Baltimore, Maryland. Each clinic is distinctive but all use the standard auricular acupuncture protocol (see Chapter 14) developed in large part by Michael Smith, MD, director of the Lincoln Hospital detoxification clinic in the Bronx, New York. I made my first observations in 1990 as a graduate student in medical anthropology while I was conducting dissertation research on the uses of acupuncture by non-Asians in New York City.[4] I was fully accepted in each of the New York clinics as a participant-observer, freely talking with patients and staff, observing treatments, and performing minor duties such as assisting the staff in the smaller (and less well-staffed clinic) with basic clerical tasks. Later, from 1995 to 1998, I spent time speaking with staff members at a detoxification clinic in Baltimore and attended a public function celebrating the anniversary of the opening of that clinic, which afforded an opportunity to become acquainted with some of the volunteers and patients. This chapter describes my findings in these settings, including reactions of staff and patients to working in such an environment, or to being treated there, as well as the manner in which they explain how the treatment works.

THE CLINIC SETTING

The philosophy of substance abuse treatment is holistic, meaning that it aims not only to alleviate a physical problem but also to address the patient's energetic, emotional, mental, social, and spiritual needs. All are viewed as interconnected and interactive, and a successful program, especially for a difficult condition such as substance abuse, may very well be more effec-

tive if several channels of intervention are used simultaneously. Typical clinics offer an array of interventions including, in addition to detoxification care, psychosocial modalities such as individual and group counseling, Narcotics Anonymous (NA) or Alcoholics Anonymous (AA) meetings, and life skills training where patients are encouraged to discuss educational and employment opportunities. Patients also may attend special groups such as those for women who are pregnant or have young children. In acupuncture detoxification clinics, practices such as Tai Chi or meditation may also be offered. In these settings, acupuncture care provides the energetic *foundation* for psychosocial care; it is the feature that permits patients to respond more effectively to psychosocial modalities, thus to "get their lives back on track."

Detoxification acupuncture in public (low-cost) clinics is also group care. Acupuncture detoxification practitioners commonly expend considerable effort to create an environment appropriate to people who may be unaccustomed to, or distrustful of, the one-on-one settings typical of private medical treatment. A common model is that of "family:" it is quite usual to observe patients sitting on chairs in a circle, listening to music, and chatting with practitioners or other patients as they rest with acupuncture needles in place. In addition to practitioners and patients, the group setting also typically includes a variety of volunteers, both in the form of students seeking acupuncture detoxification certification and of patients who have "graduated" (successfully quit substance abuse) from the acupuncture detoxification program. (The National Acupuncture Detoxification Association [NADA] offers certification for acupuncture detoxification on completion of a course, internship, and examination. Also see Chapter 14.)

Bronx Clinic

The largest of the three clinics observed was established in 1974 and situated in an extremely poor neighborhood in the Bronx, New York. A majority of the patient population was Latino, and the next largest patient group was African American. Although most patients were from the neighborhood, the clinic's fame and the fact that it also offered care for people with human immunodeficiency virus (HIV)-related problems drew people from throughout the New York metropolitan area. This clinic was completely drug-free, that is, there was no methadone maintenance program associated with it. By the early 1990s, the time of my field work, this clinic treated 200 to 300 patients each day. The staff included about 15 counselors with training specifically in detoxification ear acupuncture, and a handful of licensed professional certified acupuncturists who specialized in working with HIV-infected patients. The counselors' time was divided between intake interviews and orientations of new patients, counseling, providing auricular acupuncture treatments, and training interns and volunteers. Several counselors specialized in working with either the criminal justice or child welfare agency referrals. Most treatment was financed through Medicaid.

The work of interns and volunteers was important in maintaining a smooth flow of treatments. Interns and volunteers were usually addiction counselors or physicians, nurses, or community health workers who wished to learn the detoxification protocol and receive NADA certification. The NADA protocol calls for the insertion of four or five small needles (patients often call them "pins") at specific points on the ear. This is a simple technique, and many jurisdictions allow non-acupuncturists to administer the treatment provided they are supervised by a licensed acupuncturist or a biomedical doctor. Patients often participate in treatment by removing the "pins" themselves at the end of treatment sessions.

Although patients could receive a treatment from any number of people in the Bronx clinic, each was followed up by a primary counselor who conducted the intake interview and saw the patient on a regular basis. The intake interview consisted of a comprehensive psychosocial history that included several medical questions. The protocol for new patients consisted of daily acupuncture for 10 days, then 3 times a week for several months, and then as needed. Patients could be seen on an emergency basis before their scheduled intake interview and could be required to come to the clinic daily for 3 weeks or longer. Patients who experienced difficulty sleeping during drug withdrawal could receive a mild herbal mixture called "sleep mix" (see Chapter 14).

Each day the patient presented a urine sample, and a computerized printout of progress toward becoming completely drug-free became part of the individual's chart. The measured movement from "dirty" to "clean" urine values was used as a concrete reinforcement of progress during counseling sessions. Interestingly, traditional Chinese physicians often referred to pathological findings in terms of "dirt" (e.g., dirt in the blood). Thus the language of detoxification, in which dirty urine is a sign that further treatment is needed, coincides with the language of acupuncture.

The clinic as a community for healing and transformation is implicit in the substance abuse detoxification model. Text later in this chapter discusses how the Baltimore clinic has explicitly sought to build community. However, community building was implicit in the workings of the Bronx clinic. Each worker at the Bronx clinic was considered a part of the effort to help patients become drug-free and, as the director pointed out, to empower them. For example, the laboratory technician who had the tedious responsibility of testing the urine samples also spent time in the clinical area speaking with staff and especially with patients. Some of the counselors lived in the neighborhood from which the patient population was drawn and may have known some of the patients for years.

Aside from size (the Bronx clinic was the largest sampled), the most notable difference among the three clinics was noise level. At the Bronx clinic, announcements for meetings were called out. Cross-conversations were frequent, and many children were present. Newborns were often brought to the clinic and lay in bassinets while mothers received treatment, and some mothers held babies on their laps during treatment. The adults present, patients and staff both, managed to watch the older children even as they performed their official tasks. In addition to acupuncture treatment and NA meetings, women attended special women's groups focusing on such issues as protection from HIV infection, avoiding or escaping abusive relationships, and improving parenting skills.

When women referred by the child welfare system entered the program, they experienced a lengthy intake procedure and were given a special orientation. Some women were pregnant when they entered the program. In some cases, women had recently given birth to newborns whose urine test results were positive for illegal substances. Such children must remain in the hospital until the mother demonstrates a series of clean urine samples (although the mother is allowed to visit at feeding times). The mothers whom I met were anxious to take their children home and keep them there. This motivation resulted in significant bonding among the women as evidenced by comments such as, "I don't see my old friends any more. I just come here, go to meetings, and go home."

Brooklyn Clinic

Established in 1983, the Brooklyn clinic was in a small building on the campus of a very large metropolitan hospital. The possibility of violent crime concerned both staff and patients alike, although the few blocks from the subway to the clinic were lined with single- and two-family homes with small gardens and porches. However, these gardens and porches were secured with locked gates. The neighborhood included a large Caribbean population. The clinic served people of diverse races, religions, and ethnic groups, although African Americans predominated.

Patients entered the system somewhat differently in the three clinics, although all received referrals from the courts. In the Brooklyn clinic, referred or self-choice patients first registered with the hospital's substance abuse division and were then assigned to a primary clinic (inpatient detoxification, outpatient methadone maintenance, polysubstance abuse, or alcohol). They were then referred to the acupuncture clinic from their primary clinic.

At the acupuncture clinic, patients were required to comply with counseling. Inpatients received treatment in the same room with outpatients, some of whom began treatment as inpatients. All were advised to come daily in the beginning, then three times a week for several months; once they achieved detoxification, patients came on an as-needed basis. Payment was usually through Medicaid.

The Brooklyn clinic had a familial quality. Patients sat in large easy chairs, affording maximal comfort in a public setting. The clinic was staffed by two licensed acupuncturists who placed needles in patients' ears according to the NADA protocol. As the acupuncturists became better acquainted with their patients, other points were added to the treatment protocol. The patient rested in an easy chair for up to 40 minutes and then either removed the needles or waited for the acupuncturist to do so.

Although much quieter than the larger clinic in the Bronx, nevertheless there was a great deal of conversation about such topics as NA or AA meetings, politics, martial arts, and personal concerns. Patients freely offered advice to each other. If a staff member was receiving treatment, she or he would join in the general conversation. Once a recovering alcoholic patient and a counselor were engaged in conversation over the patient's concern that as he was also trying to stop smoking, he was eating a lot of sweets. The coun-

selor, with acupuncture needles in place, offered the observation that it was truly laudable to be able to give up alcohol and decrease cigarette smoking and reassured the patient that sometimes people replace one habit with another for a while. Thus at the detoxification clinic the social encounter and the therapeutic encounter overlap. In fact, the clinic may be viewed as a place of education as well as one of treatment.

COMMUNITY BUILDING

Because of the range of modalities offered and the group delivery setting, it is common for patient visits to detoxification clinics to last up to several hours. Because visits are also frequent and feelings of camaraderie and even ownership easily develop, the detoxification clinic can, with some effort from the staff, assume characteristics of a community. Not all clinics make this possibility overt; the Baltimore clinic, however, included the concept of "community building" in its initial design plans.

Baltimore Clinic

Baltimore's serious drug abuse problem was demonstrated in national surveys such as the Drug Abuse Warning Network.[5] For example, cocaine as a contributing factor to emergency department visits increased by 28% from 1990-1991 in the entire United States, but increased by 121% in Baltimore during the same time frame. Yet, as in other cities, treatment funds were decreasing despite the fact that treatment programs had never been adequate to deal with the problem. Detoxification acupuncture was proposed as one relatively inexpensive means to deal with this problem.

Acupuncturists from the Traditional Acupuncture Institute in Columbia, Maryland, had been using the NADA protocol to treat addicted women in Baltimore detention centers since the early 1990s. By interviewing these women, they discovered that the biggest patient concern was what to do after their jail sentence: how to maintain their freedom from drugs, how to reconnect with their families and a normal life, including paid employment. Their interviews led the practitioners to question how to combine the NADA protocol with their own intensively holistic approach to Chinese medicine, taking the whole into the Baltimore community to create a supportive environment for women leaving detention. With seed money from the Abell Foundation, in 1995 they established a Neighborhood Center that included an acupuncture detoxification clinic in a poor district of downtown Baltimore. Not coincidentally, the project was named the Community Health Initiative (CHI).

This clinic was organized somewhat differently from a clinic whose primary purpose is one of delivering health care. CHI set out, self-consciously, to build a community center *within which* was also contained an acupuncture detoxification clinic. This community center was linked by clientele and planning to local churches and other neighborhood meeting spots from the onset of planning. The intention was to serve and affect the entire community surrounding the clinic's Neighborhood Center, eventually making it an increasingly less attractive locale within which to take drugs. Patients were encouraged to bring friends, relatives, and significant others with them to the Center, all of whom were incorporated into treatment and the social life that developed around the clinic. Thus staff, patients, and significant others all join in the meditation, tai chi, Qi gong, and sign language classes at the Center. Persons affiliated with the Center also gather together on holidays, because "we're about building community." Members of the local community, even if not substance abusers, may receive acupuncture care and participate in support groups and Center educational and social activities.

The Center maintains a referral network for its substance abuse patients that includes sources of assistance with housing, education, and employment, as well as churches and Christian counseling. Those who successfully complete detoxification are invited to volunteer at the Center and sometimes are offered paid jobs. All who complete the detoxification protocol are "rewarded" by the opportunity to receive whole-body acupuncture health care and are encouraged to maintain continuing contact with the Center.

Interestingly, although certainly less intentional about their community building potential, the Bronx and Brooklyn clinics also welcomed close friends and relatives. In practice, the three clinics would not appear very different from each other in terms of their openness to community members. In many ways, the CHI program in Baltimore was a natural development of the work begun in the Bronx.

In 1998 the CHI Center was staffed with six volun-

teers who were either licensed acupuncturists or acupuncture students working under the guidance of a licensed acupuncturist, all with NADA certification. Funding comes from either individual or business donations, with a sliding fee scale of only $1 to $3 if the patient is currently unemployed. Although no one is turned away and staff members are very nurturing, they also recognize that patients should be encouraged to pay something. They need to "make a choice [of how to spend their money] compared to what they used to pay for drugs." There is no official child care program; instead, volunteers or staff simply "find someone" to be with the child as the caretaker undergoes treatment.

At the time of my visit to the Center in January 1998, approximately 60% of the patients were treated for substance abuse and 40% were receiving whole-body acupuncture. Many substance abuse patients just walk in, hearing about the clinic through other members of the community, whereas others are referred through the courts. Most patients used cocaine, heroin, or marijuana. At this clinic, staff members have found that alcoholism is more difficult to treat than drug abuse, and patients with a history of alcohol abuse must be under medical supervision; however, those with alcohol problems can be successfully treated.

In the 2½ years from April 1995 through January 1998, the clinic treated 700 patients. Attendance is somewhat unpredictable; although some patients arrive determined to complete the detoxification program, others attend for one or two sessions, drop out, and then return later to complete the program. Despite its self-concept as more of a community center than a medical clinic, patients begin their five-phase program with a heavy emphasis on treatment. To monitor response, urine samples are sent for toxicology tests, but not all decisions on a patient's progress are based on the status of urine test results. If a patient relapses, he or she may return to phase I. Regardless of the decision regarding treatment, staff members talk to patients about what happened. The concept behind counseling is that the patient assumes responsibility for his or her own recovery, and therefore it is important to discover the reason for using drugs again.

The five phases of the detoxification program are as follows:

Phase 1: Initially, the substance abusing patient comes to the clinic 5 days a week for 2 or 3 weeks. (The clinic hours are 9:30 to 11:30 AM and 5:30 to 7:00 PM Monday through Friday.) The patient receives auricular acupuncture while seated in a chair in a large open room with other patients. During treatments patients are engaged in life skills training during which they are mentored in a group setting to "move forward" with their lives. The patient is also required to attend NA or AA meetings at least three times a week (NA meetings are held at the clinic four times a week), and required to attend a weekly men's or women's support group.

Phase 2: The second phase is similar to phase 1, but the patient is only expected to attend clinic 3 or 4 days a week for a period of 2 or 3 weeks.

Phase 3: During phase 3, the intensity has decreased to only two or three treatment sessions a week.

Phase 4: This phase begins when the patient has not used illegal substances for 3 or 4 weeks. Treatment sessions occur approximately 2 days a week. This is when patients take a closer look at the question, "what *should* my life look like now?" The patient is encouraged to connect with other programs that can help with entry into the workforce (if the patient is unemployed), volunteerism, and education.

Phase 5: This phase is when patients are "getting back on their feet" and are no longer using drugs. They may be volunteers at the clinic, important to the community life and mentoring philosophies of the clinic, and providing a venue for those without funds to provide the clinic with needed services after they have received treatment at very low or no cost. At the same time, patients continue weekly treatments for general health.

In a sense, this final phase of treatment never ends. Patients are told that the program "lasts a lifetime." As they move back into the workforce, patients may return for monthly treatment and may continue to participate in the life of the clinic's community functions (e.g., meditation groups, celebrations).

LISTENING TO PATIENTS AND PRACTITIONERS

The philosophy of the Baltimore clinic is actualized in the treatment session itself. The patient enters the large treatment room and receives needles in the ear, after which he or she "chills out" for 15 or 20 minutes.

This time may also be used for meditation. The counselor spends about 10 minutes with each person individually, acting as a coach as the patient deals with life issues. Most patients are African American, although many of the volunteers are not (the director is African American). When asked how patients respond to coaching from counselors who have had different life experiences from them, the director responded saying that teaching and learning occur on both sides—for both patients and for counselors. He emphasizeed the critical nature of listening in working with patients, framing deep listening as a gift to be offered to patients: "We treat [patients] more like a family . . . you have to be here with a listening ear. That's where movement begins. . . . [I ask people] 'how is life serving you today?' In the asking of the question, I am very intent on offering deep listening."

The model for treatment described for Baltimore is a logical development of the model observed in New York City several years before the Baltimore center opened. It represents an adaptation to a smaller city that may have had more neighborhood cohesion at the location where the treatment was offered than was true for the sections of the Bronx or Brooklyn where I made my initial observations. Also, the Baltimore center was established with a far different funding structure, relying more heavily on foundation seed money, volunteerism, and donations than the hospital-based clinics. Therefore a presence in the community as a community-based center was necessary for building support. The detoxification model as developed by NADA and implemented in any setting is meant to be multimodal. One portion of the program is not considered more important than any of the others; rather the focus is on the individual person (within his or her community context) and not on the symptoms of withdrawal or the addiction itself.

DOES IT WORK?

In the nearly 10 years since I began the participant-observation study of detoxification acupuncture, the need for formal evaluation of its efficacy and long-term effectiveness has been recognized. Much of this evaluation hinges on controlled outcome studies and longitudinal research concerning recidivism. Yet, as just noted, detoxification acupuncture was never meant to be simply about placing a few needles in the ears of a patient and not offering other services. Indeed, it is one of several approaches working together to assist the patient in making a major change in the way he or she approaches life. Although controlled trials assessing whether the detoxification acupuncture potentiates the other arms of treatment (NA or AA meetings, other support groups, life skills training, and individual counseling) are certainly necessary, it is also very important to conduct qualitative studies that focus mainly on changes in quality of life and behavior, especially from the patient's point of view. Two of the broad questions that can be answered through a patient-centered interview or survey approach are "What do patients say that the detoxification acupuncture treatment does for them?" and "How do they understand the mechanism of treatment?"

In my own participant-observation study, patients revealed a range of opinions from relatively negative to markedly positive. Some patients stated that acupuncture decreased physical cravings, but this decrease was not enough to stay "clean." There was variation in experience with regard to how long it took to feel an effect from acupuncture treatment. Some said that this happened immediately, but others did not. One person said, "At first I thought it did nothing, then I noticed I did feel better." One man who tried acupuncture in the past without meetings, and meetings without acupuncture, found that, "Without my NA meetings, acupuncture would do nothing. Acupuncture can't tell me about drugs. NA can tell me about drugs because they have been there." Another opinion voiced by several patients was that church attendance was the critical component in successful treatment.

On the other hand, some detoxification patients were very pleased with the results of acupuncture, finding that it afforded much more help than they had experienced in previous attempts at becoming sober. One person with a 16-year habit (although not completely sober at the time of our discussion) found that acupuncture was helping her to have "clearer thoughts, calm down, and relax." Another, who had one prior experience with acupuncture that was not successful and had returned for 10 months at the time of our conversation, said, "Now it's part of me. It's been giving me a lot of self-confidence." This young man also credited his relationship with his counselor and tai chi lessons with these changes. Thus we return to the concept that detoxification acupuncture is an important part of a multimodal treatment in a community-based setting.

The following series of responses is from a brief, one-time survey by a colleague with the intention of exploring routes for future research. Despite their exploratory nature, these responses provide a window into the experience of patients and their reasons for staying with treatment. Table 9-1 lists the survey questions with the number responding favorably in each category. The parenthetical material denotes a follow-up question that was meant to invite more detailed narrative responses, which are presented in the text. The text also contains examples of responses by patients who were not satisfied with treatment.

Sample responses of patients who felt physically better with acupuncture treatment:

- Acupuncture helped with my addiction and with . . . an ulcer and a problem with heartburn.

TABLE 9-1

Patient Satisfaction*

Type of improvement	Are you feeling better with acupuncture care?†	Are things going better in your life?‡
Physically better	11	4
Emotionally/intellectually better	12	5
Socially better	5	9

*One-time in-clinic survey of 14 individuals receiving ear protocol detoxification acupuncture.
†What has changed for you?
‡Tell us about it.

- Symptoms of withdrawal are much reduced ... [I have a] generalized feeling of well-being and markedly less pain.
- I have more energy. My desire to do heroin is disappearing.
- I don't feel I need drugs, [and I] eat very well, walk a lot ... [and] play sports.
- [Acupuncture] curbs the craving for drugs.
- Not needing the drug as much as I was.
- [I] sleep better.
- [I] noticed a decrease in cigarette usage.

Responses of patients who felt emotionally and/or intellectually better:

- [I] no longer have to worry about my addiction.
- [It] gives me motivation to overcome my addiction ... [acupuncture] helped me realize what I've been doing to my body and helped me to do the right thing. ... [I] feel good about myself and I don't want to use anymore.
- [I have] a better outlook on myself.
- I do not have the craving for drugs I did before acupuncture care.
- I feel relaxed.
- My compulsive activities have lessened. ... [I] let go of my bad marriage. ... [And] control anger more easily.
- I feel more focused.
- I'm not chasing drugs ... I look forward to doing better because I have more to look forward to.

Responses of patients who noted improvements in social relations:

- I feel much better during my working day.
- My kids love me more and my family is happy that I'm getting help.
- I have changed my day-to-day program and look forward to getting more acupuncture treatments.
- During the time of my drugging I would get ill within a half hour of getting up. And today I can get up to do my personal hygiene, and start some household chores. ... I don't get ill for hours and I have slacked down on the usage.
- Now I'm starting back to work, which keeps me together.
- My addiction caused my performance at work to go downhill ... [Now I have] respect for my work.
- I'm back in church and doing the things I'm supposed to do and staying out of trouble.
- My relationships with family and friends are a lot better.
- Now that I am in school, I don't have to stand on the corner, and do bad things.

Examples of comments classified as dissatisfied:

- I'm feeling better, just a little. But I think I would be much better if this program would give me something for my pains.
- [Things are going better] somewhat, but a lot of my problems are personal.
- A little better, but not like it should be.

Further patient-centered interview and observational research is needed to better understand the factors that patients interpret as the benefits of acupuncture treatment for substance abuse. It does appear that most patients agree with the first description of the purpose of detoxification acupuncture that I ever heard, a statement an acupuncturist made to a rather nervous-looking patient during one of my first observation periods. The acupuncturist explained that treatment would help the patient to *calm down and sit through meetings, as she experienced less craving* than she would without it. Considering the evidence that "becoming sober"—whether from drugs or alcohol—is such a difficult process, it would seem that the auricular acupuncture approach provides a cost-effective mechanism for assisting persons as they progress through the other components of treatment.

With regard to mechanism of action, there are even fewer research findings, perhaps because the manner in which patients understand action is probably less salient to whether they continue with treatment than the question of whether treatment supports detoxification and the rebuilding of social life. Nevertheless, the question does stimulate interest in practitioners and patients alike and may shed light on how best to frame treatment to maximize compliance. An observation made early in my own participant-observation study supports the idea that patients perceive a general calming effect from acupuncture that potentiates other treatment components. Some patients were familiar with research concerning neurochemicals and were aware that needling could release these chemicals, resulting in a "mellow high." Others discussed ideas with their counselors concerning electrical energy or Qi flowing through Meridians, noting a feeling of electricity when the needle is placed on an acupuncture point. Although these ideas seemed to intrigue patients and may have added an interest in coming for treatment, it seems unlikely that the esoteric nature of acupuncture would be sufficient to promote patient retention. Rather, it is more likely that the holistic and community-based nature of the treatment was more compelling to patients as they returned and then began to see results.

SUMMARY

This chapter provides insight into the workings of public acupuncture clinics that treat addiction to illegal substances or alcohol, especially among the poor. Several issues that should be addressed through further research were also introduced and are discussed more fully in Chapter 14. Together these chapters can assist readers in decision-making concerning the appropriateness of referring patients with addictions to a setting that offers acupuncture as a part of a holistic program including group and individual support, and perhaps other activities geared toward improving community life.

References

1. Bullock ML, Culliton PD, Olander RT: Controlled trial of acupuncture for severe recidivist alcoholism, *Lancet* 1:1435-9, 1989.
2. Konefal J, Duncan R, Clemence C: The impact of the addition of an acupuncture treatment program to an existing Metro-Dade County outpatient substance abuse treatment facility, *J Addict Dis* 13:71-99, 1994.
3. Konefal J: *Acupuncture and addictions. NIH Consensus Development Conference on Acupuncture, program and abstracts,* Bethesda, Md, Nov 3, 1997, Office of the Director, National Institutes of Health.
4. Hare ML: *East Asian medicine among non-Asian New Yorkers,* [dissertation], graduate faculty of The New School for Social Research, 1992, New York.
5. Abell Foundation: Baltimore's drug problem: it's costing too much not to spend more on it, Baltimore, 1991, The Foundation.

10

A Day in the Life
Practitioners Reflect on Their Daily Lives

JANE A. GRISSMER

W. JUMBÉ ALLEN

JINGYUN GAO

PAULETTE C. HILL

ROBERT L. FELT

QI
Lingering like gossamer, it has only a hint of existence:
And yet when you draw upon it, it is inexhaustible.

TAO TE CHING[1]

SECTION 1: NOTES OF A QI TENDER

JANE A. GRISSMER

I began my work as an acupuncturist lured by my experience of a phenomenon called *Qi*. As a patient I sensed it; as a massage therapist I felt it; as a human being I stood in awe of its mystery. Twenty years later it is still a wonder to touch a point at the ankle and watch back pain ease, or touch a point on the palm of the hand and see a patient break out in a peal of laughter, or touch a point on the top of the foot and hear the patient say, "I can see more clearly."

What is this that connects the ankle to the back, the palm of the hand to laughter, and the top of the foot to the eyes? I cannot answer this question. Yet I have worked with this system long enough to know

178

that the connections are there. And that through these connections patients begin to weave themselves together, top to bottom, inside to outside, body to mind to spirit.

What is this that can move so fast? Qi is resonance; it is vibration. In my hands it is ripples on a pond or waves on a shore. Words like "gather and fill," "release and move," "sink and rise," "open and hold" are operative. Its immediacy still amazes me. I daily witness a patient's experience transform in the course of treatment. Pain gives way to ease; rage gives way to forgiveness; dryness gives way to moisture; isolation gives way to connection; stiffness gives way to flexibility, resignation gives way to hope; fatigue gives way to motivation. These shifts of being are my daily fare. They are just some of the magical moments I witness and share.

Qi is everywhere—in plants and animals and the air we breathe and the food we eat, in the beat of a heart, the flash of anger, the taste of sour, the wound that heals, the first and last breath. It is in all creation, and all creation participates in the flow of Qi. It is the movement of life within us and around us and through time. As a tender of this great Qi, I hold within myself a unique set of laws and principles by which Qi circulates and renews itself. The same laws that govern nature—the cycles of day and night and the seasons—govern my work with Qi. For my patients, I am a reminder of their participation in this great mystery and the process of healing and change. It is in this spirit of mystery and oneness that I greet my first patient of the day.

THE WHOLE PERSON

The job of the doctor of acupuncture is to see each person as whole in body, mind, spirit with every possibility of their unique being realized.

J. R. WORSLEY[2]

There is no normal in my day. There are only people seeking wholeness and aliveness. For each I ask— where is that to be found? Most begin their healing journey focused only on a symptom and most open to see that their symptom is part of a much larger construct. Joan is a breast cancer survivor who has discovered that her best insurance in this situation is to live her life fully. My contract with her is to keep her awake and alive to the movements of life through her. When she falls asleep, I help her wake up. When she

bogs down, I help her move forward. When she can't quiet down, I help her to settle. And at the moment she is beating the odds. Six years out from a bone marrow transplant, she has just finished her first year without any chemotherapy. Her oncologist is an artist too. He senses Joan, and he carefully chooses the drug regimen that is appropriate for her. Although we have never met, he and I are in partnership with Joan on her journey.

John has discovered that his stiff neck relates to the abrasive arguments he has with his wife, that his physical body tightens to protect the vulnerability he feels in his heart. I help him understand this connection and teach him to listen to his body so that he can hold himself from reaction and personal wounding when he is in the battle zone. John begins to understand himself more deeply and he begins to find a way to bring the strength of his heart forward instead of shrinking behind the contractions in his neck. He learns from this experience that body and mind are partners in the whole.

David at 48 tells me of his heart malfunctions and that if they continue he may need a pacemaker. Together we uncover that in his role as leader of an organization he has gone so far to the edge by himself that he is at risk of losing control. In learning about the heart as something broader than a mechanical device, namely that the heart is akin to the king on the throne who holds the whole of the kingdom, David discovers something about his heart—that he needs to enlist the support of family and colleagues. He learns that the wise and healthy leader knows how to rely on others.

One of the great joys of being an acupuncturist is that I dispense a wise medicine. It heals and it teaches. To use acupuncture as only technique is analogous to using a computer as only a typewriter. Its scope and possibility are so much greater. And so while I am focused on a stiff shoulder, using moxa (a warming substance placed on an acupuncture point) to kindle the flow of warmth into the area to support the healing of damaged tissue, I am also aware that these points promote the emotion of joy and that Ann is lacking laughter in her voice, is ashen in color, and is sad in emotion. And so right there we create joy together and we inquire how she can find it in her own life. As I sense her spirit moving I know her shoulder will likely follow.

For each we uncover that seamless place where body, mind, and spirit intersect. In the uncoverings and in the uniqueness of the interconnections that this system of healing offers, people rediscover themselves as whole and they learn uniquely how to balance and tend themselves.

THE SENSES

My assessment tools sound archaic in this age of technological medicine and yet ironically, simply because they are ancient, they go right to the essential nature of each person. Observing the colors on the face, hearing the sound of the voice, smelling the odor of the body, touching the 12 pulses, interacting deeply and broadly enough to know the emotional range of the patient, I quickly get in beneath all the labels as I pay attention to the subtle cues and signs. I am acutely aware of the difference between looking and seeing; between listening and hearing. I am able to discern what on the surface remains a mystery. The sensory phenomena tell me not so much the "what" of the illness but the "how" of it—the context in which the disease is occurring. Just yesterday a 65-year-old woman with a history of cancer came for her first visit. She grabbed me as I walked by, insistent to let me know that she was here and that life was at the moment a complaint for her. Before her history was taken, just by using my senses, this patient had already begun to tell me what she needed. My words to her, my presence with her, and the choice of points, were beginning to take shape.

THE MEDICINE POUCH

When I enter the treatment room I open my medicine pouch. Like many traditional healers I carry what I need with me. These are the tools that sustain the patient and me on our quest (Box 10-1).

The patient and I come together in partnership, sharing the responsibility for the outcome. I am more

of a guide than an expert in exploration of the movement of Qi within.

I cultivate myself as a healing presence. It is a lifetime of work. It requires that I evolve as a keen observer of self, of others, and of nature; that I sustain a willingness to explore and stand in my own fears, angers, joys, needs, and griefs.

I have learned that the most potent treatments are those in which technique is housed in presence, words, and touch—where I am as much an instrument as the needle itself. For instance, Sue's response to *Not at Ease* (Stomach 19) grows with the nourishment and ease that I create with her. Mindy's response to *Spirit Gate* (Heart 7) expands with the laughter and compassion I bring into the room. Nick's response to *Bright and Clear* (Gall Bladder 37) emerges with the direction and distinctions I offer. In these moments, the needle, the point, the patient, and I are one.

The acupuncture points and the Spirits they call forth grace my day. They are metaphors for our journey through life, heralding and bringing to our awareness moments along the way. At the end of the eleventh rib is *Chapter Gate* (Liver 13). It not only relieves the cramping and pain that accompanies menstrual or digestive distress but it also gives birth to a vision, opening a new course or direction in ourselves. At the bottom of the foot is *Bubbling Spring* (Kidney 1). It not only nourishes the fascia of the foot but it also taps the juice for renewed drive or generativity, where we find faith in the possibility of something new to come. On the palm of the hand is *Palace of Weariness* (Pericardium 8). It not only settles anxiety and agitation but it also opens a saddened and worn heart to renewed joy and pleasure in relationships. On the back of the knee is *Yin Valley* (Kidney 10). It not only strengthens the knees and back but it also taps the capacity for rest and quiet to gather stamina for the road ahead. Instead of arteries, organs, and bones, I more often see a village landscape of mountains, streams, valleys, ditches, gates, and palaces. These are some of the images with which I spend my day.

SPIRIT

What is the spirit? The spirit cannot be heard with the ear. The eye must be brilliant of perception and the heart must be open and attentive, and then the spirit is suddenly revealed through one's own consciousness.

BOX 10-1

Tools on Our Quest

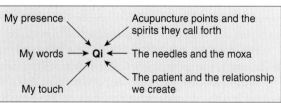

*It cannot be expressed through the mouth; only the heart
    can express*
*all that can be looked upon. If one pays close attention
    one may*
*suddenly know it but one can just as suddenly lose this
    knowledge.*
*But shen, the spirit, becomes clear to man as though the
    wind has blown away the cloud. Therefore one speaks
    of it as spirit.*

CHI PO, *The Yellow Emperor's Classic of Internal Medicine*[3]

Although some of my patients seek to heal a recently injured arm or knee, most come with chronic conditions that have worn their spirits over time as much as their bodies. I listen for the depth. How deep is the wound or injury from which the symptom is emerging? Worse than Martha's muscular pain was the resignation in life that now accompanied her. And without her spirit engaged there is little hope of her body healing. To raise a spirit that has been buried and neglected—to warm it with moxa, to kindle it with presence, to sense it begin to come alive—this is one of the greatest privileges of my day. I place five moxa on *Spirit Deficiency* (CV 8) located at the navel where we receive the vital essences and vital spirits in utero. When a baby is born there is a fresh and curious spirit for life. It is this same quality that I seek to reawaken. With fire and needle and intent and holding myself as an instrument, I watch as something more becomes possible.

I have learned that healing the spirit is critical. Without its presence the life force is weakened and vulnerable. I remember Kate's diagnosis of chronic fatigue syndrome and being on disability for the past 2 years. She had no hope of a normal life and no place to hold the devastation that she had experienced. I called on the point *One Hundred Meetings* (GV 20), at the top of the head, a gathering place of the ancestors, a spot from which flows the greatest view or vantage point a human being can have. Here the subtle energy body raises and expands our awareness to encompass the whole in which all things have their place and order. Even the most downtrodden can be lifted in spirit when they have a glimpse of the greater whole. For Kate this meant she had a meaningful context in which to hold her experience. After the use of GV 20, her treatments began to be effective and she found her way back to work and marriage.

The elegance and refinement that this system offers for working at the level of the Spirit is humbling.

Patients come with the label "depression." I need to know more. If we take the label away, what is your experience? Is it a sinking of will or desire for life, an absence of engagement or purpose, an emptiness or a longing, a lack of hope or possibility? Points such as *Spirit Burial Ground, Spirit Storehouse, Gate of Hope, Soul Door, Gate of Life, Great Deficiency,* and *Broken Bowl* assist the patient and me to breathe vitality, resiliency, and light into the dark and deadened.

NATURE

Health is a way of life.

What Season? This is a critical question in my treatment room. If it is Winter and Ann is not storing, then it is my role to assist her in aligning her way of being with that of nature. She needs to understand the importance of sleeping more for the next 3 months. If it is Spring and Dan is not finding new growth or new horizons to search, then I register concern for his overall health and well-being. I know after 20 years of practice that if we miss the movement of a Season through us, like a plant, our vitality, resiliency, and beauty are diminished. My patients have much in common with my star cactus. For years it sat in a window with low-level light and it grew only one or two small blossoms. When I placed it in a south window and it received all the sun it needed, the beauty of its blossoms was dazzling.

I assist nature and nature heals. Like a gardener I am always cognizant of the time of year and the possibilities, as well as the limitations, that each season brings. Carol was stuck in the past. At menopause and her only child now 18, she felt her life was over. She could only lament what was no longer and could find little enthusiasm for what lies ahead. She kept trying to recreate herself but nothing would take root. Her ground was filled with the dead plants and leaves of who she had been. With the arrival of Fall I sensed it was her time of opportunity. In treating *Joining the Valleys* (Colon 4), the official that "lets go of the old to make way for the new," I counseled her to clear away who she had been. I advised her to lie with a clean, empty field that would be welcome ground for new seeds and visions in the Spring. With this prescription Carol was able to place herself back in the generative cycle of life.

This is a medicine rooted in nature. Qi is nature. And when we work with Qi we must work with the laws by which it moves and flows. To do less than that—to squeeze it into any other paradigm—is to lose the power of its healing potential. In the connections of body to mind to spirit, in the alignment with nature and her cycles, in the openings to the movement of life through us, this is where the healing power of Qi is found.

References

1. Wu JCH: *Lao Tzu/Tao Te Ching*, New York, 1961, St. John's University Press, p. 9.
2. Worsley JR: Personal class notes, 1975.
3. Veith I: *The Yellow Emperor's classic of internal medicine*, Berkeley, Calif, 1949, University of California Press, p. 222.

SECTION 2: COMMITTING TO CHANGE

W. JUMBÉ ALLEN

My name is W. Jumbé Allen. I have been practicing traditional Chinese medicine (TCM) over the past 10 years in the San Francisco Bay area. This is not what I planned to do with my life, even though now it is hard to imagine a life not filled with this work. In my undergraduate days at Berkeley, I decided to combine my interests in photography and cultural diversity. I thought of myself as a visual anthropologist. Anthropology, despite its racist and colonialist roots, added legitimacy to my own desire to decipher cultural artifacts and to understand cultural outlooks that were radically different than my own. As a photographer, and then as a filmmaker, I traveled to Asia. While in the Philippines to photograph psychic healers, I worked for 2½ years on the film *Apocalypse Now*. By the end of that filming, my interest in Asian healing arts was set on course.

I went on to study in Taiwan, Hong Kong, and eventually mainland China. My appreciation for the Asian paradigms of healing grew. To my mind, what has been labelled in the United States as Chinese medicine offers a fundamental difference to Western medicine at this stage in its development. Diagnosis and treatment in Chinese medicine have the advantage of many different tools; it is customized to respond to the patient's physical environment and personal history, and honors the interplay between the physical, emotional, spiritual, and mental aspects. Thus my studies of acupuncture have always been integrated with studies of herbology, nutrition, psychology, and various movement arts, such as tai chi, Qi gong, and later Awareness Through Movement and Functional Integration.

I begin the morning with a commute across the Bay Bridge from my home in Oakland to a citywide central intake unit for substance abuse treatment in San Francisco. This public health program, Target Cities, is a 5-year federal project to assess and assign patients to appropriate treatment programs. Today I will provide a free auricular acupuncture session for many of these patients. As a co-founder of Pacific Acupuncture Associates, I have provided these daily treatments for the past 3½ years, using the National Acupuncture Detoxification Association (NADA) protocol, which is auricular treatment of 5 points in each ear (see Chapter 14).

When Target Cities first opened, patients came in one or two times for assessment and pretreatment group counseling and then were assigned to a waiting list for an appropriate program opening. These programs range from day treatment to residential settings, with various time commitments. The most difficult patients to place and those with the longest wait are those with a dual diagnosis of both drug usage and mental illness. Before the introduction of the acupuncture protocol, Target Cities found that patients frequently dropped out during the waiting period.

However, in the first week that acupuncture was added, patient retention doubled. Patients in preplacement now receive acupuncture services for as long as it takes to find placement. Patients often arrive early for treatment, staying for group counseling afterward, spending approximately 3 to 4 hours a day in the clinic, up to 5 times a week. Dependent on often unreliable public transportation schedules, they are determined not to miss their acupuncture treatment sessions.

This morning I am treating 20 men and women. Many are homeless, some have acquired immunodeficiency syndrome (AIDS) and hepatitis, many suffer from depression, schizophrenia, mania, and paranoia. Their drug use ranges from the illegal heroin, crack, cocaine, methamphetamine, and ice to the legal drugs of alcohol, methadone, and various prescription drugs. They sit in chairs arranged in a large circle. I insert five needles in both ears of each patient. The room is crowded, yet a wall of tall windows bathes the room with sunlight and provides a sense of warmth and spaciousness. A tape of Miles Davis's "Kind of Blue" is playing. The sounds of Mission Street traffic and hustling are muted. I tell them that they are in this room because they choose to be in this room. They are choosing to work on recovery.

I stimulate the auricular points for the Lung, Liver, Kidney, Sympathetic Nervous System, and Shenmen (Neurogate). The part of Chinese medicine that I can bring to them is acupuncture. The part of acupuncture that I use with them are the points for substance abuse. For the next 45 minutes, they will sit quietly, their agitation, cravings, and irritability dissipating. After treatment, several patients approach me to report the easing of tension they experience. Such testimonies are common. They claim the profundity of their experience and tell me that they are determined to return the next day and the day after.

At the end of today's session, they are a little more available, a little more alert, and a little more willing to connect with their own internal healing dynamic. Their bodies approach a state of homeostasis, what in Chinese medicine we call a state of balance between the Yin and the Yang. Today, O, who had been using speed for 14 years before acupuncture, has an announcement—he is not going to come during the December holidays as he plans to vacation "down under" in Australia where it's warm. This is great news for all of us in the room. Four years ago, O had a diagnosis of AIDS. Years of unprotected sex with multiple partners exposed him to human immunodeficiency virus (HIV). When he first started acupuncture, he was weak and tired. He had a constant cough and was often depressed and irritable. He had cashed in his life insurance policy, sure that he would not have much time to live. Yet O had the desire to stop his drug abuse. He has received acupuncture treatments 5 days a week for 9 months and he has been free of speed all that time. His health has stabilized and his pattern of intermittent hospital stays has ended. Now O takes his medications conscientiously, exercises, and pays better attention to his lifestyle. He will take a friend from our program with him to Australia. He says they'll help keep each other clean and on the path. Both plan to seek acupuncture care during their vacation and asked me for an NADA-affiliated center.

My afternoon begins in my private office elsewhere in San Francisco with another announcement: "It's a boy, 7 pounds, 9 ounces and healthy!" The new mother's voice on my office answering machine is strong and joyful. She has been my patient for the past 19 months. She came to me after the trauma of 4 miscarriages in 3 years. At that time, B was 41 years old and a respected film producer. Her hours were long and arduous. Depressed, she often could not sleep, missed meals, and was beginning to have bowel difficulties—alternating constipation and diarrhea. Allergic reactions and colds were frequent. B had planned to have a child in her late 30s. When she came to my office after the miscarriages, she recognized that her physical, emotional, and mental imbalance was preventing her from achieving her deepest desire—to have a child.

When we began to work together on her health and her quest for a child, I explained that it would require a complete examination of her modes of behavior, her attitudes, lifestyle, and her commitment to her own self. Health, I explained, is a balance between body, mind, and spirit. I would see her once a week but the real work belonged to her. She had to commit to change. Because she was in a seriously deficient condition, I advised her not to become pregnant for a minimum of half a year.

However, in the second month of treatment, she became pregnant and had another miscarriage. It would be another 7 months of weekly treatments and herbal prescriptions before her health improved enough that I could recommend that she and her husband go on a second honeymoon. The acupuncture sessions not only helped her physically but gave her balance and finally clarity. There was now enough room and strength in her life to welcome a child.

Now as I prepare to see my afternoon's scheduled clients, I reflect on the seemingly different practices of public health and private practice. Both are important to me and I see my life as always containing these two forms of healing. The meager funding of public health demands a group approach and this actually has some advantages. Most of the patients who come into the group have lost the skills to make survival decisions. My job is to weave the group together, encouraging everyone to use their various strengths to compensate for their various weaknesses. Together, the group develops a momentum. Together, they build an image of recovery and generate an excitement about getting there. Private practice, on the other hand, is a one-on-one dynamic. Here, my job is to help individual patients become more aware of how they can articulate and provide for their particular health needs. I must exercise all my training and skills to diagnose and design a particular treatment. In this setting, I have time to hear a lengthy life history, and I may suggest herbs/diet changes or exercises to accompany the acupuncture treatments. I customize the treatment to each patient, and every visit is calibrated to changes in the patient's emotional, mental, and physical environment.

Public health and private practice are both central to my life. I believe that Chinese medicine was always meant to be widely accessible. It is my pleasure to share this tradition with people whose socially marginal positions conventionally exclude them from treatment. I also enjoy the opportunity to challenge my healing skills in the depth and intimacy that is possible in private practice. While these two practices balance me as a healer exactly because they nourish me differently, I also understand these two practices as coming from the same source. My goal in both public and private practice is to bring my patients into a balance and to encourage them to listen to their own healing wisdom.

SECTION 3: *XIN DA YA:* MY THREE KEYS TO TEACHING

JINGYUN GAO*

CC: What first attracted you to acupuncture practice?

JG: That's back to 1978 [when] I started college. I graduated from high school but I didn't have a chance to go to college directly. So after 3 years of vocational school I got a chance to take the [university entrance] examination and went to a Chinese medicine university. My grandfather was a Chinese doctor so I [felt] some influence from him. But he had never taught me details. Even in college he didn't teach me. He said, "I have a lot of good formulas. But until you graduate you won't understand this." So I was always kind of curious, you know, but that was just the initial influence. I learned more and appreciated more when I went to the school. And I best appreciated [Chinese medicine] when, after 5 years of studying in the school, I graduated and became a teacher.

Even now when I'm teaching I always emphasize review, because first [you have to] study everything piece by piece, and sometimes you doubt, you question, what to know. But later, when you understand, you can put all the [pieces together] just like you play a piece of music.

CC: Did your grandfather give you some formulas after you graduated?

JG: Yeah. He gave some and I tried them and they are really good. Some, you know, some herbs he had kept a long time, almost his lifetime, like deer gall blad-

der, bile, things to cool down the Blood, to purify the Blood, to cool Heat. I tried this [gall bladder] essence he gave me.

CC: How do you mean, he gave you the essence?

JG: I just felt that he was leading me to the [most] interesting [aspects] of Chinese medicine, to know the power of the healing. And also, to see the patient recover, you feel a reward. Before [graduation, when] I saw his gall bladder, I said, "Let me have one piece to try!" And he said, "No, this is a kind of essence, you cannot have it until you understand what it's for," so he didn't let me touch. [Laughter]

CC: You finished high school and then you went to vocational school. Was that by your choice or was that the Cultural Revolution?

JG: That's the Cultural Revolution,[†] yeah. I just wanted to continue to study because a high school education was not enough for me. During that time we had Cultural Revolution we really didn't have much time to study, not enough. I wanted to continue my studies [and there was no] college, but they did have vocational school. After the Cultural Revolution there were *ten* years [worth of] students [who had not been able to go to] college, so [everyone went] together for examination, [knowing that] only 10% would get a chance to enter the school.

CC: Everyone 18 to 28 or something? And only 10% pass?

---

*In the following conversation, CC is Claire Cassidy, also a student of Dr. Gao (JG). Words in square brackets are inserted to smooth delivery in the English language.

†During the Cultural Revolution all colleges and universities were closed by the Chinese government.

JG: Yeah. Only 10% pass and only 3% to 4% enter. Ten percent pass but they only can admit maybe 3%. So we [who were admitted] really appreciated that we got a chance to go to college.

CC: And did you choose acupuncture, or was that where there was room to go?

JG: I chose chemistry actually, but they sent me to Chinese medicine university. My first choice was chemistry. I don't know why, but I really liked it in high school, seeing all the different changes, the color changes. . . . So it [would have been] totally different if I [had chosen], but then [I said to myself] "oh my grandfather is a Chinese medical doctor so [it's OK if] I get the Chinese medicine university."

CC: They knew about him? He made a request?

JG: No. No, he didn't make a request. Just by chance they chose me.

CC: Looking back for a moment, what did you do during the Cultural Revolution?

JG: Cultural Revolution, we just go follow the activities. I think when I was in third grade we started the Cultural Revolution, you know. So we [little children] just didn't know, we followed the activities. And missed some schooling.

CC: In class you mentioned being a cobbler and you made a link between being a cobbler and being an acupuncturist. Could you talk about that?

JG: Yeah. I [studied to be] a shoemaker in vocational school because I wanted to continue my study. [Shoemaking was] also not my choice. But [everyone in school was in] the same situation. We just wanted to continue school! We studied math and other practical things, electronics, and we also studied to be designers for shoes and to work in the shoe companies. We actually had a half-day study, half-day work. Then after 2 years of vocational school, I became a teacher. I like teachers, I don't know why! I have always felt teachers were important in my life. And also, I like teaching. I always [feel that] good teachers give me inspiration, and poor teachers—I always feel sorry for them. I wished I could be a teacher so I would have this kind of full feeling. So I was a [vocational school] teacher for half a year. Then I got chance to take the [university entrance] examination, so I left the vocational school and I went to college.

CC: So what's the link between making shoes and acupuncture?

JG: I would say, when I do acupuncture I always see more. [As with] shoes, you *see* the physical imagery, you *see* the shoe design, but [also] when you look at the shoe you always think about what kind of person would wear this shoe, what kind of posture, what kind of mind and figure [this person might] have. It's not just the shoe on the floor. We always put the shoe on the table, looked at it from different angles . . . and I always could *see* the person [who would] wear the shoe. Because, you know, the person [is going to] match the shoes. So when I see the patient, [think about using particular] acupuncture points, I [can] think about how the points work more vividly, how they move the Qi, how they send the energies, how they open the Channels, clear the heat, calm down the Mind. I always *feel* this kind of energy as I see the shoe. I feel this shoe is for walking, this shoe for [being] comfortable, this shoe for [being] elegant . . . just like you dress for your personality. So when I later see the points, the Channels, I always have this kind of image in my mind.

CC: Did those images come because you understand what those points do, or are they from the names of the points?

JG: Mostly from the experience. I use the points that have exactly the [right] feeling. When I think of each point's function, when I teach the points, always there is some patient's response picture in my mind, in front of me. Some people cry, some people have fullness in the chest, some people have their minds open, release this tension. [For each] point [I have a] different face in front of me. So when I [work] I really *feel,* I *try* to move the Qi, I *try* to calm you down. Each point is kind of alive in front of me, when I teach, and when I see [a patient].

CC: When you finished studying at Shanghai University of Traditional Chinese Medicine, did you become a teacher there?

JG: Yeah. I became a teacher. At that time we have our choice at graduation. So my first choice was to do study in the research lab; I wanted to do Channel study. Second choice was to be a teacher. Third choice, work in the emergency room. I liked to see acupuncture emergency room treatment of acute conditions. So much different from what I'm doing now! [Laughter] Somehow [in China] I would [treat] more physical things, but when I came out [of China] it [went] the other way! [Anyway, people] selected to be teachers must have all straight A's, all tests over 90%. [In] our class of 52 students we had 9 or 10 apply for this teacher job. Then each [had] like 20 minutes demonstration, [observed by] teachers and other students, you know, grading us. Finally only 2 people [were selected to] be teachers in the acupuncture department.

[My class was] the first to graduate, you know, after this 10 years.

CC: One of the interesting things about Chinese medicine schools is that they have lots of students who are not young.

JG: Yeah, we had totally 12 years difference, new students just graduated high school and then us, the oldest, *twelve years* difference, which makes a circling with the Chinese numbers.* So, you know, you have the [young] Rabbit and then another *big* Rabbit older than you, all in the same class, same dormitories. And sometimes it's a little hard, when you are 30 or 20, different memories, different ways to study, [ways of] thinking. [Laughing] But we all cooperated. Because we older students always appreciated that we got a chance. We caught the last training; otherwise we [would not have had] time to study.

[First semester] was not very interesting, all the Chinese stuff to study, you know, Chinese medicine. We [were assigned to] the old hall, old building, 300 to 400 students together. The teacher could recite everything, but we didn't have any detailed book to study. He just told us that he wanted to get us the *feeling.* Before you exactly know what's the Fire, what's the Metal, he wants us to get the feeling, just like music. You have to get the *sensation,* then [later on] you get detailed notes. So we all think, "oh, it's so *old!*" and sometimes we don't understand [what he means] but we *follow* his tone, repeat and repeat. *Then* we get it. Otherwise [had we started with textbooks] we wouldn't have understood. You need to get this kind of influence, you know, before you go detailed.

And we always had conflict between Western medicine† and Chinese medicine. Western medicine we [could] clearly see the stomach, liver, heart . . . but Chinese medicine was always different. You [learn that the] Liver stores the Blood in Chinese medicine; in Western medicine the spleen stores the blood. So all different functions, you know? The first year was a little bit hard but we were always laughing. We didn't laugh at ourselves [for being] stupid, you know, we laughed at Chinese medicine [for being] not settled. But later, second year, third year, [when] you really understand—we [were] laughing at ourselves.

CC: How do you mean Chinese medicine was not well settled?

JG: You see, in Western medicine you can explain. [But in] Chinese medicine you ask "why" and [the teachers] always say "Because *Nei Ching* say, because *Nei Ching* say!"* always use Nei Ching as the Bible. But *why?* Why Yin-Yang cannot be separated? *Why* Yin-Yang can transform into each other? "Because *Nei Ching* said 'Yin Yang can transform into each other' in certain conditions." They all have this philosophy and they don't have any questions! Just like, now, people ask, "Why can acupuncture relieve pain?" [And the answer a Chinese medical practitioner will give is] "Because acupuncture can remove the stagnation. Because it works." But American modern scientists try to do more research because they have questions. The Chinese doctor just says "It works!" and we don't care why! We know *how* to relieve the pain, how to treat and select points. That time [at school] we had questions, but our teacher always said "Because *Nei Ching* has this answer." [And in fact] when you get familiar with Chinese medicine, when you get used to it, then it becomes your own, and you don't have to think "why"; you *know.*

CC: How long did you practice in China?

JG: I practiced 8 years in the university and also the Long Hua (Chinese Dragon) hospital. It's an old hospital affiliated with Shanghai University of TCM.

CC: What brought you to the United States?

JG: Actually I had a chance to meet some U.S. acupuncturists [who] came to visit our school. I introduced our school and shared our research on the Channels. Then they wanted me to give a lecture here on using acupuncture to treat gynecological disorders. So I come for a visit. And Dr. Ralph Coan said he was thinking about a school.† They already had organized but hadn't got it past the Maryland Higher Education Board, so he asked me to stay another month to help the school get the curriculum done.

CC: It's been longer than a month! How long have you been here?

JG: Oh dear! [Laughing] I've been here for almost 9 years . . . this November [2000].

CC: You going to stay?

JG: Yeah, I plan to stay. That's why after [being] so

---

*The Chinese astrological calendar has 12-year cycles; each cycle is named for an animal. The older are expected to encourage and support their "little brothers and sisters."
†Biomedicine.

*Nei Ching, Yellow Emperor's Textbook of Chinese Medicine, the first textbook of Chinese medicine, assembled 2 to 4 centuries BCE.
†Ralph Coan, MD, founded the Maryland Institute of Traditional Chinese Medicine in Bethesda, Maryland, in 1991.

long separated, my family finally joined me 2 years ago. My husband and my daughter.

CC: You now have a full-time practice here in Washington, D.C. What is that like to practice in the United States?

JG: Practicing in the United States is somewhat different from in China. In China most people come in more often, like three times a week. Here people are more busy and they come once a week, every other week. They want more effective treatment with long duration. In China you usually take like 30 minutes with one patient [and see them frequently], and often after a short period of time they can be dismissed [with the condition "OK"]. Here, most people, even those you treat to wellness, want to keep [on coming]. They want [treatment] for well-being, so some people they come for years . . . for health maintenance.

CC: Because they want health maintenance and well-being. And in China they don't want that?

JG: In China most people know when they get sick it's easy to come.

CC: Here's another difference. In China people know something about acupuncture from the time they are very small children. In the United States they don't know about it until they're grown up, so it's a strange and surprising thing to them. But I take it in China it's not like that.

JG: In China it's just like medical doctor here, very popular. And we both have the [right to practice and prescribe] both* Chinese medicine and western medicine. We also have both trainings.

CC: I asked you about acupuncture but I really should be asking about Chinese medicine generally since you're also trained in herbs . . . are you also trained in tuina?

JG: Yeah. Tuina and orthopedics; tuina which is Chinese massage, and orthopedic training for the joint problems, for fractures.

CC: If you were to do a breakdown of your time when you treat patients, how much do you use acupuncture, herbs, massage, or something else?

JG: Most is acupuncture, like 70%. In the United States.† And herbs, 20% to 30%, combined with acupuncture. Few people come just for herbs.

CC: You make up your own herbal recipes?

JG: Yeah, yeah. Some I make up. Some are patent remedies if it's suitable for them; some people don't want to take the tea. So they can just have the pills to take.

CC: What do you find most rewarding about your practice in the United States?

JG: To really *see* the patient response and get a good result, not only for their physical [health], but also for their personal life, for their family, their career, all well. To be effective with them.

CC: Do you, then, follow your patients with regard to their personal lives, their family, and their career?

JG: Yeah, I do.

CC: So you give them more than a physical kind of attention. Now, if you would, tell me something about your teaching in the United States. What is that like?

JG: Because we started the school, I was one of the primary teachers and so I teach more. I try to bring all the things I teach in China in 5 years into this 3-year school, into this 3-year curriculum, so I'm always teaching more, teaching more. I think it's necessary, it's basic things they have to know. I feel students here are more enthusiastic. They are curious and they want to know all the details. They give me feedback and I get more energy. I teach a lot out of my own experience, including failures and difficult cases. I always try to share—[it's important that] students see the other side of the practice, that you may have your mistakes, you may have something more you need to know, [something you ought to] pay attention to. This also stimulates.

And teaching and practice must always stay together. When you teach you need the clinical experience to support you. When you practice you still need to keep studying, get feedback from students, try different new ways in the clinic. They all help each other, stimulate each other.

CC: It's quite a complicated thing you do. You take Chinese ideas, teach them to Americans who know nothing about China or Chinese ideas, and you teach in a foreign language . . . there are so many hurdles, barriers, to leap.

JG: So I'm like a basic translator, or interpreter. We have that in Chinese medicine, even the old literature, when you try to translate it to the modern literature, you have different languages. So my basic three key words are *Xin Da Ya. Xin* means *true* translation, loyalty to the original meaning; it's not interpretation. A precise translation—even if the words

---

*In China, students emphasize TCM or biomedicine, but all learn the elements of both systems.

†These percentages might well be reversed in China, where herbal treatment is better developed than in North America and Europe.

are not pretty they must be true to the original meaning. *Da* means explaining meanings better, deeper. You want to use better words, familiar words, rather than directly translate, find the best meaning to explain the situation. *Ya* [refers to] standard and proper performance, [whether it's] easy to accept it [when applied].

CC: So, you see your task as being a translator. You want to be loyal to the original meaning, then develop and explain it well, using a more familiar language. And then when the person sees it at work, sees it performing, the whole makes a circle and people can believe it better. OK, that's nice.

JG: Yeah. These three letters [ideographs] are my key for teaching. I want to give all the Chinese meanings but I also want people to be able to accept it. I read different translations and when I find they are away from the original meaning I always want to correct it. I want Chinese medicine to be deeply understood and explained in its original true meaning.

CC: A very difficult problem, to translate Chinese into an Indo-European language, into French, English, German, Spanish . . . it's been very hard. Do you read books in English that you think have not done a good job of translation?

JG: Not whole books, but some parts; with some words there are common mistakes. Like the meanings of the point names—mostly they find meanings in the dictionary, but some [ideographs have deeper] meanings. You need to do more study, [look at] literature, Chinese history!

CC: What is your favorite thing to do in Chinese medicine? You mentioned gynecology earlier.

JG: My practice goal is to effectively treat a wide range of cases, from the most common conditions to the most challenging. [As an example of the first kind,] I like to treat the common cold. I get very good results but not many people think they should come in for acupuncture when they have a cold. So I tell my patients my first choice is acupuncture for the common cold, for flu—they don't believe this! I say, if you catch a cold, just come here, I'll treat you! I get very good results. Because you don't want to take too many drugs to subside this fever. [Fever is] your body fighting, so you need to strengthen your defensive *Qi* to help [expel] this invading pathogenic factor. I like to see these conditions.

CC: You like to strengthen the *Qi*, the *Wei Qi*. You want to say anything more about treating the common cold?

JG: It's not just subsiding the fever. [You need to] open the Du channel, open the Yang channel to relieve the fever. [If a] headache doesn't subside, open [Du]. You know, sometimes [you even need] bleeding method or cupping to release [the blockage] rather than to just nicely cover [it up with drugs]. Release the blockage of the *Wei Qi*, release the Cold, Heat, Wind invasion, or sometimes Damp.

CC: Is there anything else you'd like to say?

JG: I'm also asked by a lot of people, "you have been teaching so many years"—you know, over five classes I've graduated now—and some people ask me, "With so many students aren't you afraid of competition, that they'll get your career?" And I say, "No, I believe acupuncture works and I believe it will become more popular when we have more good practitioners." So I really try my best to give all my knowledge, give other people experience so they can become the best acupuncturists in the world. That's why I am still teaching with abundant Qi and Blood!

SECTION 4: A COMPLETE ARMAMENTARIUM FOR PRACTICING FAMILY MEDICINE

PAULETTE C. HILL

When I became interested in practicing family medicine 25 years ago, I felt drawn to the field because of its ability to help so many. Shortly after my allopathic residency, I took a job doing physicals in an acupuncture clinic. I was allowed to observe treatments. I was very impressed with the practitioners' caring and gentle manner, so much so that I wanted to include acupuncture in my practice of family medicine. I went on to take a few weekend seminars in the field of Chinese medicine. I began to incorporate what I learned to treat a few ailments with acupuncture, and in doing so gradually realized how ill prepared I was to practice Oriental medicine. Imagine the knowledge base of someone who wished to practice allopathic medicine with a weekend degree! I then ceased all practice of acupuncture, determined that when I began again, it would be only with proper training that would give me depth in Oriental medical theory as well as technique. I went on to complete a 3-year program of studies at the Traditional Acupuncture Institute in Maryland, which offers a Masters of Acupuncture degree.

After earning my master's degree, I felt that I had a complete armamentarium for practicing family medicine. I had discovered that acupuncture could be combined with my allopathic training. With this combination I could serve patients' needs in many more ways. Since Oriental medicine tends to the body, mind, and spirit as a whole, by weaving the two systems together I felt a greater sense of fulfillment in rendering health care.

I took a position with the family practice clinic of the hospital with which I was on staff, hoping to bring acupuncture into the mainstream of family practice. Of course, I faced some difficulties. For example, noise was an issue. This was a group practice, and I wanted a space that would allow patients to transition from the noisy busyness of the clinic to a more serene environment for acupuncture. I solved this problem by being assigned to the quietest space in the clinic. A more difficult problem was that of finding a way to practice the full range of Oriental treatment. However, as the staff came to understand moxa (for point stimulation) and incense (for diagnosis of physical imbalances*) as valuable components of acupuncture treatments, they accepted my use of them.

I was happy when my colleagues began to make referrals of their most challenging patients. Today these referrals consist mainly of long-term pain conditions such as lower back pain, fibromyalgia, and migraine headaches. I also use acupuncture treatments as adjuncts to medications in treating conditions such as uncontrolled hypertension and allergies.

Because I practice both medicines, I routinely explain to new patients and educate them on the system of Oriental medicine. I let them know that allopathy focuses on disease and cure, while Oriental medicine seeks a balance of wellness within the body. Some patients drop out—they are satisfied with the biomedical disease-based system, or perhaps they are not fearless

enough to discard the safety of the familiar allopathic labels. I trust that their brief contact with me still provides some gains, even if only because they hear about other possibilities for healing.

I treasure the diagnostic skills I learned in Oriental medicine. I've found them useful even if I don't use needles. The Five Element system I learned helps me to see people in a nonjudgmental way. Instead I ask, "What color . . . sound . . . odor . . . emotion am I in the presence of?" This allows me to use observation and discovery, to see a subtle shift when I ask questions, to recognize oncoming disorder before a physical presentation, a disease, occurs. My patients who embrace the system of Oriental medicine by allowing me to offer treatments in the form of acupoint stimulation with needles or moxibustion generally come away with a feeling of well-being and a new desire to take charge of their lives. And soon they know so much more about themselves!

Acupuncture treatments complement allopathic treatments in many ways. For example, by using acupuncture one can often lower the requirement for a medication, either by reducing dosage or by decreasing the frequency with which the patient must use the drug. At the same time, I stress to patients and other health care workers that acupuncture is not a "fix-it" health delivery system. In contrast, it supports health and helps people attain "optimum" health when used on a regular basis. The allopathic system struggles to understand acupuncture partly because it is not familiar with interventions that heal before the appearance of physical manifestations. However, in the Oriental diagnostic framework, patients are taught to tune in to their inner physical voice. As they become increasingly skilled at recognizing the messages of their bodies, they can guide the acupuncture practitioner, prevent much physical disorder, and guide their own healing process.

Interestingly, allopathic practitioners faced with such a knowledgeable patient might tend to label him or her hypochondriacal. In my opinion, however, there is no better teacher of a patient's state of being than the patient's own self. This is because in our inquiries into what ails a person, we can never be truly objective. We bring our own baggage to the examination room. However, when I examine a patient using Color, Sound, Odor, and Emotion as tools to guide me into the patient's reality, I feel I am at least minimizing my own bias and maximizing my ability to see the person as he or she really is expressing life.

*Akabane test, a measure to see if Qi is flowing evenly on both sides of the body; see Chapter 8, section 2.

The physical setting in which I practice is part of the healing. For example, the comfort of the treatment table assists an acupuncture treatment. When I give comfort in simple ways, by adjusting the pillow or offering a warm blanket in a cool room, I build trust. I use soft lighting and music to bring the patient inward, able to give attention to his or her spiritual self. Moxa provides aromatherapy that also promotes arousal of the spiritual self.

This practice style also requires more time than the usual 15 minutes allotted to the primary care visit. In my view, and in my practice, the medical visit is a time for the patient to share discoveries of self that occur between visits. It provides a setting in which the patient can reflect on new ways of being with self. Some-times my task is to allow crying to take place as a clearing of past or present pains. By allowing such natural movements to take place, the next phase of healing can occur. With trust comes movement—through an illness or into a new-found security. I am rewarded when I don't have to sit as judge with a patient, but instead can allow his or her humanity to reveal itself anew at each visit.

I find numerous other rewards in this system of care. I am glad that I expanded my practice skills, and I get real joy from the warm smiles and soothing hugs that I receive from grateful patients. Appreciation is the greatest reward. It reminds me why I chose to serve in health care, and I am glad that by combining two systems I am able to offer a more diverse plan of care.

SECTION 5: LIKE A MEANDERING STREAM

ROBERT FELT

*M*y course to Chinese medical publishing was like a midwestern stream, rising unobtrusively in the north, meandering, often turning back on itself, often slow but sometimes cascading in froth and fury through some slash in the prairie landscape. The source from which it rose was an undistinguished academic career mostly dedicated to 1960's activism but graced by luck, and guided by the good will of many. Early on, I studied with Mary Youngblood and John Berryman, both Pulitzer winners; George Amberg, the founding dean of the New York University film school; and Richard Poor, a Chinese art historian whose lectures were so fascinating that I altered my intended program to take every class he offered.

Perhaps it was the mystery of bronze-age designs rooted in visions of an animistic nature, maybe it was just the simple awe of holding something so old that none would ever surely know its history, or possibly it was the pleasure of sleuthing whether an artifact was produced in the ancient past or in the pot-boiling workshop of some clever Chinese forger. But whatever the reason, the sensibilities of Asian art captivated me. When Len Jacobs, with whom I would work many times in the future, arrived in Minneapolis teaching Zen macrobiotics and Japanese massage, I became a regular.

I went to work in 1968, my first and only corporate employment. The Northwest Bank Corporation needed technical writers and I was the first one hired, apparently qualified by a thick stack of papers on European existentialism. In the next 3 years I would become one of the longest employed of a company that grew a thousandfold to become one of the largest mainframe computer centers in the world. There I learned systems analysis, programming, and statistical technique and discovered an odd talent for explaining software to "the suits" who paid our inflated salaries. The company president was a genuine mentor and arranged my training in technical and management skills. I surprised myself by enjoying a corporate culture that was rich with bright people who envisioned a world enriched by cyber-empowered science.

Nonetheless, I left. Writing manuals and businesses plans was not fulfilling, despite the exciting intellectual surround. I went freelance. I did turns as a director of news photography, photojournalist, medical manual and script writer, stringer, and freelance cinematographer. After work I helped a professor teach at what was then called the "Free University" where I renewed my studies with a Chinese expatriot who taught the *I Jing* and the rudiments of Chinese medicine. Actively studying massage, *I Jing,* and macrobiotic cooking, and succumbing to my friends' urgings, I moved to Boston to study macrobiotics.

The trip to Boston wandered through the Southwest and meandered into an isolated Mexican Indian village where I made friends with the local *brujol* (folk healer) and began to treat the local farmers' and fishermen's aches and sprains with massage, my tiny kit of acupuncture needles, and my even more diminutive knowledge. But eventually we arrived in Boston, took residence in a macrobiotic study house, and began to attend lectures.

I made a poor macrobiotic. The theory was not very satisfying. I had learned Yin-Yang as an aesthetic, a world view in which the harmony and interrelationships of all things is expressed in constant change. I understood Qi as the universal stuff that gave all creation its essential qualities and relationships. Their discussion as fixed elements seemed oddly un-Asian, as did the macrobiotic descriptions of Yin and Yang and the concentration on food rather than on naturally occurring drugs or acupuncture as medicine. Although I was attracted to the venturesome spirit of George Ohsawa, the movement's founder, his "mood of justice" was hard to locate in the dogmatism of "eating right." However, I was there, I had spent the last of my computer loot, and I needed a job. So I started washing dishes at the Seventh Inn, the brand-new, soon-to-be high-class macrobiotic restaurant. The pay was $40 a week.

The *sensei* spoke no English, I spoke no Japanese, but it took only an hour watching him work to see that he possessed a fascinating artistry and intensity. As our ability to communicate improved and I moved through his apprentice program, traditional ideas that had seemed arbitrary in the lecture hall acquired a liveliness and utility that I admired. In traditional systems one advances only through demonstrated skill. That is, exactly repeating what your teacher can do. When combined with the sense of personal duty and right livelihood, the workplace becomes a DoJo where personal development is accomplished through physical and mental exercise, even stress. In the traditional context this is known as developing and controlling your Qi.

For example, to "short order" we had to multiprocess at a very high level. One manages several dishes simultaneously, remembers a stream of shouted Japanese orders, and considers the individual arrangement of each dish prepared in kitchen temperatures well beyond comfort only by achieving a state of meditative concentration. The clarity of mind achieved is—for want of a better word—compelling, and although I had no abiding interest in being a chef, the DoJo life was appealing for its simple rigor and intense camaraderie.

The DoJo experience is rooted in personal discipline. For example, my "promotion" to head cook came on a day when my teacher simply (and deliber-

ately) did not appear. It was 5:30 AM. If someone didn't start, we would not be open at noon. If no one set the menu, the customers would be greeted with an empty page. I did the job. The master arrived at 11:55, went to the steam table (as a dozen apprentices looked for somewhere else to be), tasted everything in the traditional manner, looked at me, and said, "you like salt." No congratulations, no ceremony, just the pertinent fact.

Westerners take this story as quaint or cruel. It seems quaint to people who understand Qi as knowledge, as facts instead of actions. It seems cruel to people who believe that students must be protected from fear and failure. In a DoJo, knowledge, which is another expression of Qi, is the right action at the right time. Nothing else will do. This is the primary attribute of a strong and disciplined Qi. The martial artist must fight, the cook must present a meal, and the doctor must preserve and cure. As *sensei* put it, "theory without practice is dangerous, practice without theory is stupid." Yin and Yang, the Five Phases, all the traditional ideas lose their apparent fuzziness through consistent observation with the naked human senses. Recognizing the red of properly cooked shrimp or the red of Sinew Channel repletion are the sensory vocabulary by which to produce a fine tempura or an accurate diagnosis.

During the 3 years I worked with him closely and the 7 in which the sense of duty the DoJo life confers gave him influence over my life, I would also work for nearly a dozen different businesses, either one of his enterprises or loaned to another Japanese. I would teach hundreds of massage classes, study with everyone I could, including some of the most famous practitioners. I would spend from a few hours to a few months with Asian teachers as various as a former Japanese general visiting the American commanders he had fought in the Second World War and a priest from Japan's central Shinto shrine who traveled the world building roadside shrines meant to ensure world peace. I treated cancer patients in study houses, was a cook for a diet randomized controlled clinical trial, and was an observer and learner with herbalists, acupuncturists, and monks. I consulted natural foods companies in Europe and Canada, led the building of a restaurant in Quebec, and taught massage when short of cash to pay the rent. If life had earlier been a meandering stream, now it became a torrent in the fecund diversity of the 1970s.

Through constant interaction, these experiences contributed to developing my personal perception of

Asian thought. They also gave me a close-up view of the innards of the recently named "new age," a view that convinced me that I cared to see no more. But they also supported the events that most profoundly affected my life: meeting Martha Fielding who became my life partner, and the founding of Redwing Book Company, which would become my life work. In 1973 we opened the doors of our first bookstore on Boston's Newbury Street. It was not then the expensive haunt it is today but rather a collection of small businesses catering to, and often enough run by, the young people who inhabited the inexpensive apartments in the surrounding brownstone-lined streets.

Although I was finished with the DoJo, that experience made the rest of the so-called new age seem bereft of substance, dull, and without Qi. I had no doubt that diet, herbs, massage, and acupuncture were valuable, but the macrobiotic movement's unshakable notion that its future was linked to curing advanced degenerative diseases, and that practice could be mastered without clinical training, was more than I could accept. When I had met Yin-Yang rooted in disciplined observation and human skill, I was fascinated, sometimes truly amazed. When I met it in conversation with students, I only became angry with their teachers.

Friends who had mastered Asian languages made it clear that the information available in English was less than inadequate: it was misleading. I was beginning to understand how little acupuncture or traditional bodywork I knew, yet my steady questioning of people who knew these skills in their native contexts had given me a broader view than nearly everyone I met. Once, for example, I traveled to several acupuncture schools with a friend who had just finished 10 years with a Japanese herbalist who was respected in all of East Asia. Although every Asian I had met saw herbalism as more or less superior to acupuncture, the leaders of acupuncture schools outside of Asia held the opposite view. Some even expressed an "over my dead body" attitude toward its introduction.

It was time for study. Scholars, students, neophytes, and experts, an exciting mix of people passed through our bookstores' doors. Even if they didn't have a lot money to spend, they had a lot to say. We listened. Taking advantage of what little French I learned in Quebec, I read Soulié de Morant, Van Nigh, Chamfrault, and Garnet. Martha's management skills were already sharp, and the shelves began to fill with books on healing traditions from around the world. Our stores became centers of heartfelt and intelligent

conversation, hosting people who still remember those days with pleasure.

Traditional medicine was not our only study. Cambridge, Massachusetts, in the early 1980s was already a center of technical development and the store acquired a second focus, a crowded backroom more than filled by a noisy UNIX computer. The Harvard science center held regular meetings of the UNIX users group, and there I learned what academic computing had to offer. I met developers who, as capital poor as we were, borrowed time on our machine in trade for use of the programs they authored. I watched and learned, soon building a tool set drawn from software developers and academics. After a year of programming on the many slow days, we began our first publication as well as distribution sales to stores and schools using the software thus developed. In 1981 we sold both stores to Shambhala Publications, took the computer home, and began as full-time publishers and distributors. Thus Redwing transformed from a retail bookseller to an importer and eventually a publisher of books on healing traditions.

This was a considerable leap. Distributing books is the management of credit, a game that is easy to lose. The problems of producing books with software were more or less fully resolved, but the systems needed for mixed Chinese-English publications were as yet difficult to work with. In fact, I met few who actually believed it would ever work. Our first book project, Dr. So's books, took unexpected years because everything had to be demonstrated or recited to Dr. So—this being the only way he believed that our version would reflect his practice. Because we were distributing books and did not want to be isolated as a knock-off press, we explored new areas that were close to our personal experience. Because we knew acupuncture to be various in Korea, Japan, and China, we assumed that information about apprentice systems such as So's, or culturally adapted systems such as those found in Japan, would be welcomed. Further, thinking it would lead to better relations with the community, I accepted an invitation to apply my analytic experience as a board member of the local acupuncture school.

At my first New England School of Acupuncture (NESA) board meeting I learned that the students were on strike, divided into factions for or against TCM, as well as certain administrative decisions. The school's founder had been paralyzed during surgery and was further crippled by his Chinese-centered understanding of the crisis. Eventually he lost control of the school. Meanwhile, a small group of us decided that as local business people we could not responsibly watch NESA collapse. The community needed to achieve a workable agreement and accept a multiplicity of views. That agreement was achieved through an election of directors and slowly the school regrew, fertilized by the volunteer efforts of several key individuals. It was satisfying to contribute to the school's survival.

The experience also formalized our view of the field. During this 8 years of listening to the ideas and demands of students and faculty, as well as the opinions of intellectual and economic leaders, I acquired a deeper sense of the state of knowledge and a sense that the role of traditional medicine in China was broadly misunderstood. Even in 1985, after well-received books on TCM had been published, many matters remained controversial or were explicitly denied. TCM's genesis in China's postwar public health crisis, acupuncture's lower status relative to internal medicine,* and the dominance of biomedicine in China were never discussed in the practitioner literature and were even openly denied. This fostered an assumption that acupuncture was a sufficient replacement for biomedicine—a complete alternative. As well as reinforcing an acrimonious ideological conflict between proponents of differing styles, it emboldened those whose interest in Chinese medicine had some root in their distaste for science and technology.

One outcome of this conflict was the near disappearance of a hands-on component in training. For example, when I suggested at a faculty meeting that massage would be a useful way to teach point location, while giving students a practical feel for relative body temperatures, degrees of stiffness, and other practitioner-assessed conditions, as well as a sense for working with people, I was told that "Chinese doctors did not do manual work." There was also a more subtle disregard for attention to sensory and conceptual details. For example, the ability to distinguish subtle gradations of color is essential to something as simple as selecting and preparing food, yet the Five Phase relationships to color were memorized in acupuncture schools without even a mention of how Chinese people labeled the spectrum.

East or West, in traditional arts there is an emphasis on proper form, technique, and process to en-

sure effective learning. Whether arranging flowers, performing a martial art, preparing tempura, or physically examining a patient, step-by-step technique is often taught on at least a par with the operative theory, if not as the functional *sine qua non.* Yet the idea of cultivating Qi had all but disappeared from the Western perspective. The common understanding of Qi so emphasized spiritualizing force, so-called energy, that the self-discipline of technique as a "gong fu" or self-developmental work was, and is still, only rarely discussed.

Although we had managed to get our first book in print by 1983, and Dr. So's first book would soon follow, we had not yet understood how to integrate our view of the field and its future with a market that implicitly, and seemingly universally, pursued a different tack. This, however, would be solved by good luck. Luck took the form of a new friend, Yoshio Manaka, Japan's *dai sensei,* and an old friend from the "anti" years, Paul Zmiewski. Both would introduce us to people and ideas that would help us define our publishing goals.

Yoshio Manaka was one of the most brilliant men I have ever met. He quickly realized that Stephen Birch possessed not just the intellectual skill but also the integrity necessary to pursue an integration of Chinese and Western medical knowledge that did not depend on forcing Chinese ideas into Western molds, but on the ordering and analysis of direct clinical observations. Manaka was an ultimate dissonant. He was countering the majority trends in both the East and West by proposing Chinese medicine as a problem-solving system. Whatever the eventual adoption of Manaka's ideas, whether they survive in the West or not, his is an authentic clinically founded adaptation of traditional principles, tried and tested to a degree anyone can scrutinize in his written works. When he sent his last material for *Chasing the Dragon's Tail,* he wrote Martha that he dreamed he was a bird released from its cage; this proved a Swendeborgian prediction.

Paul Zmiewski and I had crossed paths several times but never met until my tenure at NESA. Like ourselves, Paul was uncomfortable with popular ideas of acupuncture and his own early training. His answer was to study in Taiwan. In the early 1980s many words were spent arguing the superiority of one system or another, and with TCM already dominant in the acupuncture schools, it was difficult to see any commercial access short of accepting the viewpoint of one movement or another. When Paul returned from Taiwan to finish his

---

*Formally speaking, acupuncture treats the exterior, affecting the interior indirectly; herbal medicine directly treats the interior.

dissertation, he came equipped with the idea of an "East Asian Medical Studies Center"; this would lead us toward people whose work further defined our publishing goals by providing a larger view, particularly, Paul Unschuld and Nigel Wiseman.

The idea of the East Asian Medical Studies Center was both intellectually and commercially satisfying. By providing translations of key Chinese texts we would provide a reference library to the field. Since it is hard to imagine successfully adapting anything from another culture without access to the important native-language literature, we assumed such a library would be useful to persons holding any point of view. Further, since the approach did not promote the ideas of particular individuals or groups, others could adopt it. Thus the literature might develop faster and have a greater presence. If everyone had English-language access to what the Chinese had to say about their own medicine, education would broaden. Of course, we did not fail to notice that with more participants in publishing, we could have a larger distribution catalogue, sharing the costs among a larger and less risky base of publications.

Our first step was to start distributing the list of term translations for some central Chinese medical terms. Nigel, Paul, and Andy Ellis developed the list to acquire feedback and support, as well as to further their own clinical studies. Because the potentials of a standard terminology had received little or no attention to this point, we expected that the idea would be welcomed. Anything that could lower the time and cost of creating, editing, even proofing, translations from Chinese would be useful for anyone in the trade, and a generic approach to terms could remove their interpretive weight and allow people holding different viewpoints to share a set of common understandings. The results of this effort were somewhat ironic. It failed to attract the interest of those to whom it was originally directed, but established scholars such as Nathan Sivin and Paul Unschuld were unexpectedly encouraging. Indeed, Paul Unschuld's ongoing contributions have made it more than worthwhile.* In time, Nigel's work has not only been recognized as a significant contribution but has also achieved its original intent—the development of an intellectual tool kit

that has already greatly increased the availability of clinical information direct from Chinese scholars and clinicians.*

Paul Unschuld's work is critically important to the westward acculturation of Chinese medicine. Not only has he provided translations of important works, but his insights and explanations of the intellectual foundations of Chinese medicine provide a frame of reference from which the tradition can be appropriately explored. By understanding the needs and expectations of the people who created and applied the principles of Chinese medicine, we are better prepared to avoid understanding their ideas solely from within our own context. Thus while Paul's work is only rarely a matter of clinical instruction, it is always a guide to the manner in which clinical instruction can be understood. The same is true of Nigel Wiseman's work. By providing terms and tools oriented to their sources, he has opened the gates to the vastness of Asian resources.

In Western societies change occurs when public support generates political and economic support, which together initiate social change. It is unlikely that this situation will be any different for Chinese medicine. Thus while successful treatment of significant populations is critical to public support, so too is it necessary to effectively answer skeptics, provide an unassailable scholarly foundation, and put widely acceptable evidence before the scientific community. I think, generally, that this requires an effort to look clearly at East Asian medicines in modern China and Japan, not only as sources of philosophical and clinical experience, but as examples of the social institutions where Chinese medicines coexist with biomedicine and how these systems benefit the public's health.

Although I personally doubt that Chinese or Japanese health care models will be adopted directly, examining these practices is our only source of practical information concerning the public benefits of incorporating the modern expressions of traditional Chinese medicine in today's biomedically dominated health care systems. Just as Chinese medicine suggests examining the whole person, by looking at the whole of these native systems, their reception, use, and economic impact, we will be better prepared to know the

*In addition to his many articles, Paul Unschuld's books constitute an essential body of knowledge concerning traditional Chinese medicine. These books include (in English) references 2 through 11.

*Nigel Wiseman and colleagues have produced the largest volume of Chinese medical information directly translated from known Chinese sources. These works include references 12 through 19.

value of the various parts: student selection, education, and training, as well as integration with a biomedicine that is dominant worldwide.

References

1. Manaka Y, Itaya K, Birch S: *Chasing the dragon's tail, the theory and practice of acupuncture in the work of Yoshio Manaka,* Brookline, Mass, 1995, Paradigm Publications.
2. Unschuld PU: *Medical ethics in imperial China,* Berkeley, Calif, 1979, University of California Press.
3. Unschuld PU: *Medicine in China: a history of ideas,* Berkeley, Calif, 1985, University of California Press.
4. Unschuld PU: *Medicine in China: Nan Ching—the classic of difficult issues,* Berkeley, Calif, 1986, University of California Press.
5. Unschuld PU: *Medicine in China: a history of pharmaceutics,* Berkeley, Calif, 1986, University of California Press.
6. Unschuld PU, editor: *Approaches to traditional Chinese medical literature,* Dordrecht, 1989, Kluwer Academic.
7. Unschuld PU: *Forgotten traditions of ancient Chinese medicine,* Brookline, Mass, 1990, Paradigm Publications.
8. Unschuld PU: *Learn to read Chinese,* 2 vols, Brookline, Mass, 1990, Paradigm Publications.
9. Unschuld PU: *Chinese medicine,* Brookline, Mass, 1998, Paradigm Publications.
10. Unschuld PU: *Essential subtleties on the silver sea: Yin-hai Jingwei,* Berkeley, Calif, 1998, University of California Press.
11. Unschuld PU: *Medicine in China: historical artifacts and images,* Munich, 2000, Prestel.
12. Wiseman N, Ellis A: *Fundamentals of Chinese medicine,* Brookline, Mass, 1985, Paradigm Publications.
13. Ellis A, Wiseman N, Boss K: *Fundamentals of Chinese acupuncture,* Brookline, Mass, 1988, Paradigm Publications.
14. Ellis A, Wiseman N, Boss K: *Grasping the wind,* Brookline, Mass, 1989, Paradigm Publications.
15. Wiseman N, Boss K: *Glossary of Chinese medical terms and acpuncture points,* Brookline, Mass, 1990, Paradigm Publications.
16. Wiseman N, Ellis A: *Fundamentals of Chinese medicine,* rev ed, Brookline, Mass, 1991, Paradigm Publications.
17. Wiseman N: *A Chinese English—English Chinese dictionary of Chinese medicine,* Hunan, China, 1995, Hunan Science and Technology Press.
18. Wiseman N, Feng Y: A practical dictionary of traditional Chinese medicine, Brookline, Mass, 1998, Paradigm Publications.
19. Mitchell C, Wiseman N, Feng Y: *Shang Han Lun, on cold damage,* Brookline, Mass, 1999, Paradigm Publications.

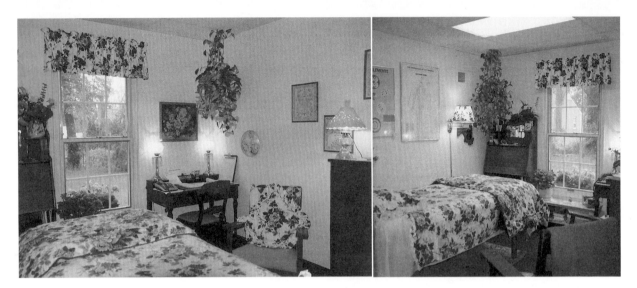

Figure 1 Acupuncturists express their personalities in their treatment rooms. In this case the practitioner chose to create a warm and homelike healing environment. Notice the Taoist emphasis on flowers and plants, the presence of natural light, the homelike sheets and pillows on the treatment table, the old wooden rocking chair for the patient to sit in while recounting her difficulties, and the framed embroideries on the walls. As in most acupuncture offices, one wall also displays acupuncture charts; on another (unseen) hang the practitioner's framed diplomas. (Courtesy Claire Cassidy.)

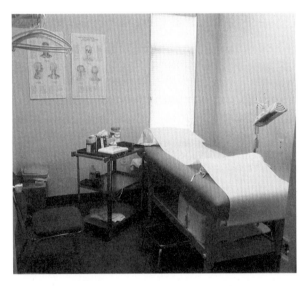

Figure 2 In marked contrast to Figure 1, this treatment room has been arranged to emphasize simplicity. The treatment table is covered with disposable paper, and both needles and the electroacupuncture machine stand ready on a strictly utilitarian table. A large sharps box can be glimpsed in the left back corner. A rack holds coats and above are a selection of cotton examination gowns. The window is shaded, and one wall displays acupuncture charts. A warming lamp waits beside the table. (Courtesy Claire Cassidy.)

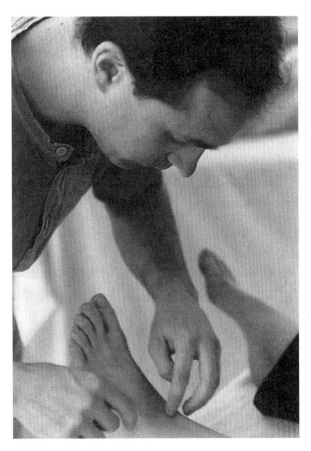

Figure 3 When treating patients, acupuncture practitioners become highly focused. Notice the attentiveness of the acupuncturist and the sensitivity of the fingers palpating for the acupoint. (Courtesy James Kegley.)

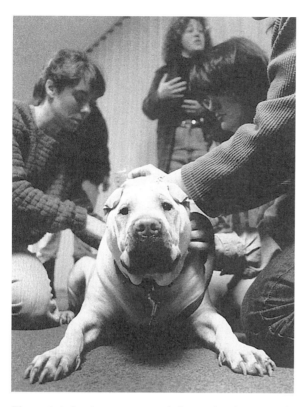

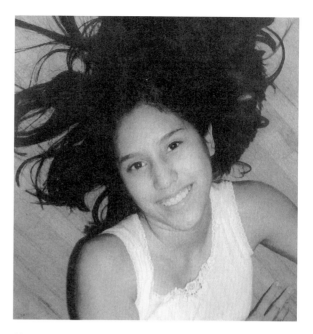

Figure 5 Shen shows best in the face. It is the spirit of life, the vitality that makes the skin glow, the eyes shine with liveliness, and the smile that connects one with another. (Courtesy Claire Cassidy.)

Figure 4 Animal acupuncture is becoming increasingly popular. Here a dog with low back pain is holding still to receive the needles. Animal acupuncturists report that animals often willingly hold still for the needles, only moving to signal that it is time to remove them. (Courtesy James Kegley.)

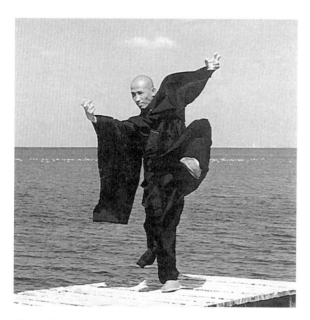

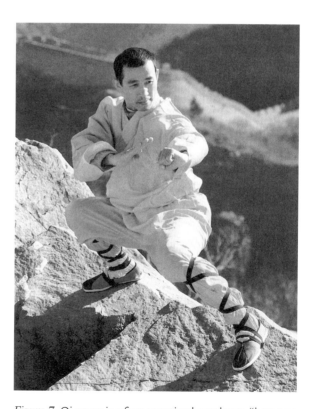

Figure 6 Master Shawn Liu in a dramatic Qi gong pose. (Courtesy Shawn Liu.)

Figure 7 Qi gong is often practiced outdoors "between Heaven and Earth." Here Qi gong Master, Shawn Liu, practices on a rock. The Great Wall of China can be glimpsed in the background. (Courtesy Shawn Liu.)

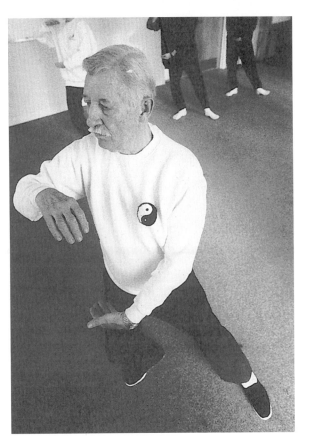

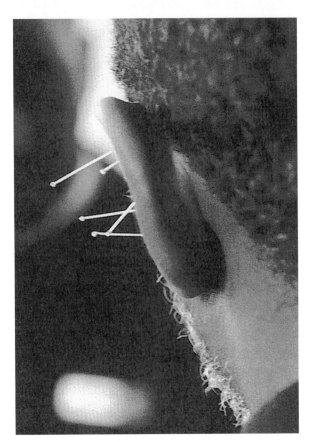

Figure 8 A major message of Chinese medicine is that one's pain response to the stress of daily life can be moderated by a daily practice of exercise and spiritual development. Qi gong offers both—a moving meditation—in one neat package. Here a man no longer young is practicing tai chi in a classroom. (Courtesy James Kegley.)

Figure 9 Five painless needles inserted in the ear can markedly reduce cravings for drugs and other substances. (Courtesy James Kegley.)

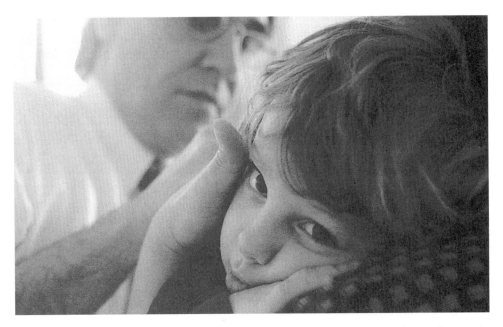

Figure 10 Children respond rapidly to acupuncture care. A child held safely by his mother receives ear acupuncture while calmly watching the photographer. (Courtesy James Kegley.)

III

RESEARCH DATA

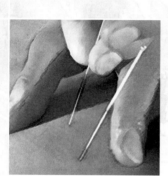

The question about Oriental medicine that provokes most research attention is "Does it Work?" In Part III, research on acupuncture is emphasized because it has received the most attention in Western settings; however, some authors of the following chapters also discuss research on herbs. The basic question can conveniently be broken into the following four aspects:

1. How does acupuncture achieve its healing effects? This question, which is best approached by laboratory scientists performing experiments, is the subject of Chapter 11. The author, Richard Hammerschlag, reviews efforts to understand the physiological effects of acupuncture from early work on pain and "gate-control theory" to recent understandings of how acupuncture modulates neurotransmitter expression.

2. Who chooses it, why, how satisfying is it, and is it cost-effective? Finding answers to these questions requires skills in the social and epidemiological sciences, including questionnaire design and interpretation. Little social research has been done so far on

Oriental medicine use and attitudes in the West. However, Chapter 12, by Claire Cassidy and Mitra Emad, both medical anthropologists, reviews data from interview and survey studies of patient attitudes and experiences with acupuncture. They identify a series of factors that help explain why patients report high satisfaction with Oriental medicine.

3. How effective or efficacious is it when compared with standard biomedical care? This comparative clinical question, which has fueled most research on Oriental medicine to date and reviews of the results, forms the majority of Part III. Although relatively little research has been performed on acupuncture compared with biomedicine, there is still a considerable body of quality work available, which the authors of Chapters 13 to 19 explore in detail. In Chapter 13, Stephen Birch reviews data on pain control with acupuncture. This topic leads the clinical research series because pain control is the best-known use for acupuncture care. Chapter 14, written by Michael Smith and James Butler-Arkow, reports on developments in using acupuncture for treatment of substance abuse. Dr. Smith's auricular acupuncture protocol for treating cocaine and opiate addiction has been so successful that many American court systems mandate it for some substance abusers. In Chapter 15, written by Kim Jobst, effectiveness data for acupuncture and respiratory disorders (especially asthma) are reviewed. Chapter 16, written by David Diehl, does the same for digestive disorders. In Chapter 17, Valentin and Luminita Tureanu focus on how Oriental medicine conceptualizes women's reproductive health and review a considerable body of research data on treating various malfunctions. Chapter 18, written by Rosa Schnyer and John Allen, discusses the treatment of mental-emotional health with acupuncture. They emphasize the care of depression, an issue that has received considerable research attention partly because biomedical approaches to depression have been only moderately successful. Chapter 19, by Margaret Naeser, reviews research on acupuncture and central nervous system dysfunction. Since biomedicine has relatively less success in treating central nervous system issues and Oriental medicine offers some novel options, the care of central nervous dysfunction is an area of rapid growth for acupuncture care.

4. How do differences in practice within the profession matter? Although not reviewed in Part III, differences in practice are briefly mentioned elsewhere in this book. This aspect concerns such issues as the significance of differences in depth, patterning, or timing of needle insertion; whether certain point combinations are more or less successful at alleviating specified symptoms; if certain herbs are best deleted from the traditional armamentarium; and similar issues. These issues are of significant interest to professional practitioners of Oriental medicine but are too technical for this text. ❧

Suggested Readings

Reviews

Diehl DL, Kaplan G, Coulter I, et al: Use of acupuncture by American physicians, *J Altern Complement Med* 3:119-26, 1997.

Eskinazi DP: National Institutes of Health technology assessment workshop on alternative medicine: acupuncture, *J Altern Complement Med* 2:1-253, 1996.

Hammerschlag R: Methodological and ethical issues in clinical trials of acupuncture, *J Altern Complement Med* 4:159-71, 1998.

Hammerschlag R, Birch S: *Acupuncture efficacy, a compendium of controlled clinical studies,* Tarrytown, NY, 1996, National Academy of Acupuncture and Oriental Medicine.

Lao L: Safety issues in acupuncture, *J Altern Complement Med* 2:27-9, 1996.

National Institutes of Health consensus panel: *Acupuncture,* Bethesda, Md, 1997, National Institutes of Health.

Stux G, Hammerschlag R, editors: *Clinical acupuncture: scientific basis,* Berlin, 2001, Springer-Verlag.

US Food and Drug Administration: Acupuncture needles no longer investigational, *FDA Consumer Magazine* 30, 1996.

Wootton JC, Sparber AG: Surveys of complementary and alternative medicine. In Micozzi M, editor: *Current review of complementary medicine,* Philadelphia, 1999, Current Medicine.

World Health Organization: *Viewpoint on acupuncture,* Geneva, Switzerland, 1979, World Health Organization.

Dental Pain

Lao L, Bergman S, Langenberg P, et al: Efficacy of Chinese acupuncture on postoperative oral surgery pain, *Oral Surg Oral Med Oral Pathol* 79:423-8, 1995.

HIV/AIDS

Burack J, Cohen M, Hahn J, et al: Pilot randomized controlled trial of Chinese herbal treatment for HIV-associated symptoms, *J Acquir Immune Defic Syndr* 12:386-93, 1996.

Galantino MLA, Eke-Okoro ST, Findley TW, et al: Use of noninvasive electroacupuncture for the treatment of HIV-related peripheral neuropathy: a pilot study, *J Altern Complement Med* 5:135-42, 1999.

Huang B-S: *AIDS and its treatment by traditional Chinese medicine,* Boulder, Colo, 1991, Blue Poppy, p. 14-33.

Shlay JC, Chaloner K, Max MB, et al: Acupuncture and amitriptyline for pain due to HIV-related peripheral neuropathy: a randomized controlled trial. Terry Beirn Community Programs for Clinical Research on AIDS, *JAMA* 280:1590-95, 1998.

Psychology

Jarrett LS: *Nourishing destiny: the inner tradition of Chinese medicine,* Stockbridge, Mass, 1998, Spirit Path Press.

Hammer L: *Dragon rises, red bird flies: psychology and Chinese medicine,* Tarrytown, NY, 1990, Station Hill Press.

Larre C, Rochat de la Vallee E: *The seven emotions, psychology and health in ancient China,* Cambridge, 1996, Monkey Press.

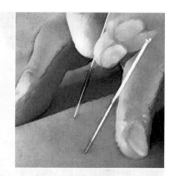

The Physiology of Acupuncture

RICHARD HAMMERSCHLAG

As noted in the preceding chapters, acupuncture is rooted in a medical tradition that differs strikingly from biomedicine. Stated simply, acupuncture is practiced from an energy-based rather than a molecular-based perspective. Its terminology, diagnostic procedures, and treatment modalities are unique, as are its fundamental views of physiology and etiology, and there is often no straightforward means to map one medicine onto the other. For example, in acupuncture theory health is equated with the free flow of energy (Qi) through an empirically defined system of Channels, notwithstanding that biomedical research has yet to anatomically identify the Channels or quantitatively detect the energy. Frequently cited evidence in defense of acupuncture theory, however, is the small proportion of acupuncture patients, including those who are treatment-naive, who are particularly sensitive to needling, and describe a propagating sensation after experiencing needling at a single acupoint. When asked to delineate the sensation, they trace a path that corresponds closely to a classical Channel.[1] This seeming paradox of sensation without anatomic representation is explored later in the chapter.

Although acupuncture is replete with concepts, such as Qi in the Channels, unfamiliar and untested in the West, the past two decades have produced sufficient evidence to indicate that its efficacy can be assessed by clinical research methods similar to those used in testing biomedical treatments. Increasing numbers of formal clinical trials, described in the following chapters, have used a variety of placebo or sham controls[2,2a] or standard care comparisons[3] to examine acupuncture efficacy for a wide range of conditions. In randomized trials, acupuncture has outperformed placebo controls (noninvasive, mock procedures) and sham needling controls (invasive but inappropriate needling), has performed at least as well as biomedical standard care, and has proved to be a beneficial adjunct to standard care.[4,4a]

As with any treatment found effective in randomized controlled trials, indications of acupuncture efficacy have prompted interest in the question, "How does it work?" The implicit assumption is that, independent of Chinese medicine's traditional explanations of acupuncture action, there must be biomedical correlates of the healing effects of needling. In response to the sensory stimuli and microtrauma of acupuncture, it seems likely that nerve pathways are activated, neurotransmitters and hormones released, local immune and circulatory responses triggered, even genes turned on or off. The present chapter surveys both the data produced and the hypotheses engendered from the testing of this assumption. It begins by examining biomedical research that has sought to define the functional substrata of Chinese medicine, the acupuncture points and Meridians. It then explores the predominant biomedical model of acupuncture, based in neurobiologically mediated responses. Within this model, the greatest attention is given to mechanisms of acupuncture analgesia. Although this emphasis reflects the preponderance of research efforts in this area, accumulating evidence of cardiovascular, gastrointestinal, and immunological effects is also reviewed. Many of these studies are discussed in light of the emerging view of acupuncture as a normalizing, homeostatic therapy. Finally, the limitations of the biomedical approach are discussed with a view toward examining what acupuncture may reveal about physiological function and dysfunction that does not yet appear in the textbooks of Western bioscience.

STRUCTURAL AND FUNCTIONAL CORRELATES OF ACUPUNCTURE POINTS

The most common technique in Chinese-style acupuncture is one in which needles are inserted at traditionally defined points, through the layers of epidermis, dermis, and fascia into the muscle to elicit the dull aching reflex sensation called *de qi* (often translated as "arrival of qi"). By contrast, in Japanese-style acupuncture, which uses the same acupoint locations and produces similar clinical effectiveness as Chinese

acupuncture, needles are most often inserted to a markedly lesser depth, usually without evoking *de qi*. If Chinese needling is predominantly intramuscular, then Japanese needling can be considered subcutaneous. These differences in depth of needling suggest that distinguishing features of acupoints, should they exist, are likely to be found in the dermal layers and fascia, the anatomical regions common to the two treatment styles.

Histological studies have yet to reveal any generally accepted evidence of unique morphological markers at the sites of traditional acupoints. Several types of known structures, however, have been found to correlate with acupoint sites, with most interest focused on the distribution of cutaneous sensory nerves. Depending on the thickness of the tissue sample, acupoint sites relative to nonacupoint regions contain greater densities of free (nonspecialized) nerve endings and cutaneous nerve branches, and a higher probability of a nerve-vessel bundle penetrating the fascia[5-7] (Figure 11-1). Even where there is no distinct layer of fascia, such as the face and scalp, nerve-vessel bundles align with classical acupoints. Thus, although Chinese medical texts assign precise locations to acupoints, the possibility remains that they are not "all-or-none" sites. Rather, they may be the sites at which, because of their relatively high density of sensory endings, the best clinical results can be obtained.

Additional correlations with acupoints include motor points (cutaneous locations overlying sites of muscle innervation),[8] trigger points (focal sites hypersensitive to palpation after trauma or muscle strain),[9] mast cells (histamine-releasing components of the immune system),[10] and gap junctions (high-conductance intercellular communication sites).[11] In light of the variety of these structures, it should be stressed that correlation does not necessarily imply identity. For example, in the study reporting a 71% correspondence between trigger points and acupoints traditionally recommended for pain management,[9] the comparison was made not on human subjects but using textbook descriptions of point locations. Furthermore, "correspondence" between a trigger point and an acupoint was defined with a seemingly overlarge 3-cm tolerance. In any case, the finding does not imply that all acupoints are trigger points.

The phenomenon of referred pain, in relation to trigger point theory, is also of interest for understanding the physiology of acupuncture. Pain is often referred from trigger points to distant cutaneous lo-

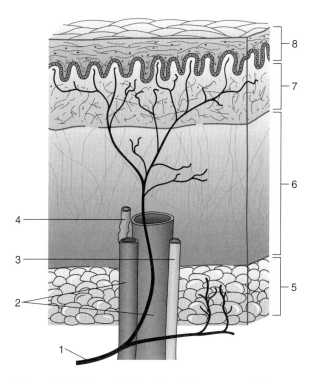

Figure 11-1 Schematic drawing of the anatomical structures proposed to underlie an acupuncture point. *1,* Nerve; *2,* veins; *3,* artery; *4,* lymphatic vessel; *5,* fascia; *6,* dermis; *7,* connective tissue; *8,* epidermis. (Modified from Heine H: *Acupunct Sci Int J* 1:1-6, 1990.)

cations in a pattern specific for each muscle or visceral organ. Such referred pain points, located by palpation, appear to be similar to what in acupuncture practice are called *ah shi* ("oh yes" or "ouch") points, locations that are searched for and needled as an additional means of suppressing pain. Correspondences between these Eastern and Western systems of diagnosing pain become more striking in light of reports that trigger points and their referred pain patterns frequently appear to follow traditional Meridian lines. As cited in Baldry,[12] 85% of patients with chronic lower back pain, when asked to indicate their sites of pain on a diagram of the human body, connected the sites by lines that corresponded to regions of acupuncture Channels.[13]

Sites of cutaneous hypersensitivity, similar to trigger points and referred pain patterns of muscles, have been recognized as originating from other tissues, including fascia and joints, as well as tendons and ligaments of the abdominal wall. Clues to the neural

mechanisms by which this pain response system operates may come from hypotheses devised to explain referred deep pain from visceral organs.

Although viscera contain relatively few nociceptive receptors that project directly to the central nervous system, these tissues appear able to recruit cutaneous nociceptive afferent neurons, in a site-specific manner, to amplify their "distress signals" to the brain (Figure 11-2, *A*). Because the recruitment of cutaneous fibers occurs by depolarization of their presynaptic terminals in the spinal cord, signals are sent to the brain in the anterograde (usual) direction and the periphery in the retrograde (reverse) direction. Signals reaching the brain are identical to those that would normally originate at nociceptive receptors in the skin, explaining why the brain may localize pain of visceral origin to peripheral sites. Signals reaching the skin trigger the local release of vasodilatory and nociceptive peptides from peripheral axon collaterals, helping to explain why tenderness and pain develop at the referred pain/*ah shi* sites (see Figure 11-2, *A*). This recruitment scheme is based on findings that spinal neurons receiving nociceptive input from the skin also respond to noxious visceral stimuli.[14] It is of particular interest in the context of acupuncture mechanisms that the needles can be seen as stimulating the viscerosomatic pathway in the reverse direction.[15] By sending neural signals from the periphery to a dysfunctional internal organ, local healing reactions—involving vasodilatation and immunomodulation—can be initiated (Figure 11-2, *B*). Systematic study of convergence in the spinal dorsal horn of afferent endings from viscera and from their referred (recruited) cutaneous afferents should yield critical information to test theories of Chinese medicine that relate peripheral acupoint sites to corresponding organ systems.

Neurophysiological mapping of somatovisceral correspondences also may help to answer a more fundamental question: With the skin so richly innervated over the whole of its surface, what enables only certain sites to function as acupoints? At least partial explanations may lie in the peripheral and central connectivity patterns of the nerve fibers associated with these sites. For example, in terms of acupuncture-induced analgesia, where needling at acupoints is clinically more effective than at nonpoint sites,[16,17] assessment is needed as to whether acupuncture-generated neural activity more effectively inhibits afferent noxious signals from reaching spinal, mid-brain, or cortical sites than do signals generated by needling adjacent nonpoint sites.

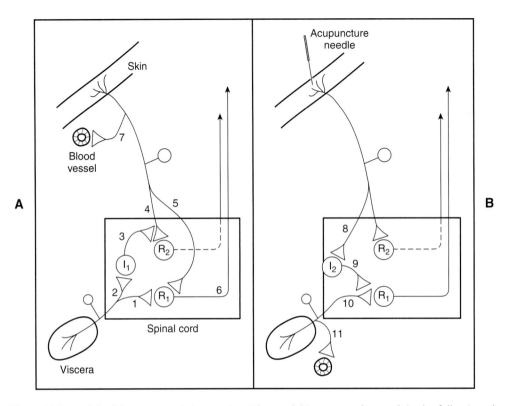

Figure 11-2 Model of viscerosomatic integration. The model is proposed to explain the following observations: (1) Visceral pain is poorly localized (subjectively) and is frequently "referred" to somatic sites that become tender (hyperalgesic); (2) spinal relay neurons are either solely somatic or are viscero/somatic (receive dual input); virtually none receive and relay exclusively visceral information; and (3) acupuncture at tender *(ah shi)* points is therapeutic for visceral pain. **A, Viscerosomatic mechanisms.** Visceral sensory neuron, carrying pain signals *(1)*, stimulates spinal relay neuron R1 but not sufficiently to fire it. Visceral neuron branch *(2)* synapses on spinal interneuron I_1 that, in turn *(3)*, synapses on the terminal of a somatic sensory neuron. This triggers an antidromic signal *(4)*, traveling toward the skin, that reaches a side branch and reverses direction *(5)* back to spinal relay neuron R_1. This convergence of somatic and visceral sensory signals is now sufficient to fire R_1, which sends a pain message to the mid-brain (thalamus) and on to the somatosensory cortex, where it is perceived as having arrived mainly from a peripheral site. Concurrently, the antidromic signal *(4)* travels to the skin where, via another branch, it triggers the release of vasodilatory and nociceptive peptides. **B, Somatovisceral mechanisms.** Just as the branches of visceral sensory neurons initiate activation of somatic sensory neurons (see Figure 11-2, *A*), so a sensory neuron branch *(8)*, in response to acupuncture, may synapse on a spinal interneuron *(I_2)* to trigger indirectly *(9)* antidromic signals in visceral sensory neurons *(10)*. This leads to the release of peptides from side branches *(11)* at or near the viscera that promote vasodilation, smooth muscle relaxation, and other healing responses. (Modified from Kendall DE: *Am J Acupunct* 17:343-60, 1989.)

BIOELECTRICAL PROPERTIES OF ACUPUNCTURE POINTS

The lack of definitive morphological descriptors notwithstanding, considerable effort has been directed at establishing that acupoints can be localized by virtue of their bioelectrical properties. In pioneering studies of the 1940s and 1950s, Niboyet[18] in France began mapping low-resistance skin points, while Nakatani and Yamashita[19] in Japan, applying the inverse of Ohm's law, were identifying high-conductance points that formed Ryodoraku or "good conductance lines." Both researchers found that the points differed markedly in electrical properties from surrounding sites and that the identified points and lines showed high correspondence to traditional Chinese acupoints and Meridians. That these findings often proved difficult to reproduce is not surprising. Measurements of electrical properties of skin are beset by numerous problems, arising from physiology as well as instrumentation. Variable amounts of sweat can shunt current away from the electrode, while uneven anatomical topography adds to the problems of differential pressure artifacts during measurements. Further, acupoints vary one from another in their intrinsic electrical characteristics and these properties alter in response to physiological and pathophysiological change.[20] Finally, measuring instruments have differing sensitivities and are not always designed to ensure constant output of current or voltage.

Many of these difficulties were overcome by the use of two devices fabricated by Becker et al[21] in the mid-1970s. By means of a 36-electrode square grid, "topographical maps" of electrical conductivity around acupoints were produced. As with a series of mountain peaks, each with its unique pattern of slopes, acupoints were observed as the high points of individually contoured conductivity fields (Figure 11-3). In separate experiments, Becker et al designed a wheel electrode that could be rolled along a traditional Meridian on the skin to produce continuous readings. Despite intrasubject and intersubject variation, the resulting conductivity profiles revealed reproducible peaks that corresponded to acupoint sites (Figure 11-4).

Modern-day battery-operated point location devices measure electrical resistance (or conductance). A sound or light in the instrument's circuit indicates sites of electrical resistance below (or conductance above) a preset threshold, or a visual meter provides a direct readout. These devices have been used in two creatively designed tests of the Oriental medicine system of ear acupunc-

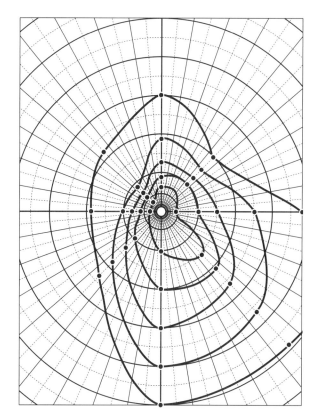

Figure 11-3 Conductance field around acupoint LI-4. By connecting points of equal conductance, an organization is revealed in which concentric lines do not cross and the overall ovoid shape is oriented with its long axis along the Large Intestine Meridian. Measurements were made with a 36-electrode square grid. (Modified from Becker RO, Reichmanis M, Marino AA, et al: *Psychoenerg Syst* 1:105-12, 1976.)

ture. Since, according to Oriental medical theory, there is a functional somatotopic projection of the body onto the ear, it is of interest to ask whether the bioelectric properties of auricular acupoints correlate with disease or dysfunction of their corresponding body sites. In a blinded assessment of patients with musculoskeletal pain, "reactive" ear points (those exhibiting at least 50 µA of electrical conductivity) corresponded to the painful musculoskeletal region of the body with a detection rate of 75%.[22] Nonreactive ear points corresponded to regions of the body with no musculoskeletal pain. Using similar blinded design and criteria, ear points traditionally designated as representing the heart were found to be "reactive" in patients with myocardial infarctions or angina at a markedly greater frequency than in healthy controls.[23]

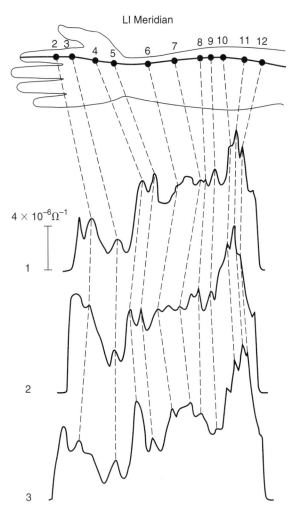

Figure 11-4 Conductance scans along the Large Intestine Meridian. Three successive scans on the same subject reveal conductance peaks that correspond to individual acupoints. Differences in scan length reflect slight changes in speed of the manually operated stainless steel wheel electrode. (Modified from Becker RO, Reichmanis M, Marino AA, et al: *Psychoenerg Syst* 1:105-12, 1976.)

BIOMEDICAL CORRELATES OF MERIDIANS

A current hypothesis, based on historical evidence from second century BCE silk scrolls, is that traditional Chinese medicine recognized the existence and therapeutic value of Meridians before detailed knowledge of acupoints.[24] Initial appreciation of Meridians may have developed as a result of the phenomenon mentioned at the start of this chapter: the propagating sensations re-

producibly reported by sensitive subjects with needling at single points.[25] The rates of these sensations, which vectorially follow the course of a Meridian, have been measured (1 to 10 cm/sec) and their responsiveness to focal changes in temperature and pressure have been documented.[26] Demonstrations of electrical coupling of successive acupoints along a Meridian[27] and reports of a variety of skin rashes following the course of Meridians[28,29] are frequently cited as providing further support for these pathways.

The question remains, however, whether peripheral modulation of propagated sensations, rashes, and electrical coupling of successive acupoints necessarily constitute evidence of physical Channels in the periphery. For example, blockade of a propagating sensation by mechanical pressure could result from a gate control-like spinal suppression of acupuncture-generated A afferent signals by pressure-generated Aδ afferent signals.

More direct evidence in apparent support of peripheral-based Meridians is that acupoint injection of technetium-99m, a radioisotope commonly used for diagnostic imaging, results in the longitudinal spread of isotope along an approximate course of a classical Meridian.[30,31] But these results have been criticized as artifacts of venous drainage,[32,33] and, in any case, should not be overinterpreted in support of Meridians until, at the least, demonstrations are forthcoming of isotope migration away from the heart and of isotope migrating preferentially along a Meridian at sites where a major vein and a Meridian diverge.

Alternative explanations of subjective Meridian phenomena seem necessary in light of reports of amputees who experience needling-induced sensations propagating along Meridians into phantom limbs.[34] As with phantom limb pain, these sensations are likely to reflect neural connectivity patterns in the spinal cord and brain. The subjective effect may be likened to that produced by a neon sign, on which a critical frequency of successive flashing lights creates the sensation that a single light is following a path around the sign's perimeter. In the case of acupuncture-induced propagating sensations, needling at a single acupoint may trigger the sequential firing of a series of spinal neurons connected by axon collaterals and interneurons. The scheme also requires that the neurons at successively higher (and lower) spinal segments, which are functionally linked in ascending and descending chains, correspond to acupoint sites along a traditional Meridian. (See Figure 11-5, based on models of Bossy[35] and Kendall.[15]) Because of the slight delays

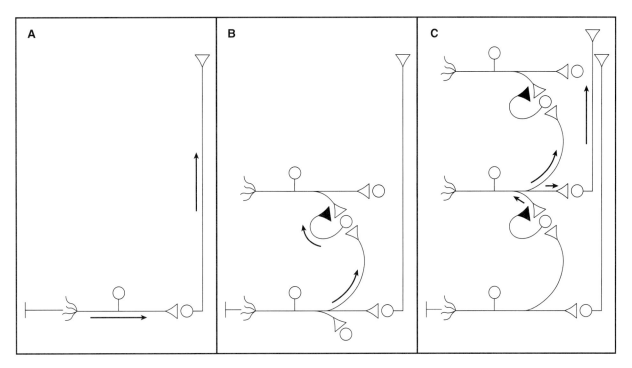

Figure 11-5 Model of "propagated sensation along the Channel" (PSC) based on central nervous system connectivity. In this model, PSC results from sequential activation of ascending and descending chains of spinal neurons. Although there is no direct experimental evidence for this theory, it is based on present knowledge of neuroanatomy and neural function. **A,** Primary sensory neuron carrying "acu-signals" makes synaptic contact with a spinal relay neuron at its same spinal level. Acu-signals are relayed to the mid-brain and cerebral cortex where their positions, as well as pricking and "de qi" sensations, are interpreted. **B,** By means of side branches (collaterals), the primary sensory neuron also make synaptic contact with spinal interneurons that, in turn, release depolarizing transmitter substances onto the presynaptic endings of specific higher- and lower-level primary sensory neurons that are otherwise positioned to carry signals from successive acupoints along the Channel (Meridian). **C,** Interneuron-triggered depolarization of sensory neuron collateral terminals initiates antidromic signals that travel back to the main nerve fiber from where they have three important destinations. *First,* the signal reverses direction and travels to its own spinal relay neuron that signals the brain, which "perceives" the signal as having originated at the "next" acupoint along the Meridian. *Second,* it reaches another branch point where it reverses direction and synapses on an interneuron at yet a higher (or lower) level, repeating the cycle just described. Because of the slight delays that occur during synaptic transmission, the signals from each successive spinal neuron in the chain reach the brain at slightly later times, giving rise to the propagated sensation that is felt to be traveling along the body surface. *Third,* the antidromic signal travels all the way to the periphery where nociceptive, vasodilatory, and immune stimulating transmitters are released (see Figure 11-2, *A*). This suggests a biomedical explanation of the therapeutic value of PSC, which Chinese medicine describes as the "arrival of qi" after distal needling. (Modified from Kendall DE: *Am J Acupunct* 17:251-268, 1989.)

imposed by synaptic transmission, the impulse initiated by each successive afferent neuron in the chain reaches the brain at a proportionately later time, giving rise to the propagated sensation. A similar theory describes the propagating sensations arising from neural activity in a higher brain center, the parietal lobe.[36] A corollary of these hypotheses is that propagating neural signals triggered by acupuncture may be a common physiological event, which only a relatively few sensitive individuals experience as conscious sensations.

The possibility of neural correlates of propagated sensations will be directly explorable once medical imaging techniques, such as functional MRI (fMRI), develop increased temporal resolution. At present, it is remarkable enough that fMRI has revealed spatially and temporally summated brain signals in response to distal needling. Manual needling of UB 67, an acupoint (on the lateral side of the little toe) traditionally included in Chinese medicine treatment for eye disorders, has been shown to activate the occipital lobe in a manner similar to that induced by direct visual stimulation.[37] Stimulation of proximal points along the same Meridian (UB 66 and 65) also activated the visual cortex, whereas needling a nonacupoint on the foot had no effect. Further fMRI studies have revealed that needling of an additional vision-related acupoint (GB 37) and two auditory-related acupoints (GB 43 and SJ 5) lead to activation in the visual and auditory cortices, respectively.[38] These findings clearly indicate that acupoints have functional representations in the central nervous system. Whether the pathway from points to brain is by means of the traditionally posited Meridians or by neural circuits is for future research to determine.

From an embryological perspective, such linear arrays of high-conductance peripheral points have been suggested to develop from so-called separatrices (lines of growth control) that play critical roles in morphogenesis.[39] Detectable alterations in bioelectric fields at these anatomical divides are indicators of developmental change[40] similar to the manner, in Chinese medicine, by which they serve as early clinical signs of physiological or pathological change. In this proposal, the Meridian system is viewed as a regulatory system that is independent of, yet constantly interacting with, the other major regulatory systems—nervous, immune, and endocrine—to monitor and adjust the organism.

BIOMEDICAL CORRELATES OF ACUPUNCTURE ACTION

From a biomedical perspective, the relatively weak anatomical evidence for acupoints and Meridians stands in contrast to the accumulating data demonstrating that insertion of fine needles at acupoints alters a variety of molecular and physiological markers. Correlates of acupuncture treatment can be grouped in two main categories: local responses to the microtrauma of needling, and distal responses mediated by sensory and sympathetic neural pathways.

Acupuncture Stimulates Local Blood Flow and Antiinflammatory Responses

Primary sensory neurons, whose receptor-rich endings in skin and muscle are likely targets of acupuncture needling, have long been known to respond to stimulation by releasing the same neurotransmitter molecules from their peripheral endings as from their central synaptic terminals. Two such molecules, the peptides substance P (SP) and calcitonin gene-related peptide (CGRP), act as peripheral vasodilators and as spinal cord transmitters. Thus it is interesting that local release of SP and CGRP has been detected in response to acupuncture stimuli that increase peripheral blood flow.[41,42] Vasomotor changes in response to manual or electroacupuncture also have been detected as increases in skin temperature[43] and as increases in microcirculation in both animals[44] and humans.[45,46] Acupuncture-induced peripheral vasodilatation is likely to result from SP and other substances released from axon collaterals acting on blood vessels, either directly or by activating sympathetic neurons (see Figure 11-2, A).

Antiinflammatory actions of acupuncture, in turn, correlate with reduced levels of histamine and prostaglandins in the inflammatory exudate,[47] suggesting that needling inhibits the local release of these substances from mast cells and nerve membranes, respectively. The question of whether these responses are unique to specific acupoints, however, was left unanswered because similar changes were detected after needling at three separate sites. Acupuncture-induced reduction of chronic inflammation may also be related to the release of pituitary adrenocorticotropic hormone (ACTH) into the circulation because increased synthesis and release of antiinflammatory adrenocortical steroids occurs after needling.[48,49] Of further interest, both studies indicated that ACTH release is not a nonspecific response to needling (e.g., a needling-related stress response) because corticosteroid increase was detected after acupuncture but not after needling of a nonpoint site.

Acupuncture Activates Peripheral Terminals of Sensory Neurons That Relay Signals to the Spinal Cord and Brain

One of the earliest indicators of acupuncture effectiveness being mediated by nerve conduction is that acupoints injected with local anesthetic become unresponsive to needling.[50,51] The question of which primary sensory neurons carry the "acu-signals" has been examined most directly by extracellular recordings from individual nerve fibers. Activity of small myelinated fibers, the Aδ cutaneous afferents and type III muscle afferents (but not the larger fibers), correlated closely with induction of analgesia in animals[52] and with analgesia onset, as well as subjective reports of the acupuncture-induced *de qi* sensation of focal achiness in human subjects.[53] The observation that acu-signals are carried by small-diameter fibers suggests that acupuncture does not produce analgesia by "gate control" mechanisms, at least not according to the original concept that input from large-diameter A fibers inhibit (close the gate on) nociceptive input carried by small-diameter C (unmyelinated) fibers at the first relay site in the dorsal horn of the spinal cord.[54]

Neural pathways by which acu-signals reach the spinal cord and brain have been mapped (mainly for acupuncture analgesia) using the same techniques developed for tracking signals initiated by the more common types of sensory stimuli such as pressure or heat. Typically, microelectrodes lowered onto the surface of discrete brain regions detect which groups of neurons become active (produce evoked potentials) or less active (are inhibited) in response to insertion of an acupuncture needle in the skin. Neurochemicals that mediate the signaling along these pathways are identified in minute samples taken from the extracellular space around active neurons, and are inferred by determining the effects of drugs known to mimic or block the suspected chemical mediators. As a result of initial findings that the opioid antagonist naloxone can partially suppress acupuncture analgesia (AcuA), the search for neural pathways of AcuA was guided by prior knowledge of brain sites mediating morphine analgesia. Also, when these AcuA studies began in the late 1970s, it was already appreciated that pain modulation occurs at multiple peripheral and central sites.

For example, neurons in the substantia gelatinosa, the dorsalmost layer of the spinal gray matter, are the sites at which peripheral nociceptive signals are first received and relayed to the brain. Electrical responses of these neurons to noxious stimuli are suppressed by acupuncture, but not in the presence of the opioid antagonist naloxone.[55] Follow-up studies[56] suggested that this spinal-level inhibition occurs by two sets of pathways, one within the spinal cord, the other descending from the mid-brain (Figure 11-6). Although pain signals are typically carried by fibers that cross the spinal cord to ascend in the contralateral spinothalamic tract (SST), acu-signals, similar to signals of other sensory modalities, ascend in fibers of the ipsilateral anterolateral tract (ALT) (see Figure 11-6). Thus spinal segmental inhibition of incoming pain signals is mediated by side branches from the ALT, whereas descending inhibition occurs by multisynaptic pathways after acu-signals have first reached mid-brain and hypothalamic sites.[56-58] In addition to the endogenous opioids (see next section), there is strong evidence that serotonin mechanisms play a role in AcuA, particularly in modulating descending inhibition from the md-brain raphe nucleus.

The relation of these analgesic neural pathways to acupuncture per se has been questioned by the well-documented phenomena of stress-induced analgesia[59] and diffuse noxious inhibitory control (DNIC), in which pain from a particular site on the body is inhibited by applying another painful stimulus at any other site on the body.[51,60] Because a considerable amount of AcuA research has been done in animals, particular care has been taken to rule out stress as a significant contributor to mechanisms attributed to acupuncture.[61,62] That DNIC is also unlikely to be a major component of AcuA can be argued based on both physiological and clinical findings. Although AcuA is mediated primarily by small myelinated fibers, DNIC is associated with unmyelinated C fibers that respond to noxious stimuli. It is also true

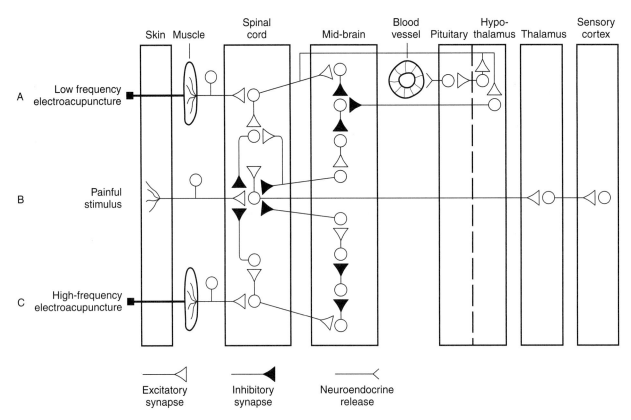

Figure 11-6 Neurophysiological model of low- and high-frequency electroacupuncture-induced analgesia. In this model, which summarizes much of the experimental findings for acupuncture analgesia, only the pathway for the sensory component of noxious stimuli reaching the brain in the spinothalamic tract is included **(B).** Low-frequency electroacupuncture **(A)** modulates incoming nociceptive signals at four levels: spinal interneurons, descending pathways originating in the midbrain (that include the periaqueductal gray and Raphe nucleus) and hypothalamus, and the circulation (involving hypothalamo-pituitary pathways). High-frequency electroacupuncture **(C)** modulates nociceptive signals at spinal and mid-brain levels. The spinal and midbrain pathways are distinct for low- and high-frequency electroacupuncture (see Figure 11-7). (Modified from Pomeranz B: Scientific basis of acupuncture. In Stux G, Pomeranz B, editors: *Acupuncture textbook and atlas,* Berlin, 1987, Springer-Verlag, p 1-34.)

that acupuncture treatment is not commonly perceived as painful. Further, as shown in controlled clinical trials, needling at acupoints is significantly more effective in moderating pain than sham needling at nonpoints.[16,17,63] Although some degree of analgesia is frequently induced by nonpoint needling, its mechanism has been differentiated from that of acupoint-induced analgesia on the basis of neural pathways and pharmacological sensitivity.[64,65]

THE ACUPUNCTURE/ ENDORPHIN CONNECTION

Anyone who has acquired even a modicum of knowledge about "how acupuncture works" knows that endorphins have been implicated in the mechanism of acupuncture analgesia.[57,66,67] But before examining the evidence in support of the acupuncture-endorphin connection, it should be noted that the term *endoge-*

TABLE 11-1

Endogenous Opioids and Antiopioids

Endogenous opioids*	Peptide length (amino acids)	Opiate receptor preference
Enkephalins	5	δ
β-endorphins	23	γ, δ
Dynorphins	11	κ
Endomorphins	4	μ
Orphanin FQ/nociceptin†	11	Orphan

Endogenous antiopioids*	Peptide length (amino acids)	
Cholecystokinin-8	8	
Angiotensin II	8	
Orphanin FQ/nociceptin†	17	
Neuropeptide FF	8	
Tyr-W-MIF-1B	4	

*See text for references.

†Acts as an opioid or an antiopioid at different sites. (Darland T, Heinricher MM, Grandy DK: *Trends Neurosci* 21:215-221, 1998.)

nous opioids, rather than *endorphins,* more broadly describes this versatile class of bioactive molecules (Table 11-1), with its three main families of polypeptides, the enkephalins, endorphins, and dynorphins, as well as the recently identified endomorphins[68] and orphanin FQ/nociceptin.[69] Each of these molecular families relays and modulates neuronal signals coding awareness of and response to pain. Because endogenous opioids attenuate pain signals at peripheral and central sites, at multiple spinal cord and brain locations, in ascending and descending pathways, presynaptically, as well as postsynaptically, it is clear that a multiplicity of studies is needed to understand how acupuncture may affect these modulators.

The possibility that AcuA is mediated by a humoral factor(s) was first suggested from cross-perfusion studies predating the discoveries of the endogenous opioids. Analgesia (detected as a delay in avoidance of a noxious stimulus) was successfully induced in animals that had not been needled but received blood or cerebrospinal fluid from animals in whom analgesia had been produced by acupuncture[70] or acupressure.[71] Similar cross-perfusions of fluid from non-needled animals did not cause analgesia in the recipients. Follow-up pharmaco-

logical studies suggested serotonin as a candidate for the transfer factor, a finding consistent with present knowledge of this neurotransmitter's role in descending pain modulation pathways in the spinal cord.

But the main implications of the cross-perfusion studies awaited the exciting discoveries of endogenous morphine-like polypeptides, announced in the mid-1970s. Several laboratories soon demonstrated that the onset of AcuA correlated with the release of one or more of the endogenous opioids. Infrared heat directed at the nose of mice or acutely induced dental pain in human subjects were each shown to be increasingly tolerated after acupuncture but not if the animal or human subjects were pretreated with the morphine antagonist, naloxone.[72,73] Independent lines of evidence, in large part from the laboratories of Jisheng Han in Beijing[57] and Bruce Pomeranz in Toronto,[66] substantiated the acupuncture–endogenous opioid hypothesis:

- A strain of mice with genetically low levels of opiate receptors develops weak AcuA in response to the same acupuncture stimuli that produce strong analgesia in mice with normal levels of receptors.
- Elevated cerebrospinal fluid and blood levels of endogenous opioids correlate with the onset of AcuA.

- AcuA is enhanced in animals pretreated with pharmacological agents that suppress enzymatic breakdown of endogenous opioids, to prolong their action.
- AcuA is suppressed after microinjection of naloxone into specific brain sites implicated in analgesic pathways.
- Cross-tolerance to AcuA is detected in animals made tolerant to morphine; cross-tolerance to morphine is detected in AcuA-tolerant animals.
- Endogenous antiopioids suppress analgesia and neuronal firing patterns induced by electroacupuncture.

Two scientific advances, the development of electroacupuncture and the production of antibodies specific to each class of endogenous opioids, added significant scope to the understanding of the acupuncture–endogenous opioid connection.

Electroacupuncture, the passage of a current of defined frequency, amplitude, and duration through wires attached to acupuncture needles, was developed to circumvent the need for continual manual manipulation of needles during long surgeries. The use of electroacupuncture in research studies[57,66] revealed that AcuA could be induced by passing current over a range from 2 to 4 Hz (low frequency) to 100 to 200 Hz (high frequency). Pretreatment with naloxone, at doses normally sufficient to block morphine (<1 mg/kg), readily suppresses low frequency but not high frequency electroacupuncture; 10 to 50 times higher doses of naloxone are required for comparable suppression of high-frequency AcuA. Based on a variety of studies, consensus formed that 2 to 4 Hz was releasing met-enkephalin and β-endorphin, whereas 100 to 200 Hz was acting through release of dynorphin and serotonin. Studies with specific opioid antagonists injected intrathecally (into the spinal cord cerebral spinal fluid) confirmed this view: low-frequency electroacupuncture appears to act predominantly through μ- and δ-opioid receptors that mediate enkephalin and dynorphin responses, whereas high-frequency electroacupuncture acts preferentially through dynorphin-activating κ-opioid receptors. Collectively, these data imply that distinct neuronal pathways mediate the analgesia induced by electroacupuncture of different frequencies.

The important clinical application of these findings is that pain suppression is best induced by alternating the frequency of electroacupuncture between high and low settings. In this manner, all three fami-

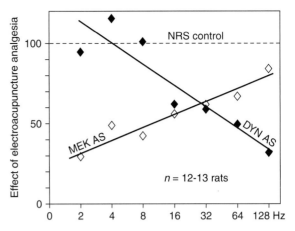

Figure 11-7 Preferential inhibition of low-frequency or high-frequency electroacupuncture by pretreatment with antisera to met-enkephalin (MEK AS) or dynorphin A (DYN AS), respectively. The log dose-response curves suggest that low-frequency electroacupuncture analgesia is mediated by enkephalin release, whereas high-frequency electroacupuncture analgesia is mediated predominantly by dynorphin release. Data are presented after normalization to the effects of pretreatment (intrathecal injection) with normal rabbit serum (NRS) (Modified from Han JS: Hndbk Exp Pharmacol 104/II:105-25, 1993.)

lies of endogenous opioids are released. Many electrostimulation devices used in acupuncture clinics now include a setting that automatically shifts the frequencies between these low and high levels.

The use of antibodies as experimental tools has provided evidence consistent with the concept of frequency-specific effects of electroacupuncture on endogenous opioids.[57] A rabbit antiserum against met-enkephalin, injected intrathecally in rats, reduced the effectiveness of 2-Hz electroacupuncture by approximately 70%, whereas it decreased 100-Hz electroacupuncture by 20%. In contrast, antiserum against dynorphin A markedly reduced the effect of high-frequency electroacupuncture with virtually no effect on the low-frequency response (Figure 11-7). All changes were assessed relative to the effects of injecting a control, preimmune rabbit serum.

Differential effects of low- and high-frequency electroacupuncture also have been demonstrated at the level of gene expression.[74] In numerous brain regions, for example, immunocytochemical studies revealed that 2-Hz stimulation increased the expression

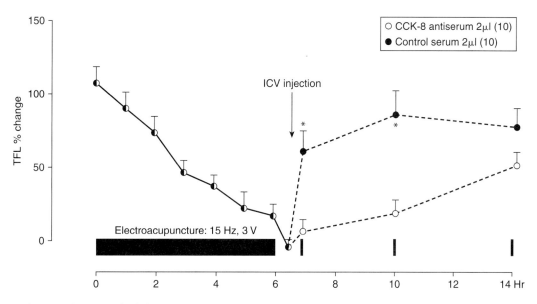

Figure 11-8 Reversal of electroacupuncture tolerance in rats by intracerebroventricular *(ICV)* injection of antiserum to cholecystokinin-8 *(CCK-8)*. The level of analgesic tolerance, developed in response to repeated electroacupuncture treatments, and recovery from tolerance were monitored by a tail-flick latency *(TFL)* assay. *$p < .01$ compared with control serum. (Modified from Han J-S, Ding X-Z, Fan S-G: *Neuropeptides* 5:399-402, 1985.)

of the messenger RNA (mRNA) for the enkephalin precursor protein with little effect on the mRNA for the dynorphin precursor. In contrast, stimulation at 100 Hz selectively increased expression of the dynorphin precursor mRNA. However, because these effects on gene expression were assayed 24 hours after electroacupuncture, they are more likely to reflect feedback regulation required to replenish stores of opioids than direct effects of acupuncture on gene expression.

An additional critical piece of the pain regulation puzzle was the discovery that the yang of endogenous opioids may be balanced by the yin of a family of endogenous antiopioids, peptides that counteract the pain-modulating action of the endorphins (see Table 11-1).[75-77,77a] Early evidence indicated that a substance with antiopiate activity was present in the brains of rats that developed tolerance to acupuncture after successive treatments.[78] Findings that the same pathway by which food consumption is *increased* by β-endorphin or morphine is used to *decrease* food consumption by the polypeptide cholecystokinin (CCK) and led to demonstrations that CCK could also antagonize opioid analgesia.[79,80] CCK-octapeptide (CCK-8), a naturally occurring brain form of the 33–amino acid poly-

peptide hormone first characterized from the gut, produces a dose-dependent suppression of analgesia induced by either morphine or electroacupuncture.[75] Further, the ability of electroacupuncture to inhibit C fiber–mediated responses of spinal dorsal horn neurons to noxious stimuli is counteracted by application of CCK-8.[81] The preliminary finding mentioned previously (that antiopioid activity is detectable in the brain of animals that become tolerant to electroacupuncture) was borne out when intracerebral ventricular injection of a CCK-8 antiserum was shown to reverse this tolerance[75] (Figure 11-8).

In this yin and yang view of pain modulation, acupuncture studies are contributing to a clinically significant hypothesis: individual variations in pain sensitivity, as well as individual responses to analgesics or to acupuncture itself, reflect differences in the balance between opioid and antiopioid peptides at pain-modulating synapses. An elegant example in support of this hypothesis is that animals characterized as poor responders to both morphine analgesia and electroacupuncture analgesia were converted to good responders by using molecular biological techniques to block expression of the gene encoding the CCK precursor protein in the brain.[82]

ACUPUNCTURE REGULATION OF CARDIOVASCULAR, GASTROINTESTINAL, AND IMMUNOLOGICAL FUNCTION

Although acupuncture, within the medical tradition it represents, treats a full spectrum of conditions, no other aspect of its clinical effectiveness has received a fraction of the physiological research attention given to pain management. It is of interest, nonetheless, to review the progress in several representative areas, including regulation of gastrointestinal, immunological, and cardiovascular function. As shown in the specific examples discussed, a common theme emerging from the research in these three areas is a clinically recognized but little-researched phenomenon of acupuncture: its ability to induce bidirectional effects, so that needling at the same acupoint can stimulate a hypo-condition or depress a hyper-condition.

Cardiovascular Regulation

Effects of acupuncture on heart rate, blood pressure, and related parameters of cardiovascular function have been examined in human subjects and in hypotensive and hypertensive animals.[83-85] In rats made hypotensive by withdrawing blood[86] or in dogs made hypertensive by intravenous infusion of epinephrine,[87] electroacupuncture at St-36 or acupuncture-like stimulation of the sciatic nerve returned blood pressure toward normal levels. In the experimental dogs, electroacupuncture also attenuated an epinephrine-induced decrease in blood flow. Pretreatment with naloxone blocked the effects of electroacupuncture, suggesting that vasodilatory effects of electroacupuncture are mediated by endogenous opioids. Similar normalizing effects of acupuncture on blood pressure and heart rate were observed in two strains of rats bred to be congenitally hypotensive or hypertensive.[83] Follow-up studies involving pharmacological pretreatment suggested that acupuncture-induced depressor effects are mediated by the release of endogenous opioid(s) and serotonin, whereas the pressor effects of acupuncture in hypotensive rats, being naloxone insensitive but attenuated by scopolamine, involve central cholinergic mechanisms.[83]

In light of the evidence supporting a homeostatic action of acupuncture, it is not surprising that studies on cardiovascular function in normal human subjects have shown either slight or nonsignificant effects on heart rate or blood pressure when the data have been examined as mean values.[88,89] A different picture can emerge, however, when effects on individual subjects are analyzed. A crossover design study (electroacupuncture at LI-4 and LI-10 versus placebo), also notable for its use of a blinded treatment assessor, revealed highly significant findings that individuals whose initial heart rates placed them in the lowest one third of the "normal" test group had increased rates after acupuncture, whereas those whose heart rates were in the highest one third experienced decreased rates.[90] Similar modulatory effects were observed for skin blood flow and the blood pressure–heart rate product (Figure 11-9). Had these sets of data been analyzed as mean effects, none of the results would have been statistically significant.

Gastrointestinal Regulation

Clinical and physiological research on digestive and other gastrointestinal disorders has been critically reviewed, with the physiological focus primarily on gastric acid secretion and gut motility.[91,92] Despite differences in research design involving acupoint selection, parameters of electrostimulation, and observation conditions, electroacupuncture has been consistently found to induce significant reductions in feeding-induced gastric acid secretion relative to control electroacupuncture (applying similar electrostimulation by needles at nonpoint sites).[93,94] In dogs, reduction in acid secretion correlated with *increases* in plasma levels of β-endorphin and somatostatin, a peptide known to inhibit secretion in a variety of endocrine and exocrine glands, and a *decrease* in plasma gastrin, a peptide hormone that stimulates secretion of stomach acid. Pretreatment with naloxone blocked the effects of electroacupuncture on acid secretion in both animals and normal human subjects, suggesting a key regulatory role for β-endorphin or other endogenous opioid. Naloxone also blocked the changes in plasma levels of somatostatin and gastrin in dogs. Acupuncture is seen as acting by means of somatic afferent and vagal efferent nerves, as well as by releasing regulatory hormones.

In the example of gastric acid secretion, acupuncture is known clinically, acting through the same acupoints, to increase acid production in cases of hyposecretion but to decrease production in conditions

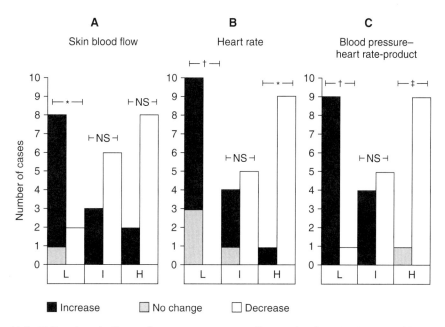

Figure 11-9 Bidirectional effects of acupuncture on cardiovascular function in normal human subjects. Skin blood flow **(A)**, heart rate **(B)**, and blood pressure–heart rate product **(C)** are presented as a function of direction of acupuncture-induced change (increase, no change, decrease) from baseline values. Data for each endpoint were divided into three equal-sized groups based on low *(L)*, intermediate *(I)*, and high *(H)* baseline values. The points of discrimination between low and intermediate baseline values, and intermediate and high values were 12 and 22 arbitrary units for skin blood flow, 57 and 66 beats/min for heart rate, and 6300 and 7750 mm Hg/min for the blood pressure–heart rate product. $*p < 0.05$; $†p < 0.01$; $‡p < 0.005$. *NS,* Nonsignificant. (Modified from Ballegaard S, Muteki T, Harada H, et al: *Acupunct Electrother Res* 18:103-115, 1993.)

of hypersecretion.[95] In this light, feeding is seen as a physiological example of a condition involving hypersecretion that the acupuncture homeostat modulates.

Results of controlled trials of acupuncture on gastric motility are less clear, with differences in research design again a confounding factor. Although a number of studies, reviewed by Li et al,[91] indicate that acupuncture has an effect significantly beyond that of nonspecific needling, more recent findings demonstrate that acupuncture markedly *stimulates* the basal level of intestinal peristalsis but significantly *reduces* peristalsis that had been experimentally accelerated by drug treatment.[96]

Immunological Regulation

Effects of acupuncture have been examined on a range of both cell-mediated immune responses (white blood cell levels, macrophage phagocytic activity, T-cell pro-

liferation and transformation, and natural killer cell cytotoxic activity) and humoral immunity (competency of B cells to engage in antibody production). Two recent reviews provide detailed summaries and critiques of these studies.[97,98]

Although it is logical, in terms of research design, to monitor specific aspects of immune function in response to acupoint needling, this approach can cause acupuncture to be regarded as a set of fine-tuned procedures that, similar to pharmacologically designed drugs, selectively affect different cell populations. An arguably more useful physiological model is to consider acupuncture as facilitating the release, and balancing the circulating levels, of the same endogenous substances (e.g., cytokines) that immune system cells use to communicate with each other and with cells of the endocrine, nervous, and other regulatory systems.[98,99]

For example, after 7 weekly individualized acupuncture treatments for lower back pain, the T lymphocytes of 10 patients showed a greater than 50%

mean increase in mitogen-induced proliferation.[100] It is also well established that β-endorphin, released into the circulation by acupuncture, enhances mitogen-stimulated T-cell proliferative responses.[98] In other studies, acupoint St-36, one of the strongest points for stimulating β-endorphin release,[101] was found to enhance natural killer cell cytotoxicity[102] and to increase T-cell function, as measured by plaque-forming activity in response to injection of foreign red blood cells.[103] In both studies, the responses to St-36 needling were significantly greater than responses to control point needling. Of added interest is that the increase in plaque-forming activity was blocked by treatment with the β-endorphin antagonist, naloxone, or the β-adrenergic blocker, propranolol. Endogenous opioid and sympathetic nervous system–mediated effects of acupuncture on immune function have been confirmed in a similar plaque-forming assay[104] and in studies of T-cell transformation.[105]

Indications of the balancing or bidirectional actions of acupuncture, discussed previously with regard to cardiovascular and gastrointestinal function, also have been detected in immune system responses. In healthy subjects, the levels of IgA (the main class of salivary immunoglobulins) appeared to increase if initial levels were low and to decrease when initial levels were high.[106]

FUTURE DIRECTIONS

Having reviewed the biomedical correlates of acupoints and Meridians, the biochemical and physiological changes associated with acupuncture analgesia, and the regulatory effects of acupuncture on the cardiovascular, gastrointestinal, and immune systems, it is of interest to identify aspects of these findings that suggest directions for future research.

For example, it is important to consider that the acupuncture–endogenous opioid connection and the mechanisms underlying the homeostatic capability of acupuncture have been proposed largely on the basis of studies using electrostimulation of the needles. From a research perspective, electroacupuncture has an obvious advantage over manual acupuncture. Descriptions of the frequency, amplitude, and duration of electrostimulation allow studies to be reproduced with a greater degree of confidence than do descriptions of the twirling, thrusting, and other traditional techniques of manual stimulation. Nevertheless, be-

cause electroacupuncture provides a more intense form of acupoint stimulation than manual needling and because the latter is the predominant technique in clinical practice, it should not necessarily be assumed that the two techniques produce similar physiological and biochemical effects.[107] Studies are needed not only to compare physiological effects of electroacupuncture with those of manual acupuncture but to examine effects of the deeper (intramuscular) style of Chinese needling relative to the shallower (subcutaneous) styles of Japanese needling.

A large proportion of physiological research on acupuncture has used either normal animals or healthy human volunteers as subjects. Accordingly, rigorous studies are needed to compare bioelectric properties of acupoints and physiological effects of needling in conditions of health versus illness.[20]

A further observation emerging from this overview of physiological research is that biomedical explanations of several areas of acupuncture results may be inadequate. For example, the mechanisms by which needling at the same acupoint(s) can return a particular physiological parameter (e.g., gastric acid secretion, antibody levels, heart rate) to normative levels from either a hypo-condition or hyper-condition are unclear. Such findings suggest that acupuncture activates a feedback system that monitors and regulates internal activities. The basic question remains whether the homeostatic actions of acupuncture are mediated by known neural and hormonal mechanisms or by a hypothetical system that is separate from but interacts with the known autonomic and humoral systems.[108,109] The possibility that acupuncture effects may not be initiated or mediated solely by neurophysiological means has potential support in preliminary reports from China of propagating sensations along Meridians (PSM) being elicited at a distance by Qigong practitioners.[110] In addition, Toyohari practitioners in Japan have decades of clinical experience using a style of acupuncture that includes noninvasive needling. In this technique, Qi is sensed through a needle held close to but not penetrating the skin at an acupoint.[111] If the efficacy of Qigong-elicited PSM and of Toyohari noninvasive needling can be demonstrated in controlled clinical trials, they will represent important approaches for exploring the energy medicine that Chinese and other Asian traditions have long described in the language of metaphor.

The recent fMRI studies, demonstrating signals in the visual and auditory cortex after stimulation of acupoints on the leg or foot that are traditionally used for eye and ear disorders, respectively[37,38] are also difficult to explain in terms of known neurobiological pathways. What is implied in these findings is that acupoint stimulation activates organ-specific brain regions, which in turn direct healing responses in the particular organ.

An additional aspect of acupuncture that merits research attention is the frequently observed long-lasting effect of treatment, as if a physiological reset mechanism has been activated. Placebo-controlled clinical trials of acupuncture for dysmenorrhea[16] and migraine[17] not only reported that acupuncture outperformed control needling at the end of the 3-month or 6-week treatment period, respectively, but that pain levels and consumption of pain medication were still significantly reduced in the acupuncture group at 1-year follow-up. This phenomenon has been discussed in terms of autonomic nervous system "conditioning"[112] and "physiological relearning,"[108] but it seems likely that systematic studies of the phenomenon will yield deeper understandings of both Chinese and Western physiology.

The one certain outcome of future research on the physiology of acupuncture is that it will significantly expand our understanding of what the renowned physiologist Claude Bernard referred to as the "internal milieu" and the equally prominent physiologist Walter B. Cannon more broadly called "the wisdom of the body."[113]

References

1. Hu Y, Qi Y-Q: The phenomenon of energy circulated in the meridian system, *Int J Chin Med* 1:7-14, 1984.
2. Lewith G, Vincent C: On the evaluation of the clinical effects of acupuncture: a problem reassessed and a framework for future research, *J Altern Complement Med* 2:79-90, 1996.
2a. Hammerschlag R: Methodological and ethical issues in clinical trials of acupuncture, *J Altern Complement Med* 4:159-171, 1998.
3. Hammerschlag R, Morris MM: Clinical trials comparing acupuncture with biomedical standard care: a criteria-based evaluation of research design and reporting, *Complement Ther Med* 5:133-140, 1997.
4. Birch S, Hammerschlag R: Acupuncture efficacy: a compendium of controlled clinical trials, Tarrytown, NY, 1996, National Academy of Acupuncture and Oriental Medicine.
4a. Stux G, Hammerschlag R, editors: *Clinical acupuncture: scientific basis,* Berlin, 2001, Springer-Verlag.
5. Ciszik M, Szopinski J, Skrzypulec V: Investigations of morphological structure of acupuncture points and meridians, *J Trad Chin Med* 5:289-292, 1985.
6. Dung HC: Acupuncture points of typical spinal nerves, *Am J Chin Med* 13:39-47, 1985.
7. Heine H: Anatomical structure of acupoints, *J Trad Chin Med* 8:207-212, 1988.
8. Gunn CC, Ditchburn FG, King MH: Acupuncture loci: a proposal for their classification according to their relationship to known neural structures, *Am J Chin Med* 4:183-195, 1976.
9. Melzack R, Stillwell DM, Fox EJ: Trigger points and acupuncture points for pain: correlation and implications, *Pain* 3:3-23, 1977.
10. Hwang Y-C: Anatomy and classification of acupoints, *Prob Vet Med* 4:12-15, 1992.
11. Zheng JY, Fan JY, Zhang YJ, et al: Further evidence for the role of gap junctions in acupoint information transfer, *Am J Acupunct* 24:291-296, 1996.
12. Baldry PE: *Acupuncture, trigger points and musculoskeletal pain,* ed 2, New York, 1993, Churchill Livingstone.
13. Macdonald AJR: *Acupuncture from ancient art to modern medicine,* London, 1982, George Allen & Unwin.
14. Milne RJ, Foreman RD, Giesler GJ, et al: Convergence of cutaneous and pelvic visceral nociceptive inputs onto primate spinothalamic neurons, *Pain* 11:163-183, 1981.
15. Kendall DE: A scientific model for acupuncture. Part II, *Am J Acupunct* 17:343-360, 1989.
16. Helms JM: Acupuncture for the management of primary dysmenorrhea, *Obstet Gynecol* 69:51-56, 1987.
17. Vincent CA: A controlled trial of the treatment of migraine by acupuncture, *Clin J Pain* 5:305-312, 1989.
18. Niboyet JEH: Étude sur la moindre résistance cutanée a l'ectricité de certains points de la peau dits "Points Chinois," *BSAC* 39:16-88, 1961.
19. Nakatani Y, Yamashita K: *Ryodoraku acupuncture: a guide for the application of Ryodoraku therapy,* Tokyo, 1977, Ryodoraku Research Institute.
20. Kawakita K, Kawamura H, Keino H, et al: Development of the low impedance points in the auricular skin of experimental peritonitis in rats, *Am J Chin Med* 19:199-205, 1991.
21. Becker RO, Reichmanis M, Marino AA, et al: Electrophysiological correlates of acupuncture points and meridians, *Psychoenerg Syst* 1:105-112, 1976.
22. Oleson T, Kroening R, Bressler D: An experimental evaluation of auricular diagnosis: the somatotropic mapping of musculoskeletal pain at ear acupuncture points, *Pain* 8:217-229, 1980.
23. Saku K, Mukaino Y, Ying H, et al: Characteristics of reactive electropermeable points on the auricles of coronary heart disease patients, *Clin Cardiol* 16:415-419, 1993.
24. Chen Y: Silk scrolls: earliest literature of meridian doctrine in ancient China, *Acupunct Electrother Res* 22:175-189, 1997.

25. Xie Y, Li H, Xiao W: Neurobiological mechanisms of the meridian and the propagation of needle feeling along the meridian pathway, *Sci China C Life Sci* 39:99-112, 1996.

26. Hu X, Wu B, You Z, et al: Preliminary analysis of the mechanism underlying the phenomenon of channel blocking, *J Trad Chin Med* 6:289-296, 1984.

27. Reichmanis M, Marino A, Becker RO: Laplace plane analysis of impedance between acupuncture points H-3 and H-4, *Comp Med East West* 5:289-95, 1977.

28. Li D: Existence of channel system as evidenced by 93 cases of skin disease appearing along the channels. In Zhang X, editor: *Research on acupuncture, moxibustion and acupuncture anesthesia,* Beijing, 1986, Beijing Press/Springer-Verlag.

29. James R: Linear skin rashes and meridians of acupuncture, *Eur J Orient Med* 3:43-46, 1994.

30. De Vernejoul P, Albarede P, Darras J-C: Etude des meridiens d'acupuncture par les traceurs radioactifs, *Bull Acad Nat Med* 169:1071-1075, 1985.

31. Kovacs FM, Gotzens V, Garcia A, et al: Experimental study on radioactive pathways of hypodermically injected technicium-99m, *J Nucl Med* 33:403-407, 1992.

32. Lazorthes Y, Esquerre J-P, Simon J, et al: Acupuncture meridians and radioactive tracers, *Pain* 40:109-112, 1990.

33. Wu CC, Chen MF, Lin CC: Absorption of subcutaneous injection of Tc-99m pertechnetate via acupuncture points and non-acupuncture points, *Am J Chin Med* 22:111-118, 1994.

34. Xue CC: Acupuncture induced phantom limb and meridian phenomenon in acquired and congenital amputees: a suggestion of the use of acupuncture as a method for investigation of phantom limb, *Chin Med J* 99:247-252, 1986.

35. Bossy J: Implication of the spinal nucleus of the trigeminal nerve in acupuncture, *Acupunct Electrother Res* 11:17790, 1986.

36. Xue C: The phenomenon of propagated sensation along channels and the cerebral cortex. In Zhang X, editor: *Research on acupuncture, moxibustion and acupuncture anesthesia,* Beijing, 1986, Science Press.

37. Cho ZH, Chung SC, Jones JP, et al: New findings of the correlation between acupoints and corresponding brain cortices using functional MRI, *Proc Nat Acad Sci U S A* 95:2670-2673, 1998.

38. Cho ZH, Na CS, Wang EK, et al: Functional magnetic resonance imaging of the brain in the investigation of acupuncture. In Stux G, Hammerschlag R, editors: *Clinical acupuncture: scientific basis,* Berlin, 2001, Springer-Verlag.

39. Shang C: Singular point, organizing center and acupuncture point, *Am J Chin Med* 17:119-127, 1989.

40. Nuccitelli R: Ionic currents in morphogenesis, *Experientia* 44:657-666, 1988.

41. Jansen G, Lundeberg T, Kjartansson J, et al: Acupuncture and sensory neuropeptides increase cutaneous blood flow in rats, *Neurosci Lett* 97:305-309, 1989.

42. Kashiba H, Ueda Y: Acupuncture to the skin induces release of substance P and calcitonin gene-related peptide from peripheral terminals of primary sensory neurons in the rat, *Am J Chin Med* 19:189-197, 1991.

43. Ernst M, Lee MHM: Sympathetic vasomotor changes induced by manual and electrical acupuncture of the Hoku point visualized by thermography, *Pain* 21:25-33, 1985.

44. Itaya K, Manaka Y, Ohkubo C, et al: Effects of acupuncture needle application upon cutaneous microcirculation of rabbit ear lobe, *Acupunct Electrother Res* 12:45-51, 1987.

45. Litscher G, Schwarz G, Sandner-Kiesling A, et al: Effects of acupuncture on the oxygenation of cerebral tissue, *Neurol Res* 20(suppl 1):S28-32, 1998.

46. Yuan X, Hao X, Lai Z, et al: Effects of acupuncture at fengchi point (GB 20) on cerebral blood flow, *J Trad Chin Med* 18:102-105, 1998.

47. Leong ML, Sin YM, Tan CH: Effect of electrical acupuncture on histamine and prostaglandins of acute inflammatory response, *Altern Med* 2:103-109, 1987.

48. Liao Y-Y, Seto K, Saito H, et al: Effect of acupuncture on adrenocortical hormone production. I. Variation in the ability for adrenocortical hormone production in response to the duration of acupuncture stimulation, *Am J Chin Med* 7:362-371, 1979.

49. Cheng R, Pomeranz B: Electroacupuncture elevates blood cortisol levels in naive horses; sham treatment has no effect, *Int J Neurosci* 10:95-97, 1980.

50. Chiang C-Y, Chang C-T, Chu H-L, et al: Peripheral afferent pathway for acupuncture analgesia, *Sci Sin* 16:210-217, 1973.

51. Pomeranz B, Paley D: Electroacupuncture hypalgesia is mediated by afferent nerve impulse: an electrophysiological study in mice, *Exp Neurol* 66:398-402, 1979.

52. German Acupuncture Society: Dusseldorf acupuncture symposium report: the scientific bases of acupuncture, *Am J Acupunct* 16:362-365, 1988.

53. Wang K, Yao S, Xian Y, et al: A study on the receptive field of acupoints and the relationship between characteristics of needle sensation and groups of afferent fibers, *Sci Sin* 28:963-971, 1985.

54. Melzack R, Wall PD: Pain mechanisms: a new theory, *Science* 150:971-979, 1965.

55. Pomeranz B, Cheng R: Suppression of noxious responses in single neurons of cat spinal cord by electroacupuncture and its reversal by the opiate antagonist naloxone, *Exp Neurol* 64:327-341, 1979.

56. Pomeranz B: Scientific basis of acupuncture. In Stux G, Pomeranz B, editors: *Acupuncture, textbook and atlas,* Berlin, 1987, Springer-Verlag.

57. Han JS: Acupuncture and stimulation produced analgesia, *Handbook Exp Pharmacol* 104/II:105-125, 1993.
58. Takeshige C, Oka K, Mizuno T, et al: The acupuncture point and its connecting central pathway for producing acupuncture analgesia, *Brain Res Bull* 30:53-67, 1993.
59. Bodnar RJ: Effects of opioid peptides on peripheral stimulation and "stress"-induced analgesia in animals, *Crit Rev Neurobiol* 6:39-49, 1990.
60. Le Bars D, Dickenson AH, Besson JM: Diffuse noxious inhibitory controls (DNIC). I. Effects on dorsal horn convergent neurones in the rat, *Pain* 6:283-304, 1979.
61. Pomeranz B: Relation of stress-induced analgesia to acupuncture analgesia, *Ann N Y Acad Sci* 467:444-447, 1986.
62. Pomeranz B, Bibic L: Electroacupuncture suppresses a nociceptive reflex: naltrexone prevents but does not reverse this effect, *Brain Res* 452:227-281, 1988.
63. Blom M, Dawidson I, Angmar-Mansson B: The effect of acupuncture on salivary flow rates in patients with xerostomia, *Oral Surg Oral Med Oral Pathol* 73:293-298, 1992.
64. Takeshige C: Differentiation between acupuncture and non-acupuncture points by association with analgesia inhibitory system, *Acupunct Electrother Res* 10:195-203, 1985.
65. Takeshige C, Luo CP, Hishida F, et al: Differentiation of acupuncture and nonacupuncture points by difference of associated opioids in the spinal cord in production of analgesia by acupuncture and nonacupuncture point stimulation and relations between sodium and these opioids, *Acupunct Electrother Res* 15:193-209, 1990.
66. Pomeranz B: Scientific research into acupuncture for the relief of pain, *J Altern Complement Med* 2:53-60, 1996.
67. Kho H-G, Robertson EN: The mechanisms of acupuncture analgesia: review and update, *Am J Acupunct* 25:261-281, 1997.
68. Zadina JE, Hackler L, Ge LJ, et al: A potent and selective endogenous agonist for the mu-opiate receptor, *Nature* 386:499-502, 1997.
69. Darland T, Heinricher MM, Grandy DK: Orphanin FQ/nociceptin: a role in pain and analgesia, but so much more, *Trends Neurosci* 21:215-221, 1998.
70. Lung CH, Sun AC, Tsao CJ, et al: An observation of the humoral factor in acupuncture analgesia in rats, *Am J Chin Med* 2:203-205, 1974.
71. Research Group of Acupuncture Anaesthesia: The role of some neurotransmitters of brain in finger-acupuncture analgesia, *Sci Sinica* 17:112-130, 1974.
72. Pomeranz B, Chiu D: Naloxone blocks acupuncture analgesia and causes hyperalgesia: endorphin is implicated, *Life Sci* 19:1757-1762, 1976.
73. Mayer DJ, Price DD, Raffi A: Antagonism of acupuncture analgesia in man by the narcotic antagonist naloxone, *Brain Res* 121:368-372, 1977.
74. Guo HF, Tian J, Wang X, et al: Brain substrates activated by electroacupuncture of different frequencies. I. Comparative study on the expression of oncogene *c-fos* and genes coding for three opioid peptides, *Mol Brain Res* 43:157-166, 1996.
75. Han JS: Cholecystokinin octapeptide (CCK-8): a negative feedback control mechanism for opioid analgesia, *Prog Brain Res* 105:263-271, 1995.
76. Takai S, Song K, Tanaka T, et al: Antinociceptive effects of angiotensin-converting enzyme inhibitors and an angiotensin II receptor antagonist in mice, *Life Sci* 59:PL331-336, 1996.
77. Harrison LM, Kastin AJ, Zadina JE: Opiate tolerance and dependence: receptors, G-proteins, and antiopiates, *Peptides* 19:1603-1630, 1998.
77a. Han JS: Opioid and antiopioid peptides: a model of yin-yang balance in acupuncture mechanisms of pain modulation. In Stux G, Hammerschlag R, editors: *Clinical acupuncture: scientific basis,* Berlin, 2001, Springer-Verlag.
78. Han JS, Tang J, Huang B, et al: Acupuncture tolerance in rats: anti-opiate substrates implicated, *Chin Med J* 92:625-627, 1979.
79. Faris PL, Komisaruk BR, Watkins LR, et al: Evidence for the neuropeptide cholecystokinin as an antagonist of opiate analgesia, *Science* 219:310-312, 1982.
80. Itoh S, Katsuura G, Maeda Y: Caerulein and cholecystokinin suppress beta-endorphin-induced analgesia in the rat, *Eur J Pharmacol* 80:421-425, 1982.
81. Liu NJ, Bao H, Li N, et al: Cholecystokinin octapeptide reverses the inhibitory effect induced by electroacupuncture on C-fiber evoked discharges, *Int J Neurosci* 86:241-247, 1996.
82. Tang N-M, Dong H-W, Wang X-M, et al: Cholecystokinin antisense RNA increases the analgesic effect induced by electroacupuncture or low dose morphine: conversion of low responder rats into high responders, *Pain* 71:71-80, 1997.
83. Yao T: Acupuncture and somatic nerve stimulation: mechanism underlying effects on cardiovascular and renal activities, *Scand J Rehab Med Suppl* 29:7-18, 1993.
84. Filshie J, White A: The clinical use of, and evidence for, acupuncture in the medical systems. In Filshie J, White A, editors: *Medical acupuncture: a western scientific approach,* Edinburgh, 1998, Churchill Livingstone, p. 225-294.
85. Longhurst JC: Acupuncture's beneficial effects on the cardiovascular system, *Prev Cardiol* 1:21-33, 1998.
86. Sun X-Y, Yu J, Yao T: Pressor effect produced by stimulation of somatic nerve on hemorrhagic hypotension in conscious rats, *Acta Physiol Sin* 35:264-270, 1983.

87. Li P, Sun F-Y, Zhang A-Z: The effect of acupuncture on blood pressure: the interrelation of sympathetic activity and endogenous opioid peptides, *Acupunct Electrother Res* 8:45-56, 1983.

88. Tayama F, Muteki T, Bekki S, et al: Cardiovascular effect of electro-acupuncture, *Kurume Med J* 31:37-46, 1984.

89. Nishijo K, Mori H, Yosikawa K, et al: Decreased heart rate by acupuncture stimulation in humans via facilitation of cardiac vagal activity and suppression of cardiac sympathetic nerve, *Neurosci Lett* 227:165-168, 1997.

90. Ballegaard S, Muteki T, Harada H, et al: Modulatory effect of acupuncture on the cardiovascular system: a cross-over study, *Acupunct Electrother Res* 18:103-115, 1993.

91. Li Y, Tougas G, Chiverton SG, et al: The effect of acupuncture on gastrointestinal function and disorders, *Am J Gastroenterol* 87:1372-1381, 1992.

92. Diehl DL: Acupuncture for gastrointestinal and hepatobiliary disorders, *J Altern Complement Med* 5:27-45, 1999.

93. Lux G, Hagel J, Backer P, et al: Acupuncture inhibits basal gastric acid secretion stimulated by sham feeding in healthy subjects, *Gut* 35:1026-1029, 1994.

94. Jin HO, Zhou L, Lee KY, et al: Inhibition of acid secretion by electrical acupuncture is mediated via beta-endorphin and somatostatin, *Am J Physiol* 271:G524-530, 1996.

95. Sodipo J, Falaiye J: Acupuncture and gastric acid studies, *Am J Chin Med* 7:356-361, 1979.

96. Iwa M, Sakita M: Effects of acupuncture and moxibustion on intestinal motility in mice, *Am J Chin Med* 22:119-125, 1994.

97. Bossy J: Acupuncture and immunity: basic and clinical aspects, *Acupunct Med* 12:60-62, 1994.

98. Blalock JE: A molecular basis for bidirectional communication between the immune and neuroendocrine systems, *Physiol Rev* 69:1-32, 1989.

99. Pert CB, Dreher HE, Ruff MR: The psychosomatic network: foundations of mind-body medicine, *Altern Ther Health Med* 4:30-31, 1998.

100. Bianchi M, Jotti E, Sacerdote P, et al: Traditional acupuncture increases the content of beta-endorphin in immune cells and influences mitogen induced proliferation, *Am J Chin Med* 19:101-104, 1991.

101. Han JS, Terenius L: Neurochemical basis of acupuncture analgesia, *Annu Rev Pharmacol Toxicol* 22:193-220, 1982.

102. Sato T, Yu Y, Guo SY, et al: Acupuncture stimulation enhances splenic natural killer cell cytotoxicity in rats, *Jpn J Physiol* 46:131-136, 1996.

103. Fujiwara R, Tong ZG, Matsuoka H, et al: Effects of acupuncture on immune response in mice, *Intern J Neurosci* 57:141-150, 1991.

104. Lundeberg T, Erikkson SV, Theodorsson E: Neuroimmunomodulatory effects of acupuncture in mice, *Neurosci Lett* 128:161-164, 191.

105. Zhao J, Liu W: Relationship between acupuncture-induced immunity and the regulation of central neurotransmitter system in rabbits. II. Effect of the endogenous opioid peptides on the regulation of acupuncture-induced immune reaction, *Acupunct Electrother Res* 14:1-7, 1989.

106. Yang MMP, Ng KKW, Zeng HL, et al: Effect of acupuncture on immunoglobulins of serum, saliva and gingival sulcus fluid, *Am J Chin Med* 17:89-94, 1989.

107. Nappi G, Facchinetti F, Legnante G, et al: Different releasing effects of traditional manual acupuncture and electroacupuncture on proopiocortin-related peptides, *Acupunct Electrother Res* 7:93-103, 1982.

108. Bensoussan A: *The vital meridian: a modern exploration of acupuncture,* Melbourne, 1991, Churchill Livingstone.

109. Manaka Y, Itaya K: Acupuncture as intervention in the biological information system (meridian treatment and the X-signal system), *J Acupunct Soc N Y* 1:9-18, 1994.

110. He Q, Zhou J, Yang B, et al: Research on the propagated sensation along meridians excited by Qigong [Abstracts 262-263]. In Second National Symposium on Acupuncture and Moxibustion and Acupuncture Anesthesia, 1984.

111. Fukushima K: *Meridian therapy: a hands-on text on traditional Japanese Hari,* Tokyo, 1991, Toyo Hari Medical Association.

112. Klide AM: A hypothesis for the prolonged effect of acupuncture, *Acupunct Electrother Res* 14:141-147, 1989.

113. Cannon WB: *The wisdom of the body,* New York, 1939, WW Norton.

What Patients Say About Chinese Medicine

CLAIRE M. CASSIDY

MITRA C. EMAD

I am a physician (MD) diagnosed with Crohn's disease. I took high doses of prednisone for months at a time with multiple side effects. Acupuncture, herbs, and [the acupuncturist's] expert and logical medical advice have kept me in general good health with what was once a debilitating disease. The disease is still active with occasional "flares" that are relieved quickly and effectively in 1 or 2 acupuncture treatments. I continue to take prednisone but at only 4 mg/day.

cupuncture was known and practiced by European Americans in North America from at least the early 19th century, enjoying brief periods of attention and popularity before once again becoming the almost exclusive specialty of Asian practitioners. Then, with increasing Western interest in Asian culture and the economic "opening up" of China beginning in the early 1970s, interest in Chinese medicine (CM) soared. The catalyst for this change is often considered to be columnist James Reston's acupuncture analgesia treatment to ease postoperative pain while he accompanied Henry Kissinger to China just before President Nixon's visit in 1971.[1] Western curiosity about how solid needles could abolish pain led to an abrupt increase in interest in acupuncture and also led researchers to new understandings about the physiology of pain (see Chapter 11). Because of this historical accident, CM as it reentered the consciousness of Westerners focused on acupuncture for pain relief; this image is still primary in many people's minds, although as this book emphasizes, CM is actually a complete health care system that offers comprehensive health care. See Engelbrecht[2] for a study of the history of acupuncture in the United States (US); for the history of acupuncture in Europe and particularly the United Kingdom (UK), see Bivins.[3]

The popularity of CM has increased steadily since the 1970s, evidenced not only by increasing numbers of schools, practitioners, and patients but also by markers of social integration such as the creation of practice and licensing laws, development of standards of use, and increasingly, insurance coverage or access to hospital privileges (see Chapter 20). Because such growth could not occur without a large and reasonably satisfied patient base, it is important to understand not only who uses CM, but also why they seek it, find it rewarding, and continue to use it.

This chapter explores these questions by using data from interview, observational, and survey studies of CM users in the United States. The first section analyzes utilization patterns. The second presents evidence that users find CM unusually satisfying and identifies some features of the medicine and its delivery that help explain this high satisfaction. A special discussion of needles and perceived pain follows. The chapter ends with a discussion of patient perceptions of biomedical care, how patients integrate CM and biomedical care, and suggestions on referral.

METHODOLOGY

This chapter reports data from three surveys of patients in the US,[4-6] from unpublished data compiled by Cassidy and Lappin,* and from several qualitative sources including in-depth interviews, participant observation, and handwritten responses to a request to "tell your own story," which were integrated into quantitative survey instruments.

The quantitative data came from three sources. Bullock et al[4] describe users of a complementary and alternative medicine (CAM) clinic in a biomedical hospital; CM was a major CAM modality at this site thus data (although not strictly comparable) from this site are included in this chapter. Cassidy surveyed data from respondents in private CM offices in multiple

*Maryland Acupuncture Society patient survey, unpublished, 1999.

sites in five US states. The Cassidy and Lappin survey did the same for multiple sites in the state of Maryland only.

The qualitative data sets consist of (1) 65 in-depth interviews of current and former patients at a faculty clinic located in an acupuncture school (Cassidy, unpublished data, 1991); (2) 460 handwritten responses collected in the 1995 survey[5] in response to a request to "describe your experience" with acupuncture care; (3) 503 "tell your own story" responses on the quantitative survey conducted in Maryland in 1999 (Cassidy and Lappin, unpublished data); and (4) 9 in-depth interviews and clinical field notes on 27 patients receiving CM care.[7]

Systematically gathered qualitative data reveal the language, issues, interpretations, and psychic investments of respondents in their experiences. Formal analysis of such individualistic materials allows them to be compared and abstracted in a search for general principles. In this chapter, reported qualitative data do not deal with isolated "anecdotes" but with coherent sets of narrative data that validly support scientific analysis.

USE OF CHINESE MEDICINE IN THE UNITED STATES

Who Uses Chinese Medicine?

As a comprehensive medical system, CM can treat all kinds of patients. In the US, because numbers of practitioners are limited and primarily located in urban locales and the practice is new to most Americans, the actual user profile is somewhat skewed. Most public clinics are funded to deliver drug detoxification; their patient census is typical of that of other drug abuse clinics and includes approximately equal numbers of men and women, a large proportion of minority patients, and people with relatively low income and moderate to low educational achievement (see Chapters 9 and 14). The profile at private and hospital clinics that expect payment from patients is considerably different (Table 12-1). At these sites, the full range of possible conditions is seen, and the modal patient is a middle-age white woman of good income and high educational attainment. A very similar pattern was reported from the UK.[8] Indeed, one of the striking features of private clinic users is that a large proportion have graduate degrees and work in professional occu-

TABLE 12-1

Demographics of Private Office Users of Chinese Medicine*

Characteristic	Responses (%)		
	1995 National survey† (N = 575)	1999 Maryland survey‡ (N = 968)	1997 Minnesota hospital survey§ (N = 760)
Female	72	80	70
European descent/white	89	NA	88
Age (yrs)			
<30	12	9	20-40 yrs: 30
30-50	64	47	40-60 yrs: 50
>50	23	43	60+ yrs: 19
Marital Status			
Single	27	21	NA
Divorced, widowed	15	14	NA
Partnered	17	13	NA
Married	40	52	NA
Education			
High school or less	6	10	18
Some college, trade school	21	14	35
Bachelor degree	22	29	23
Some graduate school, graduate degree	51	47	24

NA, Not asked on survey.
*All percentages rounded to the nearest whole number.
†Data from Cassidy CM: *J Altern Complement Med* 4:17-27, 1998. (Survey of CM patients in private offices.)
‡Data from Cassidy CM, Lappin M: Unpublished survey of CM patients in private offices.
§Data from Bullock ML, Pheley AM, Kiresuk TJ, et al: *J Altern Complement Med* 3:31-7, 1997. (Survey of users of a CAM clinic at a hospital, many of whom used CM.)

pations. As CM becomes increasingly accepted, the proportion of male users and users of younger and older ages can be expected to increase.

Why Do Patients Seek Chinese Medicine Care?

The top reasons for seeking CM care reported in the 1999 survey by the Maryland Acupuncture Society included "seeking help for a specific illness or health concern," "seeking care of my whole being," and "dissatisfied with conventional care" (Table 12-2). Of particular interest are the 38% who sought help to deal with stress, the 28% who wanted to reduce their use of prescription drugs, and the remarkable 21% who felt well and sought CM care to stay well. In other words,

one fifth of patients were using CM preventatively, a pattern quite different from the biomedical norm, which focuses on illness care.

How Long Do Patients See Chinese Medicine Practitioners?

Table 12-3 shows how long respondents to two surveys reported having seen their CM practitioners; a limited choice of check-off answers was listed. The usual pattern of intervention with a new patient consists of frequent visits, usually once or twice a week for several weeks, followed by gradual tapering of frequency to a maintenance frequency. The maintenance frequency depends on the chronicity of the patient's complaint(s) but usually results in visits every 4 to 8 weeks.

TABLE 12-2

Reasons for Choosing Chinese Medicine Care*

Reasons	1999 Maryland survey† (N = 968) (%)
Specific illness/health concern	70
Seeking care of whole being	59
Dissatisfied with conventional care	44
Needed help dealing with stress	38
Urged to go by friend or relative	36
Medical doctors could not help problem	35
Wanted to reduce use of prescription drugs	28
Basically healthy; seeking care to stay well	21
Felt something was missing from my life	14
Tried other complementary and alternative therapies without success	12

*Respondents could mark more than one of 10 options; percentages report how many selected an option and therefore do not total 100.
†Cassidy CM, Lappin M: Unpublished survey of CM patients in private offices.

TABLE 12-3

How Long and How Often Patients See Chinese Medicine Practitioners

1995 National survey (N = 575)*		1999 Maryland survey (N = 968)†			
How long?	%	How long?	%	How often in last 3 months?	%
<3 months	16	<3 months	16	Not at all	2
3-6 months	12	3-6 months	14	1-3 times	38
6-12 months	13	6-12 months	14	4-6 times	32
1-2 years	15	1-3 years	30	7-9 times	9
>2 years	44	>3 years	25	>10 times	18

*Data from Cassidy CM: *J Altern Complement Med* 4:17-27, 1998. (Survey of CM patients in private offices.)
†Cassidy CM, Lappin M: Unpublished survey of CM patients in private offices.

When the CM practitioner emphasizes keeping people healthy, practitioners offer continuing care, and then, just as with a medical doctor, patients may see an CM practitioner regularly for years. Some—approximately 39% in the 1999 survey—regard their CM practitioner as their primary care provider.

For What Conditions Do Patients Seek Chinese Medicine Care?

Table 12-4 shows data from two studies that attempted to answer this question. As implied by table data, finding accurate answers to this question is not easy. When offered a list of symptoms in a check-off style of question, as in the 1995 survey,[5,6] the most common conditions for which people report seeking treatment are "mood care" (depression, anxiety . . .) and musculoskeletal complaints. A similar pattern emerges when respondents are asked to write in answers or offered a list that includes a term such as "stress" (as in the unpublished 1999 survey). A third approach is to ask respondents to check off only one in a preferred list of "chief" or "presenting" complaints—as in the Bullock study.[4] In this case, musculoskeletal complaints were four times more frequent than the second most common complaint, "headache." The authors' category of "depression and other

TABLE 12-4

Complaints and Concerns for Which Chinese Medicine Care Is Sought

Condition	1995 National survey* (N = 575) (%)	Condition	1999 Maryland survey† (N = 968) (%)
Mood care	66	Stress/tension	35
Musculoskeletal	59	Depression/mood	16
Respiratory	40	Fatigue/energy	12
Head and neck	32	—	—
Digestive	22	Back pain	18
Urinary, male reproductive	20	Other musculoskeletal pain	21
Female reproductive	17	Arthritis	6
Infectious	13	Migraine	6
Autoimmune	13	Other headache	9
Weight problems	11	—	—
Other	44	Female concerns	10
		Gastrointestinal	9
		Allergies	8
		Asthma	9
Well care	9	Health/wholeness	9

*Modified from Cassidy CM: *J Altern Complement Med* 4:17-27, 1998. A prompted list was used. Respondents were guided by a list of specific conditions plus one of bodily systems and used both check-off and writing in of their specific concerns to complete the question. Respondents could list as many concerns or complaints as they wished. "Wellness care" was offered as a separate category. Percentages were rounded to the nearest whole number. For details for conditions within each category, refer to the article.

†Cassidy CM, Lappin M: Unpublished survey of CM patients in private offices. A recall list was used. Respondents were presented with a set of four blankcs and asked to write in "up to" four concerns of issues for which they were seeking CM care. Their terminology was later categorized by researchers into the list in the table. Percentages were rounded to the nearest whole number.

functional complaints" accounted for 215 patients or 28.3% of the total. A wide range of other complaints was also reported by smaller numbers. In the UK, Wadlow and Peringer[8] reported that musculoskeletal, neurological, and emotional disorders were the most common "presenting complaints," although a wide variety of disorders were treated.

It is probable that the list pattern is affected by the following three factors: public perception that "acupuncture is good for pain," insurance coverage that is more likely to cover musculoskeletal pain syndromes, and novices who usually do not seek CM care for acute conditions. A majority of CM users receive other forms of care for their presenting complaints before seeking CM care, a situation that implies a corollary—that the complaints that do reach CM practitioners tend to be long-lived and often recalcitrant or chronic. This pattern is likely to change in future years as the capabilities of CM become more widely known and as clinics featuring a variety of care options increase in number. Currently perhaps the most useful point to take from existing data is that patients are already using CM care to treat a very wide range of conditions and complaints, from the minor and acute to the complex and chronic.

Outcomes of Chinese Medicine Care

Do patients feel and function better with CM care? This question can be tested in numerous ways—it is the subject of Part III of this book. This chapter reports results gleaned from asking the users directly.

In the 1995 and 1999 surveys, respondents were asked to report changes in their presenting or chief complaints since receiving CM care. They were also asked specific questions about their quality of life and cost savings associated with changed use of other forms of health care since beginning use of CM care.

Table 12-5 contrasts the high-end response (patients reporting feeling much better) with the low-end

TABLE 12-5

Chinese Medicine Effectiveness Ratings in Two Surveys*

1995 National Survey (N = 575)			1999 Maryland Survey (N = 904)		
Condition (%)	Symptoms disappeared/ improved	Symptoms worsened	Condition (%)	Very effective	Mildly or not effective
Mood care (66)	93	0	Stress/tension (35)	68	3
Well care (63)	98	2	Depression/mood (16)	66	6
Musculoskeletal (59)	90	0	Fatigue/energy (12)	60	8
Respiratory (40)	86	0	Back pain (18)	55	13
Head and neck (32)	94	1	Other musculoskeletal (21)	62	11
Digestive (22)	93	0	Arthritis (6)	49	2
Urinary, male reproductive (20)	71	0	Migraine (6)	51	14
Female reproductive (17)	92	2	Other headaches (9)	47	17
Infectious (13)	97	0	Female concerns (10)	57	14
Autoimmune (13)	76	0	Gastrointestinal (9)	56	14
Weight problems (11)	61	6	Allergies (8)	54	10
Other (44)	95	1	Asthma (4)	49	16
			Health/wholeness (9)	75	0

*Respondents could report more than one complaint, thus percentages refer to percent of total who complained in the named category, and the column totals add up to more than 100%.

response to care of chief complaint(s). Because different questions were asked in the two surveys, the sources are not strictly comparable. However, the tendency identifiable in both surveys was that patients reported experiencing improvements, such as disappearance or decreased frequency of symptoms, much more often than the reverse (mild or no improvement or worsening of symptoms).

Table 12-6 reports responses to a short list of quality of life questions. CM care, as discussed in earlier chapters, tends to move bodily functioning toward the balanced or homeostatic state. This feature also means that the changes patients experience can be very broad. Thus patients commonly report not only relief of presenting symptoms but changes in other features, such as better ability to sleep or digest food, greater ability to remain well or resist illness, more stable mood, or greater ease in social interactions. Again, questions were framed somewhat differently in the two surveys but the answers were very similar. (Note that this table records only the extreme positive answers; in most cases this was the preferred option.)

Finally, both surveys attempted to determine how receipt of CM care was changing patient use of other forms of health care, including costly interventions. Table 12-7 reports these results. Both surveys indicated that, in the presence of CM care, use of other forms of health care often decreases. It is notable that in the experience of the respondents to these two surveys, CM enabled somewhat more than 50% of those for whom surgery had been recommended to *avoid* surgery. The avoided procedures included numerous major interventions such as repair of herniated disks, vertebral fusion, gall bladder removal, kidney stone removal, joint surgery, and hysterectomy.

Use of Biomedicine by Users of Chinese Medicine

Interestingly, a decrease in use of CM does not represent abandonment of other forms of care but rather an altered pattern of usage. Thus only a small minority of CM users avoid or abandon biomedicine; the majority simply use it differently. In the 1995 survey, 15% of respondents reported using only CM; 11% used CM and biomedicine; and a striking 43% used CM, biomedicine, and at least one other professional form of care that was *not* biomedical. Fifty-four percent of respondents reported consulting a medical doctor or doctor of osteopathy in the 3 months preceding the survey. In the 1999 survey, 79% reported seeing an MD

TABLE 12-6

Quality of Life Changes with Chinese Medicine Care

Statement	1995 National survey (N = 575)* "Most of the time" (%)	1999 Maryland survey (N = 904)† "Strongly agree" (%)
Feel better	76	71
Miss fewer work days	71	NA
Get along better with others	69	48
Have less pain	64	56
Can work better	64	56
Have more energy	58	53
Am more focused	58	54
Mood is more stable	NA	52
Less susceptible to illness	NA	49

NA, Not asked on survey.
*Data from Cassidy CM: *J Altern Complement Med* 4:17-27, 1998. (Survey of CM patients in private offices.)
†Cassidy CM, Lappin M: Unpublished survey of CM patients in private offices.

TABLE 12-7

Reports of Health Care Reductions and Cost Savings with Chinese Medicine Care

Issue: Reduce?	1995 National survey* (N = 575)		1999 Maryland survey† (N = 904)	
	Who responded (%)	Who said "yes" (%)	Who responded (%)	Who said "yes" (%)
Visits to biomedical doctors	58	84	77	82
Use of prescription drugs	52	79	68	73
Visits to psychotherapists	35	59	47	71
Visits to physical therapists	29	78	44	83
Avoid surgery	17	59	25	56
Coverage demands from insurance or HMO/PPO	33	77	45	69

HMO, Health maintenance organization; *PPO*, preferred provider organization.
*Data from Cassidy CM: *J Altern Complement Med* 4:17-27, 1998. (Survey of CM patients in private offices.)
†Cassidy CM, Lappin M: Unpublished survey of CM patients in private offices.

or DO in the previous 12 months. However, rather than ask what mix of professional health care providers they were seeing, this survey asked respondents to identify the profession of the person they considered to be their primary care provider. The results were interesting: 44% named a biomedical internist, 39% named their CM practitioner, and 6% named another type of professional health care provider. (Note that 11% did not answer the question.)

Bullock et al[4] reported that 70% of the patients seeking care for musculoskeletal or other pain in their

CAM clinic had consulted with biomedical physicians before seeking CAM care. However, only 50% of those who reported mood disorders, obesity, or addiction had first consulted a medical doctor. Many patients reduced visits to their medical doctor after beginning CAM, particularly if they had allergies, sciatica, or sinus problems. In summary, although current details concerning the changing face of professional health care usage in the US are limited, it is clear that users of CM also commonly use multiple other forms of health care, both of the professional and self-care varieties.

SATISFACTION WITH CHINESE MEDICINE IN THE UNITED STATES

Given the outcomes data shown previously and the high frequency with which users of CM state that their CM practitioner is the person they consider to be their primary care provider, it is not surprising that when asked directly, respondents to the surveys reported very high satisfaction with their CM care, practitioner, and even cost. Indeed, even those who stop care generally did so because their problems had disappeared or for structural reasons (patient or practitioner moved, long commute, no insurance coverage), and not because of dissatisfaction with practitioner or treatment.

Tables 12-8 and 12-9 show comparative data from two surveys. In the 1995 survey (Table 12-8), a large majority of respondents said they were "extremely" or "very" satisfied with their CM care, practitioner, and cost (on a 5-point scale, median 5 was "extremely satisfied" for care and practitioner, median 4 "very satisfied" for cost). Meanwhile, their attitudes toward biomedicine described a normal curve around "satisfied" (median score for care, practitioner, and cost was 3). The difference between these curves is statistically significant ($p < .001$).[5]

Respondents to the 1999 survey were permitted to name any of several types of practitioners to compare with their CM practitioner; 73% of the sample rated a biomedical doctor, 16% rated a chiropractor, and the remainder rated either a nurse practitioner/physician's assistant or an osteopathic doctor. A different set of questions was asked, focusing on aspects of the delivery environment. Table 12-9 shows results combining positive responses ("very positive" with "satisfied" and "strongly agree" with "agree") for questions concerning practitioner or health care setting for CM practitioner and "other" practitioner.

The comparative satisfaction with cost deserves further comment. In the 1995 survey, only 22% of users had third-party reimbursement covering CM costs; in 1999, this number had increased slightly to 25%; meanwhile, 88% had coverage for their biomedical costs. Despite or possibly because of close awareness of the cost of their care, CM patients in both surveys were largely accepting of costs or believed they received good exchange for their money. The issue of cost/benefit ratio was asked directly in the 1999 survey. Examining only the extremes of the distribution, respondents claimed a 54% "excellent" cost/benefit ratio for CM and a 25% "excellent" ratio for "other provider"; 21% reported a "poor/fair" ratio for "other provider," while only 3% reported a "poor/fair" ratio for CM.

People sometimes express surprise that patients are willing to pay out of pocket for CM care, and some potential patients claim that they will not seek CM care until it is covered by insurance. In fact, the cost of CM care is comparatively small, and users express satisfaction with the care received for their cost. What does the

TABLE 12-8

Satisfaction with Medical Care, Practitioners, and Cost (1995 Survey) *

1995 National survey (N = 575)	Extremely/very satisfied (%)	Satisfied (%)	Not very/ not at all satisfied (%)
Care			
Chinese	89	11	1
Biomedical	31	36	33
Practitioner			
Chinese	91	8	1
Biomedical	44	33	23
Cost			
Chinese	67	25	5
Biomedical	26	37	37

*Data from Cassidy CM: *J Altern Complement Med* 4:17-27, 1998. (Survey of CM patients in private offices.)

CM patient buy? First, the cost of a single treatment varies from about $30 US to $90 US, depending on region of the country and rural versus city office location. For this fee, patients spend 30 to 60 minutes in direct contact with their practitioner, both talking and receiving hands-on care. Diagnosis and treatment occur more or less simultaneously, and often the patient can feel a lessening of symptoms even while receiving moxibustion or resting with needles in place. When herbs are to be taken, the prescription is discussed and often delivered on the spot. Education of the patient is ongoing because patient and practitioner converse as an aspect of treatment. When the session ends, often the patient writes a check and hands it directly to the practitioner while making another appointment. Even in large offices, usually only one person intervenes between the practitioner and the patient (e.g., a receptionist). In technical terms, this form of care is "patient-centered." Such care involves a relatively high intensity of verbal and touch contact with a single caregiver, and this in turn means that the patient receives, along with medical care, a sense of being in a relationship, even in partnership (see box on p. 71). This characteristic of CM care is very rewarding to patients as hundreds of reports attest.

Underlying reports of satisfaction are patient perceptions that the care is effective and desirable. The text now turns to features of CM that patients find most desirable.

What Patients Say Chinese Medicine Does

Patient perceptions of what CM does for them can be conveniently summarized under four headings (Table 12-10). The table was constructed from formal analysis of hundreds of narratives offered in interviews or in response to open-ended questions on surveys.[5,6,7]

Theme 1: Relief of Disorders, Complaints, or Symptoms

Theme 1 refers to both physical and emotional/spiritual symptoms, complaints, or both. Narratives report decreases in frequency, intensity, or duration of presenting complaints. More subtly, many narratives refer to "discovering" complaints they had previously ignored or simply not been aware of, for which, in turn, they received help.

TABLE 12-9

Satisfaction with Medical Care and Practitioners (1999 Survey) *

	Chinese medicine practitioner (%)	"Other" medical practitioner (%)
Practitioner		
Helps me feel better about myself as a person	99	61
Sees me on time for appointments	97	68
Motivates me to take care of myself	98	69
Spends enough time with me to understand the problem	99	71
Is friendly and interested in me personally	100	80
Really listens to me and tries to understand my concerns	99	81
Answers my questions clearly and completely	99	86
Health Care Setting		
Length of time in office spent waiting to see practitioner	99	62
Ease of getting appointment	98	71
Amount of time with practitioner during visit	99	72
Comfort and ambience of treatment setting	99	82
Office hours	98	86
Office location	96	87

*Cassidy CM, Lappin M: Unpublished survey of CM patients in private offices.

TABLE 12-10

Survey Respondents: What Chinese Medicine Care Does for Them

Themes	Patient perceptions
1. Relieves or reduces complaints, symptoms, discomfort	Physical, psychological, spiritual, social
2. Improves sense of wellness, improves coping function	Sense of calm, relaxation, ease; Fewer "colds," stronger immune system, speedier healing from trauma; Reduced dependence on prescription drugs; Expanded effects of care: relief of nonprimary complaints
3. Permits enjoyment of delivery environment	Feel close to practitioner; Enjoy office visits; Feel "whole" self is being treated
4. Improves sense of self-efficacy, individual empowerment	Increased self-awareness and self-efficacy; Changed lives

Theme 2: Improved Sense of Wellness, Improved Coping Function

A host of "secondary" gains from CM care are often difficult to formally measure yet help explain the high frequency of patients reporting a general sense of "feeling better" or "having a stronger immune system," or "am better able to control my emotions," "feel more whole and centered," and similar remarks.

An important and potentially measurable feature of enhanced wellness is the often reported reduction in use of prescription drugs.

Theme 3: Enjoyment of the Delivery Environment

Many patients simply report "liking" CM care; those who elaborate on this theme often single out their practitioner and her or his listening and teaching as factors in making visits meaningful and empowering. For example, in reporting their experiences, patients often say "we decided" or "we addressed"—referring to their sense of working in partnership with their practitioner (see box on p. 127). Another reason for enjoying the delivery environment often cited by patients is that of feeling as if their "whole" person is being addressed (i.e., not part by part, but all at once). In oral interviews, patients also often remark on the peaceful, or homey, atmosphere of acupuncture offices. Although offices vary widely, many consciously encourage a sense of tranquility or ease by, for example, offering views of parkland from the treatment table or decorating with homelike pictures, rocking chairs, and plants (see Photo Essay after Chapter 10).

Theme 4: Improved Sense of Self-efficacy, Individual Empowerment

Theme 4 is perhaps the single most important outcome for patients, although it is difficult to measure formally and is rarely discussed in the medical literature. A term emerging from recent scholarship in psychology, *self-efficacy,* has been described by Myla and Jon Kabat-Zinn[9] as "[An] inner quality of confidence, built upon repeated experiences of successfully achieving a desired effect. . . . Many studies show self-efficacy to be the single strongest factor predicting health and healing, an ability to handle stress, and the ability to make healthy life-style changes."

Much of our interview and written-response material includes statements of newly established or renewed self-efficacy concomitant with CM care. Patients report increases in self-awareness and body awareness and a sense of empowerment, especially in the arena of making important changes in lifestyle, self-care, and occupation. Another point often cited by patients is that they have learned the difference between wanting a "fix" or a "cure" and taking a realistic view of their condition; in this case they find themselves more able to accept physical limitations on daily life while also successfully maintaining a high level of emotional, social, and spiritual wellness.

Narrative Database

Excerpts from our narrative database follow. In addition to identifying the themes as they are sounded in these narratives, other features should be noted. First, the tone of these stories, while heartfelt, is generally calm and analytical. Few respondents in these studies expressed extreme or highly emotional attitudes to either CM or biomedicine. Second, some patients are very ill when they seek CM care, sometimes with multiple presenting complaints. Others seek the care to stay well. Third, patients bring many different conditions for CM care. This underlines the point that CM offers *comprehensive* health care.

The fourth point is implied by the breadth of these themes but is so important that we discuss it further. The results of CM care typically extend well beyond relief of the presenting complaint(s). CM has *expanded effects* because it does not treat "diseases" or local conditions, but instead addresses the homeostatic balance of the whole organism in its environment. Not only does this medicine conceive malfunction in dynamic physiological terms, but practitioners also consider it within their domain to train and teach patients, and to make lifestyle recommendations. By judicious choice of acupuncture points, herbs, and other modalities, practitioners say they can enhance the ability of patients to learn and to make lifestyle changes. It is common for patients to report ways in which they have "turned their lives around" in the presence of CM. They also often remark on the importance of their practitioner in engaging this turnaround.

The following excerpt from a woman with chronic incapacitating headaches illustrates this point about the expanded effects of care:

I immediately loved acupuncture—it made me feel better and my mood elevated. Also I became very creative—it sparked my muse. I know that sounds nebulous and nonmedical . . . but acupuncture truly appeared to do this for me. I don't have a lot of money and I would not have continued to come all this time if I hadn't gotten results. The results don't always translate into the relief of a specific physical symptom. The results are less tangible but just as obvious—I feel better.

In this case there is relief of the presenting symptom—headache pain. In addition, her mood improved, which can be attributed to acupuncture (e.g., release of mood-enhancing neurotransmitters; see Chapter 11) or might be attributed to relief from experiencing less pain. The "nebulous" component, an increase in creativity, could equally be attributed merely to relief, but—and this is an important point—it is the sort of result that CM practitioners say they can specifically promote. In fact, CM is typically just as much concerned with relieving "nebulous" symptoms such as

confusion, indecisiveness, intensity (workaholism), or hyperalertness as it is concerned with relieving physical symptoms.

This single report features themes 1, 2, and 4 of the four themes found in Table 12-10. Multiple themes feature in many of the reports. A selection of narratives and the themes they illustrate follows.

 Narrative Database Excerpts

Asthma: Relief of Symptoms and Improved Wellness
I have had allergic bronchial asthma for 21 years. Acupuncture has greatly reduced my use of prescription inhalation medication.

Auto Accident: Relief of Symptoms and Empowerment
I was involved in a [car accident] in 1994. I began treatment immediately of pain killers, muscle relaxers, and anti-inflammatories. Physical therapy relieved about 60% of my muscle tension and cervical strain [but when] I stopped I began to experience incredibly painful headaches and neck strain. My doctor . . . prescribed an antidepressant (used for migraines) but she failed to understand that I was having muscle tension headaches. I ended up in the emergency [room] . . . was written off of work for 6 weeks, prescribed more painkillers, muscle relaxers, and anti-inflammatories and told to go back to physical therapy. I then went to another doctor [who] gave me the option of physical therapy and antiinflammatories or acupuncture. I went to one acupuncture session and was relieved almost 100% for 2 days. I canceled my physical therapy and did not fill my prescription. I am on my second treatment of acupuncture and plan to continue until my pain subsides and disappears for good.

High Blood Pressure: Relief of Symptoms, Improved Wellness, and Empowerment
I was refused life insurance coverage [because of] high blood pressure and weight. My MD prescribed medication that made me sleepy and nauseous. I had constant diarrhea and fatigue. I began acupuncture and stopped all medications. Within 3 months my blood pressure was normal and it has stayed that way for 8 years. My weight has not changed much but I am free of chronic diarrhea and my overall health is vastly better. I "discovered" my addiction to alcohol and found acupuncture helpful in supporting my recovery from that, too. I now have life insurance, too.

Bunions: Relief of Symptoms and Increased Wellness
After bilateral bunion surgery I was in severe pain and experienced awesome swelling every day. Since I had to

work . . . I began treatments of acupuncture and was amazed at pain reduction and lessening of swelling even when I remained on my feet mowing lawns.

Sinus Headaches and Fibromyalgia: Relief of Symptoms, Improved Wellness, and a Changed Life

I was having sinus headaches and infections from October to April. Went to the medical doctor who prescribed antibiotics—one more powerful than the next— did not relieve the infection. One month in acupuncture and infection was gone—Have had about 3 mild infections in past 3 years. I ached all over with fibromyalgia. Thought I would be in a wheelchair before I was 60 (am 54 now). Medical doctor prescribed pain killers and increased the dosage until I felt like a zombie. Since acupuncture: prescription dosage down to minimal amount and pain lessened by 70% to 80%. Dramatic results!

Rheumatoid Arthritis: Relief of Symptoms and Improved Self-efficacy

I feel like I've had very positive results. The thing that I have experienced is that I'm not having inflammation in the way that I did before. The acupuncture keeps the inflammation under control and it helps with pain management. Sometimes the pain is much more tolerable, especially in my feet. I leave appointments and I am generally "pain better." I don't know that I'll ever be "pain free" in my life.

Endometriosis: Relief of Symptoms

The most significant changes were the pain before my period and the typical premenstrual symptoms like breast tenderness and bloating and crankiness. Within a month and a half to 2 months of treatment, I would say 60% of my symptoms were gone: breast swelling and tenderness, headaches, the clotting. I used to have huge clots. I'm not bleeding as heavily as I was before acupuncture.

Behavioral Problems: Relief of Symptoms

We were desperate for help with our son's behavior/emotional problems. It wasn't a parenting problem and we took him to a good psychologist with no results. He also had moderate virally triggered asthma and some allergies. We researched alternative treatments and tried a chiropractor/naturalist who does allergy desensitization, with minimal results and a rather high cost. The acupuncture treatment has had dramatic results for a much more reasonable cost, and we are very relieved, even though we have to come from Virginia to Maryland for the treatments.

Vertigo: Relief of Symptoms and Enjoyment of Delivery Environment

I had seen four MDs with a vertigo problem that I suffered with for 6 weeks. My acupuncturist was the only doctor who understood the problem in a holistic sense, fixed the problem, and is helping me to correct the underlying causes.

Knee Problems: Relief of Symptoms, Improved Wellness, Improved Self-Efficacy, and Enjoyment of Delivery Environment

I began seeing an acupuncturist . . . for continuing knee problems though I had had arthroscopy and major surgery. The acupuncture treatments helped my knees within 2 months. I began to get stronger in every way (more energy, clearer skin) and enjoyed my visits with my new doctor (discussions of Chinese medicine, lots of individualized attention). I began to use acupuncture/herbs for everything from colds to stomach aches to hormonal problems.

Smoking Cessation: Relief of Symptoms, Increased Wellness, Enjoys Visits, and Feels Empowered

[I came in] desperate need of quitting smoking. I came to him 2 times a week for 13 weeks—quit smokes and caffeine. I continue to see [him] for other things . . . once every 3 months . . . I just love it. I always feel so good. I'm more in tune with my body and . . . have more awareness in other things I would normally do that damage my body.

Chronic Pain: Improved Wellness and Self-Efficacy

I now judge my life differently. Success is not being pain free—but not having to take pain medication and being able to be out of bed some.

Endometriosis: Relief of Symptoms, Improved Wellness, and Self-Efficacy

Before acupuncture I set about doing what I wanted kind of ignoring my body and its conditions . . . if it was hurting I either took pills or just proceeded forth. Upon finally coming for acupuncture (after two laparotomies) there has been incredible movement on all, each and every, aspect of my life. These days I am paying attention to my body. My period has evened out. I still have some cramps. Previously I would take up to eight 200 mg ibuprofen. Now two a day is a lot. I am now up to the challenge: it is no longer happening to me, I am happening with it.

Chronic Colds: Improved Wellness

[Even my family] noticed it. The fact that last winter I had anywhere from seven to eight colds, and they would last 2 or 3 weeks. Whereas this winter I've had one cold. It was in October, and it lasted me 2 days and I was back on track.

Mind, Body, Spirit: Improved Wellness

My level of wellness after treatments is the most important criterion I have for evaluating my acupuncturist. I don't mean just symptomatic relief, but mind and body and spirit health. ❧

Paraplegic: Improved Wellness
I am a T-12 paraplegic. It is hard to say whether acupuncture has saved me any health care expenses as I have had regular acupuncture treatment since I got out of the rehab hospital. It is part of my regular health care. I depend on my acupuncturist to take care of my spirit and my energy.

A Sense of Balance: Relief of Symptoms, Improved Wellness and Self-Efficacy, and Enjoyment of Delivery Environment
Acupuncture treatment helped me stay well for a long time. While going through a difficult time a few years ago where I had three surgeries and multiple infections, treatment was the one place that I got help seeing the causes and interactions of these so-called *separate* problems. I cannot say "a cure" was the result, but acupuncture treatment certainly reminds me when I am taking poor care of myself, and it helps me regain a sense of balance and perspective. It has been the one place where my mind and body and emotions do not feel disconnected, each from the other, during a course of treatment.

Feels Heard: Improved Wellness, Enjoyment of Delivery Environment, and Improved Self-Efficacy
This acupuncturist really listens. . . . I feel better, less hyper and yet buoyant. He sees me as a whole person and I am also encouraged to help myself in various ways (e.g., exercise).

Knee Injury: Relief of Symptoms, Improved Wellness and Self-Efficacy, and Enjoyment of Delivery Environment
I started seeing an acupuncturist for a skiing knee injury and have since (10 years) used acupuncture as my primary health care. I have no dramatic story—just consistent good health. I believe the real gift of acupuncture is not the cure—though that is important—but the maintenance of balance it provides.

Eczema: Enjoyment of Delivery Environment
There's something about her [the acupuncturist] that's nurturing. I go into that place and I immediately feel better. She gives off this energy that just makes you feel better. I mean I could go to sleep there and be happy as a lark! After being stressed out, I go in there and feel so relaxed. I've got someone here who'll think about me instead of me thinking constantly.

Trusting Relationship: Enjoyment of Delivery Environment and Improved Self-Efficacy
The most important part of acupuncture is the trusting relationship I have with my practitioner, and the fact that it has made me much more aware of my body and its relationship to my spirit.

Partnership: Enjoyment of Delivery Environment and Improved Self-Efficacy
I like my caregiver/practitioner very much. . . . It is a partnership and I must do my part without expecting to be healed by being passive.

Self-Awareness: Improved Self-Efficacy
It's just such a new concept that your body knows what's wrong with it; it's just a matter of how to make your body talk! I think I've become more in tune with my body. I'm becoming more aware of my health and that I have to eat and I have to relax and not take things so seriously.

Mental Focus: Improved Wellness and Self-Efficacy
I feel happier and more focused. I recently changed jobs and I am really happy with my work. I feel that acupuncture has made a huge difference in my ability to make these changes.

AIDS: Relief of Symptoms, Improved Wellness, and a Changed Life
I feel that there has been an awakening in my body. My pain decreased to no pain. T4 (CD4) count increased 100 points in 3 months. Energy that was not there for some time, rejuvenated, so that life can be looked at from the right angle. New Human!

Addiction: A Changed Life
I was a multiple addict at the end of the road with all the consequences that implies for professional life and personal happiness. [With acupuncture] I am making an extraordinary comeback on all fronts. ❧

WHAT ACUPUNCTURE NEEDLING IS LIKE

CM delivers care by several modalities, of which acupuncture needling is the most common in the US and Western Europe. Several kinds of needles are used, as described in Chapter 4. That chapter also discusses clean needle technique and provides data on the frequency of needling adverse events. This chapter examines the experiential side of needling: what do the needles feel like to patients, and do they hurt?

Many first-time patients express fear of needles or concern about whether the needles will hurt or not:

Of course you can't help but wonder, how's this going to be? This person's going to poke needles in my body. How painful is this going to be? What's it going to be like?

I was terrified of needles when I started but had heard acupuncture was effective with depression/anxiety. I love my acupuncturist so much that while I'm still not thrilled with needles, I continue to go back because of trust and respect.

My intense fear of needles and fear of pain from acupuncture needles prevented me from seeking acupuncture for several years. However, after explaining this to my practitioner, she was extremely understanding, sensitive, caring, and supportive, and helped me overcome my fears of needles.

Culturally, Westerners associate needling with hypodermic injections and sharp pain. Even television journalist Bill Moyers, during filming of acupuncture treatments in Beijing for his PBS documentary, *The Mystery of Chi,* remarked "It hurts *me!*" when a patient receiving needling treatment reassured him, "It doesn't hurt."

For many patients, their concern with needling pain undergoes a transformation similar to the transformation toward self-efficacy previously described. The very notion of what constitutes pain seems to shift. This shift can be constituted as a movement from an experience of *physical pain* to one of *sensation.* One patient's narrative offers an informative example. This narrative is from a patient with congenital kidney problems.

I had never tried acupuncture and I was curious about it. I wanted to learn what map of the body Chinese medicine worked with . . . [My practitioner] placed needles right over the kidneys; I felt an engulfing pain in my kidneys. It made me very doubtful of my capacity to work [on my health] this way. . . . Subsequent treatments were not as painful. If he put a needle in, I could feel a pain all the way up my leg. [It told me] where I was in my body. That sensation located something within my body which I didn't know, I wasn't familiar with. This coursing of this Qi, feeling it there, I could work with it, not tense up or reject it; it was a very interactive experience. . . . There's so much more to learn about your body and we do it through sensations. These are not all pleasurable, but there is a certain pleasure in understanding, in knowing how something works.

Acupuncture treatment for this patient allows her to undergo an experience with and through her body that fundamentally changes her experience of pain. What she refers to as *pain* at the beginning of her story ("I felt an engulfing pain" . . . "I could feel a pain all the way up my leg"), changes into *sensation* ("That sensation located something within my body" . . . "There's so much to learn . . . and we do it through sensations") as her narrative progresses. Her word choices, although unconscious, indicate a transformation in her experience. By the end of her narrative, she talks about *non-pleasurable sensations* and distinguishes these from *pain.*

Acupuncturists themselves carefully teach patients to distinguish between different needling sensations. As a Minnesota acupuncturist explained:

The main thing is do you feel a sharpness, . . . a sticking, a needle sticking in your body? [The patient says], "Oh, that's painful," and I say, "Does it feel like a needle? Does it feel like a burning or a pointing?" And [the patient says], "Oh, no, no, no. It feels like it's really aching." Well that's Qi. I don't consider that to be pain. But I think it's the limitations of the English language. Anything that's uncomfortable is immediately "pain."

Thus patients are guided into the sensations associated with a *Qi response:* a dull, aching, spreading sensation, sometimes a tingling, or the sense of a current of energy. These sensations, when they become familiar to patients, are not at all painful and can be deeply relaxing.

Generally most long-term patients of acupuncture care note a deep level of relaxation made possible by acupuncture needling. Some clients explicitly seek acupuncture care in order to achieve an experience of intense relaxation.

I enjoy the treatments themselves, because I get really relaxed. A lot of times I feel a lot better, kind of cleansed a bit. . . . I enjoy lying there with needles in me. It sounds sort of silly. But it's so relaxing, and I feel like, well, I don't have to meditate today. I feel like I'm doing something good for myself that way.

When [my practitioner] would do the points in my abdomen, I felt like my organs and muscles and connective tissue were just kind of sinking and relaxing. And just able to be healed. [It felt] very open with lots of space in there instead of contracted and tight.

Patients generally emerge revitalized from these states of deep relaxation during acupuncture treatments.

WHAT CHINESE MEDICINE PATIENTS THINK OF BIOMEDICINE

As noted earlier in this chapter, although users of CM are generally very satisfied with the care, they usually do not abandon other medicines, including biomedicine. In the case of biomedicine, two kinds of narratives are common. In the first, the long path to CM care is detailed through reports of failed care in other systems, especially biomedicine because it is the dominant health care system in the Western world. These reports support the widely reported assumption that people seek CM care "when they've come to the end of the road." This pattern is well known to CM practitioners. It is in such cases that one is most likely to find angry or dismissive remarks about biomedicine, yet, these remain in the minority.* For example, three patients reported the following:

> I really feel like I am known as a whole being with my acupuncture practitioner—not just a symptom that needs a quick fix like an antibiotic prescription.

> The atmosphere with an acupuncturist is generally less rushed. Also you usually can talk to them on the phone to ask questions without having to go through staff people whose job is to get you off the line without "bothering" the doctor. In the case of my gynecologist, I like her/hate her staff!

> It's funny how much it can help to get advice from someone who's *not* determined to tell you that you have a problem. My therapist wanted to put me on antidepressants. My cardiologist told me that my heart palpitations were nothing serious and couldn't be helped anyway. My gynecologist was concerned but couldn't stop my yeast infections. My acupuncturist gave me some hints about diet and sleeping, some helpful advice about life, and some needles—*now* where are all of my problems? Almost gone!

Another excerpt also reflects the "long path" model; we offer this narrative because of its last line. It is worth remembering that patients are enlivened simply by feeling that they are being cared for in ways that make good sense to them:

> Last winter I began to experience an onslaught of physical as well as mental problems. For the physical problems I saw doctors, nutritionists, naturopathic doctors, gynecologist, and dermatologists. I had blood tests, a sonogram, x-rays, urine tests, and numerous physical exams and treatments. *Nothing* worked. I was severely depressed. I was considering seeing a psychiatrist when I heard about acupuncture. I related to the idea of healing the mind, body, and spirit as a whole. Since I have started treatment, I have regained a spirit that I thought was lost forever. I have been given energy and a will to live and be strong. I still have a ways to go, as we are trying to get at the root of all my problems. It's very exciting.

The second pattern is perhaps more interesting because it reflects efforts by patients, and sometimes by practitioners (e.g., automobile accident narrative), to

efficiently use more than one system of medicine to enhance wellness. Occasionally, we even hear of patients creating teams of practitioners who, working together, help the patient feel and function better. Of course, the team that a patient builds may—or may not—resemble what a biomedical doctor traditionally thinks of as a team. See Berman et al[10] and Diehl et al[11] for studies of American medical doctors' attitudes to alternative and complementary medicine.

In the following excerpt, a woman with osteoporosis has good self-efficacy and created a team in her own mind, but we cannot tell if she has shared this perception with her various practitioners.

> After the bone density test, I began to read extensively at a library of medicine open to the public. Reading about alternative medicine such as acupuncture made me feel better about myself and more hopeful than traditional medicine articles. The more I read, the more I realized, I knew I could be in charge of my own treatment using traditional and alternative doctors as my consultants.

In their 1993 article, Eisenberg et al[12] reported that fewer than half of patients using nonbiomedical forms of medicine told their medical doctors. This proportion is sure to rise if medical doctors remember to ask their patients, in a friendly and nonjudgmental manner, if they are using CM or other forms of alternative medicine. The asking also opens the door to proactive team-building.

Another survey respondent, who has both systemic lupus and multiple sclerosis, reports using multiple medicines, plus a series of self-care modalities, although she does not state that her practitioners actively work together. Her use of biomedicine continues but shows a new pattern—it is primarily used for diagnosis.

> During all this time, I have continued to see an acupuncturist, a psychotherapist, and a rheumatologist to follow laboratory studies. I have had visits to a neurologist and nephrologist who have offered corticosteroids, but I have refused. I have also been doing visualization, guided imagery, and meditation on a regular basis.

Another respondent also implies that his use of biomedicine is primarily diagnostic:

> I have a high regard for my MD. However, I take any chance to avoid prescription drugs and procedures.

Three more examples of team work follow. These are cases in which the patient integrated biomedical and Chinese medical care, although only in the last case is it clear that acupuncturist and MD were working together.

---

*Themes that echo through such critiques are discussed in greater detail in Chapter 7.

At the age of 55 I have had trouble with weight most of my life. Since being diagnosed with type II diabetes I have had trouble keeping my sugars and weight down. Five weeks ago I started on the protein power diet by the Doctors Eaders [sic]. At the same time I started acupuncture to help with dieting and stress. The outcome so far is 12 pounds easily and a drop of over 100 points in my sugars. I need the acupuncture to keep the emotional strongholds in check.

When I realized I needed surgery, perhaps a hysterectomy to eliminate fibroid tumors, I scheduled the hysterectomy. Not feeling quite right about it, I sought to heal myself through "alternative means," including more frequent visits to my acupuncturist. (This was *before* I had children.) With my acupuncturist's wisdom and help, I came to see that I needed to have surgery and chose to have only the fibroids removed, a more serious surgery, actually, than the hysterectomy. Anyway, my doctors were amazed at how quickly I healed and recovered my energy. Today, I have two beautiful children. I believe acupuncture tended my spirit, emotions, *and* body, enabling me to use what Western medicine had to offer my body, while I stayed healthy and recovered quickly in all aspects of my life!

My acupuncturist practices in my medical doctor's office. Both are cutting-edge in their thinking.

REFERRING BIOMEDICAL PATIENTS FOR CHINESE MEDICINE CARE

The following text highlights some points from the preceding discussion to help practitioners identify candidates among their patient populations who would be most likely to respond positively to CM care. Chapter 20 discusses the issue of referral for CM care in detail. Likely candidates for CM care may include the following:

- Patients with long treatment histories who do not seem to respond well to biomedical care, or for whom multiple trials of interventions have not yielded success; practitioner or patient may be becoming frustrated with the lack of progress.
- Patients who dislike or resent taking drugs, or who are unusually sensitive to pharmaceuticals.
- Patients who want to "try something else" before having surgery.
- Patients with a range of relatively nonspecific complaints that seem to affect several body systems and yet, by laboratory tests, have little "wrong."
- Patients who want to be active participants in their care, who seek to be educated, who demand to be more "in charge" of their care. Some of these may be among a practitioner's "noncompliant" patients.
- Patients who want holistic care, who respond to messages concerning their emotional or spiritual health, or frame their concerns in spiritual or social terms.
- Patients who the practitioner might consider referring to a psychotherapist, but who do not quite fit the picture of needing psychotherapy.
- Patients who have an energetic imbalance.

References

1. Reston J: Now about my operation in Peking, *New York Times* July 26, 1971, pp 1, 6.
2. Engelbrecht C: *The rise and decline of needling (acupuncture): innovation, reinvention, decision frame, and communication,* San Diego, Calif, 1993, University of California at San Diego (dissertation).
3. Bivins R: *The needle and the lancet: British acupuncture and the cross-cultural transmission of medical knowledge (China),* Cambridge, Mass, 1997, Massachusetts Institute of Technology (dissertation).
4. Bullock ML, Pheley AM, Kiresuk TJ, et al: Characteristics and complaints of patients seeking therapy at a hospital-based alternative medicine clinic, *J Altern Complement Med* 3:31-7, 1997.
5. Cassidy CM: Chinese medicine users in the United States. I. Utilization, satisfaction, medical plurality, *J Altern Complement Med* 4:17-27, 1998.
6. Cassidy CM: Chinese medicine users in the United States. II. Preferred aspects of care, *J Altern Complement Med* 4:189-202, 1998.
7. Emad M: *Feeling the qi: emergent bodies and disclosive fields in American appropriations of acupuncture,* Houston, 1998, Rice University (dissertation).
8. Wadlow G, Peringer E: Retrospecitve survey of patients of practitioners of traditional Chinese acupuncture in the UK, *Complement Ther Med* 4:1-7, 1996.
9. Kabat-Zinn M, Kabat-Zinn J: *Everyday blessings, the inner work of mindful parenting,* New York, 1997, Hyperion, p 171.
10. Berman BM, BK Singh, Lao L, et al: Physician's attitudes toward complementary or alternative medicine: a regional survey, *J Am Board Fam Pract* 8:361-6, 1995.
11. Diehl DL, Kaplan G, Coulter I, et al: Use of acupuncture by American physicians, *J Altern Complement Med* 3:119-26, 1997.
12. Eisenberg DM, Kessler RC, Foster C, et al: Unconventional medicine in the United States, *N Engl J Med* 238: 246-52, 1993.

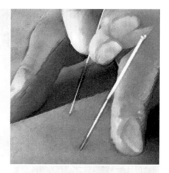

Treatment of Pain by Acupuncture

STEPHEN BIRCH

HISTORY AND BACKGROUND

Problems of pain and the need for treatments of pain are universal. Currently, pain is the most common reason for physician visits in the United States, with an estimated 80% of all visits related to pain.[1-4] It is estimated that 10% of Americans have painful conditions that are present for more than 100 days a year.[5,6] Lower back pain and headaches are the most commonly presented problems. Approximately 11.4% of all physician visits are for lower back pain,[5] and as many as 13.7% of all males and 27.8% of all females report relatively frequent headaches.[7,8] Chronic muscle pain is also very common and occurs in approximately 10% of the US population.[5]

The reported costs of physician visits, health care, work loss, and compensation for pain-related prob-

lems are enormous. In the late 1980s, it was estimated that lower back pain alone costs the United States $16 billion per year in related expenses,[5,9] which means that the total cost of pain-related problems in the United States probably exceeds $100 billion annually. These trends in the prevalence and costs of pain also are found in other countries, with profiles similar to that of the United States. There is strong interest on the part of health care practitioners, governments, and the insurance industry in finding effective and inexpensive pain treatments.

The historical literature on acupuncture contains a wealth of descriptions of the treatment of numerous pain conditions from more than 22 centuries and many countries spanning all major continents. (For an overview of the history of acupuncture, see references 10 and 11.) The earliest major treatise on acupuncture, the *Huang Di Nei Jing (The Yellow Emperor's Classic of Internal Medicine,* circa 200 BCE) is no exception. The 41st chapter of the *Su Wen (Fundamental Questions),* the first of the two books that comprise the *Nei Jing,* is devoted to the treatment of lower back pain; more than 20 different types are described with treatments offered for each.[12] Today modern traditional Chinese literature describes from 3 to as many as 19 different types of back pain.[13] The treatment of headaches also can be found in the early literature. Chapter 24 of the *Ling Shu (Spiritual Pivot),* the second of the two *Nei Jing* books, describes six types of headache[14]; the *Zhen Jiu Da Cheng (Great Compendium of Acupuncture and Moxibustion,* published 1601) describes treatment for more than 10 types of headache,[15] whereas modern traditional Chinese texts describe treatment of from 4 to 10 types of headache.[16-19] Acupuncture has and continues to be commonly used for the treatment of pain in East Asia. A brief review of two modern texts from China found the treatment of at least 20 different common pain conditions described,[16,20] and the modern Japanese literature includes many books specializing in the treatment of pain.[21,22]

Although the practice of acupuncture has many historical traditions,[10,23] there has always been a clearly defined literature base focusing on the treatment of pain. With the introduction of acupuncture to the West starting in the seventeenth century, a strong emphasis on the treatment of pain also emerged. In the late nineteenth- and early twentieth-century descriptions of acupuncture in the Western medical literature, the primary focus was on the alleviation of pain. For example, acupuncture was recommended by Sir William Osler for the treatment of back and sciatic pain in his *Principles and Practice of Medicine.*[11] When acupuncture became more well known at the beginning of the current cycle of interest (the fourth cycle in the West according to Skrabanek[24]) after James Reston's now famous *New York Times* description of his pain relief with acupuncture after an appendectomy, the focus again went to the use of acupuncture for pain. A recent study estimated that approximately 1 million Americans used acupuncture in a 1-year period; the primary reason for seeking treatment was probably pain[25] (see Chapter 12).

However, pain is a very subjective phenomenon and has always been somewhat difficult to research and understand. Thus when acupuncture appeared in the headlines in the early 1970s, it was natural that it would be considered not only as a potentially useful

treatment of pain, but also as a potentially useful tool in pain research.[10] In the early 1970s when the Chinese government began to showcase the analgesic and anesthetic uses of acupuncture for minor and major surgical procedures, the Western scientific community began to use acupuncture as a tool in the race to understand the elusive problem of pain. After a slow start in Japan in the mid-1960s,[10,26,27] controlled clinical trials of acupuncture began in the West in the 1970s; these were primarily pain studies. In addition, a large body of physiological research was initiated to understand the analgesic effects of acupuncture, which led to major discoveries about the actions and mechanisms of acupuncture[28,29] (see Chapter 11).

Recognition of the analgesic effects of acupuncture has extended into mainstream medical practice and reimbursement outside China. For example, in Japan the government has approved a list of six pain conditions for which insurance reimbursement can be sought after standard therapy has failed. Although the list does not appear to evidence-based,[30] these conditions are whiplash, lower back pain, neuralgia, rheumatism, cervicobrachial syndrome, and periarthritis of the shoulder.

In 1979 the World Health Organization (WHO) published a list of 43 different medical conditions for which acupuncture was reportedly effective, including 14 pain conditions.[31] Some confusion continues regarding this list. It represents a discussion of conditions for which acupuncture has often been used,[10] but it was not approved by the WHO.[31-33] Box 4-2 lists these conditions, but this information should be interpreted judiciously.

Current practice of acupuncture in pain relief is based mainly on patient choice, clinical judgment, and political influences, but validation of pain conditions for which acupuncture is effective will increasingly rest on clinical trial studies. In surveys of the use of alternative or complementary therapies such as acupuncture, pain is clearly among the principal reasons for consulting an acupuncturist.[34,35] Acupuncture has acquired a reputation among the general population and medical practitioners as being effective for treating pain.

This chapter begins with an overview of the clinical encounter, followed by a detailed review of clinical trials research of acupuncture in the treatment of pain. In the discussion of clinical trials, it quickly becomes evident that methodological issues render interpretation of much of the data difficult. Yet despite technical difficulties, the weight of the research indicates that acupuncture in the treatment of pain is promising or specifically effective.

THE PATIENT ENCOUNTER

Treatment of Back Pain

The following is a fictionalized account of the acupuncture experiences of a 58-year-old man who had been treated by an acupuncturist in Minnesota and was now being treated by another acupuncturist in the Boston area. It is quite typical of patients who present for acupuncture treatments and indicates how treatments are used for the relief of chronic symptoms that have a clear and probably irreversible underlying component, in this case, mild degeneration with bone spur formation in the lumbar spine.

Mr. Smith presented for acupuncture to treat his chronic lower back pain. He had had lower back pain intermittently for the past 12 years. During the first 7 years he tried physical therapy, trigger point injections, acetaminophen, ibuprofen, and cortisone shots with no long-term results. He had been told that his pain was related in part to lumbar muscle spasm and in part to mild degeneration with bone spur formation on the lumbar spine. He underwent acupuncture treatments intermittently for approximately 5 years while living in Minnesota, with good results. Recently arrived in the Boston area, he had a flare-up of the pain and wanted to begin acupuncture treatments again.

His immediate impression of care was that the acupuncturist was doing something quite different than had been done by the acupuncturist in Minnesota. In Minnesota, the acupuncturist had asked many questions and examined his radial pulses and the tongue. The treatment involved insertion of needles primarily into the lower back and legs and occasionally into points on his arms. Mr. Smith usually felt the needles quite distinctly, and about half the time had additional electrical stimulation added to the needles in his lower back. When he had asked the acupuncturist for a diagnosis, he was told that he had Stagnation in the lower back region, with weak Spleen Qi. However, the acupuncturist in Boston asked different questions, did not look at his tongue, spent more time examining the radial pulses, and also palpated the abdomen and chest regions, finding several

tender points. The needling started on the hands and feet and was quite different than before, using much shallower needling techniques that Mr. Smith barely felt. He also had needles inserted shallowly into his abdomen, lower back, and shoulders; instead of electrical stimulation, heat was added on the lower back. He left the office with two small needles inserted and taped onto the lower back region at very tender points. When he asked for a diagnosis, he was told that his Liver and Kidney channels were weak, and that there was a general condition of weakness in all the Yang channels.

Mr. Smith experienced the same pain relief in Boston as he had in Minnesota. On visiting the acupuncturist again, he asked about his treatment plan. He was told that he should try a course of six treatments; if no clear improvements occurred he should stop treatment, but if clear changes occurred, then they would develop a plan in terms of frequency and number of treatments. Mr. Smith also noticed that the treatments with the acupuncturist in Boston seemed to vary more from week to week than those in Minnesota. He found that his mild irritable bowel symptoms, stiff shoulders, and occasional achy knees improved with the acupuncture treatments, just as they had in Minnesota. In the initial visits he had forgotten to tell the acupuncturist about his mild bowel disturbance. On questioning the acupuncturist, Mr. Smith learned that it was quite common for seemingly unrelated symptoms to improve during the treatments. Sometimes patients even reported improvements of symptoms they had never expected, such as sleep problems, feelings of anxiety, and so forth. As he adapted to his new city, Mr. Smith was able to manage his pain basically the same as when in Minnesota. He needed 8 to 12 treatments a year to stay relatively free of pain and did not need to take analgesic medicines such as acetaminophen or ibuprofen.

This patient's experiences with chronic pain and an irreversible underlying problem are quite typical and can be used to preview some delivery characteristics that become issues of research design in clinical trials. First, note that treatments can vary from practitioner to practitioner and from treatment session to treatment session. This variation is related to many factors: the training and preferences of the acupuncturist, complex cultural factors, the conditioning of prior experiences, and others. Although it may seem strange that different diagnostic patterns were identified by the two acupuncturists, it helps to view diagnostic labels as dynamic and as stepping stones in the selection of treatment rather than as references to materially different pathologic conditions (see Chapters 2, 4 and 7).[10,36] Second, note how many treatments are commonly used for this problem, the expansion of response to ameliorate complaints other than the presenting complaint, and the use of needles both at the site of pain and at other parts of the body. The surveys on the prevalence and use of alternative medicine conducted by Eisenberg et al found that acupuncture was used more frequently per year than other therapies, suggesting a use of the therapy beyond the original problem for which treatment was first sought.[34] Third, note the use of acupuncture as an episodic yet ongoing therapeutic option for this patient. It is not uncommon for patients who experience good results with acupuncture to use it subsequently as a first line of defense in flare-ups of chronic pain conditions. Traditional systems of acupuncture, such as those practiced by these two acupuncturists, use a two-pronged approach to patient assessment and treatment selection.[10,23] The first targets correction of disturbances in the overall condition of the patient ("the root"); the second targets relief of symptoms ("the branch").

As shown in the following text, few clinical trials of acupuncture for chronic pain have reflected actual clinical practice. Many trials have tested forms of acupuncture significantly less complete than usual clinical practice.

CONTROLLED CLINICAL TRIALS OF ACUPUNCTURE FOR PAIN CONDITIONS

Clinical trial studies of acupuncture began in the mid-1960s. Sodo Okabe and Haruto Kinoshita of Japan conducted the first controlled clinical trials of acupuncture in 1966.[26,27] The first clinical trial of acupuncture published in English appeared on MEDLINE in 1973.[37] To date, more than 300 clinical trials of acupuncture have been published; more than half are pain-related trials.

These studies covered a broad range of conditions.[38] Some studies examined the effects of acupuncture on experimentally induced pain.[39-41] The majority of studies examined the efficacy of acupuncture in chronic pain; only a few explored its effects on acute pain.

Many uncontrolled studies have explored treatment of various pain conditions including osteoarthritis of the knees, back pain, neck pain, whiplash, painful crises of sickle cell anemia, cancer pain, peripheral neuropathy, and headache.[42-50]

There also have been numerous controlled studies of acupuncture in the treatment of pain. Tables 13-1 and 13-2 indicate the primary pain conditions and principal controlled studies for each (trials to 1998

TABLE 13-1

Clinical Trials of Acupuncture for Musculoskeletal and Neurological Pain

Pain conditions	Trials (No.)
Low back pain[51-54]	20
Sciatica[55-57]	3
Tension headache + migraine[58-62]	19
Neck pain[63-65]	10
Cervicobrachial syndrome[66]	1
Shoulder pain[67,68]	6
Facial pain[69-72]	4
Tennis elbow[73-75]	3
Carpal tunnel syndrome[76]	1
Knee pain[77,78]	2
Postherpetic neuralgia,[79,80] acute herpetic neuralgia[81]	3
Peripheral neuropathy[82]	1
Fibromyalgia + myalgia[83]	3
Reflex sympathetic dystrophy[84]	1
Plantar fasciitis pain[85]	1
Arthritis[86-88]	17
More than one location of pain, including musculoskeletal pain[89,90]	14

TABLE 13-2

Clinical Trials of Acupuncture for Other Pain Conditions

Pain condition	Trials (No.)
Surgical and postsurgical dental pain[91,92]	4
Postsurgical pain[93,94]	5
Renal colic[95]	1
Dysmenorrhea[96]	1
Sore throat[97]	1
Angina[98,99]	4
Chronic pancreatitis[100]	1
Pain associated with endoscopy procedures[101,102]	2

only). Table 13-1 lists the main musculoskeletal pain conditions for which controlled clinical trials have been conducted, the approximate number of trials in each area, and some of the important studies in each. Table 13-2 lists the nonmusculoskeletal pain conditions for which controlled clinical trials have been conducted, the approximate number of studies in each area, and some of the important studies in each. Some studies are somewhat difficult to interpret because they either did not include sufficient detail,[103] were abstracts,[104,105] or were studies that tested nonacupuncture techniques, such as lasers[106] or surface electrical stimulation.[107,108] Another factor clouding the interpretation of some studies occurs when the study simultaneously tests a particular neurophysiological model of action by administration of naloxone (which blocks endorphin action) or other chemicals that act on the nervous system.[109,110]

A number of research models have been used in the scientific study of the clinical efficacy of acupuncture. In studies incorporating control groups, acupuncture treatment usually was compared with one of the following "control" situations:

1. No treatment control group[93]
2. Wait-listed control group[51,86]
3. Standard therapy control group:
   - Physical therapy[64,104,111]
   - Transcutaneous electrical nerve stimulation (TENS)[112-114]
   - Medication[73,95,102,115]
   - Combination of standard therapies[52,78]
4. Mock-TENS control group[53,87,116,117]
5. "Suggestion" control group[118]
6. "Sham acupuncture" control needling control group
   - "Sham acupuncture"[83,101,119]
   - "Sham acupuncture" plus injection lidocaine, naloxone[109,110]
7. "Minimal acupuncture" control needling control group:
   - At nonacupuncture points[61,69]
   - At irrelevant acupuncture points[63]
   - At same acupuncture points[65,74]
8. "Sham" or "minimal" acupuncture control needling plus medication or placebo control groups[60,65]
9. Noninvasive needling control group[62,91]

These general research models have been discussed by several authors.[120-127] Models 1 and 2 compare treatment with doing nothing. Model 3 compares the treatment with usual care treatments that are routinely used for the same condition. Usually this is done as a simple comparison. Sometimes the acupuncture is added to usual care treatments so that the additional effects of acupuncture can be compared with usual care treatments.[52] Model 4 uses a novel placebo-control design model, but it is not accepted by all researchers.[128] Model 5 is a unique model that has not been used by other research groups. Models 6 and 7 are models that attempt to control for placebo effect. The control treatments vary according to location of stimulation, intensity of stimulation, or both, and each model uses an invasive control needling procedure. Model 8 is a complex model that combines elements of models used in models 6, 7, or 9 with a routine drug placebo-control testing model. Model 9 is similar to models 6 and 7 except that noninvasive control needling procedures are used, with assessments determining the validity of the control.

METHODOLOGICAL ISSUES IN DESIGNING STUDIES OF ACUPUNCTURE

Since the early 1980s a number of reviews have evaluated these clinical trials testing the efficacy of acupuncture for pain.[25,125,127-131] These reviews and other literature evaluations[124,132,133] have agreed that the methodological quality of the pain studies is poor, raising many questions about the efficacy of acupuncture in the treatment of pain,[134] the ability to interpret the results of the studies, or both.[125,128,133,135]

The following problems in clinical trials of acupuncture are very important:

- *Inadequate sample size.*[129,133] Insufficient numbers of patients are enrolled in the studies to afford significant results, introducing bias against showing that acupuncture works.
- *Inadequate treatment given.*[120,136,137] In many studies, insufficient treatment was administered for the study to be considered a fair test of treatment. In a review of 34 controlled studies of acupuncture for head, neck, and back pain, Birch found that none could be clearly said to have administered adequate treatment.[121,138]
- *Use of inappropriate "sham" or "placebo" control needling.*[120,136] In many studies incorporating some type of control needling, quite inappropriate treatments were given, some being more like the treatment for which they were designed to control.[136]
- *Inadequate long-term follow-up.*[128] In the treatment of chronic pain, follow-up of at least 3 months after

cessation of treatment is important; otherwise the clinical significance of the results cannot be properly assessed.

- *Inadequate blinding and/or assessment of blinding of patients.*[63] In studies where control needling is used as the control treatment, it is almost impossible to conduct a true double-blind study of acupuncture. Therapy is administered by acupuncturists who know what they are doing, to patients who are not supposed to know what treatment they are receiving. It is therefore vital that assessments be made of patients' beliefs and perceptions about what treatments they are receiving; otherwise it is not possible to really claim a placebo control[63,139] (see Chapter 19). Most studies using a control needling treatment arm did not make such assessments and thus are difficult to clearly interpret.

The following clinical trials are presented to understand these problems in context. The first trial is selected to illustrate how these problems undermine interpretation of the results of the study. The next studies are selected because they illustrate application of some of the different research models, and because they are examples of better studies.

Example 1: Acupuncture Treatment of Lower Back Pain[140]

In this trial, 30 patients in whom conventional therapies for their chronic lower back pain with lumbar disk involvement had failed were randomly assigned to receive "real acupuncture" or "sham acupuncture." Each patient received a course of three treatments. In the "real" treatment, four needles were inserted, manipulated, and then electrically stimulated. The points of insertion were actual acupoints claimed to be commonly used for lower back pain. In the "sham" treatment, four needles were inserted into nonacupoints and were not manipulated but did have the same electrical stimulation. Each patient was reevaluated after the three treatments. The authors found no significant difference between the treatments, concluding that they "were unable to differentiate any benefit for low back pain in excess of the placebo effect and suggest that much of the improvement in pain syndromes associated with acupuncture may be on the basis of the placebo effect."

Critique

1. Too few patients were recruited to achieve statistical significance.[129] Pilot studies are usually required to determine the required number of patients in such a study.

2. The "real" treatment was completely inadequate. Four needles were inserted on 3 occasions, but literature reviews have found that a minimum of 10 needles on 10 occasions is the minimum adequate treatment, with more required for optimal treatment.[121,137] Further analyses have found that an "approximately adequate treatment" using stimulation of six loci in each of six sessions is significantly associated with a positive treatment effect.[25] In addition, neither of the (bilateral) acupoints stimulated in this study is commonly used for lower back pain, and one is not mentioned at all for back pain in a major review of the literature.[13]

3. The "sham" treatment was inappropriate as a control in this study. It involved the stimulation of non-acupoints, which, without pilot data, is tantamount to stimulating points about which nothing is known. In fact, they could have been important loci in the treatment of lower back pain.[120] Electrical stimulation was also added, making it likely that the total stimulus given was comparable to the "real" treatment, for which this was considered a placebo control.[120,136]

4. No follow-up was conducted at some date after the end of treatment assessment; thus any clinical significance was lost.

5. No credibility or other measures were conducted making it impossible to realistically know whether blinding was successful or to discuss placebo controls in this study.

This study is a typical example of poorly designed and conducted trials in acupuncture. Not only do the conclusions of the authors not follow from the study, but it is likely that this was not a test of acupuncture for lower back pain. To make a comparison with the testing of a new pharmaceutical: one would not consider a test analgesic drug administered at the wrong dose, for an inadequate period of time, for the wrong condition, to have been properly tested. It would not improve the interpretive power of the test were this test drug also contrasted, under the rubric of "placebo control," with an unknown active analgesic delivered at unknown strength. ∾

Example 2: A Controlled Trial of Acupuncture Treatment of Migraine[61]

In this trial, 30 patients were randomly assigned to receive a course of test or control acupuncture treatments. In each test course, six acupuncture treatments were administered at eight points indicated for migraine; in each control course, treatments employed eight non-acupoints. In the former, appropriate manipulations of the needles were given; in the latter, the needles were inserted shallowly with no manipulation. Pain assessments and consumption of medications were made at baseline, at the end of treatment, and at 4 and 12 months after completing treatment. Credibility of the treatments was assessed during the treatment phase. The author found a significant difference between the two treatments in favor of the test acupuncture treatment in pain reduction, use of medications after treatment, and at 4- and 12-month follow-up. Treatments were equally credible.

Critique. Despite its small sample size, the study found significant differences. Conducting a pilot study before would have been better to determine sample size requirements. The test treatment satisfied the approximately adequate minimal requirements.[137] The control treatment should have been tested first in a pilot study, but because of the use of both nonacupoints and minimal stimulation, it was reasonable to expect larger differences in treatment effects than found in the back pain study in Example 1, in which the same electrical stimulation was given in both treatment groups. Long-term follow-up measures were made, establishing the clinical significance of the findings. Credibility was measured, thus establishing comparability of placebo-related effects in the two treatment groups. However, more elaborate forms of assessments are probably necessary to be completely convincing.[63] ๑

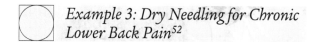

Example 3: Dry Needling for Chronic Lower Back Pain[52]

In this study, 56 patients undergoing rehabilitation for their chronic lower back pain with little progress were randomly assigned to receive either continued standard therapy or continued standard therapy plus acupuncture therapy. The acupuncture was tailored to each individual patient according to the nature of the pain and response to treatment. Variable numbers of acupoints were treated in a variable number of sessions. Needle manipulation, often with electrical stimulation of the needles, was routine. Assessments involved both pain assessment and whether the patient had returned to work; assessments were made at 12 and approximately 27 weeks after beginning the treatments. Of those who had acupuncture treatment, 18 of 29 patients had returned to their original or equivalent jobs and 10 to lighter employment. Of the 27 who did not receive acupuncture, only 4 returned to their original or equivalent jobs, with 14 to lighter employment.

Critique. No efforts were made to control for placebo in this study. Instead this study design allowed researchers to examine the effects of the addition of acupuncture in terms of overall function and return to work. It is important in such studies that reasonably large sample sizes be used to ensure against bias in favor of the test treatment;

this study had a larger sample size than the previous studies. It is not possible to state clearly whether adequate acupuncture was administered because actual treatments were not described. However, given the average number of treatment sessions (7.9), it is likely that most patients received at least the approximately adequate minimum treatment. Sufficient long-term assessment was made to establish clinical significance of the results. No efforts were made to control for placebo; thus comments cannot be made on its role in treatment outcome. This study illustrates assessment of more pragmatic questions about the effectiveness of acupuncture and shows what was probably a large cost savings because of the addition of acupuncture in the rehabilitation program, an important finding for health care payers and policy makers. ๑

Example 4: Acupuncture Treatment of Severe Knee Osteoarthrosis[86]

In this study, 29 patients with severe osteoarthritis of the knee, each awaiting arthroplasty surgery, were randomly assigned to receive either a course of acupuncture treatment immediately or 9 weeks later (a wait-list design). Treatment consisted of the insertion and manipulation of six needles in each of six sessions. Patients were evaluated after completing treatment, and if desired could receive further acupuncture up to 50 weeks after beginning of the study. Medication consumption was assessed, and various pain and objective measures were made at baseline and at 4, 8, 12, 16, 36, and 48 weeks. Significant pain relief and improvement in objective symptoms were found compared with the wait-listed group. There were significant improvements on all measures after all patients had received treatment. Seven of the 29 patients were able to cancel—and did not need—the planned surgery for their osteoarthritic knees, at an average cost savings of $9,000 US per procedure.

Critique. This study made no effort to control for placebo effects. Instead it compared acupuncture with no acupuncture and then the overall effects of acupuncture on this group of patients, who acted as their own controls. Sample size was relatively small, and a pilot study would have been useful to ensure adequate sample size; however, the results were quite clear on all measures. The study probably administered the approximately adequate minimum treatment on all patients, and with the additional treatments given to 17 of the patients, adequate treatment was probably administered. Long-term follow-up was done, establishing the clinical significance of the treatment. Blinding of patients was not necessary in this study but was necessary on the part of those making assessments. This is a good study design to establish that acupuncture can be effective for patients with osteoarthritic knees that require surgery. It should be followed up with a larger study using more elaborate controls to better understand the role of the acupuncture treatment. However, it was significant that in this small study more than $60,000 US was saved in surgical costs. It is very unlikely that the administration of the acupuncture for this small group of patients would have been this costly. Thus it appears that substantial cost savings were obtained, an important finding for health care payers and policymakers. ❧

LITERATURE REVIEWS AND META-ANALYSES

An overall sense of the effectiveness of acupuncture in the treatment of pain conditions requires examination of the major reviews and meta-analyses of published studies. Several reviews of the pain clinical trials have been conducted. Depending on the criteria of the reviewers, acupuncture has been found to demonstrate some efficacy for pain, or to have little to no efficacy for pain. In addition, it is difficult to interpret the data from the studies because of their many methodological limitations. However, given these somewhat confusing findings, there is an overall sense that acupuncture has demonstrated effectiveness in the treatment of chronic pain conditions.

In their 1986 evaluation of 28 controlled studies for pain of multiple origins, Richardson and Vincent[130] concluded that the "commonly occurring immediate success rate of 50% to 80% is greater than might be expected if the effects of acupuncture were mediated entirely by placebo-related factors," and that "there is good evidence from controlled studies for the short-term effectiveness of acupuncture in relieving clinical pain in each of the areas we examined" but inadequate measurement of long-term effects.

Patel et al's meta-analysis of acupuncture for the treatment of chronic pain examined 14 studies that met their criteria for inclusion, concluding that "results favourable to acupuncture were obtained significantly more often than chance alone would allow."[131]

Ter Reit et al's meta-analysis of 55 chronic pain studies focused on the quality of the studies rather than the clinical results because of the heterogeneity of the studies examined. Thus, strictly speaking, it was not a meta-analysis. They developed a list of 18 criteria for evaluating the studies, concluding "no studies of high quality seem to exist. Therefore at this moment no definitive conclusions on the efficacy of acupuncture in the treatment of chronic pain can be drawn."[128]

In his 1993 analysis of 12 well-controlled studies for pain, Vincent concluded "acupuncture may be effective for some types of chronic pain, but the results are equivocal in many cases"; however, "disappointingly little has been achieved by literally hundreds of attempts to evaluate acupuncture. Major methodological flaws are apparent in the vast majority of studies."[125]

Hammerschlag and Morris evaluated the quality of 23 controlled studies that compared acupuncture with biomedical standard care[124]; 16 of these studies were for the treatment of pain. Their analysis found that the quality of the majority of studies was generally poor, concluding that their analysis "indicates a generally low level of research design and reporting."

After presentations on acupuncture in April 1994 to a panel of US Food and Drug Administration (FDA) experts, five submissions of evidence for the efficacy of acupuncture were made to seek reclassification of the acupuncture needle from a class III, experimental to a class II, safe and effective device.[141] The submission on pain included discussion of 37 studies covering pain of many origins.[142] After these submissions the FDA concluded that:

. . . the clinical studies . . . included in the petitions constitute valid scientific evidence in support of clinical effectiveness of acupuncture needles for the performance of acupuncture treatment. However reference to a specific disease, condition, or therapeutic benefit requires additional valid scientific evidence in the form of well-controlled prospective clinical studies.[135]

In perhaps the broadest and possibly most important review of evidence from acupuncture studies, the US National Institutes of Health (NIH) held a special consensus development conference on acupuncture in early November 1997. At this conference a group of experts presented general information about acupuncture, data supporting the physiological mechanisms of action of acupuncture, and the data from clinical trials covering a broad range of conditions. Five separate presentations were given on studies in the treatment of pain.[143] These data were evaluated by an independent panel of experts. After examining needle or "sham" acupuncture controlled studies, they concluded that "there is clear evidence that needle acupuncture is efficacious" in four conditions, including postoperative dental pain, and that "there are reasonable studies" for a number of "diverse pain conditions such as menstrual cramps, tennis elbow and fibromyalgia."[143] After examining studies that compare acupuncture with standard biomedical therapies, they concluded "one of the advantages of acupuncture is that the incidence of adverse effects is substantially lower than that of many drugs or other accepted medical procedures used for the same conditions." The panel mentioned postoperative pain, myofascial pain, and lower back pain as conditions that compare favorably for acupuncture. In addition, they listed carpal tunnel syndrome, osteoarthritis, and headache as conditions for "which the research evidence is somewhat weaker, but for which there are clinical reports."[143] This is probably the broadest list of pain indications for which acupuncture research has been judged as good or at least promising; see the left column of Table 13-3.

It is obvious that researchers interpreting the clinical trials of acupuncture for pain have had difficulties because of common methodological problems. Nonetheless, this does not mean that acupuncture does not work; rather, there is some difficulty reaching clear statistically valid conclusions. In fact, in studying the clinical trials, there is a very obvious sense that acupuncture was effective in the majority of studies. To make such general comparisons, differentiation is needed between studies wherein acupuncture was compared with sham or placebo treatment in an effort to control for placebo effects and studies in which acupuncture was compared with standard therapies. In the former, acupuncture must show better results than the control treatments to be considered effective; in the latter, acupuncture should perform as well as or better than the standard therapy to be considered effective. Tables 13-4 and 13-5 present general comparison of 35 controlled studies on the effectiveness of acupuncture for head, face, neck, and lower back pain.[121,138] Nineteen (95%) of the 20 studies that used a sham or placebo design found acupuncture to be more effective than the control; in 9 studies, the effect was significant (Table 13-4). Thirteen (87%) of the 15 studies that used standard therapy as the control treatment found acupuncture to be as or more effective than the standard therapy (Table 13-5). This trend can be found throughout the clinical trial literature. It is evident that some effect occurs and acupuncture is reducing pain in these studies. Better designed studies are needed to yield clear answers regarding the relative efficacy of acupuncture compared with different control treatments for the range of pain conditions for which acupuncture is commonly used.

TABLE 13-3

NIH Consensus Panel List of Pain Conditions for Which Evidence Exists for the Efficacy of Acupuncture

Pain Conditions	
Effective or promising evidence	Some promising evidence
Pain from dental surgery	Sciatica
Postoperative pain	Facial pain (especially from temporomandibular disorder)
Myofascial pain	Neck pain
Pain from osteoarthritis	Shoulder pain
Lower back pain	Cervicobrachial syndrome
Migraine	Knee pain
Tension headache	Pain associated with endoscopy procedures
Tennis elbow (epicondylitis)	Renal colic
Fibromyalgia	Reflex sympathetic dystrophy
Carpal tunnel syndrome	
Dysmenorrhea	

TABLE 13-4

Relative Efficacy of Acupuncture Compared with Invasive or Noninvasive Control Treatments for Head, Face, and Neck Pain

Type of pain	Significantly more effective	More effective but not significant	Not more effective
Headache	Hansen, 1985[59] Vincent, 1989[61] White et al, 1996[62] Jensen et al, 1979[144]	Dowson et al, 1985[116] Tavola et al, 1992[119] Henry et al, 1985[145] Vincent et al, [146]	Baust, 1978[147]
Face pain	Hansen, 1983[69]	—	—
Neck pain	Petrie, 1983[148]	Thomas et al, 1991[65] Petrie, 1986[117] Matsumoto et al, 1974[149]	— —
Lower back pain	McDonald et al, 1983[53] Lopacz, 1979[118] Duplan et al, 1983[150]	Mendelson, 1983[110] Edelist, 1976[140] Emery, 1976[151]	—

TABLE 13-5

Trials on the Relative Efficacy of Acupuncture Compared with Standard Therapy in Head, Face, and Neck Pain

Type of pain	As effective as standard therapy	Not as effective as standard therapy
Headache	Ahonen et al, 1983[58] Hess et al, 1991[60] Loh et al, 1984[115] Doerr-Proske, 1985[152] Carlsson, 1990[153]	Carlsson, 1990[111]
Face pain	Johansson et al, 1991[70] List et al, 1991[71] List, 1992[72]	Raustia, 1985[154]
Neck pain	Loy, 1983[64]	
Lower back pain	Gunn et al, 1980[52] Fox, 1976[112] Laitinen, 1976[113] Lehmann, 1976[114] Ghia, 1976,[155]	

SUMMARY

In studying the research literature on the efficacy of acupuncture in the treatment of pain, one can find a multitude of methodological problems. These problems do not indicate that acupuncture does not work, rather they cloud judgments about the relative efficacy and clinical significance of the results from most of these studies. The task of collecting and evaluating the results of the numerous studies has proven difficult, leading to the conflicting conclusions. There is an obvious need for more methodologically sound studies.

Applying very strict scientific standards, few studies can be included in meta-analyses of the efficacy of acupuncture for pain; consequently the results are not very convincing. However, if a pragmatic assessment is made by comparing results from the various acupuncture clinical trials with results from biomedicine in the treatment of pain, the acupuncture studies fare well. Indeed, biomedicine experiences many problems in the management and treatment of pain. Not only have results in conventional medical research often not been better than those found in the acupuncture studies, but many of the conventional therapies routinely used in the treatment and management of pain are problematic with relatively high side effect profiles. Acupuncture, on the other hand, has a very low side effect profile, especially when compared with common conventional therapies.[156] An independent panel of experts at the NIH consensus development conference considered these factors when they reached their conclusion that acupuncture is a clinically significant treatment.

Although the extent of clinical effectiveness of acupuncture in different pain conditions requires further research, the promising results and low side effect profile make it a valuable tool in the treatment and management of pain.[143] Furthermore, as recommended by the panel, it should be recognized that the full potential of acupuncture has yet to be unlocked in clinical trials, as problems with adequacy of treatment and the lack of studies testing acupuncture as actually practiced have barely been addressed.[143]

Currently, scientific evidence shows acupuncture to be effective or promising in the 11 pain conditions listed in Table 13-3. There is additional promising scientific evidence in a number of other pain conditions (see right column in Table 13-3). More studies are needed in all areas. As use of acupuncture increases, it is probable that increased familiarity with the practice will encourage more and better scientific assessment, which in turn will fuel more efficient utilization.

References

1. Bresler DE: *Free yourself from pain,* New York, 1979, Simon & Schuster.
2. Koch H: *The management of chronic pain in office-based ambulatory care: national ambulatory medical care survey. Advance data from vital and health statistics,* No. 123 (DHHS Publication No. PHS 86-1250), Hyattsville, Md, 1986, Public Health Service.
3. Turk DC, Meichenbaum D, Genest M: *Pain and behavioral medicine,* New York, 1983, Guildford Press.
4. Turk DC, Melzack R: The measurement of pain and the assessment of people experiencing pain. In DC Turk, Melzack R, editors: *Handbook of pain assessment,* New York, 1992, Guildford Press.
5. Hanson RW, Gerber KE: *Coping with chronic pain,* New York, 1990, Guildford Press.
6. Osterweis M, Kleinman A, Mechanic D, editors: *Pain and disability: clinical, behavioral, and public policy perspectives,* Washington, DC, 1987, National Academy Press.
7. Blanchard EB, Andrasik F: *Management of chronic headaches,* New York, 1985, Pergamon Press.
8. Dupuy HJ, Engel A, Devine BK, et al: *Selected symptoms of psychological stress* (US Public Health Service publication No. 1000, Series 11, No. 37), Washington, DC, 1977, National Center for Health Statistics.
9. Frymoyer JW: Back pain and sciatica, *N Engl J Med* 318:291-300, 1988.
10. Birch S, Felt R: *Understanding acupuncture,* Edinburgh, Churchill Livingstone (in press).
11. Lu GD, Needham J: *Celestial lancets,* Cambridge, 1980, Cambridge University Press.
12. Liao SJ: Acupuncture for low back pain in Huang Di Nei Jing Su Wen, *Acupunct Electrother Res* 17:249-58, 1992.
13. Birch S, Sherman K: Zhong Yi acupuncture and low back pain: traditional Chinese medical acupuncture differential diagnoses and treatments for chronic lumbar pain, *J Altern Complement Med* 5:412-25, 1999.
14. Anonymous: *Ling Shu Jing. The ling shu text,* Taipei, 1978, Chung Hwa Book Company.
15. Yang J-z: *Zhen Jiu Da Cheng,* Taipei, 1982, Da Zhong Guo Tu Shu Publishing.
16. Qiu ML: *Chinese acupuncture and moxibustion,* Edinburgh, 1993, Churchill Livingstone.
17. Shanghai College of Traditional Chinese Medicine: *Zhen Jiu Zhi Liao Xue,* Hong Kong, Shao Hua Cultural Service Publishing.
18. Wiseman N, Feng Y: *A practical dictionary of Chinese medicine,* Brookline, Mass, 1998, Paradigm Publications.
19. Wu Yan, Fischer W: *Practical therapeutics of traditional Chinese medicine,* Brookline, Mass, 1997, Paradigm Publications.
20. Cheng XN: *Chinese acupuncture and moxibustion,* Beijing, 1987, Foreign Languages Press.
21. Debata A: *Diagnosis and treatment of sciatica for the private practitioner acupuncturist,* ed 4, Yokosuka, 1990, Idono Nippon Publications.
22. Takaoka M: *Acupuncture treatment of pain for physicians: key points for intradermal needle therapy,* ed 5, Yokosuka, 1988, Idono Nippon Publications.
23. Birch S: Diversity and acupuncture: acupuncture is not a coherent or historically stable tradition. In Vickers AJ, editor: *Examining complementary medicine: the sceptical holist,* Cheltenham, 1998, Stanley Thomas, pp. 45-63.

24. Skrabanek P: Acupuncture: past, present, and future. In Stalker D, Glymour C, editors: *Examining holistic medicine,* Cheltenham, 1998, Stanley Thomas, pp. 181-96.

25. Ezzo J, Berman BM, Hadhazy VA, et al: Is acupuncture effective for the treatment of chronic pain: a systematic review, *Pain* 86(3):217-25, 2000.

26. Shichido T: Clinical evaluation of acupuncture and moxibustion, *Ido no Nippon Journal* 623:95-102, 1996.

27. Tsutani K, Shichido T, Sakuma K: *When acupuncture met biostatistics.* Presented at the Second World Conference of Acupuncture and Moxibustion, Paris, 1990.

28. Pomeranz B: Scientific basis of acupuncture. In Stux G, Pomeranz B, editors: *Basics of acupuncture,* ed 2, Berlin, 1991, Springer-Verlag, pp. 4-55.

29. Pomeranz B: Scientific research into acupuncture for the relief of pain, *J Altern Complement Med* 2:53-60, 1996.

30. Watanabe H, Tsutani K: Personal communication, 1997.

31. World Health Organization: Use of acupuncture in modern health care, *WHO Chronicle* 34:294-301, 1980.

32. World Health Organization: *The role of traditional medicine in primary health care,* WPR/RC36/Technical Discussions, September 12, 1985.

33. World Health Organization: *A proposed standard international acupuncture nomenclature. Report of a WHO scientific group,* Geneva, 1991, World Health Organization.

34. Eisenberg DM, Kessler RC, Foster C, et al: Unconventional medicine in the United States; prevalence, costs, and patterns of use, *N Engl J Med* 328:246-52, 1993.

35. Eisenberg DM, Davis RB, Ettner SL, et al: Trends in alternative medicine use in the United States 1990-1997: results of a follow-up national survey, *JAMA* 280:1569-75, 1998.

36. Tsutani K, Birch S: Evaluating complementary and alternative diagnostics (in preparation).

37. Scarognina P, Gardiol E, Lanza U, et al: The value of chemical pre-anesthesia in acupuncture anesthesia, *Am J Chin Med* 1:143-50, 1973.

38. Birch S, Hammerschlag R: *Acupuncture efficacy: a compendium of controlled clinical trials,* New York, 1996, National Academy of Acupuncture and Oriental Medicine.

39. Anderson DG, Jamieson JL, Man SC: Analgesic effects of acupuncture on the pain of ice water: a double-blind study, *Can J Psychiatry* 28:239-44, 1974.

40. Chapman CR, Chen AC, Bonica JJ: Effects of intrasegmental electrical acupuncture on dental pain; evaluation by threshold estimation and sensory decision theory, *Pain* 3:213-27, 1977.

41. Mayer DJ, Price DD, Rafii A: Antagonism of acupuncture analgesia in man by the narcotic antagonist naloxone, *Brain Res* 121:368-72, 1977.

42. Ballegaard S, Meyer CN, Trojaborg W: Acupuncture in angina pectoris: does acupuncture have a specific effect? *J Intern Med* 229:357-62, 1991.

43. Berman B, Lao LX, Greene M, et al: Efficacy of traditional Chinese acupuncture in the treatment of symptomatic knee arthritis: a pilot study, *Osteoarthritis Cartilage* 3:139-42, 1995.

44. Carlsson CPO, Sjolund BH: Acupuncture and subtypes of chronic pain: assessment of long-term results, *Clin J Pain* 10:290-95, 1994.

45. Junnilla SY: Long-term treatment of chronic pain with acupuncture. Part 1, *Acupunct Electrother Res* 12:23-36, 1987.

46. Lewith GT, Turner G, Machin D: Effects of acupuncture on low back pain and sciatica, *Am J Acupunct* 12: 21-32, 1984.

47. Strauss S: Acupuncture therapy in the treatment of chronic head, neck and neck related pain, *J Trad Chin Med* 5:13-8, 1985.

48. Strauss S: Acupuncture for head and neck pain, *Aust Fam Physician* 16:302-3, 1987.

49. Stux G: Migraine treatment with acupuncture and moxibustion, *Acupunct Sci Int J* 1:16-8, 1990.

50. Yuen RW, Vaughan RJ, Dyer H, et al: The response to acupuncture therapy in patients with chronic disabling pain, *Med J Aust* 1:862-5, 1976.

51. Coan R, Wong G, Ku SL, et al: The acupuncture treatment of low back pain: a randomized controlled treatment, *Am J Chin Med* 8:181-9, 1980.

52. Gunn CC, Milbrandt WE, Little AS, et al: Dry needling of muscle motor points for chronic low-back pain, *Spine* 5:279-91, 1980.

53. MacDonald AJR, Macrae KD, Master BR, et al: Superficial acupuncture in the relief of chronic low back pain, *Ann R Coll Surg Engl* 65:44-6, 1983.

54. Molsberger A, Winkler J, Schneider S, et al: Acupuncture and conventional orthopedic pain treatment in the management of chronic low back pain: a prospective randomised and controlled clinical trial (in press).

55. Kinoshita H: Zakotsushinkeitsu shokogun no taisuru shinkyu sayo, *Kokusai Shinkyu Gakkai J* 15:76-95, 1966.

56. Kinoshita H: Rinsho shiken kara mita ho sha no kento, *Nippon Shinkyu Chiryo Gakkai J* 20:6-13, 1971.

57. Kinoshita H: Boshinkeishi wo zakotsu shinkeitsu ni oyoshita rinsho shiken, *Nippon Shinkyu Chiryo Gakkai J* 32:4-13, 1983.

58. Ahonen E, Hakumaki M, Mahlamaki S, et al: Acupuncture and physiotherapy in the treatment of myogenic headache patients: pain relief and EMG activity, *Adv Pain Res Ther* 5:571-76, 1983.

59. Hansen PE, Hansen JH: Acupuncture treatment of chronic tension headache—a controlled cross-over trial, *Cephalgia* 5:137-42, 1985.

60. Hesse J, Mogelvang B, Simonsen H: Acupuncture versus metoprolol in migraine prophylaxis: a randomized trial of trigger point inactivation, *J Intern Med* 235:451-56, 1994.

61. Vincent CA: A controlled trial of the treatment of migraine by acupuncture, *Clin J Pain* 5:305-12, 1989.

62. White AR, Eddleston C, Hardie R, et al: A pilot study of acupuncture for tension headache, using a novel placebo, *Acupunct Med* 14:11-5, 1996.

63. Birch S, Jamison RN: A controlled trial of Japanese acupuncture for chronic myofascial neck pain: assessment of specific and nonspecific effects of treatment, *Clin J Pain* 14:248-55, 1998.

64. Loy TT: Treatment of cervical spondylosis—electroacupuncture versus physiotherapy, *Med J Austral* 2:32-4, 1983.

65. Thomas M, Eriksson SV, Lundeberg T: A comparative study of diazepam and acupuncture in patients with osteoarthritis pain: a placebo controlled study, *Am J Chin Med* 19:95-100, 1991.

66. Kinoshita H: Keiwan shokugun no taisuru boshinkeishi no rinshoteki kenkyu, *Nippon Shinkyu Chiryo Gakkai J* 27:61-71, 1978.

67. Berry H, Fernandes L, Bloom B, et al: Clinical study comparing acupuncture, physiotherapy, injection and oral anti-inflammatory therapy in shoulder-cuff lesions, *Curr Med Res Opin* 7:121-6, 1980.

68. Moore ME, Berk SN: Acupuncture for chronic shoulder pain, an experimental study with attention to the role of placebo and hypnotic susceptibility, *Ann Intern Med* 84:381-4, 1976.

69. Hansen PE, Hansen JH: Acupuncture treatment of chronic facial pain—a controlled cross-over trial, *Headache* 23:66-9, 1983.

70. Johansson A, Wenneberg B, Wagersten C, et al: Acupuncture in treatment of facial muscular pain, *Acta Odontol Scand* 49:153-8, 1991.

71. List T, Helkimo M, Andersson S, et al: Acupuncture and occlusal splint therapy in the treatment of craniomandibular disorders. I. A comparative study, *Swed Dent J* 16:125-41, 1991.

72. List T, Helkimo M: Acupuncture and occlusal splint therapy in the treatment of craniomandibular disorders. II. A one year follow-up study, *Acta Odontol Scand* 50:375-85, 1992.

73. Brattberg G: Acupuncture for tennis elbow, *Pain* 16:285-88, 1990.

74. Haker E, Lundeberg T: Acupuncture treatment in epicondylalgia: a comparison study of two acupuncture techniques, *Clin J Pain* 6:221-26, 1990.

75. Molsberger A, Hille E: The analgesic effect of acupuncture in chronic tennis elbow pain, *Br J Rheumatol* 33:1162-65, 1994.

76. Naeser MA, Hahn KK, Lieberman B: Real vs sham laser acupuncture and microamps TENS to treat carpal tunnel syndrome and worksite wrist pain, *Lasers Surg Med* 8(Suppl):7-15, 1996.

77. Maruno SD: Shitsu kansetsu sho ni taisuru tsuden chiryo no hikaku, *Nippon Shinkyu Chiryo Gakkai J* 25:52-4, 1976.

78. Wang LQ, Wang AM, Zhang SD: Clinical analysis and experimental observation on acupuncture and moxibustion treatment of patellar tendon terminal disease in athletes, *J Trad Chin Med* 5:162-66, 1985.

79. Lewith GT, Field J, Machin D: Acupuncture compared with placebo in post-herpetic pain, *Pain* 16:361-68, 1983.

80. Rutgers MJ, van Romunde LKJ, Osman PO: A small randomized comparative trial of acupuncture versus transcutaneous electrical neurostimulation in post-herpetic neuralgia, *Pain Clin* 2:87-9, 1988.

81. Nielsen SE, Valentin N, Lewinski A: Treatment of acute herpes zoster with acupuncture and sympathetic blocks. A controlled study, *Ugeskr Laeger* 138:2305-09, 1976.

82. Shlay JC, Chalmers K, Max MB, et al: Acupuncture and amitriptyline for pain due to HIV-related peripheral neuropathy: A randomized controlled trial, *JAMA* 280:1590-95, 1998.

83. Deluze C, Bosia L, Zirbs A, et al: Electroacupuncture in fibromyalgia: results of a controlled trial, *Br Med J* 305:1249-52, 1992.

84. Ernst E, Resch KL, Fialka V, et al: Traditional acupuncture for reflex sympathetic dystrophy: a randomised, sham-controlled, double-blind trial, *Acupunct Med* 13:78-80, 1995.

85. Vrchota KD, Belgrade MJ, Johnson RJ, et al: True acupuncture vs. sham acupuncture and conventional sports medicine therapy for plantar fasciitis pain: a controlled, double-blind study, *Int J Clin Acupunct* 2:247-53, 1991.

86. Christensen BV, Iuhl IU, Vilbek H, et al: Acupuncture treatment of severe knee osteoarthrosis. A long-term study, *Acta Anaesth Scand* 36:519-25, 1992.

87. Dickens W, Lewith GT: A single-blind, controlled and randomised clinical trial to evaluate the effect of acupuncture in the treatment of trapezio-metacarpal osteoarthritis, *Complement Med Res* 3:5-8, 1989.

88. Takeda W, Wessel J: Acupuncture for the treatment of osteoarthritic knees, *Arthritis Care Res* 7:118-22, 1994.

89. Godfrey CM, Morgan P: A controlled trial of the theory of acupuncture in musculoskeletal pain, *J Rheumatol* 5:121-24, 1978.

90. Junnila SYT: Acupuncture therapy for chronic pain. A randomised comparison between acupuncture and pseudoacupuncture with minimal peripheral stimulus, *Am J Acupunct* 10:259-62, 1982.

91. Lao L, Bergman S, Langenberg P, et al: Efficacy of Chinese acupuncture on postoperative oral surgery pain, *Oral Surg Oral Med Oral Pathol Oral Radiol Endod* 79:423-28, 1995.

92. Sung YF, Kutner MH, Cerine FC, et al: Comparison of the effects of acupuncture and codeine on postoperative dental pain; *Anesth Analg Curr Res* 56:473-78, 1977.

93. Christensen PA, Noreng M, Andersen PE, et al: Electroacupuncture and postoperative pain, *Br J Anesth* 62:258-62, 1989.

94. Mast R, Schoch T, Scharf HP: Acupuncture against postoperative pain after total knee replacement: a placebo-controlled trial on immediate effects, *Aktuel Rheumatol* 20:131-34, 1995.

95. Lee YH, Lee WC, Chen MT, et al: Acupuncture in the treatment of renal colic, *J Urol* 147:16-18, 1992.

96. Helms JM: Acupuncture for the management of primary dysmenorrhea, *Obstet Gynecol* 69:51-6, 1987.

97. Gunsberger M: Acupuncture in the treatment of sore throat symptomatology, *Am J Chin Med* 1:373-40, 1973.

98. Ballegaard S, Pedersen F, Pietersen A, et al: Effects of acupuncture in moderate, stable angina pectoris, *J Intern Med* 227:25-30, 1990.

99. Richter A, Herlitz J, Hjalmarson A: Effect of acupuncture in patients with angina pectoris, *Eur Heart J* 12:175-78, 1991.

100. Ballegaard S, Christophersen SJ, Dawids SG, et al: Acupuncture and transcutaneous electric nerve stimulation in the treatment of pain associated with chronic pancreatitis, *Scand J Gastroenterol* 20:1249-54, 1985.

101. Cahn AM, Carayon P, Hill C, et al: Acupuncture in gastroscopy, *Lancet* 28:182-83, 1978.

102. Wang HH, Chang YH, Liu DM: A study in the effectiveness of acupuncture analgesia for colonoscopic examination compared with conventional premedication, *Am J Acupunct* 20:217-21, 1992.

103. Yue SJ: Acupuncture for chronic back and neck pain, *Acupunct Electrother Res* 3:323-24, 1978.

104. Ahonen E, Hakumaki M, Mahlamaki S, et al: Acupuncture and physiotherapy in the treatment of tension neck patients: pain relief and EMG activity, *Pain* 13(Suppl 1):S278, 1981.

105. Boureau F, Luu M, Kisielnicki E: Effects of transcutaneous nerve stimulation (TNS), electrotherapy (ET), electrocacupuncture (EA) on chronic pain: a comparative study, *Pain* 13(Suppl 1):S277, 1981.

106. Ceccherelli F, Altafini L, LoCastro G, et al: Diode laser in cervical myofascial pain: a double-blind study versus placebo, *Clin J Pain* 5:301-04, 1989.

107. Cheng RSS, Pomeranz B: Electrotherapy of chronic musculoskeletal pain: comparison of electroacupuncture and acupuncture-like transcutaneous electrical nerve stimulation, *Clin J Pain* 2:143-49, 1987.

108. Hackett GI, Seddon D, Kaminski D: Electroacupuncture compared with paracetamol for acute low back pain, *Practitioner* 232:163-64, 1988.

109. Lenhard L, Waite PME: Acupuncture in the prophylactic treatment of migraine headaches: pilot study, *N Z Med J* 96:663-6, 1983.

110. Mendelson G, Selwood TS, Kranz HK, et al: Acupuncture treatment in chronic back pain: a double-blind placebo-controlled trial, *Am J Med* 74:49-55, 1983.

111. Carlsson J, Fahlcrantz A, Augustinsson LE: Muscle tenderness in tension headache treated with acupuncture or physiotherapy, *Cephalalgia* 10:131-41, 1990.

112. Fox E, Melzack R: Transcutaneous stimulation and acupuncture: comparison of treatment for low back pain, *Pain* 2:141-48, 1976.

113. Laitinen J: Acupuncture and transcutaneous electric stimulation in the treatment of chronic sacrolumbalgia and ischialgia, *Am J Chin Med* 4:169-75, 1976.

114. Lehmann TR, Russell DW: Efficacy of electroacupuncture and TENS in the rehabilitation of chronic low back pain patients, *Pain* 26:277-90, 1986.

115. Loh L, Nathan PW, Schott GD, et al: Acupuncture versus medical treatment for migraine and muscle tension headaches, *J Neurol Neurosurg Psychiatry* 47:333-37, 1984.

116. Dowson DI, Lewith GT, Machin D: The effects of acupuncture versus placebo in the treatment of headache, *Pain* 21:35-42, 1985.

117. Petrie JP, Hazleman BL: A controlled study of acupuncture in neck pain, *Br J Rheumatol* 25:271-75, 1986.

118. Lopacz S, Gralewski Z: Evaluation of the results of low backache by acupuncture or suggesting (preliminary report), *Neurol Neurochir Pol* 13:405-09, 1979.

119. Tavola T, Gala C, Conte G, et al: Traditional Chinese acupuncture in tension-type headache: a controlled study, *Pain* 48:325-29, 1992.

120. Birch S: Testing the clinical specificity of needle sites in controlled clinical trials of acupuncture, *Proceedings of the Second Society for Acupuncture Research,* 1995, Society for Acupuncture Research, pp. 274-94.

121. Birch S: *An exploration with proposed solutions of the problems and issues in conducting clinical research in acupuncture* [dissertation], Exeter, United Kingdom, 1997, University of Exeter.

122. de la Torre CS: The choice of control groups in invasive clinical trials such as acupuncture, *Frontier Persp* 3:33-7, 1993.

123. Hammerschlag R: Methodological and ethical issues in clinical trials of acupuncture, *J Altern Complement Med* 4:159-71, 1998.

124. Hammerschlag R, Morris MM: Clinical trials comparing acupuncture with biomedical standard care: a criteria-based evaluation of research design and reporting, *Complement Ther Med* 5:133-40, 1997.

125. Vincent CA: Acupuncture as a treatment for chronic pain. In Lewith GT, Aldridge D, editors: *Clinical research methodology for complementary therapies,* London, 1993, Hodder and Stoughton, pp. 289-308.

126. Vincent C, Lewith G: Placebo controls for acupuncture studies, *J R Soc Med* 88:199-202, 1995.

127. Vincent CA, Richardson PH: The evaluation of therapeutic acupuncture: concepts and methods, *Pain* 24:1-13, 1986.

128. Ter Reit G, Kleijnen J, Knipschild P: Acupuncture and chronic pain: a criteria-based meta-analysis, *J Clin Epidemiol* 43:1191-9, 1990.

129. Lewith GT, Machin D: On the evaluation of the clinical effects of acupuncture, *Pain* 16:111-27, 1983.

130. Richardson PH, Vincent CA: Acupuncture for the treatment of pain: a review of evaluative research, *Pain* 24:15-40, 1986.

131. Patel M, Gutzwiller F, Paccaud F, et al: A meta-analysis of acupuncture for chronic pain, *Int J Epidemiol* 18:900-6, 1989.

132. Ernst E: Acupuncture research: where are the problems? *Acupunct Med* 12:93-97, 1994.

133. Lytle CD: *An overview of acupuncture,* Washington, DC, 1993, U.S. Department of Health and Human Services, Public Health Service, Food and Drug Administration, Center for Devices and Radiological Health.

134. National Council Against Health Fraud: Acupuncture: the position paper of the National Council Against Health Fraud, *Clin J Pain* 7:162-66, 1991.

135. Alpert S: FDA letter—reclassification order, docket No. 94P-0443, acupuncture needles for the practice of acupuncture. In Birch S, Hammerschlag R, editors: *Acupuncture efficacy: a compendium of controlled clinical trials,* New York, 1996, National Academy of Acupuncture and Oriental Medicine, pp. 76-8.

136. Birch S: Issues to consider in determining an adequate treatment in a clinical trial of acupuncture, *Complement Ther Med* 5:8-12, 1997.

137. Stux G, Birch S: Proposed standards of acupuncture treatment for clinical studies. In Stux G, Hammerschlag R, editors: *Scientific bases of acupuncture in basic and clinical research,* Berlin, 2000, Springer Verlag.

138. Birch S: *Overview of the efficacy of acupuncture in the treatment of headache, face, and neck pain,* Presented at the Consensus Development Conference on Acupuncture, Bethesda, Md, Nov 3-5, 1997.

139. Vincent CA: Credibility assessment in trials of acupuncture, *Complement Med Res* 4:8-11, 1990.

140. Edelist G, Gross AE, Langer F: Treatment of low back pain with acupuncture, *Can Anaesth Soc J* 23:303-06, 1976.

141. Eskinazi DP, Jobst KA: National Institutes of Health office of alternative medicine—Food and Drug Administration workshop on acupuncture (editorial), *J Altern Complement Med* 2:3-6, 1996.

142. Birch S, Hammerschlag R, Berman BL: Acupuncture in the treatment of pain, *J Altern Complement Med* 2:101-24, 1996.

143. Acupuncture: NIH consensus development panel on acupuncture, *JAMA* 280:1518-24, 1998.

144. Jensen LB, Melsen B, Jensen SB: Effect of acupuncture on headache measured by reduction in number of attacks and use of drugs, *Scand J Dent Res* 87:373-80, 1979.

145. Henry P, Baille H, Dartigues F, et al: Headaches and acupuncture. In *Updating in headache,* Berlin, 1985, Springer Verlag.

146. Vincent CA: The treatment of tension headache by acupuncture: a controlled single case design with time series analysis, *J Psychosom Res* 34:553-61, 1990.

147. Baust W, Strutzbecher H: Akupunkturbehandlung der migraine in doppelblindversuch, *Med Welt* 29:669-73, 1978.

148. Petrie JP, Langley GB: Acupuncture in the treatment of chronic cervical pain. A pilot study, *Clin Exp Rheumatol* 1:333-35, 1983.

149. Matsumoto T, Levy B, Ambruso V: Clinical evaluation of acupuncture, *Am Surg* 41:400-05, 1974.

150. Duplan B, Cabanel G, Piton JL, et al: Acupuncture et lombosciatique a la phase aigue: etude en double aveugle de trente cas [Acupuncture and sciatica in the acute phase. Double-blind study of 30 cases], *Sem Hop* 59:3109-14, 1983.

151. Emery P, Lythgoe S: The effect of acupuncture on ankylosing spondylitis, *Br J Rheumatol* 25:132-33, 1986.

152. Doerr-Proske H, Wittchen HU: Ein muskel-und gefaborientiertes entspannungsprogramm (SEP) zur behandlung chronischer migrainepatienten: Eine randomisierte klinische vergleichsstudie [A muscle and vascular oriented relaxation program for the treatment of chronic migraine patients. A randomized clinical comparative study], *Z Psychosom Med Psychoanal* 31:247-66, 1985.

153. Carlsson J, Rosenhall U: Oculomotor disturbances in patients with tension headache treated with acupuncture or physiotherapy, *Cephalgia* 10:123-29, 1990.

154. Raustia AM, Pohjola RT, Virtanen KK: Acupuncture compared with stomatographic treatment for TMJ dysfunction. 1. A randomized study, *J Prosthet Dent* 54:581-85, 1985.

155. Ghia JN, Mao W, Toomey TC, et al: Acupuncture and chronic pain mechanisms, *Pain* 2:285-89, 1976.

156. Lytle CD: Safety and regulation of acupuncture needles and other devices. Presented at the NIH Consensus Development Conference on Acupuncture, Bethesda, Md, 1997, Nov 3-5, 1997.

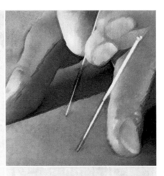

Acupuncture in the Treatment of Addictions

MICHAEL O. SMITH

JAMES C. BUTLER-ARKOW

For over 3000 years, acupuncture has been an important modality of Chinese medicine. Today, in over 1300 programs worldwide, including the United States and Europe, acupuncture is used as a technique to curb substance abuse. A substantial body of clinical evidence supports this application of acupuncture. Studies have demonstrated that auricular acupuncture can minimize the impact of withdrawal symptoms from alcohol, cocaine, and opiates such as morphine and heroin. In addition, acupuncture reduces the craving that often occurs with the use of addictive substances.

In treating drug addictions, auricular acupuncture is the modality generally used. Needles are inserted to a depth of approximately ⅛ inch into specific points located on the external ear. Auricular acupuncture is a nonverbal, nonthreatening first-step intervention that has immediate calming effects. It is a safe and cost-effective procedure that has gained increasing acceptance from US agencies responsible for overseeing substance abuse treatment.*

THE DEVELOPMENT OF ACUPUNCTURE TO TREAT SUBSTANCE ABUSE

In 1973, Hong Kong neurosurgeon, H. L. Wen, first reported successfully using acupuncture to treat symptoms of addiction withdrawal.[1] Wen observed opium addicts who had undergone surgery followed by elec-

---

*Discussion of the NADA auricular protocol for treating drug addition forms the bulk of this chapter. Use of body acupoints to treat other addictions is briefly discussed in the Appendix to this chapter.

troacupuncture (needles connected to a low-voltage alternating current) to relieve postoperative pain. Coincidentally, Wen discovered that these addicts found that they experienced fewer withdrawal symptoms, an observation he confirmed in subsequent clinical studies.

Lincoln Hospital, now the Lincoln Medical and Mental Health Center, pioneered the use of acupuncture to treat drug and alcohol addiction in the United States. Lincoln is a public facility operated in the impoverished south Bronx by New York City. It has performed more than 500,000 acupuncture treatments in the past 20 years in its substance-abuse division, a state-licensed treatment program. In 1974, the clinic began by using the method Wen had discovered, applying a weak electrical stimulation through a needle to the "Lung Point" on the ear.[2] (Auricular acupoints are frequently named after organs or functions that they have been observed to influence.) Patients who participated in the clinic's electroacupuncture program reported feeling more relaxed, having less opiate withdrawal symptoms, and being able to take part in longer periods of psychotherapy.

Subsequently, Dr. Michael Smith and his Lincoln Center colleagues discovered that simple, manual needling produced a more prolonged effect than electrical stimulation. Patients who were given manual acupuncture once a day found their symptoms were relieved throughout the day. Moreover, clinicians discovered that the manual needling caused cravings to abate, particularly those for alcohol and heroin—an effect that had never been described previously. Then, over a period of years, after extensive clinical research and experimentation, the clinic developed a five-point ear acupuncture protocol.

A New Class of Practitioner

Since 1990, more than 3000 substance-abuse clinicians have been trained to provide acupuncture through the substance-abuse program at the Lincoln Clinic, which works in conjunction with the National Acupuncture Detoxification Association (NADA). NADA was established in 1985 to train and certify substance abuse clinicians in using auricular acupuncture as a detoxification method. One of NADA's missions is to promote the use of the Lincoln model nationwide, and to ensure that acupuncture detoxification facilities and programs maintain rigorous standards. In a 70-hour apprenticeship-based training pro-

 NADA Clearinghouse

NADA Clearinghouse offers a wide range of articles and videotapes and information on training and certification. Contact:

NADA Clearinghouse
Box 1927
Vancouver, WA 98662

gram, licensed or certified acupuncturists teach the location of the ear points and the techniques for inserting the needles. This approach enables acupuncture to be integrated with existing medical and psychosocial services in a convenient, flexible, and cost-effective manner.

Clinicians who have completed the 70-hour training program are called *Acupuncture Detoxification Specialists* (ADSs). Statutes authorizing ADSs have passed in several states (including New York, Virginia, Texas, Connecticut, Indiana, and Missouri), as well as Germany and Hungary. In many other cases, state medical boards or other authorities have established special provisions allowing ADSs to treat patients with the five-point ear protocol.

THE NADA FIVE-POINT PROTOCOL

The protocol utilizes some combination of five specific auricular acupoints to treat most substance abuse disorders.* Not all points are used on all patients, and in clinical practice the treatment is tailored to fit the individual patient's needs on a given day (Figure 14-1). A standard Chinese textbook in translation[3] summarizes these points as follows:

1. *Sympathetic point* has a strong analgesic and relaxant effect on internal organs, relieves pain associated with ulcers and stomach spasm, dilates blood vessels, and treats sweating. This point is often used to treat conditions related to disruption of

---

*Different systems of auricular acupuncture (e.g., French and Chinese) locate auricular points differently. Unless otherwise noted, points discussed in this chapter are located according to Chinese methods.[3]

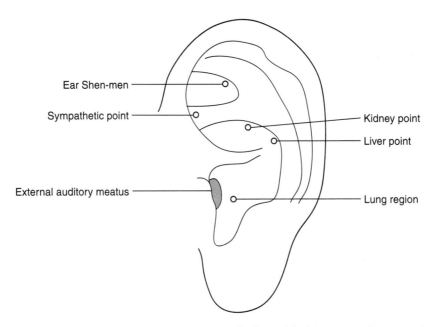

Figure 14-1 Ear with five ear detoxification points marked. Modified from Mao-liang Q, editor: *Chinese acupuncture and moxibustion,* Edinburgh, 1993, Churchill Livingstone.

the autonomic (both sympathetic and parasympathetic) nervous system and is an important point in anesthesia.

2. *Ear Shen-men "(Spirit Gate") point* (also known as "neurogate") is used for neuropsychiatric disorders (hysteria, psychosis, and so on) and has sedative, analgesic, and antiallergy effects. This point is indicated in hypertension, coughing, and itching symptoms, regulates excitation and inhibition of the cerebral cortex, and is an important point in anesthesia.

3. *Lung point* is indicated in various respiratory disorders, rhinitis, mutism, night sweats, spontaneous sweating and is used in anesthesia; since it is large, it is marked as a region.

4. *Liver point* is used for acute and chronic hepatitis, arthritic pain, neuralgia, headache, vertigo, stomach gas and pain, and to move stagnation.

5. *Kidney point* is the strengthening point and is beneficial to the cerebrum and hematopoietic system. It is used for amnesia, neurasthenia, vertigo, headache, lassitude, electrolyte imbalance, and gynecological and genitourinary diseases.

As previously discussed, Chinese medicine conceives of the organs in substantially different ways than biomedicine and assigns psychological, as well

as physiological, function to them. This model proved useful in choosing which points to use when treating addiction. For example, Chinese medical theory associates the Lung with the grieving process, the Liver with resolving aggression, and the Kidney with willpower and rebirth.

The value of using one standard group of acupuncture points became clear over time. Patients responded better when acupuncture treatment was administered quickly without a self-conscious, diagnostic prelude. The basic five-point protocol seemed to be equally effective for different drugs of abuse and at different stages of treatment. Since acupuncture produces a homeostatic response (see Chapter 11), it was not necessary to adjust the formula for mood swings, agitation, or lack of energy.

Bringing Balance to "Empty Fire"

From a Chinese medical perspective, the basic NADA protocol makes sense because addicts tend to be emotionally and physically depleted. A healthy person is said to possess a balance of "water," or calm inner tone, and "fire," or extroverted activity. When a patient lacks a calm inner tone, a condition known as Empty

Fire *(xu huo)* results, wherein the "fire" principle is said to burn out of control and become a heated aggressiveness. This Empty Fire condition, representing an illusion of power, results in more desperate chemical abuse and senseless violence. Indeed, the aggressiveness that many addicts show may be confusing, and cause one to conclude that the treatment goal should be to "put out the fire" pharmacologically. Addicts themselves take this approach when they resort to using highly sedating drugs. Acupuncture, by contrast, helps to restore patients' inner calm and control, thus reducing their aggressive behavior, and minimizing their withdrawal symptoms.

The treatment of Empty Fire is illustrated by the example of a single mother who enrolled in the Lincoln Clinic program. She had given birth to four children before she turned 18 and had a long history of impulsive child abuse and substance addiction. She had never been given a chance to grow and mature herself. When she began the Clinic program, she was extremely hostile toward her counselor and highly jittery. In the first interview, she focused entirely on the pressures and problems of raising her children and talked of little else. After just one acupuncture treatment, however, she reported that she felt "like a changed person." In her subsequent interview, which proved to be much more constructive and detailed than the first, she told her counselor, "My kids said I didn't act the same at all." She continued in treatment, and the Lincoln program staff was very enthusiastic about her new calm and constructive outlook.

Herbal medicine also has proved useful in calming the addicted patient's "fire." In conjunction with acupuncture treatment, Lincoln clinicians use an herbal formula called "sleep mix." The tea is made up of inexpensive herbs, including peppermint, chamomile, yarrow, skullcap, hops, and catnip. All of these herbs are commonly used in Europe to treat stress and insomnia, and are believed to calm the nervous system, stimulate blood circulation, and promote the elimination of waste products and toxins by the body. The herbal formula is taken as a tea on a nightly basis or frequently during the day as symptoms indicate. Sleep mix is presently used in a number of addiction treatment settings, and is particularly appropriate for the management of alcohol withdrawal symptoms. Patients receiving benzodiazepine treatment, the standard pharmacological treatment for alcohol withdrawal, will often voluntarily refuse this medication if sleep mix is available.

Mindset and Treatment Setting

At the Lincoln Clinic, patients have needles placed in three to five points in each ear for about 45 minutes. A large group setting enhances the acupuncture effect, in addition to enabling the treatment of many patients at the same time. Experience has shown that patients who are treated individually (or in small groups) tend to be self-conscious and easily distracted. However, if the group consists of at least six patients, the clients experience enhanced relaxation and relief from their withdrawal symptoms.

The procedure is nearly painless and causes the rapid onset of a gratifying sense of relaxation. On first exposure, most patients express fear of the pain of needle insertion and are confused by the idea that little needles can cope with their big problems. This fear is easily solved by letting prospective patients observe the actual process of treatment. It is a mistake to rely on leaflets and verbal explanations.

The atmosphere of the treatment room should be adjusted to fit varying clinical circumstances (see Chapter 9). Programs with a significant number of new intakes and/or socially isolated patients do well to use a well lighted room and allow a moderate amount of conversation in order to minimize alienation and encourage social bonding. On the other hand, programs with relatively fixed clients who relate to each other frequently in other group settings succeed when they dim the lights and minimize conversation to limit distraction. Background music is often used in the latter circumstance.

Although nearly painless, acupuncture may cause patients to experience a few temporary sensations. During a treatment, patients sometimes feel a local warmth and tingling in the region where the needles were inserted. They may also experience momentary electrical sensations or a sense of heaviness in other parts of their bodies. Some patients have reported feeling sleepy for a short period of time after their initial treatments. This reaction is a normal part of the process of recovering from an addiction. A few patients incur a brief headache near the end of their treatment sessions. In rare situations, the patient has a "needling reaction," in which he or she has sensations of dizziness or lightheadedness and may faint during the treatment or when getting up afterwards (a reaction seen occasionally in other medical settings).

In virtually every substance abuse program, sterile, disposable needles are used. Upon removal, the needles are immediately discarded in a sharps container. Because bleeding occasionally occurs, acupuncturists take standard precautions to prevent exposure to the patient's blood. In a large group, a useful approach is for patients to remove and count the needles themselves.

"Relaxed but Alert"

In the group setting used in the Lincoln Clinic model, each patient appears comfortable in his or her own space; the quiet 45-minute period is conducive to personal reflection and self-assessment. As one patient put, "I sat and thought about things in a slow way like I did when I was 10 years old." Acupuncture treatment promotes awareness of various relaxing bodily processes. Patients gradually gain confidence that their minds and bodies can function in a more balanced and autonomous manner. After just a few treatments, most substance abusers who receive acupuncture treatment come to realize that the technique works largely by revealing their own internal capabilities—capabilities that they can realize without adding external chemicals.

Patients often describe detoxification acupuncture as a unique kind of balancing experience: "I was relaxed but alert" and "I was able to relax without losing control." For many substance abusers, such an experience is both unusual and welcome. Indeed, the perception that a person can be both relaxed and alert is rather unusual in Western culture. We are used to associating relaxation with somewhat lazy or spacey behavior and alertness with a certain degree of anxiety. Yet the relaxed and alert state is basic to the concept of health in all Asian culture. Acupuncture generally encourages a centering, focusing process that is also typical of meditation and yoga. Patients who are depressed or tired say that they feel more energetic. Therapists report that patients are "able to listen" and "remember what we tell them." Restless, impulsive behavior is greatly reduced, yet so are discouragement and apathy. It is a balancing, centering process.

Detoxification patients initially respond best to acupuncture that is administered quickly, without a great deal of discussion, examination, or other preliminaries. The absence of such verbal communication and interpersonal action is especially valuable at a time when the patient may be experiencing acute physical withdrawal symptoms (e.g., aching, headache, nausea, sweating, muscle cramping, and cravings), as well as intense anxiety and/or depression. As treatment progresses and acute symptoms abate, acupuncture helps patients deal with more long-standing issues of fear and social isolation. As they develop greater calmness and confidence, patients are able to enter gradually into more positive psychosocial interactions.

As one example, consider a female patient who was six months pregnant and addicted to crack cocaine. She showed up one day anxious and nervous at a NADA-run clinic. "I can't tell you much about myself," she told the staff, "because my husband is out in the street with a baseball bat, and he'll hit me in the knees if I say too much." The program provided an emergency acupuncture treatment and conducted a simplified admissions interview. Two weeks later, the patient brought her husband in and said, "This is my husband; he doesn't have a drug problem, but he is nervous. Can you help him?" Both of them received acupuncture that day. The woman needed a protective environment in which she was not vulnerable to her husband's physical abuse; he needed a nonthreatening treatment setting in which he was not subjected to verbal questioning or challenges. The whole process was so supportive and calming that the husband was able to begin trusting his wife and encouraging her detoxification.

Immediate Needs, Long-Term Responsibility

The duration of acupuncture treatment depends on many factors. Inpatient programs stress acupuncture in the beginning for detoxification and stabilization; before discharge it is used to allay separation anxiety. Outpatients in a drug-free setting typically receive acupuncture for 1 to 3 months on an active basis. About 10% of these outpatients will choose to take acupuncture for more than one year if possible.

Easy access and better retention encourage the outpatient management of difficult patients with less need for additional drugs or services. One can select times for hospitalization more appropriately. An outpatient continuum also facilitates primary health care management for AIDS, tuberculosis, and sexually transmitted diseases (STDs). Acupuncture is used in a large proportion of AIDS prevention and outreach programs in New York and London, as well as other cities. These facilities include needle exchange and harm reduction programs; recovery readiness and pretreatment programs, as well as health service providers for HIV positive and AIDS patients.

In treating addictions, acupuncture is most often used in conjunction with group rehabilitation programs such as Alcoholics Anonymous and Narcotics Anonymous. Acupuncture provides an excellent foundation for both of these well-established 12-step recovery programs, with which it has much in common. Participation in both is independent of diagnosis and level of recovery. Both have a "one-day-at-a-time" philosophy. In both components of treatment, participants draw on the collective strength of the group and gain comfort and inspiration from others who are managing their recovery well. Both approaches are simple, reinforcing, nurturing, and convenient, and both emphasize self-responsibility in the recovery process.

Substance abuse patients are characteristically oriented to the present. Unfortunately, conventional treatment efforts tend to focus on assessment of past activities and planning for the future. Because patients are preoccupied by present sensations and problems, they often feel alienated and resentful that therapists cannot focus on their immediate needs. Acupuncture is one of the only ways that treatment staff can respond to a patient's immediate needs without using addictive drugs. Therapists can meet patients in their present-time reality, validating their needs and providing substantial relief. Once a comfortable day-to-day reality support is established, we can approach past and future issues with a better alliance with the patient.

CONTROLLED STUDIES

The selection of appropriate controls in placebo design experiments presents a challenging problem. At the Lincoln Clinic, during the trial-and-error search for a more effective ear acupuncture formula for addiction treatment, it became clear that a large number of points had some effect on acute withdrawal symptoms. Ear acupuncture charts developed both by Chinese and Western researchers identify all areas on the anterior surface of the ear as active treatment locations. Using "sham" acupuncture as a control is actually an effort to use relatively ineffective points, in contrast to the conventional use of ineffective sugar pills in pharmaceutical trials. "Sham" points are usually located on the external helix or rim of the ear. Margolin and colleagues[4,5] investigated various sites used as sham points and concluded that the helix region is probably the least active in terms of evoking the "acu-

puncture response" seen in addiction settings. To summarize, sham-controlled studies tend to generate false negatives (type II errors) rather than false positives (type I errors).

Despite the caveats regarding experimental design noted above, a number of controlled studies support the conclusion that acupuncture's effectiveness in facilitating abstinence with alcohol, opiate, and cocaine abusers is not due to a simple placebo effect. Seven published studies involving animal subjects (mice or rats) indicate that electroacupuncture (EA) reduces opiate withdrawal symptoms with morphine-addicted subjects.[6] These studies examined experimental and control animals with regard to typical signs of rodent opiate withdrawal symptoms such as hyperactivity, "wet dog" shakes, and teeth chattering. Each of these studies noted significantly fewer withdrawal signs with subjects receiving EA relative to controls. In addition, several studies noted significant differences between experimental and control subjects in post-EA hormonal and beta endorphin levels.

A number of controlled studies have been conducted on human subjects, using various modified versions of the NADA five-point protocol. An important conclusion from such studies is that acupuncture enhances patients' participation in addiction treatment programs. Washburn[7] reported that opium addicted individuals receiving correct-site acupuncture showed significantly better program attendance relative to subjects receiving acupuncture on sham sites. Patients being treated for cocaine addiction remained in treatment longer when acupuncture was part of the protocol.[8]

Two placebo-control studies provide strong support for using acupuncture to treat alcoholics. Bullock and colleagues[9] studied 54 chronic alcohol abusers randomly assigned to receive acupuncture either at points related to addiction or at nearby sham points. Subjects were treated in an inpatient setting but were free to leave the program each day. Throughout the treatment and follow-up period, experimental subjects showed significantly better outcomes regarding attendance, self-reported need for alcohol, self-reported drinking episodes, and rate of readmission to a local detoxification unit for alcohol-related treatment. Bullock et al[10] replicated the above study using a larger (N = 80) sample over a longer (6-month) follow-up period. Twenty-one out of 40 patients in the treatment group completed the eight-week treatment as compared with only one out of 40 controls. Significant differences favoring the experimental group were again noted. Experimental subjects self-reported half as many drinking episodes as control subjects, and were readmitted to the local detoxification unit at half the rate of control subjects.

By contrast, another study[11] found no significant results in using acupuncture to treat alcoholics. This study used smaller treatment groups and less frequent treatment compared to the research by Bullock and colleagues.[10] Although the results did not rise to the level of statistical significance, the acupuncture group did show the best outcome on seven of eight measures reported.

Chronic cocaine/crack users receiving acupuncture showed a significant decrease in cocaine metabolite levels as measured by urinalysis.[12] Subjects (N = 150) were randomly assigned to receive auricular acupuncture either at correct sites or nearby sham sites. Self-report measures showed a significant tendency with both groups toward decreased cocaine consumption, from a pretreatment average of about 20 days per month to a posttreatment average of 5 days per month. Urinalysis profiles showed decreased cocaine usage by both groups, with the experimental group's measured usage significantly less than that of the control group.

Konefal and colleagues[13] found that substance-abusing patients treated with three different protocols of acupuncture showed significantly different outcomes, as measured by urinalysis, depending on the protocol received. Subjects (N = 321) with various substance abuse problems were randomly assigned to one of three groups: a one-needle auricular treatment protocol using the shen men point; the NADA five-point protocol; or the NADA five-point protocol plus selected body points for self-reported symptoms. All groups showed an increase in the proportion of drug-free urine tests over the course of treatment. Subjects with the single needle protocol, however, showed significantly less improvement compared to the other two groups.

More recent research by Bullock and colleagues showed no significantly different outcomes between cocaine-addicted patients assigned to receive conventional psychosocial therapy alone and those also receiving acupuncture.[14] The authors pointed out that the study's design did not reflect real-world delivery of acupuncture treatment and cautioned against evaluating acupuncture based solely on such studies without "consideration of several difficult methodological issues encountered by those involved in acupuncture substance abuse research."

In a study that closely duplicated real-world delivery of acupuncture detoxification therapy, a group of researchers at Yale University[15] found that cocaine-dependent, methadone-maintained patients receiving NADA-based treatment were significantly more likely to avoid cocaine use than those assigned to control groups. Subjects (N = 82) were randomly assigned to receive either the NADA protocol, a needle-insertion control (using relatively inactive points on the helix of the ear), and a no-needle relaxation control (using relaxing video images and music). Treatments were provided five times weekly for 8 weeks, and cocaine use was assessed by three-times weekly urine toxicology screens. Patients in the acupuncture treatment group were significantly more likely to provide cocaine-negative urine samples relative to both the relaxation control (odds ratio 3.41) and the needle-insertion control (odds ratio 2.40).

CLINICAL APPLICATIONS

Acupuncture is used in numerous and diverse treatment settings. Because of an emphasis on blinded, placebo- or sham-controlled studies, not many outcome reports have been published, although this situation seems to be changing. Unless otherwise noted, these outcomes are based on clinical experiences at Lincoln Hospital or personal observation of other programs made by the lead author.

As controlled research (cited previously) has shown, acupuncture is demonstrably successful in discouraging recidivism and encouraging program participation. Detoxification programs of many types report substantial reduction in their recidivism rates when acupuncture is used.

In a large, retrospective cohort study on clients discharged from publicly funded detoxification programs in Boston, researchers found that clients who received outpatient acupuncture treatment were significantly less likely to be readmitted for detoxification within 6 months, compared to those receiving conventional, short-term residential treatment.[16] Using multivariate models, the study compared four free-standing short-term residential detoxification programs (with an average length of inpatient stay of 1 week) with three outpatient acupuncture detoxification programs (with an average duration of treatment of 1 month). The former were used by a total of 6907 clients, and the latter by 1104 clients. The outcome measure was whether clients were readmitted for detoxification (of any type, either residential or acupuncture) during the first 6-month period in which they were at risk for relapse.

The study found that acupuncture clients were less likely to be readmitted to detoxification treatment compared to residential clients, with an odds ratio of 0.71. (In other words, the odds that an acupuncture client was readmitted to treatment were 71% of the odds that a residential detoxification client was readmitted.) Since the former group differed from the latter group in terms of many of the covariates, the authors identified a subsample of both groups that was similar in terms of baseline characteristics and reran the multivariate analysis. For this subsample, similar results were found, with an odds ratio of 0.61. The authors conclude that acupuncture detoxification is a valuable component of a substance abuse treatment system, and is "particularly useful when residential detoxification beds are in short supply, for it allows some of the demand for detoxification to be met on an outpatient basis."

Examples of acupuncture's beneficial contribution to substance abuse treatment are numerous. Hooper Foundation (Portland, Oregon) cited a decrease from 25% to 6% in comparison to the previous nonacupuncture year. Kent-Sussex (in Delaware) reported a decrease in recidivism from 87% to 18%. Substance Abuse Recovery (Flint, Michigan) noted that after a year of acupuncture-based treatment, 83% of a group of 100 General Motors employees (most of whom had attempted treatment in the past, with frequent relapses) were productive workers, free of drugs and alcohol. Of the General Motors group, all of the 17% who failed had had less than five program visits during the entire year; of those who succeeded, nearly three-quarters continued to attend AA and NA meetings after completing the treatment program. Programs specifically designed for adolescents, such as the Alcohol Treatment Center in Chicago and a Job Corps–related program in Brooklyn, have shown retention rates comparable to adult programs.

It should be noted that certain medications—methadone, corticosteroids, and benzodiazepines—seem to suppress part of the acupuncture effect. Although patients taking these medications in substantial quantity are positively affected by acupuncture, they seem to respond more slowly and clearly show less relaxation during treatment. Nevertheless, acupuncture is an effective treatment for secondary addiction in high-dose methadone patients and is helpful to alcoholics receiving benzodiazepine treatment.

Acupuncture is also widely used to treat adrenal suppressed patients who need to be weaned off corticosteroid medication. (This may suggest that while part of the initial relaxation response is endorphin- and steroid-dependent, there are deeper, more important mechanisms that relate to a different type of process.) Preliminary research[17] suggests that buprenorphine does not suppress the effects of auricular acupuncture.

Opiate Addiction

Opiate addiction was first treated by Dr. Wen in Hong Kong and has been treated at Lincoln Hospital since 1974. Acupuncture provides nearly complete relief of acute observable opiate withdrawal symptoms within five to 30 minutes. This effect lasts for 8 to 24 hours, and its duration increases with the number of serial treatments provided. Patients often sleep during the session and may feel hungry afterward. Acutely intoxicated patients, after receiving acupuncture, will behave in a much less intoxicated manner after the session. Surprisingly, these patients are gratified by this result, in contrast to patient reports of discomfort after Narcan administration.

In acute detoxification settings, acupuncture for opiate addiction is typically administered two to three times daily. Alternatively, it may be administered only once a day with clonidine or methadone on an outpatient basis. Many patients do well on once daily acupuncture because they taper their illicit opiate usage over a 3- to 4-day period. Typically, patients who receive acupuncture are twice as likely to complete the recommended duration of opiate detoxification programs. Given acupuncture's success with abuse of illicit opiates, it seems likely that it would be beneficial in tapering prescription narcotics as well.

Methadone Maintenance

Methadone maintenance patients benefit from acupuncture in a number of different settings. Methadone, a potent synthetic narcotic, is effective for treating addiction to heroin and other narcotics. It suppresses withdrawal symptoms, causes no euphoria, and enables recovering addicts to lead relatively normal, productive lives. But it is also an addictive drug, and withdrawal from methadone is notable for unpredictable variations in symptoms and significant malaise after withdrawal. Acupuncture seems to reduce secondary symptoms of methadone use (e.g., sweating, constipation, and sleep problems), and its calming and confidence-boosting effects are especially valuable during the progression from methadone to abstinence. Acupuncture's most important contribution to methadone maintenance programs is reduction of secondary substance abuse, primarily involving alcohol and cocaine, even in patients with minimal motivation.[18] Patients on any dosage level of methadone will respond to acupuncture, although methadone does appear to suppress part of the acupuncture effect.

From 1974 to 1978, Lincoln Hospital used methadone and acupuncture together. During that period, several hundred methadone maintenance patients were detoxified with tapered doses of methadone and acupuncture. Lincoln staff observed that patients were much more comfortable and confident in the acupuncture setting than with methadone alone, exhibiting decreased hostility and increased compliance. Even though patients regularly complained about withdrawal symptoms, there were very few requests for dosage increase and a substantial drop in requests for symptomatic medication.

Cocaine and Crack Cocaine Addiction

Acupuncture has been recognized as an important innovation in treating cocaine and crack addictions, conditions for which no major pharmaceutical treatments exist. The Lincoln Clinic operates the largest outpatient program for crack cocaine patients in the world, with some 400 patients attending the program on a regular basis. About 60% of new crack-dependent patients give a series of clean urine tests within several weeks of entering treatment and more than 65% complete the first 3 months of treatment.

Acupuncture patients report more calmness and reduced craving for cocaine even after the first treatment. The acute psychological indications of cocaine toxicity are visibly reduced during the treatment session, an effect that is sustained for a variable length of time. As with opiate detoxification, the duration of acupuncture's beneficial effects after treatment is in direct proportion to the number of treatments received. After three to seven 45-minute treatments, patients report a nearly continuous anticraving effect as long as acupuncture is received on a regular basis.

Researchers at Yale[18] followed 32 cocaine-dependent, methadone-maintained patients who received an 8-week course of auricular acupuncture for the treatment of cocaine dependence. Half completed the study, and 44% achieved abstinence, defined as providing cocaine-free urine samples for the last 2 weeks of the study. Abstainers reported decreased depression, a shift in self-definition, decreased craving, and increased aversion to cocaine-related cues. Post-hoc comparisons to pharmacotherapy with placebo, amantadine (AMA), and desipramine (DMI) revealed a significantly higher abstinence rate for acupuncture (44%) than for placebo (13%) or AMA (15%) but not significantly higher than for DMI (26%).

The beneficial effects of acupuncture in cocaine treatment often lead to dramatic increases in retention of cocaine patients. Women in Need, a program located near Times Square in New York, reported the following outcome figures in their treatment for pregnant crack-using women:

1. Patients with conventional outpatient treatment averaged 3 visits per year.
2. Patients who took acupuncture in addition to conventional treatment averaged 27 visits/year.
3. Patients who participated in an educational component in addition to acupuncture and conventional treatment averaged 67 visits/year.

Since patients averaging 3 visits per year would be unlikely to participate in an educational component, it seems likely that acupuncture treatment created a foundation for patients' successful participation in the educational component.

Addictions to Other Illicit Drugs

Methamphetamine abuse patients experience similar dramatic improvement. Hooper Foundation, the public detoxification hospital in Portland, Oregon, reported 5% retention of methamphetamine users before the introduction of acupuncture, compared to a remarkable 90% retention after adding acupuncture to their protocol. Patients demonstrated increased psychological stability and reported decreased craving.

At the Lincoln Clinic, marijuana abuse has also been curbed with acupuncture treatment. Primary marijuana abusers experience a prompt reduction in craving; they also report improved mental well-being. Secondary marijuana abuse is usually eliminated in the course of detoxification of the primary, "harder" drug (e.g., cocaine).

Alcohol Addiction

As with opiate detoxification, retention of alcohol detoxification patients generally increases by 50% when an acupuncture component is added to conventional settings. Some alcoholics who receive acupuncture actually report an aversion to alcohol. Woodhull Hospital in Brooklyn reported that 94% of the patients in the acupuncture supplement group remained abstinent as compared to 43% of the control group who only received conventional outpatient services. These results are in accordance with the often-quoted Bullock study previously described.

Directors of the acupuncture social setting detoxification program conducted by the Tulalip Tribe at Marysville, Washington estimate a yearly savings of $148,000 due to fewer referrals to hospital programs. Inpatient alcohol detoxification units typically combine acupuncture and herbal "sleep mix" with a tapering benzodiazepine protocol. Patients show stable vital signs, and report few symptoms and better sleep. One residential program in Connecticut noted a 90% decrease in Valium use when herbal "sleep mix" alone was added to their protocol.

Maternal Substance Abuse

Pregnant women who abuse drugs are at high risk for delivering toxic, low-birth-weight infants, who generally begin life with many developmental difficulties and health risks. These women need a drug-free form of treatment, as well as one that addresses their other prenatal needs. Since 1987, the Lincoln Clinic has been treating more than 100 pregnant cocaine users per year, with a high number of positive outcomes.

Lincoln patients have regular visits with a nurse-midwife and receive specific education and counseling relative to pregnancy and child care. At the time of delivery, 90% of women in the Lincoln program are free of drugs. The average birth weight for babies at Lincoln with more than 10 maternal visits is 6 pounds 10 ounces. The average birth weight for less than 10 visits is 4 pounds 8 ounces, which is typical of high-risk cocaine mothers. There is a high correlation between clean toxicologies, retention in the clinic program, and higher birth weights. Seventy-six percent of pregnant intakes are retained in long-term treatment and give birth to nontoxic infants. Other obstetrical programs have adopted similar programs with beneficial results.

Female patients are frequently trapped in destructive and exploitative relationships and consequently will have special difficulty with any therapeutic relationship. Acupuncture-based addiction treatment emphasizes patients' recovery of their own self-worth, and thus encourages them to become drug-free out of intrinsic motivation and not only for the sake of the baby. The supportive treatment atmosphere makes it relatively easy for patients to keep children with them during treatment activities. Continuation of treatment can help patients cope with the difficult postpartum period and all the stresses of parenthood.

Criminal Justice Related Services

The well-known "Drug Court" program in Miami, Florida uses the same acupuncture-based model commonly used in addictions. This program diverts 2000 felony drug possession arrestees into treatment each year. More than 50% of these patients eventually graduate the program on the basis of providing 90 consecutive negative toxicologies over the period of a year or more. Despite minimal access to outside funding, Drug Court diversion and treatment programs have been established in more than 100 settings nationwide. The majority of the Drug Court programs use acupuncture as a primary component of their protocol.

Another essential component is an objective measure of success in detoxification. Frequent urine testing provides just such an objective, nonpersonalized measure, one that can be accepted by all parties equally. In this system, the counselor is the "good cop" and the urine machine is the "bad cop." The counseling process can be totally separated from the process of judgement and evaluation. Thus discipline is separated from the difficulties of interpersonal relationships. Within this context, discipline or leniency by judicial authority can lead to constructive rather than escapist behavior. Positive toxicology results are used primarily to require a more prolonged or intense commitment to treatment.

Acupuncture is also being used in more than two dozen jails and prisons in the US and abroad. In Santa Barbara, California, women who received acupuncture were found to be 50% less likely to be rearrested after being released from the county jail. In a maximum security prison in Oak Park Heights, Minnesota, sex offenders who received acupuncture on a regular basis showed a significant reduction in anger and violent intrusive sexual fantasies as compared to a control population.[19]

Coexisting Mental Health Problems

During the past 20 years at Lincoln Hospital, clinicians have noted numerous effects of acupuncture on mentally ill, chemical-abusing (MICA) patients. Agitated patients routinely fall asleep while receiving acupuncture. Chronic paranoid patients have a higher than average retention rate. Clinicians report many examples of grossly paranoid MICA patients making special efforts to access acupuncture treatment, without projecting paranoid ideation on the treatment (despite being floridly psychotic otherwise). These patients experience a gradual reduction in psychiatric symptoms, as well as a typical reduction of craving and withdrawal symptoms.

Psychotropic mediation does not interact with acupuncture. Patients should remain on psychotropic medicines while using acupuncture, since the improved level of compliance that correlates with acupuncture often makes the process of medication more reliable and effective.

A recent pilot program* used acupuncture according to the Lincoln model in the public mental health system in Waco, Texas with a goal of the reduction in the rate of rehospitalization. Highly disturbed, noncompliant, chronically dual-diagnosed patients were deliberately selected for this trial. Rates of hospitalization dropped from 50% to 6% in the group of 15 patients. Harbor House, a residential program for MICA patients in the Bronx, reported a 50% reduction in psychiatric hospitalization in the first year of acupuncture utilization. The number of patients who left treatment during their first month in the program dropped by 85%.

Acupuncture has an obvious advantage in the treatment of MICA patients because it can be used for a wide variety of substance abuse and psychiatric problems. MICA patients have particular difficulty with bonding and verbal relationships. Acupuncture facilitates the required lenient supportive process; but at the same time, it provides an acute anticraving treatment that is also necessary. The use of acupuncture can resolve the contradictory needs of MICA patients. More work needs to be done to evaluate and understand these data.

SUMMARY

Addictions are a primary problem affecting modern society and are associated with many other public health problems. High rates of addiction are directly or indirectly associated with high crime rates and high rates of illness and injury. In many communities today, drug abuse is so rampant that it threatens to overwhelm the limited resources that are available to deal with it. Less acute but still serious are the problems with obesity and nicotine, and alcohol addiction that pervade all strata of society. In such a social context, acupuncture offers a compassionate, convenient, noninvasive, and cost-effective foundation for psychosocial rehabilitation.

Acupuncture can play a role in all steps of the recovery process, from relieving unpleasant withdrawal symptoms to reducing craving, overcoming dependence on chemical substances, and taking steps toward long-term social and emotional recovery. The ultimate aim of any addiction treatment is for participants to achieve "street sobriety." That means that those who were once hooked on harmful substances are able to adopt a positive, drug-free lifestyle, despite the continuing presence of drugs in their environment. With acupuncture, patients are able to utilize their innate healing capacities to rediscover the intrinsic self-motivation to lead healthy and productive lives.

*Manuscript report by Michael O Smith, MD.

APPENDIX: AURICULAR ACUPUNCTURE

JAMES C. BUTLER-ARKOW

As noted in the preceding chapter, Chinese medicine identifies certain patterns (such as Empty Fire) as underlying addictive disorders. Chinese medicine has long sought to treat such patterns with various modalities. Auricular acupuncture is a comparatively recent development in the treatment of addiction. Although auricular acupuncture has received the most attention in treating addictions, some clinical evidence (particularly from China) suggests that certain body acupuncture points may also be effective, particularly in smoking and overeating. Certain body acupuncture points have been incorporated in some of the substance abuse studies cited.[10,16]

Nicotine Addiction

Acupuncture is frequently used to treat nicotine addiction in office-based practices and many other outpatient settings.[20] The standard five-point protocol may be used, or just the Lung Point. Additional auricular points used include the "Hunger" and "Mouth" Points. To engage a sustained effect, a "press needle" may be inserted on the ear. Press needles are shaped like a thumb tack. They lie flush to the ear, and patients are encouraged to tap them gently 3 minutes at a time, three times a day. The needles are left in place for up to a few days (but not longer owing to the risk of infection). Treatment continues over a period of 1 to 2 months.

In China, body acupuncture in addition to auricular acupuncture is a standard treatment in smoking cessation. Points used include *Yingxiang*, LI 20, *Hegu*, LI 4, *Zusanli*, ST 36, *Taichong*, Liv 3, and *Baihui*, GV 20. These points have also been used in the treatment of other substance abuse disorders such as opiate addiction.[21,22] Moderate-to-strong stimulation is recommended.

Another useful nonauricular acupoint that has been used is the so-called *sweet point,* or *Tién Mi.*[23,24] A heavy smoker at the time, Dr. J. Olms discovered the

point by needling his wrist with the intention of treating a cough, only to find that his desire to smoke had vanished. Subsequently, Olms reported clinical success using this point, which has been adopted by Chinese practitioners as well. The point is located in a minute depression near the wrist, about 0.4 units dorsal and slightly distal to LU 7 *(Lieque),* and about one unit proximal to the border of the anatomical snuffbox, the center of which is LI 5, or *Yangxi* (Figure 14-2). It is located by pressing with a small probe or hemostat until the tender depression is found.

In a randomized, single-blinded study on smoking cessation, researchers in Norway found a significant reduction in tobacco consumption using acupuncture.[25] Long-time smokers (N = 46) consuming an average of 20 cigarettes per day were randomly assigned to receive body and ear acupuncture either at correct or sham sites. Those receiving acupuncture at correct sites reported consuming an average of 7 cigarettes per day, compared to the control group that consumed 13; serum concentrations of tobacco metabolites also dropped significantly more for the treatment group. Of those in the treatment group, 31% stopped smoking altogether, compared with 0% of the control group.

Treatment of heavy smokers often produces dramatic results. The effect is not immediate, however, so patients may continue to smoke after the insertion of the needles. Though their skepticism is usually quite evident at the beginning of treatment, patients tend to experience a sudden aversion to smoking about 4 to 10 hours after the insertion of the needles. Typically, they will put out a cigarette just after lighting it. Patients simply feel no desire to smoke, without the experience of withdrawal symptoms—an effect lasting as long as the needles are in place. Whether they can continue their abstinence after the treatment period ends depends on their motivation and willpower. The primary advantage of acupuncture in quitting smoking is that it encourages a rapid reduction in nicotine use, which most habituated smokers can easily tolerate in the early stage of treatment. Such initial success, in turn, often enhances the course of the entire treatment process.

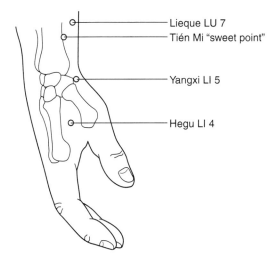

Figure 14-2 Hand and wrist with craving point marked. From Mao-liang Q, editor: *Chinese acupuncture and moxibustion,* Edinburgh, 1993, Churchill Livingstone.

Lieque LU 7
Tién Mi "sweet point"
Yangxi LI 5
Hegu LI 4

Obesity

Acupuncture's utility in treating obesity has been reported in a few Western clinical studies. Patients who received electrical nerve stimulation at certain ear acupoints ("Shen-men" and "Stomach") lost significantly more weight than the control group in a placebo-design, randomized, double-blinded study.[26] However, another study found no effect when only auricular acupressure was used.[27] Auricular acupuncture has been used also in conjunction with a high-protein diet.[28] Interestingly, the latter researchers reported that treatment longer than about 20 minutes actually reduced appetite in some patients, whereas shorter treatment simply seemed to calm the urge to binge (which was the goal of this program, as patients were encouraged to eat plenty of meat). Overall, these studies suggest that in promoting weight loss, relatively strong stimulation is desirable (e.g., electrical stimulation or long duration of needle retention).

As a rule, Chinese acupuncturists, unlike those in Western countries, do not shy away from relatively strong stimulation of needles when they feel it is warranted. This fact—combined with the high accessibility of acupuncture treatment in China—probably accounts for the widespread acceptance there of acupuncture as a treatment for obesity. As with smoking, a standard protocol includes both body and ear points. Body points include *Zusanli* ST 36, *Tianshu* ST 25, *Sanyinjiao* SP 6, *Zhongwan* CV 12, *Pishu* B 20, *Weishu* B 21, and *Fenglong* ST 40. Ear points are similar to those used in China for smoking cessation.[23] Although a search of Chinese-language literature revealed virtually no controlled studies, there are dozens of clinical reports, including use of the "sweet point."[24]

In addition to the calming and centering effects that have been observed with auricular acupuncture, various specific mechanisms have been suggested for their putative effects on appetite. Stimulation of rat auricular regions corresponding to those commonly used to help people lose weight evoked potentials in the hypothalamic satiety center[29] and was also associated with loss of weight by rats; stimulation of other auricular zones had no effect. Human subjects wearing ear clips (i.e., acupressure devices) on the "Hunger" Point showed a significant slowing of gastric peristaltic waves, which would produce a prolonged sensation of fullness; researchers suggested that this effect could be mediated by the auricular branch of the vagus nerve.[30]

References

1. Wen HL, Cheung YC: Treatment of drug addiction by acupuncture and electrical stimulation, *Asian J Med* 9:139-141, 1973.

2. Omura Y, Smith MO, Wong F, et al: Electro-acupuncture for drug addiction withdrawal, *Acupunct Electrother Res* 1:231-233, 1975.

3. O'Connor J, Bensky D, translators: *Acupuncture: a comprehensive text,* Seattle, 1985, Eastland Press.

4. Margolin A, Avants SK, Chang P, et al: A single-blind investigation of four auricular needle puncture configurations. *Am J Chin Med* 23(2):105-114, 1995.

5. Margolin A, Avants S, Birch S, et al: Methodological investigations for a multisite trial of auricular acupuncture for cocaine addiction: a study of active and control auricular zones, *J Subst Abuse Treat* 13(6):471-481, 1996.

6. Brewington V, Smith MO, Lipton D: Acupuncture as a detoxification treatment: an analysis of controlled research, *J Subst Abuse Treat* 11(4):289-307, 1994.

7. Washburn AM, Fullilove RE, Fullilove MT, et al: Acupuncture heroin detoxification: a single-blind clinical trial, *J Subst Abuse Treat* 10:345-351, 1993.

8. Otto KC, Quinn C, Sung Y-F: Auricular acupuncture as an adjunctive treatment for cocaine addiction, *Am J Addict* 7:164-170, 1998.

9. Bullock ML, Umen AJ, Culliton PD, et al: Acupuncture treatment of alcoholic recidivism: a pilot study, *Alcohol Clin Exper Res* 11(3):292-295, 1987.

10. Bullock ML, Culliton PD, Olander RT: Controlled trial of acupuncture for severe recidivist alcoholism, *Lancet* 24:1435-1439, 1989.

11. Worner TM, Zeller B, Schwartz H, et al: Acupuncture fails to improve treatment outcome in alcoholics, *Drug Alcohol Depend* 30:169-173, 1992.

12. Lipton DS, Brewington V, Smith MO: Acupuncture for crack-cocaine detoxification: experimental evaluation of efficacy, *J Subst Abuse Treat* 11(3):205-215, 1994.

13. Konefal J, Duncan R, Clemence C: Comparison of three levels of auricular acupuncture in an outpatient substance abuse treatment program, *Altern Med J* 2(5): 1995.

14. Bullock ML, Kiresuk TJ, Pheley AM, et al: Auricular acupuncture in the treatment of cocaine abuse: a study of efficacy and dosing, *J Subst Abuse Treat* 16(1):31-38, 1999.

15. Avants SK, A Margolin, TR Holford, et al: A randomized controlled trial of auricular acupuncture for cocaine dependence, *Arch Int Med* 160:2305-2312, 2000.

16. Shwartz M, Saitz R, Mulvey K, et al: The value of acupuncture detoxification programs in a substance abuse treatment system, *J Subst Abuse Treat* 17(4):305-312, 1999.

17. Margolin A, Avants SK: Should cocaine-abusing, buprenorphine-maintained patients receive auricular acupuncture? Findings from an acute effects study (in process citation), *J Altern Complement Med* 5(6):567-574, 1999.

18. Margolin A, Avants KS, Chang P, et al: Acupuncture for the treatment of cocaine dependence in methadone-maintained patients, *Am J Addict* 2(3):194-201, 1993.
19. Culliton P, Leaf L: Personal communication, 1996.
20. Smith MO, Brewington V, Culliton P: Unpublished manuscript, 1996.
21. Zhang E, editor: Chinese acupuncture and moxibustion. In *A practical English-Chinese dictionary of traditional Chinese medicine,* Publishing House of Shanghai College of Traditional Chinese Medicine, 1990, Shanghai, China, pp 570-74.
22. Zhang E: Personal communication based on review of Chinese-language literature, 1999.
23. Olms JS: How to stop smoking: effective new acupuncture point discovered, *Am J Acupunct* 9(3):257-260, 1981.
24. Olms JS: Increased success rate using new acupuncture point for stop-smoking program, *Am J Acupunct* 12(4):339-343, 1984.
25. He D, Berg JE, Hostmark AT: Effects of acupuncture on smoking cessation or reduction for motivated smokers, *Prev Med* 26(2):208-214, 1997.
26. Richards D, Marley J: Stimulation of auricular acupuncture points in weight loss, *Aust Fam Physician* 27(suppl 2):S73-77, 1998.
27. Allison DB, Kreiblich K, Heshka S, et al: A randomized placebo-controlled clinical trial of an acupressure device for weight loss, *Int J Obes Relat Metab Disord* 19:653-658, 1995.
28. Niemtzow RC, Little JR, Matanga MA, et al: A high-protein regimen and auriculomedicine for the treatment of obesity: a second clinical observation, *Med Acupunct* 2(10):21-25, 1998.
29. Asamoto S, Takeshige C: Activation of the satiety center by auricular acupuncture point stimulation, *Brain Res Bull* 29(2):157-164, 1992.
30. Choy DS, Eidenschenk E: Effect of tragus clips on gastric peristalsis: a pilot study, *J Altern Complemen Med* 4(4):399-403, 1998.

Suggested Readings

Ackerman RW: *Acupuncture as treatment for substance abuse and its application during pregnancy,* Vancouver, 1995, NADA Clearinghouse.

Brumbaugh A: *Transformation and recovery: a guide for the design and development of acupuncture-based chemical dependency treatment program,* Santa Barbara, Calif, 1993, Still Point Press.

Cassidy C: Chinese medicine users in the United States. I. Utilization, satisfaction, medical plurality, *J Altern Complemen Med* 4(1):17-27, 1998.

Eory A: Society for Acupuncture Research: discussion, 1995.

Guidepoints: *Acupuncture in recovery,* a monthly newsletter, 7402 NE 58th Street, Vancouver, WA 98662.

Hammerschlag R: Methodological and ethical issues in clinical trials of acupuncture, *J Altern Complemen Med* 4(2):159-71, 1998.

Konefal J, Duncan R, Clemence C: The impact of the addition of an acupuncture treatment program to an existing metro-Dade County outpatient substance abuse treatment facility, *J Addict Dis* 13(3):71-99, 1994.

Margolin A, Avants SK, Kleber HD: Rationale and design of the Cocaine Alternative Treatments Study (CATS): a randomized, controlled trial of acupuncture, *J Altern Complemen Med* 6(4):405-418, 1998.

Mitchell ER: *Fighting drug abuse with acupuncture,* Berkeley, 1995, Pacific View Press.

Oleson T: *Auriculotherapy manual,* 1998, Health Care Alternatives, Inc.

Smith MO: *Nature of Qi,* Society for Acupuncture Research: proceedings, 1995.

Smith MO: Lincoln Hospital Acupuncture Drug Abuse Program: testimony presented to the National Institute of Health, Office of Alternative Medicine and the National Wellness Coalition, May 21, 1993.

Smith MO, Kahn I: An acupuncture program for the treatment of drug addicted persons, *Bull Narcot* 40(1):35-41, 1988.

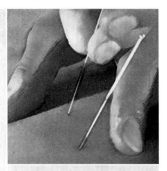

15

Treating Respiratory Disease with Acupuncture

KIM A. JOBST

Acupuncture has been used for millennia in China, Tibet, and elsewhere in Asia to treat pulmonary conditions such as asthma, tumors, tuberculosis (TB), viral pneumonias, pneumothoraces, and pleural effusions. Today, professional acupuncturists around the world daily treat the common cold, sinusitis, bronchitis, asthma, allergies, and other respiratory system disorders.

However, randomized clinical trial (RCT) research to evaluate the effectiveness of acupuncture in pulmonary disease has been largely confined to the three lung conditions evaluated in this chapter: bronchial asthma, chronic bronchitis, and chronic disabling breathlessness due to chronic obstructive pulmonary disease (COPD). Acupuncture care is a good choice as an adjunct to biomedical care in many cases, based on published reports on these topics.

First, to place this discussion in context, Chinese medicine (CM) and biomedical approaches to chronic pulmonary disease are compared. Then the many methodological issues are examined that make clinical research on acupuncture difficult both to do and to evaluate. I conclude with some suggestions for referral of patients.

This chapter is adapted from the expert evidence presented to a panel convened jointly by the Food and Drug Administration (FDA) and the National Institutes of Health (NIH) to evaluate the efficacy and safety of acupuncture in 1994 and subsequently in more detail in 1997.[1,2]

Establishing the Safety and Effectiveness of Interventions

To establish the safety and effectiveness of any intervention we need evidence on the following issues.

1. Is there significant amelioration or even "cure" of the condition and/or symptoms? For example, (a) do patients report improvement in symptoms and quality of life? (b) Is there a measurable and durable impact on symptoms from the practitioner's point of view? (c) Are there verifiable subjective and objective changes?

2. Is there improved patient management as in diminishing or ceasing medication, physiotherapy, or other interventions?

3. Is there sufficient safety for the patient and practitioner and an acceptable side-effect profile?

4. Is there a desirable cost to benefit ratio?

These questions have been asked of only a few of the many pulmonary disorders that Chinese medicine treats clinically. But for those few (bronchial asthma, chronic bronchitis, and chronic disabling breathlessness), evidence discussed in this chapter indicates that acupuncture facilitates criterion 1a substantially, 1b potentially, and 1c variably. It appears to reduce the need for pharmacological medication (criterion 2) and fulfills criterion 3. Criterion 4 has yet to be adequately tested. Thus acupuncture as an adjunct in the treatment of asthma and respiratory disease might prove safer than prolonged allopathic maintenance therapy alone. ∾

HOW CHINESE MEDICINE AND BIOMEDICINE VIEW AND TREAT RESPIRATORY DYSFUNCTION

Prevalence, and Problems with Definition in Biomedicine

The lack of universally accepted biomedical definitions for respiratory diseases has hindered both communication and research. According to the American Thoracic Association (1962), asthma and chronic bronchitis are defined as follows:

Chronic bronchitis: a clinical disorder characterized by excessive mucus secretion in the bronchial tree, manifested by chronic or recurrent productive cough. Arbitrarily, these manifestations should be present on most days for a minimum of 3 months in a year and for not less than 2 years.

Asthma: a disease characterized by an increased responsiveness of the trachea and bronchi to various stimuli, manifested by a widespread narrowing of the airways that changes in severity either spontaneously or as a result of therapy. Bronchial hyperresponsiveness may be defined as a 20% fall in the forced expiratory volume in 1 second (FEV_1) in response to methacholine or histamine provocation at a dose of less than 9 μmol. Usually the symptoms

and physical findings are completely relieved by the administration of bronchodilator drugs. During episodes of asthma, bronchial narrowing leads to one or more of the following alterations in respiratory function with the degree of dysfunction depending upon the severity of the bronchial obstruction:

1. Diminished vital capacity (VC), forced and peak expiratory flow rates (maximum mid-expiratory flow rate [MMFR], peak expiratory flow rate [PEFR], FEV_1) and maximal voluntary ventilation

2. Increased airway resistance (Raw)

3. Increased residual lung volume (RV)

4. Abnormal intrapulmonary gas mixing causing hypoxemia and hypercarbia (diminished PaO_2 and increased $PaCO_2$)

Because there are several acceptable measures of the presence of asthma and the definition of bronchitis is so flexible, it is difficult to get accurate prevalence figures for these conditions. However, overall prevalence is higher in children and is rising, as is asthma mortality.[3-5] Prevalence figures for asthma have increased to up to 12% in Australian children, with lower figures for Europe and the United States (US). In the United Kingdom (UK) the number of cases of asthma diagnosed in children was estimated at 36,650 in 1979 and rose to 93,277 in 1991. The mortality from asthma varies between 0.5 to 3.0 per 100,000, with almost 2000 deaths from acute asthma in the UK in 1988, a figure that has now fallen below 1500.[5] Both mortality and morbidity appear to correlate positively with regular maintenance medication use.[6,7]

Chronic bronchitis is widely prevalent throughout the world. A conservative estimate reveals that 8% of males and 3% of females aged between 40 and 65 years suffer from chronic bronchitis in the UK where it is the single most common cause of lost working days.[5,8] For both conditions there can be little doubt that these represent substantial underestimates.

The Chinese Medicine View of Respiratory Disorders

Both CM and biomedicine are derived from sophisticated cosmologies and have their own well-established languages, a point that has been developed elsewhere in this book. The CM model is functional and often employs daily-life metaphors.

In the physiological terms of CM, the functional Lung includes not only the anatomical lung and bronchioles but also the nose and related parts, the skin, and the hair of the body (not head). The emotion associated with the Lung is the kind of sadness that is best characterized as grief. The Lung's actions are also reflected in the strength of the voice and in the quality of speech, the quality of the pores and of sweating, and the success of moisturization of the whole body. The Yin Lung is paired with the Yang Large Intestine, and one can say that the Lung is in charge of "taking in" while the Large Intestine is in charge of "letting go." What the Lung "takes in" is "pure Qi"—the air we breathe is a form of Qi. This Qi is combined by the Lung with the purified "food Qi" sent from the Spleen; together these form Zong Qi, which nourishes the Heart and then travels everywhere in the body, nourishing the whole. Importantly, the Lung sends Qi to the surface of the body, where it is known as Wei Qi—its task is to protect the outside of the body from invasion by external pernicious factors. The Lung also has a special relationship with the Kidney—together they regulate the passage of water through the body, including by regulating sweating. One of the tasks of the Kidney is to "grasp" the Qi of the Lung and anchor it deeper in the body. The Lung, Spleen, and Kidney are three Yin Organs that are in special relationship to each other. Recalling the Five Phases chart (see Chapter 2), note that in terms of the ordinary direction of flow of energy in the body, the Spleen is the "mother" of the

Lung, while the Lung is the "mother" of the Kidney. It is not surprising that people with weak Spleen function have Lung symptoms, whereas those with weak Lung function express Kidney symptoms. The emotion associated with Spleen malfunction is a kind of obsessive anxiety and worry, and that associated with the Kidney is fear. The remaining Yin Organs—Heart and Liver—can also affect the Lung and express themselves via respiratory symptoms.

Applying these general characteristics of the Lung and its relationships to the analysis of disorder: People who suffer frequent "Wind invasions" (e.g., the common cold, bronchitis, sinusitis, respiratory allergies) have weak Wei Qi (i.e., the Lung is not tending the periphery successfully). The character of their complaint varies, depending on additional factors such as the presence of Heat, Cold, Damp, or Dry and chronicity. Reversible bronchospasm—asthma—is recognized to have at least two origins, one primarily centered in the Lung (associated with difficulty breathing out) and the other a result of Kidney Qi deficiency (associated with difficulty breathing in because the Kidney is not grasping the Lung's Qi). Wheezing can occur in other circumstances as well (e.g., when the heart's pumping action is weak and allows fluid to accumulate). A damp (weak) Spleen creates phlegm, which is stored by the Lung—usually to its detriment.

For example, the condition called TB in biomedicine is recognized as fitting the pattern of Lung Yin deficiency with Empty Heat in CM. This condition presents as a feverish disease that consumes Yin and results in weight loss, with pores opening at inappropriate times (afternoon and night sweats), and a dry cough with little sputum or bloody sputum. Many good textbooks of CM contain in-depth discussions of the Lung and associated Disharmonies.[9-11]

According to the CM perspective, health is a result of and reflects the presence of a harmonious balance of energies within an individual, and treatment of any respiratory disharmony involves returning the body to harmony. The immediate tasks are to move Qi and Blood, resolve Phlegm, strengthen the Exterior (the Wei Qi), and expel pernicious influences. Symptomatically, the practitioner tries to relieve cough, breathlessness, pain, fatigue, weakness, fever, grief, fear, and anxiety; support bodily resistance; and enhance the sense of connectivity of the individual to self and to society. These ends are sought not only by using acupuncture and moxibustion but also by diet, physical and breathing exercises, herbal remedies, meditation, and lifestyle changes. Although most

Western research focuses only on acupuncture, there are a variety of modalities within CM. Patients typically receive care that includes several modalities. For example, patients with asthma are not only treated with acupuncture and moxibustion but are also prescribed herbal remedies formulated to control wheezing, clear sputum, and strengthen Wei Qi; are recommended or taught breathing and meditative exercises (tai chi, qi gong), physical exercises particularly helpful for respiratory complaints (walking, swimming); and are given lifestyle guidance on diet, rest, and avoidance of asthma triggers.

The Biomedical Approach to Respiratory Disorder

Compared to the CM description of the respiratory system, the biomedical is technical, chemical, molecular, and focused on pharmaceutical intervention even though this is not the sole interventive strategy.

In brief, the biomedical physiological model of the lung and in particular the control of breathing states that the autonomic nervous system is central to the regulation of breathing and respiration and is itself influenced by both intrinsic (conscious control) and extrinsic factors. Although without sympathetic innervation, bronchial smooth muscle can be affected by both exogenous and endogenous catecholamines acting on beta-2 adrenoceptors, as well as by cyclic-AMP and adenylcyclase. Cholinergic innervation extends throughout the bronchial tree with its release causing increased bronchial smooth muscle tone. Atropinic drugs (muscarinic antagonists) may therefore be useful in treatment. Additionally, central nervous system involvement supports the suggestion that gentle exercise, yoga, breathing exercises, meditation, and compassionate care may profoundly influence the perception, experience and expression of breathlessness.[12-14] All of these interact to affect respiration and offer a complex psychophysical axis about which to devise treatment.

In both asthma and chronic bronchitis, acute attacks of breathlessness may be induced and relieved by psychological intervention.[15-21] Patients with asthma and/or chronic bronchitis experience the subjective sensation of breathlessness that results in varying degrees of functional and/or physical disability. While this may reflect patients' inherent or acquired ventilatory sensitivity to carbon dioxide (CO_2), it may also reflect perceptual differences that are independent of ventilation.[22] Indeed, the perception of breathlessness bears only a crude direct relation to objective spirometric indices of lung function. Paradoxically, therefore, severe breathlessness may accompany relatively minor objective spirometric abnormalities and vice versa.[8,23,24] To the researcher, this means that while there may be significant changes in subjective symptoms, they may not be accompanied by equivalent changes in spirometric indices and vice versa. This situation creates a considerable challenge to making objective assessments and evaluations of studies.

The mainstays of biomedical treatment are oral or inhaled bronchodilators (such as beta-2 sympathomimetic adrenergic agonists), anticholinergic inhaled agents (such as ipratropium bromide), inhaled, ingested or parenteral corticosteroids, and other antiinflammatory or membrane stabilizing agents (such as disodium cromoglycate). Methylxanthines such as theophylline, antibiotics for current infection, and more recent and controversial immunosuppressive agents such as cyclosporine may also be used. In severe crises, recourse to sedation, artificial ventilation, and intensive care may be required. The majority of patients with asthma are maintained on regular, inhaled sympathomimetics and corticosteroids that may be augmented during exacerbation or before exercise. These treatments are not without their side effects (Table 15-1). At this point, it is important to remember that it is against this biomedical pharmaceutical standard that acupuncture must be evaluated.

Biomedicine does offer some nonpharmaceutical therapeutic guidance in respiratory disease. For example, it is now well established that drinks and foods containing sulfur dioxide may precipitate bronchoconstriction in those with bronchial hypersensitivity, so asthmatics are given lists of food to avoid. Allergen hygiene (e.g., of the home) is also encouraged, since it is known that endogenous histamine, prostaglandins, and leukotrienes can adversely affect bronchial smooth muscle tone.[21]

Parallels between Chinese Medicine and Biomedicine

According to biomedicine, a disease is defined by a particular parameter or causal agent (e.g., reversible airways obstruction for bronchial asthma) or a causal organism for infection. In CM, however, the "disease" is often only one component of a disharmony comprising a constellation of factors defined in terms of

TABLE 15-1

Side-Effect Profile of Mainstay Allopathic Pharmaceutical Treatments for Bronchial Asthma Contrasted with the Side-Effect Profile of Acupuncture Treatment

Biomedical Side-Effects Profile

Corticosteroids	Beta-2 agonists/sympathomimetics
Diminished immunity	Tremor
Altered blood glucose control/diabetes	Headache
Hypertension	Cardiac arrhythmias and arrest
Mental psychological changes	Hypokalemia
Skin changes, especially thinning and easy bruising	Sudden death
Diminution in bone density/osteoporosis	Deterioration of breathlessness; paradoxical bronchospasm
Peptic ulceration	Autonomic side-effects: vasoconstriction and vasodilation,
Hoarseness of voice	sweating, palpitations, hypertension and hypotension,
Candidiasis of mouth/throat	cold extremities
Adrenal suppression	Hypersensitivity reactions
Myopathy	Psychiatric effects: anxiety, paranoia, panic
Possible growth suppression in children	

Side-Effect Profile of Acupuncture

Relatively rare (negative)	Very rare (negative)*	Common (positive)
Vasovagal episode on needle insertion, transient	Pneumothorax (at least 8 cases)	Warmth
Nausea	Hepatitis B	Relaxation
Anorexia	Granuloma formation (1 case Japan)	Well-being
Ear ache	Cardiac tamponade (1 case Japan)	More energy, more "vital"
Local skin irritation, pruritus		Confidence
Aching, inflammation		Stronger
Exacerbation of breathlessness fatigue		

*See Chapter 4.

the flow of Qi. The complete symptom picture reflects and reveals the complex interaction of Qi, the Organs, and the patient's response to the environment. So, for example, reversible airways obstruction—asthma—is but one component of a broader symptom complex.

There are striking similarities in the two approaches. In biomedicine, reversible airways obstruction can be due to many different things: it may originate in the lungs or heart (e.g., in congestive cardiac failure or left ventricular failure), it may be extrinsic (allergen sensitive) or intrinsic (cryptogenic), or it may originate from the liver (e.g., carcinoid tumors), the immune system (eosinophilia infection), or within the central nervous system, the mind, or the psyche. Compare this with CM, in which asthma may be caused by,

among others, Heart dysfunction, Liver dysfunction, Lung dysfunction, Spleen or immune dysfunction, and Kidney or CNS dysfunction. There are diagnostic and therapeutic consequences to each of these categories in both systems. Where there are still differences, they appear to relate to the more subtle CM energetic terms and signs such as pulse character, tongue appearance, skin, and other changes. Even the energetic differences are beginning to disappear as biomedicine increasingly grasps the concept of bodily unity through better understanding of the relationships between brain function, neurochemistry, physiology, and "mind," rendering distinctions between "functional" (i.e., "of the mind") and "organic" (i.e., physical or chemical) conditions out of date. In fact, experienced biomedical practitioners increasingly conclude that the best treatment for lung disease is practiced within a holistic biomedical paradigm that does not look at the lungs in isolation and is not wholly reliant on pharmaceutical drugs.

METHODOLOGICAL ISSUES IN RESEARCH ON PULMONARY DISEASE AND ACUPUNCTURE

Numerous methodological challenges face those who wish to examine the efficacy or effectiveness of acupuncture in pulmonary disease using RCT designs. In this section, several of these designs are examined to set the scene for the critical evaluation that comes in the next section.

What Constitutes Efficacy and Safety?

The researcher looking at acupuncture's role in the treatment of respiratory diseases must evaluate issues of both safety and efficacy. However, since different audiences have different ways of evaluating their care, designing high quality research takes considerable care and subtlety. Questions such as the following play a role:

- What do patients say is effective for them? Do they feel better, do more, or experience meaningful lifestyle changes connected with treatment?
- What do biomedical and acupuncture practitioners themselves consider evidence of effectiveness?
- Are "objective" and/or "subjective" parameters affected? For example, has acupuncture treatment led to a change in medication usage; is there a change in the patient's subjective experience of well-being and capacity, and if so, is it lasting?
- Is it appropriate to interpret the increasing numbers of patients seeking acupuncture treatment as indirectly reflecting efficacy?
- Is efficacy reflected in the cost of treatment or its impact on other costs?
- How can emotional cost/benefit ratios be evaluated or quantified?
- What are acceptable levels of side-effects; how is this to be evaluated and by whom?

There are no simple answers to these questions but I hope that findings offered in this chapter will provoke not only appropriate referral of patients but also further exploration of methodological issues.

The latter issue looms large in all acupuncture research. Indeed, it is unfortunate that the vast majority of published clinical studies provide insufficient information for objective assessment (see Chapters 13 and 19). This is well shown in the recent Cochrane review of acupuncture in asthma,[25] which can be interpreted in different ways. The authors state in their conclusion that "it is not yet possible to make recommendations to patients, their physicians or acupuncturists on the basis of the data currently reported. Given the increasing use of acupuncture by the public, there is an urgent need for quality research which should take into account the complex nature of acupuncture as a treatment modality." This conclusion is based on analysis of data that fulfills the restricted criteria for entry into the Cochrane format. When looking at this same data more broadly and with better attention to model fit issues,* as in this chapter, it is equally possible to interpret it in quite another way, without twisting or misrepresenting it. The conclusion then can be as follows: "Current published evidence reveals no reason to withhold acupuncture as a safe and potentially effective treatment in patients with bronchial asthma and chronic obstructive lung disease. Further, more appropriately designed studies are urgently required."

Models and Parameters

If the efficacy of acupuncture in pulmonary disease is to be established, then optimal practice must be evaluated, just as allopathic treatment trials would only be adequate if optimal assessment, dosage, administration, and timing were employed. But what is optimal practice of acupuncture? There are at least two issues here. The first concerns the technical aspect of acupuncture practice, and the second is the fact that it

---

*"Model fit" is an aspect of validity that demands that a system be studied using the rules of its own logic and technology.[26] In our case, this would mean that acupuncture when tested in RCTs should be delivered in ways that are fair to the practice—e.g., real needles, in real points, for sufficient periods of time, with individualized care, and not in isolation, since acupuncture is but one of several modalities normally offered patients. A lack of model fit is clearly an issue in evaluating clinical trials research studies, because virtually none assess acupuncture *in the context of its own theory or according to the rules of its own practice.*

is not practiced in isolation but is embedded in a whole medicine. In normal practice its use is combined with the use of other techniques and modalities. Thus in designing and evaluating research we must not only consider if the acupuncture technique is appropriate and adequate, but also whether our measures reflect actual practice. At present, only two clinical studies have considered the latter issue.[2,27]

Another issue is how we are to measure the impact or evaluate the impact of acupuncture on respiratory function and pulmonary disease. In this chapter we use the following parameters:

- Alteration and amelioration of abnormal baseline values in chronic cases
- Alteration of spirometry during an acute attack
- Prior prophylactic protection and/or bronchodilation after methacholine- or histamine-induced bronchoconstriction as a model for an acute asthmatic attack
- Prophylaxis or bronchodilation either before or after exercise-induced asthma
- Alteration in drug requirements, attack frequency, symptom control, and severity in chronic asthmatics
- Changes in subjective experience and well-being and changes in activities of daily living

Research Design Issues

Clinical trials designs—most of them originally developed for use in the evaluation of pharmaceuticals—contain traditional components that do not necessarily "work" as expected when applied to the assessment of acupuncture. These features are intended to minimize the influence of perception, preference, and bias of various kinds and include randomization of subjects to intervention types, blinding of participants, and use of placebo interventions.

Research Designs
The following includes research designs actually used in pulmonary disease research on acupuncture.
- A triple blind (TB) trial design in the context of acupuncture refers to one in which the practitioner, the patient, and the evaluators are all blinded. Such a design is not possible if needling is used but would be possible using TENS or laser stimulation.
- This chapter uses the convention that a double

blind (DB) study is one in which both the patients and the evaluators are blind to treatment (9 studies reviewed in the next section).
- A single blind (SB) design is one in which only the patient is blinded to the treatment protocol (5 studies reviewed in the next section).
- An unblinded (UB) or nonblinded study is effectively an open study. Often no control intervention is used, and all participants know that acupuncture of some sort is being used (three studies reviewed in the next section).
- The terminology offered to the NIH/FDA review[1] is used throughout the chapter. Thus "sham/placebo true point" or SP (TP) refers to the use of designated real acupuncture points on the acupuncture meridians but not thought by the investigators to be indicated in the condition being treated.
- "Sham/placebo nonpoints" or SP (NP) are not designated real acupuncture points on the meridians in any of the classical CM texts. Such locations are often chosen 2 to 3 cm distant to the true point or in adjacent dermatomes.
- Acupuncture treatment that utilized the same designated true point(s) for each subject in a formulaic fashion is referred to as real symptomatic acupuncture or RA (SA). Such formulary prescription ignores the central tenet of CM acupuncture that point selection should be specific to each individual case and each treatment episode.
- When CM principles of diagnosis and treatment are employed, the acupuncture is referred to as real Chinese Traditional Medicine acupuncture or RA (CTM). Only one of the 17 studies in the next section fulfilled such criteria.[34]
- *Da qi*—the CM needling sensation—refers to the sensation of aching, heaviness, or tingling, often with a sense of contraction around the needle, that according to the classical CM texts indicates the "capture of the meridian energy" or adequate "access" to the point. It is important to note that in the fullest CM practice, *da qi* is not required at every point on every occasion.

Blinding
How can you blind a practitioner who manually inserts needles in specific points? How can you blind a patient to the insertion of a needle? Indeed, blinding presents a considerable problem in the evaluation of

acupuncture practiced according to CM principles. Efforts to resolve this issue have involved a great deal of creativity—the use of blind evaluators, "sham" points, "placebo" stimulation, and so forth.

If, however, as CM insists, point location, the method of needle insertion and manipulation, and the "state" or intention of the practitioner are key ingredients to optimal treatment, the practitioner cannot by definition be blinded. In this sense, acupuncture using needle insertion is akin to surgery for the purposes of trial design. Thus the usual solution to achieving double blind design in acupuncture research is then to use a blind evaluator design (but see a novel "blind practitioner" model described in Chapter 19).

On the other hand, patients can be blinded if they are naive to point location and technique and cannot discern "real" from "placebo/sham" treatments. There is some loss to normal practice here, for acupuncture patients become more responsive to treatment over time—a "dosage" effect no research has yet addressed. The crucial significance of this has been illustrated by Reilly and Taylor using their "overall progress interactive charts" (OPICS) in a triple blinded trial of homeopathy in asthma. What this work showed is that knowledge of trial design alone may be sufficient to influence outcome.[28] If subjects are requested to stop routine allopathic interventions prior to experimentation, particularly if the group is significantly impaired as in one of the studies,[29] it is naive to think (as Yu and Lee imply) that they will have no idea that the intervention is designed to affect their symptoms! Equally, it defies credibility that ethical approval could be gained if "the patients were not told anything about acupuncture and had no knowledge of possible effects." These issues are less critical if the subject of inquiry is the effectiveness of acupuncture as an intervention, including its capacity to mobilize the placebo, nonspecific, or "self-healing" response on measures of breathlessness.

Placebo Intervention

If a placebo is defined as an inert intervention acting as a control for the active intervention, then clearly a true placebo cannot be found for acupuncture. This is because acupuncture involves not only a distinct sensation but also puncture of the skin to a depth of between 3 mm and 3 cm or more in some places, with subsequent needle manipulation. These features render the selection of a comparable placebo for controlled trials virtually impossible, particularly since there is abundant evidence that skin puncture alone can affect pain threshold, perception, and well-being with quantifiable physiochemical changes peripherally and centrally.[23,30-32]

At best a sham procedure mimicking true acupuncture can be employed. So far no procedure has been found that causes the same sensation as acupuncture without necessitating piercing the skin. All the controlled studies reviewed in this chapter used sham procedures. Either SP (TP) or SP (NP) were chosen with needles inserted to varying depths, stimulated either manually, electrically, with or without moxibustion, and with or without evoking *da-qi*.

The fact that every study involved needle insertion of some sort has crucial implications for interpretation, which are often ignored or misunderstood. One of these concerns is that nonspecific and minimal needling using SP (NP) give rise to quantifiable subjective and objective effects with central and peripheral neurochemical changes (i.e., they are not true inert placebos).[23,30-35] There is considerable debate as to how much this "nonspecific" needling phenomenon contributes to the overall acupuncture effect.

Equally, if not more, important to acupuncture evaluation is the activity of points chosen for sham/placebo needling. Researchers not versed in the principles of CM have often inadvertently selected points that are "active sham points" (SP [TP]) (i.e., points that according to CM will have an effect over and above nonspecific needling at SP [NP]s). This error was made in 10 of the studies we reviewed and means that these studies have actually compared two active treatments for asthma (RA [SA] vs SP [TP]). This makes it impossible to measure the effect of acupuncture per se, since there is no inactive placebo control against which to compare.

The consequence of this error—essential to understand when trying to evaluate the evidence concerning the effects of acupuncture—is that results of such studies do not constitute either true negatives or true positives, since a true placebo has not been employed. In our discussion, we designate such results as positive/negative.

However, the combined result of both sham/placebo true point and real symptomatic acupuncture treatments (RA [SA] + SP [TP]) can be compared against baseline or qualification period values. This approach can provide some idea of the efficacy of the overall interventions (acupuncture treatment) and a comparison between them, but it is not possible to derive an objective evaluation of specified acupuncture alone because of the lack of a true placebo. What is most interesting about the evaluation of these studies once this is understood is that they indicate that although there is no statistically significant difference between the two treatments in many cases (i.e., RA [SA] vs SP [TP] = no significant difference), it is evident that "acupuncture treatment" leads to a significant change from baseline (i.e., RA [SA] + SP [TP] vs baseline = significantly different).[2] Where this pertains, the outcomes are referred to as equivocal, using "positive/negative" in the tables since no definite conclusion can be drawn from them, other than that needle insertion in a regulated manner can improve both quality of life and spirometric indices. A truly inert placebo is possible only if subliminal electroacupuncture or laser stimulation are used.

Individualization

CM demands individualized assessment, point selection, and manipulation (with or without moxibustion) in each case and at every visit (full history and examination, pulses, tongue diagnosis, skin signs, etc). This feature has two downstream implications. The first is that two biomedically identical cases of asthma (airways reversibility, age of onset, attack rate, symptom scores, spirometry, etc.) may be treated entirely differently in CM. The second is that from visit to visit, and in response to current conditions, treatment changes. Neither of these features presents insuperable problems for RCT evaluation, but—if one is interested in assessing the effect of acupuncture as practiced—it does prohibit the use of uniform point-formulas. Such formulas were, however, used in the large majority of published trials. So far, only two studies in respiratory disease have been conducted according to CM principles[27,33] and only the latter fulfilled both CM and biomedical criteria.

Allopathic Medication

The level 1a Cochrane evaluation evidence for the efficacy of biomedical intervention in asthma and the possibility of fatal consequences of inadequately treating acute asthma, make it ethically and medicolegally unacceptable to authorize the cessation of maintenance medication for more than a few hours before acupuncture treatment. However, the effects of sympathomimetics, corticosteroids, cromoglycate, and other drugs may diminish the apparent efficacy of acupuncture since similar mechanisms of action appear to be involved in their action.[36] For example, both sympathomimetics and corticosteroids affect adenylcyclase, cyclic-AMP, and glucose metabolism, and the same is true of acupuncture. Acupuncture stimulates cortisol release, giving rise to raised serum cortisol levels, as well as affecting the reactivity of leukocytes to leukotriene challenge.[6,33,36-41] Thus treatment with corticosteroids may mask the effect of acupuncture in clinical trials, which some investigators acknowledge.[36,42]

Duration to Onset of Action

Since it is evident that acupuncture involves similar mechanisms of action to allopathic immune modulators, it may well be that time for any effect to be demonstrated after treatment may be longer than that allowed in most studies (as little as hours in some cases). Experienced acupuncture clinicians expect that the effects of acupuncture will take time to develop and will accumulate, typically over weeks, months, and finally, years. Sustaining an adequate protocol over weeks or months is a challenging exercise to even the most seasoned researchers, yet those who wish to assess acupuncture well must provide an adequate "dosage" of the therapy. After all, both corticosteroids and cromoglycate take days to exert a sustained effect on airway constriction, whereas bronchial hyperresponsiveness and allergen removal may take weeks or even months to achieve maximum benefit. Research on these is designed to adjust for this fact. The same rule should apply in acupuncture research.

Crossover

Crossover design trials depend on the intervention ceasing action after a relatively short period. For a pharmaceutical with clear metabolic effects, "washout" can be accurately measured. But for an intervention that modifies the energetics of the body, the rate of hormonal and neurotransmitter production, and the client's experience of himself or herself, can a true washout period be specified? Many feel that even when a long washout period is provided, the possibility of prolonged duration of action and carry-over effects of treatment with acupuncture make the crossover design problematic or impotent.

RESEARCH RESULTS

Selecting the Studies

A search of the literature in English revealed 25 articles reporting clinical assessments of the effectiveness or efficacy of acupuncture in treating pulmonary disease (Table 15-2). Of these 25 studies, 17 met our criteria and were evaluated for this chapter. We examine only those studies in which needles have been used to puncture the skin, in two cases involving the use of additional electrical stimulation. Studies using transcutaneous electrical nerve stimulation (TENS), laser stimulation, or acupressure were excluded.

Among the 25, many were poorly reported, although 11 were of high quality.* Rejected studies included 5 of particularly poor quality[27,41,49,50,51]; of these, 4 were positive in favor of acupuncture and one negative, but this used laser point stimulation.[49] The negative study was conducted double-blind, one was single-blind but included insufficient data for interpretation,[51] two studies employed no blinding,[27,41] and one was descriptive and objectively uninterpretable.[50] All five were studies of acupuncture in bronchial asthma, one also including many other conditions labeled "endocrine and other conditions."[50] Of the latter, seven were clinical trials, one was a criteria-based metaanalysis of the literature,[47] two were systematic reviews,[2,44] and one was a Cochrane meta-analysis.[25] Of the full set, sixteen were selected for further evaluation on the basis of their design and clinical relevance.† One of these[29] investigated two separate conditions (acute asthma and histamine-induced bronchoconstriction) making a total of 17 "situations" to be analyzed in the 16 studies.

Kleijnen's criteria based meta-analysis[47] (see Table 15-2) included 13 studies up to 1989. Kleijnen and his

colleagues concluded that most studies were of poor quality, with insufficient sample size, poor follow-up, poorly documented medication use and interventions given, and poorly reported subjective symptoms. Unfortunately these analysts did not assess the studies from a CM perspective. This biased the analysis against one of the most important methodological issues (i.e., the way in which patients are assessed, which points are prescribed and used, and the duration and follow-up of the cases). Their bias may not have altered the scores given to many of the studies, but some were better than described and the negativity of this report limited attention to methodological issues discussed here for some years.

Linde[44] and Jobst[2] both performed systematic reviews of the literature on acupuncture in pulmonary disease. Linde looked at 15 trials and considered 5 to be unequivocally positive, one negative, and 8 showing no difference between acupuncture and "placebo" acupuncture.[44] This analyst also concluded that the trials were of poor quality, noting the heterogeneity of treatments which were not based on CM treatment guidelines and commenting on the variable quality and detail of the reporting of the methods used in the studies evaluated.

The review by Jobst[2] looked at 21 studies, analyzing data from 16 and finding 10 to be positive, 3 negative, and 3 equivocal using the same criteria described in this chapter. Many similar conclusions to those of Kleijnen[47] and Linde[44] were described, but the most important aspect of this review was the attention drawn to the significant impact of using sham-true points (SA [TP]) on the analysis of outcomes, ultimately rendering the analysis of the efficacy of acupuncture more significant because in many cases two different treatments for respiratory disease are used instead on one (see below).

Linde et al[25] used the Revman Cochrane software to perform a Cochrane review—analyzing the seven studies found by Linde and Jobst that could be entered. Of these, two were positive, and 5 showed no difference between sham and real acupuncture. Only one paper had been written in such a way that all the data could be fully analyzed. Again, the authors comment on the generally poor quality of design and reporting and draw particular attention to the problem of "active" sham points.

Table 15-3 summarizes ten studies that studied acupuncture in bronchial asthma, including 3 studies

Text continued on p. 287

---

*References 2, 25, 33, 34, 42-48.
†References 29, 33, 34, 42-46, 48, 49, 53-59.

TABLE 15-2

Acupuncture in Pulmonary Disease: Studies Reviewed

Study (no. patients)	Subject	Outcome
Wen, 1973* (6)	Status asthmaticus	POSITIVE Spirometry: FEV_1 ↑ 45%, FVC ↑ 12.5%, FEV_1/FVC ↑ 30%, PEFR ↑ 49.7% Subjective: significant improvement within 4 hours Attack rate: ↓ <50% Sleep: improved Medication: ↓ >30% Excellent study: data and patient reports support TCM theory, e.g., warmth, energy, etc
Yu and Lee, 1976 (20)	Bronchial asthma: 20 pts Histamine challenge: 4 pts	POSITIVE Isopren>acupuncture>sham: FEV_1, FVC; $0.05 > p < 0.025$ ↓BP; $p > 0.05$ ↑Heart rate; $p < 0.05$ $Paco_2$; ↓ $p < 0.05$ Histamine: NS
Berger, 1977 (12)	Asthma	POSITIVE SGaw: 9/12 ↓ >30% Subjective improvement significant in SA + S (TP) Changes last at least 2 hours Data indicates should wait at least 10 minutes for spirometry
Tashkin, 1977† (12)	Methacholine-induced asthma	POSITIVE Isoproterenol>acupuncture>saline>sham Objective: SGaw, Raw, Vt, FEV, ↑ 14% MMFR; all $p < 0.05$ No change autonomics: BP, heart rate, respiratory rate
Virsik, 1980 (20)	Bronchial asthma	POSITIVE Subjective: acupuncture>sham $p < 0.05$ Objective: SGaw, FEV_1, PEFR, RV, VC; all $p < 0.05$
Dias, 1982‡; see Marcus, 1982, Hayhoe, 1982 (20)	Chronic bronchial asthma	POSITIVE/NEGATIVE Sham>real $p < 0.01$; PEFR Subjective ↑ + *both* groups Medication: ↓ in 13/20, ↑ 4/20, no change in 3/20

Additional analysis for entries in **bold** can be found in Tables 15-3 and 15-4.

AQLQ, Asthma Quality of Life Questionnaire; *beta-*2, beta-2 sympathomimetic bronchodilators; *BP,* blood pressure; *COPD,* chronic obstructive *GWB,* general well being; *LAI,* leukocyte adherence inhibition; *MMFR,* maximum mid-expiratory flow rate; *MOD BORG,* modified Borg score; *NP,* rate; *po,* by mouth; *pts,* points; *RA,* real acupuncture; *Raw,* airway resistance; *Rrs,* respiratory resistance; *RV,* residual volume; *Rx,* treatment; *S,* sham capacity; *Vtg,* thoracic volume at functional residual capacity; *WSA,* Weekly Severity of Asthma Score.

*Significant improvement.

†Best studies from either Chinese medical and/or biomedical perspectives.

‡Real vs sham = NS but (real + sham) vs baseline = significantly different.

Design	Medication	Acupuncture type	Problems

Uncontrolled
Ear pts only
Included
  electrostimulation
	Not clear,
	  probably
	  beta-2 +
	  steroids
		SA
		2 ear pts
		Ear "lung" × 2
			Unblinded; would have benefited from more
			  analysis of data.

Single blind
S (TP + NP) vs SA
  vs beta-2 agonist
	Incomplete
	  data, 12 on
	  steroids
		SA formula 2 pts
		St 36 × 1
		Ding chuan × 2
			Blinding (improbable), "sham" point often
			  indicated for asthma in TCM; large data overlap
			  for 2 groups; poor description of point
			  selection; positioning of needles; 1 × Rx only.

Single blind
S (TP) vs SA
	Not given	SA formula 9 pts
		UB 13, UB 15,
		  UB 17, *Ding chuan*,
		  Lu 1, CV 17
			Blinding, inadequate information given, raw data
			  not given, no controls, pts used not given
			  (inferred from diagram).

Double blind
S (NP) vs SA vs
  beta-2 +
  crossover
	Incomplete
	  data, 3 on
	  steroids
		SA formula 6 pts
		CO 4 × 2, *Ding chuan*
		  × 2, St 36 × 2,
		  Lu 7 × 2, GV 14
		waiting chuan
			Wide age range, wide range age of onset of
			  symptoms.
			Stats should have used nonparametric methods.
			  Inclusion/exclusion criteria not given.
			No stats on beta-2 vs SA given.
			No *da qi* at S (NP) sites.

Single blind
S (NP) vs SA
	Not given	SA formula 6 pts
		Lu 1 × 2, Lu 7 × 2,
		  UB 13 × 2, CV
		  17, CO 4 × 2
		Ear × 2
			Patients, methods, data insufficient for repeating
			  or inferential stats.
			Stats should have used nonparametric methods.
			1 × Rx only.
			Impressive results but very poorly reported.

Double blind
S (TP) vs SA
	↓Beta-2, franol,
	  ephedrine
	Steroids not
	  mentioned;
	  amounts not
	  given
		SA formula 3 pts
		Ding chuan × 2, Lu 7
		  × 2, CV 22
			Breathing exercises included in some and not
			  controlled for or described compliance.
			Methods poorly reported: not repeatable.
			Homogeneity poor (age, duration of Rx +
			  symptoms, etc).
			Stats should have used nonparametric methods.
			Inconsistent number of Rx for the different
			  patients.

pulmonary disease; *DSA,* Daily Severity of Asthma Score; *FEV₁,* forced expiratory volume in one second; *FVC,* forced vital capacity; *GH,* growth hormone; nonacupuncture point; *NS,* not statistically significant; *O₂ cost,* oxygen cost score; *PaCO₂,* partial pressure of carbon dioxide; *PEFR,* peak expiratory flow acupuncture; *SA,* symptomatic acupuncture formula; *SGaw,* airway conductance; *SOB,* shortness of breath score; *TP,* true acupuncture point; *VC,* vital

Continued

TABLE 15-2

Acupuncture in Pulmonary Disease: Studies Reviewed—cont'd

Study (no. patients)	Subject	Outcome
Takishima, 1982* (10)	Acute asthma	POSITIVE Rrs $p < 0.01$ and correlates with significant subjective improvement (20/26 Rx and 5/10 patients) Very interesting objective changes
Landa, 1982 (2500)	Asthma + other conditions	POSITIVE Report many parameters assessed but little objective data Blood cortisol: normalized 50 pts; serum GH: normalized 50 pts urinary steroids: normalized 36 pts; trypotophan exchange: normalized 81 pts; physical + immunology: normalized, etc
Chow, 1983‡ (16)	Exercise induced asthma	POSITIVE/NEGATIVE NS difference between sham + real *but* both confer significant protection over baseline; >50% improvement in 1/3 pts
Christensen, 1984 (17)	Chronic bronchial asthma	POSITIVE Both showed changes, but acupuncture>sham DSA, WSA, PEFR, puffs beta-2, IgE all, $p < 0.05 + p < 0.01$ Medication: clear ↓ puffs beta-2 Very interesting results
Sliwinski, 1984 (57 entered; 36 completed)	Chronic bronchitis (3 years Rx)	POSITIVE ↓Medications particularly steroids (63.8% stopped steroids) Stop all drugs 19.5% 16.7% ↓ steroids, 13.9% ↓ in dose >60% Spirometry reported significant but no data given
Tashkin, 1985† (25)	Bronchial asthma	NEGATIVE But trend in subjective, objective + medications to improvement Rigorous study
Shao, 1985 (111)	Bronchial asthma, asthmatic bronchitis, and asthmatic bronchitis with emphysema	POSITIVE Spirometry + medication ↓; $p < 0.001$ 48 marked improvement, 61 improved, 2 no change Interesting attempt to quantify contribution of specific pts

Additional analysis for entries in **bold** can be found in Tables 15-3 and 15-4.

AQLQ, Asthma Quality of Life Questionnaire; *beta*-2, beta-2 sympathomimetic bronchodilators; *BP,* blood pressure; *COPD,* chronic obstructive *GWB,* general well being; *LAI,* leukocyte adherence inhibition; *MMFR,* maximum mid-expiratory flow rate; *MOD BORG,* modified Borg score; *NP,* rate; *po,* by mouth; *pts,* points; *RA,* real acupuncture; *Raw,* airway resistance; *Rrs,* respiratory resistance; *RV,* residual volume; *Rx,* treatment; *S,* sham capacity; *Vtg,* thoracic volume at functional residual capacity; *WSA,* Weekly Severity of Asthma Score.

*Significant improvement.

†Best studies from either Chinese medical and/or biomedical perspectives.

‡Real vs sham = NS but (real + sham) vs baseline = significantly different.

Design	Medication	Acupuncture type	Problems
Single blind S (TP/NP) vs SA vs beta-2	Not given	SA 1 pt St 10	Blinding. Complex protocol. Sham procedure active according to TCM. 1 × Rx only. Confused patients with Rx in analysis.

Descriptive	Not given	TCM but questions
		  on how and what
			Anecdotal.
			Interesting results but *not* a scientific study.
			No relevant data given (e.g., TCM but ?needles,
			  ?laser, ?herbs, etc.)

Single blind
Ear S (TP) vs SA
	Beta-2
	  cromoglycate
	  steroids not
	  mentioned
		SA single ear point
		  bilaterally
			Data interpretation: both types of ear acupuncture
			  confer protection.
			Specificity of pts dubious.
			Needs further study.
			Sham pts possibly better than "real."

Double blind
S (NP) vs SA +
  electro
Included
  electrostimulation
	Only at least 4
	  puffs beta-2;
	  never steroids
	  or
	  cromoglycate
		SA formula 4 pts
		CO 4 × 2, *Ding chuan*
		  × 2, UB 13 × 2,
		  CV 17
			Blinding: only real acupuncture patients had
			  electrostimulation, controls did not.
			Different needle depths for real + sham.
			Real worse than sham before Rx.
			Incomplete data; no baseline values given.

Cohort	Steroids po +
	  im, mucolytics
	  antibiotics,
	  beta-2,
	  xanthines,
	  sedatives
		SA formula 9 pts
		GV 14, GV 9, Ex 17
		  × 2, UB 17 × 2,
		  TH 15 × 2
		CO 4 × 2, GV 12,
		  CV 17, UB 13 × 2
			Uncontrolled evaluation.
			Raw data missing.
			No reasons for 15 drop-outs given.
			Data not analyzed on intention to Rx.

Double blind
S (NP) vs SA x-over
	Steroids beta-2,
	  xanthines
	  cromoglycate,
	  19 on oral
	  steroids
		SA formula 6 pts
		CO 4 × 2, ST 36 ×
		  2, GV 14, Lu 7 ×
		  2, *Ding chuan* × 2
		waiting chuan
			Blinding: no placebo response is improbable.
			Insufficient data on diary use.
			Stats should also have analyzed individual changes
			  with nonparametric stats.
			Insufficient power.

Uncontrolled
Some +
  moxabustion;
  some + cupping
	Not given	TCM + formula
		  baseline 3 pts
		UB 13 × 2, GV 14,
		  UB 12 × 2, Lu 5,
		  Lu 9, CV 12,
		  St 36, Bl 23, CV 4,
		  Ki 3
			Uncontrolled.
			Not enough data.
			Statistics dubious.
			Study should be expanded and written in more
			  detail.

pulmonary disease; *DSA,* Daily Severity of Asthma Score; FEV_1, forced expiratory volume in one second; *FVC,* forced vital capacity; *GH,* growth hormone; nonacupuncture point; *NS,* not statistically significant; O_2 *cost,* oxygen cost score; $PaCO_2$, partial pressure of carbon dioxide; *PEFR,* peak expiratory flow acupuncture; *SA,* symptomatic acupuncture formula; *SGaw,* airway conductance; *SOB,* shortness of breath score; *TP,* true acupuncture point; *VC,* vital

Continued

TABLE 15-2

Acupuncture in Pulmonary Disease: Studies Reviewed—cont'd

Study (no. patients)	Subject	Outcome
Jobst, 1986†; see Jobst, 1987 (26)	COPD Chronic disabling breathlessness (COPD + some reversible airways disease)	POSITIVE Walking distance + subjective $p < 0.01$ Spirometry NS but trend to improvement + trend in blood gases Only study with true TCM Rigorous study Excellent discussion
Fung, 1986† (19)	Exercise-induced asthma	POSITIVE Beta-2>real>sham>none FEV_1, PEFR: $p < 0.01$ Rigorous study Excellent discussion
Mitchell, 1989†‡ (31 entered; 2 withdrew)	Chronic bronchial asthma	POSITIVE/NEGATIVE Both real and sham ↑ (i.e., [SA +S(TP)] > baseline $p < 0.0003$) Real = sham = ↑ but no attacks in RA group, + 4 in sham PEFR ↑ $p < 0.0003$, ↓ medication $p < 0.04$, ↓ symptoms $p < 0.04$, ↑ PEFR variation $p < 0.0005$ Important, rigorous study
Choudhury, 1989 (10)	Bronchial asthma	POSITIVE Spirometry: FEV% 7/10 significant ↑, PEFR ↑ 14% in 9/10 Subjective; significant improvement Medication: 8/10 stopped all Rx
Tandon, 1989‡ (16)	Histamine challenge	NEGATIVE NS + no change in all indices FVC, FEV_1, Histamine Challenge, DCO = NS
Sternfield, 1989 (9)	Extrinsic bronchial asthma	POSITIVE ↓Medication in all patients, all stopped steroids: significant LAI: significant Spirometry: NS

Additional analysis for entries in **bold** can be found in Tables 15-3 and 15-4.

AQLQ, Asthma Quality of Life Questionnaire; *beta-2,* beta-2 sympathomimetic bronchodilators; *BP,* blood pressure; *COPD,* chronic obstructive *GWB,* general well being; *LAI,* leukocyte adherence inhibition; *MMFR,* maximum mid-expiratory flow rate; *MOD BORG,* modified Borg score; *NP,* rate; *po,* by mouth; *pts,* points; *RA,* real acupuncture; *Raw,* airway resistance; *Rrs,* respiratory resistance; *RV,* residual volume; *Rx,* treatment; *S,* sham capacity; *Vtg,* thoracic volume at functional residual capacity; *WSA,* Weekly Severity of Asthma Score.

*Significant improvement.

†Best studies from either Chinese medical and/or biomedical perspectives.

‡Real vs sham = NS but (real + sham) vs baseline = significantly different.

Design	Medication	Acupuncture type	Problems
Double blind S (NP) vs TCM	All medication maintained, but which medication not listed, changes not given	TCM individualized 2-12 pts	Pts not given.
Double blind S (TP) vs SA	On beta-2 po + aerosol only; no steroids.	SA formula 3 pts RA: *Ding chuan* × 2, Lu 6 × 2, Ki 3 × 2 S (TP): SI 14 × 2, PC 4 × 2, GB 39 × 2	Sham pts can be used in TCM Rx. Demographic data missing. 1 × Rx only.
Double blind S (TP) vs SA	Beta-2: po, aerosol; xanthines, cromoglycate, 6 on steroid aerosol	SA formula 4 pts SA: CV 17, *Ding chuan* × 2, Li 3 × 2, UB 13 × 2	Sham pts active in asthma. Homogeneity. Raw data for inferential statistics lacking. Some missing data. S (TP): Sp 8 × 2, GB 37 × 2, Ki 9 × 2
Uncontrolled Unblinded Cohort Electroacupuncture Included electrostimulation	Not detailed, but steroids used	SA formula 7 pts GV 20, CV 17, CV 22, CV 12, CO 4, CO 11, UB 13	Open, nonblinded study. No controls. No statistics on lung function indices.
Double blind S (TP) vs SA crossover (laser)	Beta-2, xanthines, cromoglycate, 15/16 on aerosol steroid	SA formula 4 pts SA: CV 17, *Ding chuan* × 2, Lu 6 × 2, Lu 7 × 2	Blinding: no response in either group is suspicious; ? blinding. Sham pts "active" according to TCM. Placement of *Ding chuan* incorrect. Histamine Challenge too soon after Rx. S (TP) GB 24 × 2 St 25 × 2 TH 5 × 2
Unblinded	Maximum bronchodila-tors, 4 on steroids	SA formula 7 pts GB 20 × 2, GV 14, LI 11 × 2, St 36 × 2, SP 6 × 2, Ki 7 × 2, *Ding chuan* × 2 + 4 pts, Lu 1 × 2, CV 17, CV 22, Lu 9 × 2	Poorly reported. Unblinded. Inadequate Rx information given to differentiate between formulas.

pulmonary disease; *DSA*, Daily Severity of Asthma Score; *FEV₁*, forced expiratory volume in one second; *FVC*, forced vital capacity; *GH*, growth hormone; nonacupuncture point; *NS*, not statistically significant; *O₂ cost*, oxygen cost score; *Paco₂*, partial pressure of carbon dioxide; *PEFR*, peak expiratory flow acupuncture; *SA*, symptomatic acupuncture formula; *SGaw*, airway conductance; *SOB*, shortness of breath score; *TP*, true acupuncture point; *VC*, vital

Continued

TABLE 15-2

Acupuncture in Pulmonary Disease: Studies Reviewed—cont'd

Study (no. patients)	Subject	Outcome
Tandon, 1991‡ (15)	Chronic bronchial asthma	POSITIVE/NEGATIVE 5 SA improved, 5 S(TP) improved, 5 no difference No raw data on FEV_1, PEFR, inhaler use, etc
Biernacki, 1998 (23)	Stable bronchial asthma	POSITIVE SA improved AQLQ Medication significantly reduced in SA group No change in PEFR or spirometry
Kleijnen, 1991† (18 studies)	Asthma + breathlessness	POSITIVE/NEGATIVE Included all types acupuncture 18 methodological criteria: overall 8 positive, 5 negative but with score <50, 5 negative 3 positive
Linde, 1996† (15 studies)	Asthma + breathlessness	POSITIVE/NEGATIVE Included all types acupuncture 5 positive, 1 negative, 8 no difference
Jobst, 1996† (21 studies)	Asthma + breathlessness	POSITIVE Included all types acupuncture 16 met criteria: overall 10 positive, 3 negative, 3 equivocal

Additional analysis for entries in **bold** can be found in Tables 15-3 and 15-4.
AQLQ, Asthma Quality of Life Questionnaire; *beta-2,* beta-2 sympathomimetic bronchodilators; *BP,* blood pressure; *COPD,* chronic obstructive *GWB,* general well being; *LAI,* leukocyte adherence inhibition; *MMFR,* maximum mid-expiratory flow rate; *MOD BORG,* modified Borg score; *NP,* rate; *po,* by mouth; *pts,* points; *RA,* real acupuncture; *Raw,* airway resistance; *Rrs,* respiratory resistance; *RV,* residual volume; *Rx,* treatment; *S,* sham capacity; *Vtg,* thoracic volume at functional residual capacity; *WSA,* Weekly Severity of Asthma Score.
*Significant improvement.
†Best studies from either Chinese medical and/or biomedical perspectives.
‡Real vs sham = NS but (real + sham) vs baseline = significantly different.

Design	Medication	Acupuncture type	Problems
Double blind S (TP) vs SA crossover LASER	Beta-2, xanthines, all inhaled steroids	SA formula 9 pts SA: SP 6 × 2, St 36 × 2, Lu 9 × 2, CO 11 × 2, CV 17, CV 22, *Ding chuan* × 2, UB 13 × 2 Ear: lung + asthma S (TP): GB 34 × 2, Li 8 × 2, Li 14 × 2, SI 3 × 2, SI 6 × 2, UB 18 × 2, UB 25 × 2 Ear: uterus + bladder	Blinding. Sham pts "active" according to TCM. No raw data about patients. Symptom scores not elucidated. Methods unclear. No information on attack frequency, allergen sensitivity, etc.
Double blind SA vs S (NP) Crossover	–	SA formula ? Number of pts	Inadequate treatment; only once and then evaluate at 2/52 (= in 2 weeks). Remarkable changes despite the protocol.
Review Criteria based metaanalysis	Not relevant	Various	Arbitrary but excellent. No weighting for TCM criteria. No query of authors of studies about whether judgments correct.
Review Systematic	Not relevant	Various	No allowance for use of active sham pts.
Review Systematic	Not relevant	Various	Highlights for first time problem and effect of using active sham pts.

pulmonary disease; *DSA,* Daily Severity of Asthma Score; *FEV$_1$,* forced expiratory volume in one second; *FVC,* forced vital capacity; *GH,* growth hormone; nonacupuncture point; *NS,* not statistically significant; *O$_2$ cost,* oxygen cost score; *Paco$_2$,* partial pressure of carbon dioxide; *PEFR,* peak expiratory flow acupuncture; *SA,* symptomatic acupuncture formula; *SGaw,* airway conductance; *SOB,* shortness of breath score; *TP,* true acupuncture point; *VC,* vital

Continued

TABLE 15-3

Acupuncture Trials in Bronchial Asthma

	Acute attack				Chronic symptoms					
	Yu and Lee, 1976	Takishima, 1982	Virsik, 1980	Christensen, 1984*	Choudhury, 1989*	Wen, 1973	Mitchell, 1989†‡	Dias, 1982†	Tashkin, 1985§	Biernacki, 1998
Rx duration	1 × Rx	1 × Rx	1 × Rx	5/52	10/52	4+/52	12/52	1-6/52	8/52	4/52
PEFR	(?)		+	+	+	+	+	+		–
FEV$_1$	+		+		+	+				–
Medication				+	+	+	+	+	Trend	+
Subjective symptoms (well-being)	+	+	+	+	+	+	+	+	Trend	+
Others	↓PaCO$_2$ ↓Wheeze, etc ↑FVC	↓Rrs	↑SGaw ↑VC ↓RV	IgE ↓DSA ↓WSA	↑FEV% ↑VC ↑FVC	↑FVC	↓Symptom score ↓PEFR fluctuation		Trend subjective symptoms (well-being) + medication only	AQLQ positive
Overall outcome	Positive	Positive	Positive	Positive	Positive	Positive	Positive/negative	Positive/negative	Negative	Positive
Design	SB	SB	SB	DB	UNB	UNB	DB	DB	DB	DB

Overall results: 2/5 DB = positive; 2/5 DB = equivocal; 1/5 = negative; 3/3 SB = positive; 2/2 UNB = positive.

AQLQ, Asthma Quality of Life Questionnaire; beta-2, beta-2 sympathomimetic bronchodilators; BP, blood pressure; COPD, chronic obstructive pulmonary disease; DB, double blind; DSA, Daily Severity of Asthma Score; FEV$_1$, forced expiratory volume in one second; FVC, forced vital capacity; GH, growth hormone; GWB, general well being; LAI, leukocyte adherence inhibition; MOD BORG, modified Borg score; NP, nonacupuncture point; NS, not statistically significant; O$_2$ cost, oxygen cost score; PaCO$_2$, partial pressure of carbon dioxide; PEFR, peak expiratory flow rate; RA, real acupuncture; Raw, airway resistance; Rrs, respiratory resistance; RV, residual volume; Rx, treatment; S, sham acupuncture; SA, symptomatic acupuncture formula; SB, single blind; SGaw, airway conductance; SOB, shortness of breath score; TP, true acupuncture point; UNB, unblinded; VC, vital capacity; Vtg, thoracic volume at functional residual capacity; WSA, Weekly Severity of Asthma Score.

* Included electrostimulation.

†Real vs sham = NS but ([real + sham] vs baseline) = significantly different.

‡Significant improvement.

§Best studies from either Chinese medical or biomedical perspective.

of acute attacks,[26,29,53] and 7 studies of chronic asthma.*

Table 15-4 shows data on the remaining 7 studies. Of these, two studies[29] investigated the effect of acupuncture on histamine-induced bronchoconstriction and examined acupuncture both before and after, whereas Tandon[48] looked at its effect only before histamine challenge. One study[43] looked at the effect of acupuncture on methacholine-induced bronchoconstriction, when acupuncture was given only after methacholine administration. Two studies of acupuncture in exercise-induced asthma were found, one used body points alone,[33] and one also used ear points.[55] One study[34] looked at chronic disabling breathlessness and some patients having evidence of reversible airways obstruction; this is the only one of the 17 studies that fulfills CM principles. Finally, one study looked at acupuncture effectiveness in the care of chronic bronchitis.[57]

In summary, a limited amount of clinical trials and review data on acupuncture and pulmonary disease exists and the quality varies. However, although there is an obvious need for more high quality clinical trials, the results of these studies are sufficient to support CM clinical experience that acupuncture is useful in the care of pulmonary disorders such as asthma, bronchitis, and COPD.

Acupuncture in Acute Bronchial Asthma

The three single blind studies are all positive for acupuncture (see Table 15-3). Yu and Lee[29] and Virsik[53] found significant changes in FEV_1; Yu and Lee[29] also finding significant concomitant changes in FVC, $PaCO_2$, and wheeze. Virsik[53] found changes in PEFR lasting the full 2 hours over which it was monitored, with a diminution in residual volume, improved VC and airway conductance. However, the study is poorly documented and does not permit inferential statistics. In Takishima's study,[46] respiratory resistance (Rrs) was evaluated but no other spirometric indices. Autonomic functions such as ECG, skin temperature, and plethysmography were monitored but revealed no change. This study is hard to interpret. A combination of SP(TP) and SP(NP) was used, and protocol involved

three separate different interventions, which could have interacted. A significant fall in Rrs and three different physiologically significant responses to beta-2 sympathomimetic challenges emerged. The sham/placebo involved deep needle insertion so it cannot have been without effect, raising doubt about the effectiveness of blinding because the authors report no response in that group. It does not, however, negate the overall importance of this particular study.

Acupuncture in Chronic Bronchial Asthma

Of the seven studies summarized in Table 15-3 (five double blind, two unblinded), four were unequivocally positive,[48,56,58,59] one negative,[42] and two equivocal.[45,54]

Tashkin's negative double-blind study[42] is one of the few rigorously conducted and reported studies involving both a run-in period and crossover design, as well as assessment of subjective and objective parameters (diaries, symptoms, physical examination, medication, spirometry, plethysmography, and so on). There was a trend toward improvement in lung function and symptomatology that did not reach statistical significance. The cases were moderately severely disabled and the patient population far from homogeneous (age ranged from 8 to 70 years and duration 3 to 45 years). The fact that only 25 patients took part and a crossover design was employed may have compromised power.

Significant changes in PEFR, reduced medication usage, and improvement in symptoms were reported in all the other studies. Christensen's five-week trial revealed evidence of immune system alteration after acupuncture with a significant drop in serum IgE in the real (SA) group, although the ranges were extremely wide (42 to 2000 IU/L) in both groups.

Dias's study[54] is seriously methodologically compromised. Breathing exercises, well known to affect airways resistance and reactivity,[6] were part of the protocol, although not specified or controlled for in the trial design. No mention is made of why or how the exercises were taught or performed. Controls were given different numbers of needles. SP (TP)s are indicated in certain forms of respiratory disease in TCM, and the treatment length for the SP (TP) and RA (SA) groups were very different. The population was inhomogeneous in all respects with no information about inclusion or exclusion criteria given. The study

---

*References 42, 45, 48, 52-54, 58, 59.

TABLE 15-4

Acupuncture Studies in Exercise-, Histamine-, and Methacholine-Induced Bronchoconstriction and Chronic Bronchitis/Breathlessness

Condition	Chronic bronchitis/breathlessness		Exercise-induced asthma			Histamine-induced asthma		Methacholine induced-asthma
	Jobst, 1986*	Sliwinski 1984	Chow 1983†	Fung, 1986‡	Yu and Lee, 1976	Tandon, 1989	Tashkin, 1977‡
Rx duration	3/52	3 years	1 × Rx	1 × Rx	1 × Rx	1 × Rx	1 × Rx
PEFR	Trend	+	?	+	−		+
FEV$_1$	Trend	+	±	+	−	−	+
Medication		+	?				
Subjective symptoms (well-being)	+	+	?	?			
Others	Walking distance, SOB, O$_2$ cost, MOD BORG, GWB, trend PaO$_2$/PaCO$_2$		MMFR↑	FVC↑	No effect	FVC	↑FVC ↑SGaw ↓Raw ↑Vtg ↑MMFR All $p < 0.05$
Overall outcome	Positive	Positive	Positive/negative	Positive	Negative	Negative	Positive
Design	DB	UNB	SB	DB	SB	DB	DB

Overall results: 3/4 DB = positive; 1/2 SB = equivocal; 1/1 UNB = positive.

AQLQ, Asthma Quality of Life Questionnaire; *beta-2*, beta-2 sympathomimetic bronchodilators; *BP*, blood pressure; *COPD*, chronic obstructive pulmonary disease; *DB*, double blind; *DSA*, Daily Severity of Asthma Score; *FEV$_1$*, forced expiratory volume in one second; *FVC*, forced vital capacity; *GH*, growth hormone; *GWB* general well being; *LAI*, leukocyte adherence inhibition; *MMFR*, maximum mid-expiratory flow rate; *MOD BORG*, modified Borg score; *NP*, nonacupuncture point; *NS*, not statistically significant; *O$_2$ cost*, oxygen cost score; *PaCO$_2$*, partial pressure of carbon dioxide; *PEFR*, peak expiratory flow rate; *RA*, real acupuncture; *Raw*, airway resistance; *RV*, residual volume; *Rx*, treatment; *S*, sham acupuncture; *SA*, symptomatic acupuncture formula; *SB*, single blind; *SGaw*, airway conductance; *SOB*, shortness of breath score; *TP*, true acupuncture point; *UNB*, unblinded; *VC*, vital capacity; *Vtg*, thoracic volume at functional residual capacity; *WSA*, Weekly Severity of Asthma Score.

*Significant improvement.

†Real vs sham = NS but (real + sham) vs baseline = significantly different.

‡Best studies from either Chinese medical and/or biomedical perspectives.

compared two treatments and found that both required less medication, 6/10 RA (SA) vs 7/10 SP (TP), reaching statistical significance in the sham (TP) group, and overall 13/20 requiring less medication. This significant finding was nevertheless reported to be negative.

Although marred by missing data, Mitchell and Wells's study[45] is rigorous. However, SP (TP)s are used and highly significant differences from baseline were found for both the RA (SA) and SP (TP) groups in subjective and spirometric indices. No statistically significant difference was observed between them, but there were no episodes of asthma in the RA (SA) group and four in the SP (TP) group. Changes were sustained over 36 weeks, the most impressive being morning PEFRs ($p <0.002$), daily PEFR fluctuation ($p <0.0005$), and a marginal diminution in medication use. Thus acupuncture (RA [SA] + SP [TP]) produced highly significant improvements sustained for over 6 months. Mitchell and Wells recognize that these results may simply reflect improved compliance as a result of monitoring and the possibility that both combinations of points may be actively treating the asthma.

Both Choudhury and Wen and Chau report unblinded studies, but both represent practical clinical realities. Choudhury used electroacupuncture on 10 acupuncture naive patients in Nigeria (racial mix not given, 9 extrinsic, 1 intrinsic asthma, duration 2.5 to 60 years). Nine had a decreased attack rate after the first session and 8 were able to come off all medication after 10 treatments. VC improved in 7, with an increase in FEV_1 over 13.6% in 9, and substantial subjective improvements.

Wen and Chau's study[48] from Hong Kong is startling. It remains a mystery that it has not yet been repeated anywhere. Six acupuncture-naive cases of status asthmaticus were treated with electro-auriculopuncture once or twice daily for 30 to 60 minutes during hospitalization, initially daily and then at longer intervals after discharge. Symptom severity, attack frequency, and medication use were significantly improved in all. One patient in status asthmaticus was effectively treated with acupuncture alone for the first 48 hours. There was a mean 45% increase in FEV_1, 49.7% increase in PEFR, and 12.5% increase in FVC after 30 minutes. These improvements lasted up to 24 hours with cumulatively improving lung function and bronchial reactivity so that the number of days of distress reported by patients was reduced by 50% compared with conventional therapy. Bronchodilator dose was reduced

by over 33% in those followed for at least 3 months. All patients reported significantly fewer side effects after auriculopuncture with increased well-being; in particular, sensations of warmth as well as more effective, longer lasting relief of breathlessness, reflecting what CM refers to as "enlivenment of Chi," which is both practice- and practitioner-dependent (see Table 15-1). The authors draw attention to the simplicity of the technique and the importance of correct needle placement and training. Within the CM paradigm, a well-trained acupuncturist can enhance well-being not only because of good technique but also because training implies a state of well-being and vitality and a knowledge and practice of health in the practitioner. Such studies therefore lend support to the wider issues of CM.

Acupuncture in Exercise-Induced Asthma

Both trials of acupuncture in exercise-induced asthma came from the same medical unit in Hong Kong and involved children only (Tables 15-2 and 15-4).[32,55] The first showed no significant difference between the real (SA) and sham-treated patients using auriculopuncture. However, 25% of the children had at least 90% protection and a third had over 50% protection from a drop in FEV_1 when treatment was stopped, and there was a 32% difference in the fall in FEV_1 after real (SA) needle insertion compared to none. The conclusion therefore that acupuncture confers no protection against exercise-induced asthma is erroneous. It is also noteworthy that controlling temperature and humidity in the trial setting was ignored, since these are factors that play a significant role in airways reactivity. The second study[32] was much improved and used body acupuncture points. However some of the sham (TP) points are indicated for treating asthma in CM texts. Here, bronchodilators conferred maximal benefit on FEV_1 and PEFR, with real (SA) yielding a significant improvement when compared with both baseline and sham (TP). The SP (TP) did confer protection but much less than real (SA). The discussion offers an excellent proposition as to potential mechanisms of action involving cyclic AMP, endogenous opiates mediating diminished ventilatory drive, load compensation, muscle fatigue, and cholinergic stimulation via the neurocutaneous reflex.

Acupuncture in Histamine-Induced Bronchoconstriction as a Model for Asthma

Both studies looking at the effect of acupuncture on histamine-induced asthma yielded negative results (see Table 15-4); one study was single blind[29] and one study was double blind.[49] In Yu and Lee's study[29] 4 of 20 patients underwent histamine challenge, and acupuncture whether before or after histamine made no impact on FEV_1 or FVC. Stimulating only one point, *Ding chuan,* either immediately before or 10 minutes after histamine challenge is almost certainly unlikely to produce any effect for all the reasons already discussed, including the unreality of artificially provoking asthma to "see if acupuncture will work." Furthermore, the location of *Ding chuan* used (3 cm lateral to TI) appears to have been inaccurate (1.5 cm lateral to TI in the classical texts). Tandon's study[49] of 16 cases, double blind and with a crossover design, used histamine challenge given immediately after acupuncture treatment with evaluation of FVC, and FEV_1. Again, the sham points chosen are potentially active in asthma, but neither was found to have any impact and there was no significant difference between them. However, the mean difference in dose of histamine required to produce a 20% drop in FEV_1 from baseline was ten times greater (0.1 mg/mL vs 0.012 mg/kg) in the real (SA) group than the sham (TP) group, possibly due to stabilization of bronchial hypersensitivity by acupuncture. Unfortunately, the acupuncture-histamine interval is not given. The small number of patients and crossover design mean that the trial was very probably underpowered, and the use of averaged symptom scores may have masked significant individual changes, as were found in the study by Jobst et al.[34]

Acupuncture in Methacholine-Induced Bronchoconstriction

Tashkin's study[43] (see Table 15-4) is one of the most interesting studies in the literature. The study was conducted double blind with 12 subjects and compared real (SA), sham (NP), and beta-2 bronchodilator therapy. It showed a range of significant effects on spirometry at intervals after treatment that followed methacholine challenge. It is one of the very few studies to use real nonpoints as sham. The greatest reversal of bronchoconstriction was from the sympathomimetic isoproterenol, but real (SA) conferred significantly greater advantage over nebulized saline or no treatment. Changes in airway conductance were statistically significant, lasting at least for 2 hours during which assessment was performed.

Acupuncture in Chronic Bronchitis and Chronic Disabling Breathlessness

The single study of acupuncture in chronic bronchitis[57] is uncontrolled and unblinded (see Table 15-4) but pertains to real clinical practice and was sustained over 3 years. Fifty-one patients were enrolled but 15 dropped out, although no reasons are cited. Weekly treatment was given on and off in alternating blocks of 2 to 3 months with significant reductions in medications shown in the 36 who completed the trial; 63.8% eliminating all steroid use, with 16.7 % substantially reducing and 19.5% stopping all medication. Although no data are given, the authors claim there were significant physical changes. This is also the only study specifically to report an exacerbation of symptoms before improvement in some, which is a phenomenon well described in CM texts, but rarely if ever in the biomedical literature.

Only one study in the acupuncture and respiratory disease literature currently fulfills criteria for CM acupuncture, with individual case assessment and point formulation at each episode and a double blind protocol.[58] Sham (NP)s were employed after discovering that SP(TP)s led to real and significant changes in the pilot phases, and the study included a baseline qualification period and strict randomization. A statistically significant improvement in all subjective indices, including well being (the only parameter to change significantly under sham treatment), was found, in addition to significant improvement in 6 minute walking distance and activities of daily living (oxygen cost score), although none of the spirometric indices reached statistical significance. A change in ventilation/perfusion dynamics was indicated by the trend to reduced PaO_2 and $PaCO_2$ found, similar to that seen after administering methylxanthines. This study demonstrates unequivocally that CM acupuncture can be evaluated and that it can make a significant impact in the most difficult COPD cases: those patients moderately to severely disabled by breathlessness and airways obstruction.

Acupuncture and Medication Use

Data on medication use were available from 12 of the 17 studies reviewed.* After acupuncture treatment of whatever sort, 11/12 studies (92%) in which it could be evaluated, yielded significant reductions in medication use. In the remaining study,[43] a clear trend toward reduction is described. Medication reduction is particularly impressive in other studies.[45,48,57,58] These studies are all close to what is encountered in routine CM office settings. The significance of these data is readily apparent in the light of the increase in mortality and morbidity found in association with maintenance drug therapy in asthma and the considerable side-effect profile of bronchodilator and corticosteroid medication (see Table 15-1).

The Experience of Breathlessness and Well Being After Acupuncture

The subjective responses of patients as outcome measures are of great importance, especially in pulmonary disease where both subjective and objective variables intricately interact to influence perception, well being, and the experience of and response to breathlessness.† Significant subjective improvement was found in 9/10 studies in which it was documented in bronchial asthma, the tenth showing a clear trend toward improvement.[42] The same is true of the studies of chronic bronchitis and chronic disabling breathlessness. However a formal protocol for assessing subjective improvement was used in only four studies,[34,42,45,56] and only the latter three measured the impact of these changes on what the patients could actually do. Thus in 11/12 studies (92%) the subjective experience of symptom severity and well being was significantly improved. The true potential of acupuncture in this context, especially in relation to long-term follow-up and application, has yet to be exploited.

*In the histamine-, methacholine-, and exercise-induced asthma cases, the three acute asthma studies, and a study[33] of chronic disabling breathlessness, change in medication was not reported.
†References 6, 7, 17-20, 24, 34.

Side Effects and Adverse Events

The 17 studies embraced 343 subjects, of whom 7 or 8 reported mild symptoms that may have been side effects of their acupuncture treatment. Among these, three vasovagal episodes were reported with only one dropout,[29,45,49] two had earaches insufficient to require dropout or cessation of treatment,[55] one reported mild nausea,[33] and one or two reported minimal dizziness, nausea, and anorexia.[48] In Sliwinski's trial,[57] 15 withdrew, some cases having an exacerbation in response to treatment, which then improved. However, it is not clear whether the 15 cases withdrew due to exacerbations or not. This is the only study to report exacerbation. It is a phenomenon widely documented in the CM literature, with admonitions to prepare patients for it, and indicating that it heralds a favorable response. Thus at the very worst only 7% reported side effects/adverse events (23 cases, including the 15 for whom inadequate information is given). All were negligible according to the reports and it is not possible to discover from them why those who dropped out did so. The debate about the adverse event profile of acupuncture has been somewhat stirred in recent years,[60] but it is clear that despite the very rare serious and in some cases fatal events reported, the overall profile of acupuncture compares extremely favorably with orthodox allopathic prescribing in routine practice where thousands die every year as a result of mistakes.[61]

The Effect of Acupuncture in Bronchial Asthma

For the most part, acupuncture, although effective, is less immediately effective than beta-2 bronchodilator inhalation. However, Wen[48] (open study) and Takishima[46] (single blind) document instances of equivalence. It should also be noted that this is the experience of many working in acupuncture clinics where asthma is a staple part of the therapeutic diet. However, one should not ignore the fact that none of the double-blind studies found such an effect, which is also in no way to negate the significance of the other findings. After all, it is still unclear what exactly in the consultation and treatment brings this about, especially since so many of the point formulae are flawed as discussed above, and the whole framework of CM care is rarely assessed.

TABLE 15-5

Acupuncture in Pulmonary Disease: Overall Positive and Negative Outcomes*

Study type	Number	Positive	%	Negative	%	Positive/ negative	%	Positive + positive/ negative	%
Double blind	9	5	56	2	22	2	22	7	78
Single blind	5	3	60	1	20	1	20	4	80
Unblinded	3	3	100					3	100
TOTAL	17	11	65	3	18	3	18	14	82

*Trial design in 16 studies critically evaluated.

Table 15-5 summarizes the data. Of the 17 studies discussed, 4/8 of the double-blinded studies showed a clear positive effect in favor of acupuncture (50%), 2 (25%) were clearly negative, and 2 (25%) studies were equivocal (i.e., the results of RA [SA] vs SA [TP] were not significantly different, but the combined results of both were significantly different from baseline in favor of acupuncture). Four of the 6 single-blinded studies showed positive outcomes in favor of acupuncture (67%), one negative, and one equivocal. All 3 studies without blinding were positive. Thus 11/17 (65%) were unequivocally positive, 3 (18%) showed that acupuncture had no impact, and 3 (18%) were equivocal.

Viewing acupuncture as a whole by combining the positive effect over baseline of the equivocal studies with those that are clearly positive yields an impressive overall positive impact on symptoms or spirometric indices of 82%.

REFERRAL

There are few if any contraindications to acupuncture treatment of asthma and respiratory disease. For the vast majority, including those on large doses of medication such as long-term maintenance steroids, there is much to be gained from a trial of acupuncture by a well-qualified CM practitioner. At worst patients will experience something new and at best may find that they feel and function better and can come off medications altogether in time.[48,57]

An important caveat is to remember that untreated asthma can kill and that just because a person is not wheezing does not mean that he or she is not at risk. Therefore patients should understand that even if acupuncture may help them eventually reduce or come off pharmaceuticals, they should not be in a hurry to achieve this goal and should do so with the continued guidance of their biomedical practitioner. Professional acupuncturists understand this point very well, and most welcome the chance to work in co-operation with a physician.

Some special points that should be noted follow:
1. Chinese medicine practitioners rarely needle children before the age of 7 to 9 years. Younger children are successfully treated with massage and acupressure.[11,62]
2. Patients in the middle of an asthmatic attack often display tight thoracic muscles. Although needling is likely to be done distant to the thorax, it is always delivered with particular care in the thoracic region.
3. Although needling causes very small wounds, even those on anticoagulants need not fear if their clotting is well controlled and regularly monitored.
4. Acupuncturists are trained to recognize and treat vasovagal episodes, so even sensitive or fatigued patients and those prone to hypotension can be treated.

SUMMARY

In 1974, Bonica[63] called for the collection of objective scientific evidence about acupuncture. As reviewed in this book—Chapter 11 on physiology, Chapter 12 on patient attitudes and experiences, and Chapters 13 to 19 on clinical research—much has been learned. However, there is still a long way to go on all fronts. Particularly, there is the huge task of educating the biomedical professions as to the significant consequences of erroneous trial design, inappropriate point selection, inadequate time to onset of action, and inappropriate outcome measures.

Much of the work from the past 30 years has used inferior methodology. A most significant aspect of this is that some of the most careful studies have yielded misleading results by failing to evaluate acupuncture "on its own terms" as this chapter has sought to highlight. Nowhere is this better evidenced than in the Cochrane metaanalysis that concludes that there is no evidence on which to recommend acupuncture for the treatment of asthma or respiratory disease. In the light of the analyses presented in this chapter and elsewhere,[2] we prefer to conclude that there is no evidence *not* to recommend acupuncture for the treatment of respiratory disease based on the Cochrane metaanalysis. Indeed, existing data show acupuncture to be a useful and extremely safe method of ameliorating the experience of breathlessness and improving quality of life and activities of daily living. As clinicians, we must decide whether we wish to describe the cup as half full or half empty.

Thus there is clear evidence that acupuncture treatment in bronchial asthma and chronic disabling breathlessness may have a beneficial effect on both subjective and objective indices of lung function. The majority of studies reveal that acupuncture therapy may be used in addition to conventional biomedical management of asthma. Indeed, the study by Wen[48] of acupuncture in status asthmaticus suggests that acupuncture treatment should be more widely represented in routine respiratory medicine.

However, the paucity of well-designed studies from both the CM and biomedical points of view prevents definitive conclusions from being drawn other than endorsing the need for further well-designed trials. Both Linde[25,44] and Jobst[2] call for studies to represent more closely what happens in routine clinical practice, to involve careful point selection, to be mindful of the potential of sham effects and point selection, to compare acupuncture treatment with routine medications and management strategies in pragmatic trials and case studies, and to document data in a format that allows entry into the Cochrane software. They also call for assessment of cost effectiveness, since we already have limited evidence that acupuncture treatment enables a reduction in maintenance allopathic medication, particularly corticosteroids. This might significantly reduce the cost of care, quite apart from the benefit of improved well-being, easier breathing, and willingness and ability to work.

A new study[64] reports success in utilizing acupuncture in the treatment of allergic asthma. This study measured numerous immunomodulatory parameters in addition to standard respiratory function tests. The outcome of this study supports the arguments advanced in this chapter and further endorses the potential for acupuncture to provide benefit for patients with respiratory disease.

An admonition is necessary here. It is perhaps important to reflect on how the assumptions of biomolecular science methodology, when applied in a culturally insensitive manner (as in the case of point selection in studies of acupuncture), may lead to misrepresentation. No self-respecting chest physician would take a trial of assessment and treatment in asthma seriously if the practitioner concerned had only spent a week learning chest medicine. Yet the equivalent of this is what has been done in some trials of acupuncture, reinforcing how such methodology can be far from benign when misapplied. Additionally, acupuncture is but one of many modalities used conjointly by CM practitioners treating asthma. Its true value therefore may multiply when used in the traditional context, which includes herbs, diet, tai chi, meditation, and so on.

There is no doubt that acupuncture is a safe and effective procedure in the hands of professional practitioners.[60] It is very likely that the integration of acupuncture into management programs for asthma and respiratory disease may render its allopathic treatment less toxic and more effective.

References

1. Eskinazi DP, Jobst KA, editors: NIH technology assessment workshop on alternative medicine: acupuncture, *J Altern Complement Med* 2(1):1-256,1996.
2. Jobst KA. Acupuncture in pulmonary disease: issues of safety and efficacy, *J Altern Complement Med* 2(1):179-207, 1996.
3. Crane J, Burgess C, Pearce N, et al: Asthma deaths in New Zealand, *Br Med J* 304:1307, 1992.
4. Evans R et al: National trends in the morbidity and mortality of asthma in the US. Prevalence, hospitalization and death from asthma over two decades 1965-1984, *Chest* 91(6 suppl):65S-74S, 1987.

5. Lung and Asthma Information Agency: *Trends in asthma mortality in the elderly: fact sheet,* St Georges Hospital Medical School, London, 1992, Department of Public Health Sciences.

6. Lane DJ, Lane TV: Alternative and complementary medicine for asthma, *Thorax* 46:787-797, 1991.

7. Lane DJ: What can alternative medicine offer the treatment of asthma? *J Asthma* 31(3):155-162, 1994.

8. Benson MK: Chronic bronchitis, emphysema and COAD. In Weatherall DJ, Ledingham JGG, Wartrell DA, editors: *Oxford textbook of medicine,* ed 2, Oxford, 1988, Oxford University Press.

9. Maciocia G: *The practice of Chinese medicine: the treatment of disease with acupuncture and Chinese herbs,* Edinburgh, 1994, Churchill Livingstone.

10. Ross J: *Acupuncture point combinations, the key to clinical success,* Edinburgh, 1995, Churchill Livingstone.

11. Scott J, Barlow T: *Acupuncture in the treatment of children,* ed 3, Seattle, 1999, Eastland Press.

12. Looney GL: Acupuncture study, *JAMA* 228:1522, 1974.

13. Nagarathna R, Nagendra HR: Yoga for bronchial asthma: a controlled study, *Br Med J* 291:1077-1079, 1985.

14. Singh V et al: Effect of yoga breathing exercises (Pranayama) on airway reactivity in subjects with asthma, *Lancet* 335:1381-1383, 1990.

15. Rosenthal RR, Wang KP, Norman PS: All that is asthma does not wheeze, *N Engl J Med* 13:372, 1975.

16. Luparello T et al: Influences of suggestion on airway reactivity in asthmatic subjects, *Psychosom Med* 30:819-825, 1968.

17. McFadden ER et al: The mechanism of action of suggestion in the induction of acute asthma attacks, *Psychosom Med* 31:134-143, 1969.

18. Spector S, Luparello TJ, Kopetzky MT, et al: Response of asthmatics to methacholine and suggestion, *Am Rev Resp Dis* 113:43-50, 1976.

19. The enigma of breathlessness (editorial), *Lancet* 19(i):891-892, 1986.

20. Shapiro AK, Morris LA: The placebo effect in medical and psychological therapies. In Garfield SL, Bergin AE, editors: *Handbook of psychotherapy and behaviour change,* New York, 1978, Wiley.

21. Woolcock AJ: Asthma. In Weatherall DJ, Ledingham JGG, Wartrell DA, editors: *Oxford textbook of medicine,* ed 2, Oxford, 1988, Oxford University Press.

22. Adams L et al: Breathlessness during different forms of ventilatory stimulation: a study of mechanisms in normal subjects and respiratory patients, *Clin Sci* 69:663-72, 1985.

23. Burns BH, Howell BJL: Disproportionately severe breathlessness in chronic bronchitis, *Quart J Med* 38:277-94, 1969.

24. Acupuncture, asthma and breathlessness (editorial), *Lancet* ii:1427-1428, 1986.

25. Linde K, Jobst KA, Panton J: *Acupuncture for chronic asthma,* Cochrane database of systematic reviews (2):CD000008, 2000.

26. Cassidy CM: Social science theory and methods in the study of alternative and complementary medicine, *J Altern Complemen Med* 1(1):19-40, 1995.

27. Shao J, Ding Y: Clinical observation on 111 cases of asthma treated by acupuncture and moxibustion, *J Trad Chin Med* 5:23-25, 1985.

28. Reilly D, Taylor M: Developing integrated medicine: report of the RCCM research fellowhip in complementary medicine, University of Glasgow, 1987-1990, *Comp Ther Med* 1:1-50, 1993.

29. Yu DC, Lee SP: Effect of acupuncture on bronchial asthma, *Clin Sci Mol Med* 51:503-509, 1976.

30. Smith G, Chian HT, Regina EG: Sensory effects of acupuncture and placebo acupuncture (abstract No: 628), *The Pharmacologist* 6:301, 1974.

31. Bressler DE, Kroening RJ: Three essential factors in effective acupuncture therapy, *Am J Chin Med* 4:81-86, 1976.

32. Stux G, Pomeranz B: *Acupuncture: textbook and atlas,* Heidelberg, 1988, Springer Verlag.

33. Fung KP, Chow OKW, So SY: Attenuation of exercise induced asthma by acupuncture, *Lancet* ii:1419-1422, 1986.

34. Jobst KA et al: Controlled trial of acupuncture for disabling breathlessness, *Lancet* ii:416-419, 1986.

35. Lewith GT, Machin D: On the evaluation of the clinical effects of acupuncture: concepts and methods, *Pain* 16:111-127, 1983.

36. Kim SS: The mediator theory of acupuncture and its practical application in bronchial asthma and myaesthenia gravis, *Am J Acupuncture* 9(2):101-116, 1981.

37. Lee DZ, Sun AY: Effect of acupuncture on synaptosoma (Na+, K+)-ATPase. *Neurochem Res* 9(5):669-678, 1984.

38. Kuan TK et al: The effect of needle stimulation of Acupuncture Loci Tienshu (of 25) Chung Wan CV 12) on the immune response in sensitized mice against experimental cholera, *Am J Chinese Med* 14:73-85, 1986.

39. Lao YY et al: Effect of acupuncture on adenocortical hormone production. I. Variation in the ability for adrenocortical hormone production in relation to the deviation of acupuncture stimulation, *Am J Chinese Med* 7:362-371, 1979.

40. Nappi G et al: Different releasing effects of traditional manual acupuncture and electro-acupuncture on proprio-cortin related peptides, *Acupunct Electrother Res* 7:93-104, 1982.

41. Sternfield M et al: The role of acupuncture in asthma: changes in airways dynamics and LTC4 induced LAI, *Am J Chin Med* 17:129-134, 1989.

42. Tashkin DP et al: A controlled trial of real and simulated acupuncture in the management of chronic asthma, *J Aller Clin Immunol* 76:855-64, 1985.

43. Tashkin DP et al: Comparison of real and simulated acupuncture and isoproterenol in methacholine-induced asthma, *Ann Allergy* 39:379-87, 1977.

44. Linde K et al: Randomised clinical trials of acupuncture for asthma: a systematic review, *Forsch Komplemantarmed* 3(3):148-155, 1996.

45. Mitchell P, Wells JE: Acupuncture for chronic asthma: a controlled trial with six months follow up, *Am J Acupuncture* 17:5-13, 1989.

46. Takishima T et al: The bronchodilating effect of acupuncture in patients with acute asthma, *Ann Allergy* 48:44-49, 1982.

47. Kleijnen J, Ter Riet G, Knipschild P: Acupuncture and asthma: a review of controlled trials, *Thorax* 46:799-802, 1991.

48. Wen HL, Chau K: Status asthmaticus treated by acupuncture and electro-stimulation, *Asian J Med* 9:191-195, 1973.

49. Tandon MK, Soh PFT: Comparison of real and placebo acupuncture in histamine induced asthma: a double-blind crossover study, *Chest* 96:102-105, 1989.

50. Landa NM, Fadeeva MA: Acupuncture effect on reactivity of hormonal systems of children suffering from bronchial asthma, pollinosis and atopic dermatitis, *Br J Acupunc* 15:3-8, 1982.

51. Berger D, Nolte D: Acupuncture in bronchial asthma: body plethysmographic measurements of acute bronchospasmolytic effects, *Alt Med East West* 5:265-269, 1977.

52. Tandon MK, Soh PFT, Wood AT: Acupuncture for bronchial asthma? A double-blind crossover study, *Med J Australia* 154:409-412, 1991.

53. Virsik K et al: The effect of acupuncture on pulmonary function in bronchial asthma, *Progr Respir Res* 14:271-75, 1980.

54. Dias PLR, Subramaniam S, Lionel NDW: Effects of acupuncture in bronchial asthma: preliminary communication, *J Roy Soc Med* 75:245-248, 1982.

55. Chow OKW et al: Effect of acupuncture on exercise-induced asthma, *Lung* 161:321-326, 1983.

56. Christenson PA et al: Acupuncture and bronchial asthma, *Allergy* 39:379-385, 1984.

57. Sliwinski J, Matusiewicz R: The effect of acupuncture on the clinical state of patients suffering from chronic spastic bronchitis and undergoing long term treatment with corticosteroids, *Acup & Electrotherap Res* 9:203-215, 1984.

58. Jobst K A, Chen J H, Hext A: Review of acupuncture for bronchial asthma: a double-blind crossover study, *Comp Med Research* 1992;6:57-58.

59. Biernacki W, Peake MD: Acupuncture in treatment of stable asthma, *Respir Med* 92(9):1143-1145, 1998

60. MacPherson H: Fatal and adverse events from acupuncture: allegation, evidence and the implications, *J Altern Complement Med* 5(1):47-56, 1999.

61. Lazarou J, Pomeranz BH, Corey PN: Incidence of adverse drug reactions in hospitalised patients. A meta-analysis of prospective studies, *JAMA* 279(15):1200-1205, 1998.

62. Chen JH, Jobst KA: Childhood asthma: traditional Chinese medicine, *Comp Ther Med* 2:138-139, 1994.

63. Bonica JJ: Therapeutic acupuncture in the Peoples Republic of China: implications for America medicine, *JAMA* 228:1544-1551, 1974.

64. Joos S, Schott C, Zou H, et al: Immunomodulatory effects of acupuncture in the treatment of allergic asthma: a randomized controlled study, *J Altern Complement, Med* 6(6):519-525, 2000.

Suggested Readings

Aldridge D, Pietroni PC: Clinical assessment of acupuncture in asthma therapy: discussion paper, *J Roy Soc Med* 80: 222-224, 1987.

Bodner G, Topilsky M, Greif J: Pneumothorax as a complication of acupuncture in the treatment of bronchial asthma, *Ann Allergy* 51:401-403, 1983.

Calehr H: Acupuncture treatment of the asthmatic patient, *Am J Acupuncture* 1:41-45, 1973.

Carroin H, Epstein BS, Grand B: Complications of acupuncture, *JAMA* 228:1552-1554. 1974.

Chronic bronchitis, asthma and pulmonary emphysema: a statement by the committee on diagnostic standards for non-tuberculous respiratory diseases, *Am Rev Resp Dis* 85:762-768, 1962.

Corbett M, Sinclair M: Acu- and pleuro-puncture, *N Engl J Med* 17:167-168, 1974.

Dias PLR: Effects of acupuncture in bronchial asthma (reply to Marcus P), *J Roy Soc Med* 75:670, 1982.

Donnelly WJ, Spykerboer JE, Thong JH: Are patients who use alternative medicine disatisfied with orthodox medicine? *Med J Australia* 142:539-541, 1985.

Fuller JA: Acupuncture (letter about experience with 42 cases and 14 conditions), *Med J Australia* 31:340-341, 1974.

Fung KP: Acupuncture and asthma (letter), *Lancet* i:857, 1987.

Goldberg I: Pneumothorax associated with acupuncture, *Med J Australia* 1:941-942, 1973.

Hayhoe S: Effects of acupuncture in bronchial asthma (letter re: study by Dias), *J Roy Soc Med* 75:917,1982.

Jobst KA et al: Acupuncture for respiratory disease (letter), *Lancet* i:802,1987.

Kent G P et al: A large outbreak of acupuncture-associated Hepatits B, *Am J Epidemiol* 127:591-598, 1988.

Lewith GT, Kenyon JN: Physiological and psychological explanations for the mechanism of acupuncture as a treatment for chronic pain, *Soc Sci Med* 19(12):1367-1378, 1984.

Marcus P: Effects of acupuncture in bronchial asthma (letter re: study by Dias and reply), *J Roy Soc Med* 75:670, 1982.

Mazal DA, King T, Harvey J, et al: Bilateral pneumothorax after acupuncture, *N Engl J Med* 302:1365-1366, 1980.

Millman BS: Acupuncture: context and critique, *Ann Rev Med* 28:223-234,1977.

Platts-Mills TAE et al: Reduction of bronchial hyperreactivity during prolonged allergen avoidance, *Lancet* 2:675-678, 1982.

Ritter HG, Tarala R: Pneumothorax after acupuncture, *Br Med J* 26: 602-603, 1978.

Stack BHR: Pneumothorax associated with acupuncture, *Br Med J* 1:96, 1975.

Urban S, Bangha O, Kristufek P: Changes in breathing pattern in asthma after acupuncture, *Br Europ Phys* 19(3):49, 1983.

Veith I: Acupuncture (editorial), *JAMA* 228:1577-1578, 1974.

Vincent CA, Richardson PH: Acupuncture for some common disorders: a review of evaluative research, *J Roy Coll Gen Prac* 37:77-81,1987.

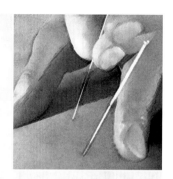

Oriental Medicine for Digestive Disorders

DAVID L. DIEHL

$\mathscr{A}$cupuncture and herbal medicine have a long history of use for gastrointestinal (GI) disorders. However, it is only recently that rigorous clinical studies and basic research data have supported this positive clinical impression. For example, acupuncture treatment for nausea is one of the most extensively researched and proven techniques in the whole body of clinical research in acupuncture for any indication.

This chapter reviews some of the indications for traditional Chinese medicine (TCM) in GI disease, conditions commonly treated, and research that has been done in this area. Finally, some suggestions on which patients to refer for TCM management are given. TCM is one style of Oriental medicine practice that follows standard "point prescriptions" and/or selects points based on the "pattern of illness." GI illnesses are treated by all styles of Chinese medicine, al-

though others will not be discussed in this chapter. For details, see Moss[1] on five-element theory, Helms[2] on French energetics theory, or Denmai[3] on Japanese meridian theory. Chapter 2 briefly discusses the various styles. Table 16-1 reviews potential applications of TCM for digestive disorders.

WHICH GASTROINTESTINAL PROBLEMS CAN BE TREATED WITH TRADITIONAL CHINESE MEDICINE?

TCM has been used for the entire range of GI disorders. A comprehensive review of the acupuncture literature has revealed studies of acupuncture treatment for a number of conditions.[4] Similarly, herbal medicine has been used for many GI disorders.

TABLE 16-1

Potential Applications of Traditional Chinese Medicine for Digestive Diseases

Condition	Biomedical therapy	TCM therapy	PRCT	Likeliness of usage*
Nausea and vomiting	IV antiemesis	PC 6 *(Neiguan)* acupuncture	Yes	5+
Irritable bowel syndrome	Anticholinergics, newer 5HT3 antagonists	Herbal medicine, acupuncture	Yes	4+
Postoperative ileus	Nasogastric suction, "tincture of time"	Acupuncture	Yes	3+
Ulcerative colitis	Corticosteroids, 5-ASA products	Herbal medicine	No	3+
Chronic viral hepatitis	Interferon, other antivirals	Herbal medicine	No	3+
Analgesia for endoscopy	IV benzodiazepines, IV opiates	Preprocedure acupuncture	Yes	2+
Gallstones	Surgery	Herbs, acupuncture	No	1+
Common bile duct stones	ERCP	Auricular acupuncture, herbs	No	1+
Acute appendicitis	Surgery, antibiotics	Acupuncture	No	1+

5HT3, 5-Hydroxytryptamine type 3 receptor; *5-ASA,* 5-aminosulfasalicylic acid; *ERCP,* endoscopic retrograde cholangiopancreatography; *PRCT,* prospective, randomized, controlled trial; *TCM,* traditional Chinese medicine.
*Likeliness of usage of the TCM alternative by biomedicine, 5+ very likely, 1+ not likely.

In some cases, using biomedicine is probably more efficient, since this medicine also can be successfully applied to treating a wide range of disorders of the GI system. For example, eradication of the bacterium *Helicobacter pylori* with antibiotics is the most efficient treatment for recurrent peptic ulcer disease (PUD). It is more efficient than prolonged use of herbal medicine and acupuncture, which have also been reported to be used for PUD. Similarly, although acupuncture and herbs can and have been used for acute appendicitis, surgery remains the mainstay for management of this disorder.

Nevertheless, Chinese medicine offers advantages in some situations, particularly in the care of conditions that allopathic medicine treats less successfully. These include the functional bowel disorders (e.g., irritable bowel syndrome), some cases of inflammatory bowel disease (ulcerative colitis and Crohn's disease), and chronic liver disease.

Functional Bowel Disorders

Management of functional bowel disorders (FBDs) often presents a real challenge to the gastroenterologist. The FBD most commonly encountered is irritable bowel syndrome (IBS). The treatments that are available are frequently nonspecific, and as any practitioner who has managed IBS knows, these available treatments often lack effectiveness. However, Chinese herbalists have been treating functional bowel disorders for centuries with considerable success, and Chinese herbs are routinely used for IBS.

FBDs are conditions affecting the nerves and smooth muscle of the gut. There may be a significant influence from descending neural pathways from the brain, which may be why stress often makes GI symptoms worse. The symptoms associated with FBD may be quite varied, and several symptoms may coexist in the same patient. Symptoms typically include abdominal pain in various locations, abdominal bloating, and changes in bowel habits. Different patterns of FBD may coexist, such as IBS and nonulcer dyspepsia (NUD). Nonintestinal symptoms, such as dysmenorrhea, fatigue, bladder symptoms, and poor sleep patterns, commonly occur with FBD symptoms.

FBDs are very common disorders that affect up to 15% of adults. The range of these disorders includes:

IBS
NUD
Noncardiac chest pain
Globus sensation ("plum-pit symptom" in Chinese medicine)

Bloating syndromes
Functional diarrhea
Unclassified functional bowel disease

Many people do not seek biomedical care for their symptoms but instead manage their symptoms with over-the-counter remedies. In these conditions, the results of clinical testing, such as blood tests, x-rays, computed tomography (CT) scans, and endoscopic evaluation, are typically normal. These results lead some clinicians to tell their patients that "the problem is all in your head." Frustration is experienced on both sides. The clinician is frustrated about the patient's continued symptoms that are not being helped by the proffered therapy, and the patient is frustrated by the lack of successful treatment and the clinician's disbelief in the reality of his or her symptoms. In some cases pharmaceuticals may help symptoms, but none address the root cause, and in many patients, these drugs are ineffective. CM may offer another set of treatment options for FBD.

Inflammatory Bowel Diseases: Crohn's Disease and Ulcerative Colitis

The inflammatory bowel diseases (IBDs) are immune-mediated conditions of the small intestine and colon. Exact causes are still unknown. Ulcerative colitis (UC) affects the large intestine, whereas Crohn's disease can affect the large intestine, the small intestine, or both. Unlike the FBDs, a diagnosis is generally easy to make, since colonoscopic examination and barium x-rays are almost always significantly abnormal. Both diseases (particularly UC) carry an increased risk of colon cancer after the patient has had the condition for more than a decade.

Immunosuppression with corticosteroids and other agents and use of aminosalicylates has remained the mainstay of therapy for UC and Crohn's disease for decades. More recently, the availability of tumor necrosis factor-alpha (TNF-α) antibody infusions has expanded the therapeutic armamentarium for management of IBD. However, patients remain dependent on steroids or have frequent relapses despite therapy. Another therapeutic modality would be welcome in the management of some of these stubborn cases. There are data regarding management of UC with Chinese herbal medicine that make this an area worthy of further study.

Chronic Viral Liver Diseases: Hepatitis B and C

Chronic viral hepatitis is one of the most common chronic infectious diseases known to humankind. Patients with chronic viral hepatitis, especially hepatitis B, carry a significantly increased risk of primary cancer of the liver (hepatocellular carcinoma [HCC]; also known as hepatoma). In fact, HCC is the most common cancer in humans. Aside from cancer, chronic viral hepatitis also can progress to cirrhosis and liver failure and is not a rare cause of death. Hepatitis B is endemic in Asia; hepatitis C has gained more attention for its increasing prevalence in the West.

The advent of injectable medication (interferon alpha-2b [INF-α2b] therapy, and more recently, INF-α2b combined with oral ribavirin) has given hepatologists more treatment options for chronic viral hepatitis. However, this mode of treatment is expensive and often toxic and may not be available to hepatitis patients in many parts of the world. In addition, this treatment is not very efficacious. In the United States, public awareness and concern regarding hepatitis C is growing. As a result, Americans are becoming more interested in alternative treatments for chronic viral hepatitis.

Because of the high prevalence of hepatitis B in China, it is not surprising that there is extensive clinical experience with the herbal treatment of this condition. In years to come, widely accepted clinical outcome markers, such as clearance of hepatitis B early antigen (HBeAg) from the blood and clearance of hepatitis B surface antigen (HBsAg), will be needed to document clinical response.[5] Recently, treatment of hepatitis C with herbal formulas has been attempted, and quantitative polymerase chain reaction (qPCR) of viral load (HCV-RNA qPCR) has been used as a marker of response.[6]

With the increasing prevalence of and public attention to hepatitis C, there has been a recent push to look at TCM therapy for chronic hepatitis.

TRADITIONAL CHINESE MEDICINE APPROACH TO GASTROINTESTINAL DISORDERS

In TCM, the essence of diagnosis lies in the identification of "patterns of illness."[7] The pattern is arrived at by combining elements from the patient's symptoms, other features noted on the review of systems, and data from physical signs, including pulse quality and tongue appearance. With this data, the nature of the patient's *pattern of disharmony* is identified, and treatment is directed at resolving the disharmony and bringing the body back into homeostasis (Table 16-2) (see Chapters 2 and 7).

Questions asked during a TCM diagnosis are sometimes different from those asked during a biomedical diagnosis. To identify the diagnostic pattern of a patient with a biomedical diagnosis (e.g., UC), the practitioner will ask many detailed questions including: Is there undigested food in the stool? Is there a burning sensation during defecation? At what time of day is the diarrhea worse? Is the smell of the diarrhea very strong? Is it urgent? What makes the condition better or worse? Are spasms relieved after defecation? Other questions concern the patient's energy, emotional well-being, sleep, and body temperature. Assessment of the patient's tongue and pulse quality may provoke additional questions. The pattern of disharmony identified by this diagnosis typically indicates both an immediate and an underlying condition.

The terminology of Chinese medicine diagnostic patterns is expressed according to different perceptions than those of biomedicine and sounds foreign to the ears of allopathic practitioners who are unfamiliar with TCM. For example, two common GI diagnostic patterns are *Spleen Qi Deficiency with Dampness* and *Liver Qi Stagnation* (see Table 16-2). A look at the component symptoms, however, shows them to be familiar. Thus Spleen Qi deficiency presents with anorexia, diarrhea, undigested food in the stool, lassitude, weak pulse in the Spleen position, and often a swollen wet tongue showing tooth marks along the edges and a thick white coating. Liver Qi Stagnation presents in many forms but typically includes a sensation of bloating in the hypochondriac region, borborygmus and flatus, a plum-pit sensation in the throat, headache, irritability, constipation or diarrhea, a string-taut pulse pattern, especially in the Liver position, and a tongue with redness along the edges.

A basic tenet of TCM is that treatment should be tailored to the individual patient based on clinical presentation. Different patients may have the same biomedical diagnosis but different TCM diagnoses. For example, five patients with a biomedical diagnosis of ulcerative colitis may have varying TCM diagnoses, and all five might receive different acupuncture treatments or herbal formulations. For further information on this topic, the reader is directed to several excellent books[7-10] and Chapters 2 and 7.

Commonly Used Acupuncture Points for Digestive Disorders

There are over 400 described acupuncture points. They are named by their relationship with one of 14 meridians, their functions on the ear or scalp, or their

TABLE 16-2

Common Traditional Chinese Medicine Diagnoses for Selected Gastrointestinal Disorders

Biomedical diagnosis	Traditional Chinese medicine pattern diagnoses
Irritable bowel syndrome	Stagnant Liver Qi invading the Spleen
	Damp-Heat in the Intestines
	Spleen Qi and/or Yang Deficiency
Ulcerative colitis	Damp-Heat in the Intestines
	Liver/Spleen Disharmony
	Spleen Qi Deficiency
	Spleen Yang Deficiency
	Blood Stasis
Chronic viral hepatitis	Damp-Heat in the Liver and Gallbladder
	Liver/Spleen Disharmony
	Liver and Kidney Yin Deficiency
	Blood Stagnation
	Spleen and Kidney Yang Deficiency

*Many patients have a combination of diagnoses. Recall that Spleen, Kidney, and Liver are functional Organ systems and have different connotations from the biomedical use of these terms.

special uses, as in the case of the newer "extra" points. The selection of acupuncture points to treat a condition may be done in a variety of ways, depending on the style; the underlying goal is always to bring the disordered body back into balance.

Rogers has abstracted a large body of published articles on acupuncture treatment and has entered the frequency of citations for the acupoints used into a computerized database.[11] A review of his database and general impressions from published studies suggest that commonly used acupoints for GI diseases are located in the following locations (Figure 16-1):

Paravertebrally in a dermatomal relationship with the GI organs (Back Shu points on the Urinary Bladder Meridian).
Over the abdomen, also in relation with the GI organs (Front Mu points, Ren (Conception Vessel) points, and other points).
On the extremities at well-known points (e.g., St 36 *Zusanli*, Sp 6 *Sanyinjiao,* and the Lower He-Sea points on lower leg; P 6 *Neiguan* on the inside of the wrist).
On the ear (auricular points).

Herb Selection and Gastrointestinal Dysfunction

TCM employs both patent combinations and individualized herbal prescriptions in treating disorders. As with pharmaceutical preparations, many common patented combinations are available over the counter. To create individualized prescriptions, the practitioner performs a diagnostic analysis and then selects groups of herbs that not only have individual effects but also create synergistic effects when used in combination (see Chapter 5).

RESEARCH DATA ON TRADITIONAL CHINESE MEDICINE AND GASTROINTESTINAL DISORDERS

There are few good studies of TCM for any GI condition. A plethora of case reports, including some reports that involve hundreds of patients, strongly suggest the potential clinical benefit of TCM but may not be convincing enough to biomedicine, which prefers evidence from prospective, randomized, controlled trials (PRCTs).

The lack of such studies is easy to understand. First, the concept of a placebo-controlled trial is not a historical part of Chinese medicine. The idea of giving a patient a placebo instead of active treatment for a condition is an equally foreign concept. As a result, it is only during the last few years, influenced by the evidentiary rules of biomedicine, that these trials have been attempted in TCM. Second, clinical trials demand validated outcomes measures, and only recently have some of these measures become available for studying disorders such as functional bowel disease. Third, designing valid research with nonbiomedical interventions such as acupuncture or herbs demands new approaches, and this point has been only slowly realized[12] (see Chapters 11, 12, 13, 15, and 19).

Nevertheless, properly performed PRCTs showing a positive effect of TCM exist in the following areas:

Antiemesis
- Chemotherapy-associated
- Motion-induced
- Postoperative
IBS (single herbal medicine study)
Acupuncture analgesia for endoscopy (several acupuncture studies)
Postoperative ileus

Clearly better PRCTs are necessary. At the same time, we currently have sufficient evidence to make it reasonable to use acupuncture and selected herbs to treat GI conditions that are not well-managed by biomedicine.

Effects of Acupuncture on the Physiology of the Digestive System

Abundant evidence exists in the scientific literature to suggest a physiological basis for the effects of acupuncture on the GI tract. Studies have been done in both animal models and humans demonstrating effects on gut motility and gastric acid secretion. The body of this literature therefore points to a true effect of the needling (with or without electrical stimulation) rather than just a placebo effect.

Gastrointestinal Motility and Sensation
Controlled animal and human studies have shown an effect of acupuncture on gastric and intestinal motility. Different methodologies have been used for assessing effects, such as implanted strain gauges (in

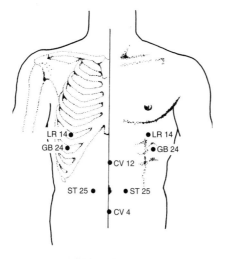

Abdominal points

Point	*"Mu"* (Gathering) Point of:	Level of Nerve Root
*ST 25	Large intestine	T10-T11
*CV 12	Stomach	T8-T9
CV 4	Small intestine	T12-L1
LI 14	Liver	T8-T9
GB 24	Gall bladder	T7-T8

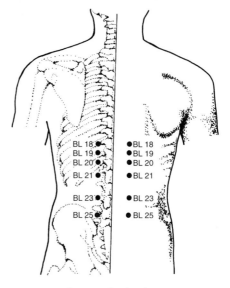

Paravetebral points

Point on Bladder (BL) Meridian	*"Shu"* (Transporting) Point of:	Level of Nerve Root
BL 18	Liver	T9-T10
BL 19	Gall bladder	T10-T11
BL 20	Spleen	T11-L12
BL 21	Stomach	T12-L1
BL 23	Kidney	L2-3
BL 25	Large intestine	L4-5

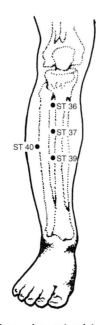

Lower leg, anterolateral

Point on Stomach (ST) Meridian	Traditional Function
*ST 36	Lower He-Sea point of Stomach meridian
ST 37	Lower He-Sea point of Large Intestine meridian
ST 39	Lower He-Sea point of Small Intestine meridian
ST 40	Luo-connecting point of Stomach meridian

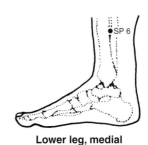

Lower leg, medial

*SP 6   Innervation level L4

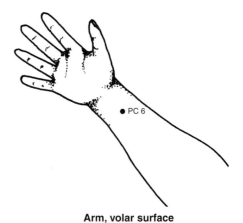

Arm, volar surface

*PC 6   Median nerve (C6-C7)
(also referred to as
"Master of the Heart" (MH) 6)

Figure 16-1 Commonly used acupuncture points for digestive conditions. *Designates one of the five most commonly used points.

animal models), manometry, endoscopic observation of antral motility, and fluoroscopic observation of barium passage. Acupuncture effects on electrical activity in the gut have been measured with implanted electrodes (electromyogram [EMG]), and with surface electrical measurements (electrogastrogram [EGG]).

Li et al[13] summarized the effects of acupuncture on motility, EMG, and EGG. They concluded that active acupuncture has a significantly greater effect than placebo acupuncture for gastric motility, with incomplete data on small bowel motility. Restoration of disrupted interdigestive migrating motor complexes (MMC) has been noted. A self-regulating or homeostatic action has been reported,[14] with inhibitory or stimulatory effects being dependent on initial motility.

Gastric Acid Secretion

The effect of acupuncture on acid secretion has been examined in animal models as well as in humans (Figure 16-2). These studies have examined the effect of acupuncture on basal acid output (BAO), stimulated acid output (maximal acid output [MAO]), and vagus nerve mediated acid output (sham feeding). In one PRCT on human volunteers,[15] electroacupuncture (although not sham acupuncture, simple acupuncture, or "laser acupuncture") reduced vagally stimulated acid secretion. Another randomized, placebo-controlled

study[16] showed that electroacupuncture decreased BAO compared with sham acupuncture but had no effect on pentagastrin-stimulated MAO. This effect was blocked by pretreatment with intravenous (IV) *naloxone* (an agent that blocks the effects of endogenous opioids).

Similar effects were seen in animal studies. In animal models, cannulas can be placed directly into the animal's stomach, and acid secretion can be precisely measured. Electroacupuncture can inhibit acid secretion by as much as 75%. This effect coincides with significant changes in hormones that are known to be involved in the physiology of acid secretion, including somatostatin, gastrin, vasoactive intestinal peptide, and β-endorphin.[17] Other investigators[18] showed increases in gastric bicarbonate secretion and decreased acid secretion. These effects were blocked by both local anesthetic and anticholinergic agents at the acupoints. These findings suggest a neural reflex that involves cutaneous receptors and the vagus nerve.

Clinical Uses of Acupuncture for Digestive Disorders

Antiemesis

Clinical benefit of acupuncture or acupressure has been shown in nausea and emesis associated with chemotherapy, postoperative state, optokinetic stimulation, and pregnancy. Typically, the well-known "antinausea point" P 6 (*Neiguan,* Pericardium-6, Master of the Heart-6) has been used. Local anesthesia (intradermal and subcutaneous infiltration with 1% lidocaine) at P 6 block the antiemetic effect of electroacupuncture stimulation of this point.[19]

Dundee has carried out many of the PRCTs in the use of PC-6 antiemesis. He has summarized the clinical usefulness of PC-6 antiemesis[20] and has also raised the possibility of self-administered transcutaneous electrical nerve stimulation (TENS) at PC 6 for antiemesis. TENS for this indication has been used at a frequency of 10 to 15 Hz with amplitude suited to patient tolerance—typically in the mA range.

Recently, a prospective, sham-needle controlled trial of acupuncture for emesis associated with chemotherapy was carried out in 30 patients.[21] This study was unique in that the patients included for study received a very aggressive chemotherapeutic regimen before autologous bone marrow transplantation. This chemotherapy regimen is especially emetogenic and thus was a challenging test of the efficacy of

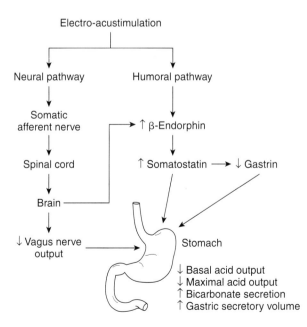

Figure 16-2 Mechanism of effect of electro-acustimulation on decreasing gastric acid secretion.

acupuncture. Electroacupuncture at PC 6 and ST 36 (4 Hz for 20 minutes daily between 7 and 9 AM for 5 days) was used, with results compared to sham acupuncture (minimal acupuncture with mock electrostimulation at nearby control points near LU 7 and GB 34). Clinical outcomes that were followed included nurse-recorded vomiting episodes and patient self-rated nausea and global quality of life measures using a previously validated symptom diary. The number of emesis episodes over 5 days was lower for subjects receiving specific acupuncture than for those receiving either nonspecific acupuncture or no acupuncture ($p = 0.02$). Nausea severity and quality of life measures were also more favorable in the specific acupuncture group.

Another recent report studied acupuncture in preventing postoperative nausea and vomiting.[22] Eighty-one patients scheduled for gynecological laparoscopic surgery were randomly assigned to an acupuncture group (with manual stimulation at PC 6) or a control group (no needling). Bandages were placed at the wrist after surgery in both groups to maintain patient blinding. Acupuncture was found to decrease the incidence of nausea and vomiting in the recovery room and also after discharge. The authors also analyzed the incidence of nausea and vomiting in patients with a history of previous postoperative nausea and vomiting and/or motion sickness. Acupuncture was found to be useful even in this group of patients.

Vection-induced motion sickness is an interesting model to test the effect of acupuncture on nausea. In this experimental model, subjects are seated inside a rotating metal cylinder that has a striped pattern on the inside, which induces "motion sickness" (stomach discomfort, nausea, and vomiting) and is associated with an increase in measurable gastric myoelectrical activity as measured by the EGG from 3 cycles per minute (cpm) to 4 to 9 cpm. This effect has been referred to as *tachygastria*. In a carefully controlled study using this model, Hu et al[23] studied the effects of electroacupuncture, sham acupuncture, or no acustimulation on the clinical manifestations of motion sickness and changes on the EGG. Also, experiments were performed on Chinese subjects in addition to Caucasian and African-American subjects because of concerns that results might be influenced by the placebo effect or caused by a unique response of Chinese subjects. In this study, the acustimulation group reported fewer symptoms of motion sickness than the sham-acustimulation or control groups, and tachygastria was also less. Caucasian and African-American subjects benefited as much as the Chinese subjects.

Postoperative Gastrointestinal Dysmotility

An intriguing possible clinical application is the use of acupuncture in cases of postoperative ileus or gastric atony after vagotomy. A positive effect has been noted in case reports in humans and animals. In a prospective, randomized trial, Liu and Zhao[24] examined the effects of acupuncture at ST 36 and SP 6 given 12 to 24 hours postoperatively on 39 abdominal surgical patients. Time to first passage of stool (and serum liver tests) improved significantly. Xunshi[25] performed a prospective, randomized study of 100 patients after laparotomy (gastrectomy or cholecystectomy) using tender points on the hand. Points in the real acupuncture group were needled manually 30 to 40 minutes daily until flatus occurred. The treatment group passed flatus at an average of 42 hours postoperatively compared with 92 hours for the control group.

Kabanov et al[26] used acupuncture in 220 patients with purulent peritonitis to try to restore motor function of the stomach and intestines. Although this study was not randomized, a single session of acupuncture improved patients with local peritonitis, whereas 100 patients with diffuse peritonitis needed 2 to 3 sessions for clinical effect. Twenty patients in the diffuse group showed no effect. Wu et al[27] analyzed 250 gastrectomy patients, noting advantages of using acupuncture in preventing the need for routine gastric decompression and allowing earlier refeeding.

Analgesia in Gastrointestinal Endoscopy

In the United States and much of the industrialized world, "conscious sedation" with pharmaceutical agents is the standard for GI endoscopic procedures. In other countries, unsedated endoscopy is more common. Five prospective randomized studies demonstrate the efficacy of acupuncture as analgesia for endoscopic procedures, such as upper endoscopy (gastroscopy) and colonoscopy. The methodology for these studies is good; two are sham-needle controlled,[28,29] and three compare acupuncture with IV premedication.[30-32] Taken together, these reports suggest that acupuncture analgesia is effective for both upper endoscopy and colonoscopy and in most cases gives results similar to IV sedation. Although this approach does not provide the depth of analgesia and the anamnestic response to benzodiazepine anesthesia (which usually occurs during sedated endoscopy), it may find a role in providing another option for analgesia when a patient undergoes an unsedated endoscopic examination.

Clinical Uses of Herbal Medicine for Digestive Disorders

The following are three main areas in gastroenterology where TCM herbal formulations may have a potentially large impact on disease management:

IBS
Inflammatory bowel disease (UC and Crohn's disease)
Chronic viral liver disease

In difficult cases of these conditions but also in less severe patients, Chinese herbal medicine may fill an important niche.

Herbal Medicine for Irritable Bowel Syndrome

Bensoussan et al[33] described a blinded PRCT of the use of Chinese herbal medicine for IBS. A total of 116 patients who fulfilled the Rome criteria for IBS were recruited during an 18-month period. One group received a standard herbal formula consisting of 20 different herbs designed, according to TCM, to regulate and improve bowel function. A second group received individually tailored formulations that were modified at various stages of treatment (a classical TCM approach), and the third group received a placebo. The gastroenterologist, the Chinese herbal practitioner, and the patient did not know to which group they were assigned. The success of blinding patients to treatment was tested at regular intervals throughout the treatment. Outcomes that were followed included change in total bowel symptom scale (BSS) scores, global improvement assessed by patients and gastroenterologists, and change in the degree of interference in life caused by IBS symptoms as assessed by patients.

There was a significant difference between the mean total BSS scores as assessed by patients and physicians, with patients in either treatment group (standardized or individualized herbal combination) responding significantly better compared with patients receiving placebo. No significant differences were noted between standardized and individualized herbal treatment groups. There was also improvement in global improvement scores as assessed by patients

and physicians for the treatment groups as compared with placebo.

Although the standardized herb group performed slightly better than the individualized herb group, the study suggests that the individualized therapies may work better over the long term. Results of the BSS administered to patients 14 weeks after the completion of the study showed that only the individualized herb group maintained improvement. In the individualized herb group, 75% of patients stated that they felt improvement, compared with 63% of patients in the standardized herb group and 32% in the placebo group. As far as adverse effects of the herbs, two patients withdrew from the trial due to discomfort associated with the treatment (GI discomfort in one patient and headaches in another). Liver function tests were obtained from all study participants after 8 weeks of treatment and showed no abnormalities.

This study is notable for the scientific rigor with which it was performed. Other studies in the literature are lacking in appropriate methodology, although positive results of herbal medicine may be observed. For example, in a 1986 study, 120 patients with chronic diarrhea caused by IBS were given an herbal combination.[34] The study design, although prospective, was not randomized, and insufficient details regarding blinding were included. The authors reported that 67.5% of patients had sustained normalization of bowel movements at 1-year follow-up. Thirty-one percent of patients showed improvement, whereas only 4.2% showed no change in symptoms.

Herbal Medicine for Ulcerative Colitis

Chen has done numerous studies using a formulation of 11 Chinese herbs to treat UC.[35,36] In a number of studies published by his group, initial response rates typically exceeded 60%, and recurrence rates at 6 months or 1-year follow-up were low (approximately 10%). Response was also evaluated by colonoscopy and measurement of immune markers. Some of the studies that were done at Chen's institution were randomized, with some study participants receiving standard therapy with sulfasalazine and hydrocortisone. Unfortunately, exact details of the randomization protocol and issues related to blinding were not completely described. In addition, standard outcomes measures used by clinical research groups working in the field of IBD were not used in this study.

Other intriguing results have been observed in the United States with the use of standard herbal combinations for IBD. In some cases, patients who were steroid dependent could be tapered off their medication when Chinese herbal therapies were instituted. Preliminary results indicate that patients with UC respond more favorably than patients with Crohn's disease. Gaeddert has described other herbal combinations that may be of benefit in managing IBD.[37] It would be useful to undertake PRCTs based on these encouraging preliminary results.

Herbal Medicine for Chronic Liver Disease

A large body of research has documented "hepatoprotective" effects of certain herbal extracts. The largest body of information is available for silymarin,[38] which is derived from the milk thistle plant (Silybum marianum). The active constituent is silybin, which has been shown to exert hepatoprotective effects and also shows usefulness in the management of acute and chronic hepatitis. Although silymarin is not technically a Chinese herb, it is commonly combined with Chinese herbs to treat chronic liver disease.

Other plants that are commonly used for herbal treatment of chronic liver disease include gan cao (licorice root), wu wei zi (schisandra fruit), dan shen (salvia root), hu zhang (bushy knotweed root and rhizome), yu jin (Curcuma), nu zhen zi (ligustrum), pu gong ying (dandelion), ban lan gen (isatis root), and yin chen hao (capillaris). There are intriguing and exciting basic, animal, and clinical data regarding the beneficial effects of these substances on liver function. Other plant extracts have been investigated for their potential helpful effects. As mentioned earlier, clinical pattern recognition is most often used as a basis for selecting an herbal therapy.

There are limited data regarding effectiveness of viral clearance, since viral quantitation is a more recent development. However, clearance of antibody over a limited follow-up period (3 to 6 months) has been reported. Batey et al[6] studied 40 patients with hepatitis C in a randomized, blinded, and placebo-controlled trial of a Chinese herbal combination (CH-100). There was a significant reduction in alanine transaminase (ALT) levels over the 6-month study period (with normalization in four patients); however, no patient cleared the virus as determined by qPCR.

Suppression of hepatic fibrosis by herbal combinations is another treatment outcome that would potentially have significant benefit. To date there are no allopathic therapies that can accomplish this effect. In rat models of liver fibrosis (dimethylnitrosamine-induced liver injury), a Chinese herbal formula known as Sho-saiko-to (commonly used by Japanese Kampo medical doctors) was shown to be beneficial in decreasing hepatic levels of collagen and improving markers of lipid peroxidation.[39]

Prevention of HCC arising in patients with cirrhosis is another area that has attracted the attention of clinicians interested in the therapeutic use of herbal medicine. One report from Japan used Sho-saiko-to in a prospective, randomized study of 260 patients followed for 5 years.[40] Cumulative incidence of HCC was lower and survival was better in the treated group, particularly in those patients without hepatitis B surface antigen.

Research on herbal medicine is a rapidly moving front. A National Institutes of Health (NIH)-funded Complementary Medicine Center at Hennepin County Medical Center in Minneapolis has recently won approval from the United States Food and Drug Administration (FDA) to test a Chinese herbal combination for chronic hepatitis C.[41] This will be an important trial to rigorously test the effectiveness of an herbal combination for this disease. Other groups have proposed herbal combinations based on TCM differentiation combined with acupuncture, Qi Gong, and Chinese dietary therapy.[42]

The Issue of Potential Hepatotoxicity of Chinese Herbal Medicine

Without question, herbal medicine, including Chinese herbal combinations, is safer than pharmaceutical agents. Herbal medicines have less profound immediate effects on physiology and work more gradually. For most herbal formulations, practitioners have long-standing experience with both the individual plants and the combination of plants used in the formulas. In addition, Chinese herbal theory designs formulas to minimize potential side effects of any one herb.

The safety of giving herbal medication to patients who already have preexisting liver disease is an important concern; however, hepatotoxicity in this situation has not been reported. Some GI reactions have been noticed, including nausea, bloating, diarrhea, and constipation. In addition, excessive intake of licorice root may cause a hyperaldosteronemia-like syndrome. However, it appears to be very rare at commonly prescribed doses.[43]

There have been reported cases of hepatotoxicity of herbal medicines. However, it is not fair to implicate herbal medicines in general as being hepatotoxic. Most cases of hepatotoxicity can be traced to the use of plants that contain pyrrolizidine alkaloids.[44] Examples of such plants include germander, comfrey, and chaparral. Use of these substances is uncommon in Chinese herbal formulas, and these substances are never used as "single agents." Almost all of the cases of hepatotoxicity with pyrrolizidine-containing plants were from overuse or overdose of extracts or teas from one plant, not combination formulas.

Several cases of hepatotoxicity have been reported with a patent formula called *Jin Bu Wan*.[45] This patent medicine contains the single active ingredient levotetrahydropalmitine, which is present in the plant genera *Stephania* and *Corydalis*. The active ingredient is structurally similar to the pyrrolizidine alkaloids, which may be the mechanism of toxicity.

Another potential source of hepatotoxicity of Chinese herbal medicine is the surreptitious addition of a potentially hepatotoxic medication (acetaminophen, for example) to "patent medicines." There have been several cases reported of these patent medicines containing pharmaceuticals (e.g., diazepam in a herbal sleeping aid or prednisone in a herbal arthritis pill; see Chapter 5). The inclusion of these substances is not an accepted practice, but misleading labeling by unscrupulous manufacturers has led to this occurrence.

Contamination of herbal medication by pesticides and heavy metals is also a possibility. However, no cases of hepatotoxicity have been described by this mechanism. Drug-herb interaction is another possible cause that should be considered. Inclusion of herbal substances that increase activity of the P450 system may cause problematic interactions between herbal medications and pharmaceuticals. Again, no clear incidences of hepatotoxicity have been described in the literature related to this mechanism.

The following are keys to avoiding hepatotoxicity from Chinese herbal medicine:

- Receive herbal prescriptions only from qualified herbalists.
- Avoid herbs containing pyrrolizidine alkaloids or other known hepatotoxins.
- Use only herbs from trustworthy manufacturers that are unlikely to contain misidentified herbs, toxic substances, or pharmaceuticals.
- Take herbal compounds only in the recommended doses, which typically have a long history of safe use. A philosophy of "if a little is good, a lot is better" can be dangerous.

REFERRAL FOR MANAGEMENT OF GASTROINTESTINAL PROBLEMS

After excluding the presence of a more serious condition, clinicians who conclude that FBD alone accounts for their patients' symptoms may want to refer them to a professional practitioner of Oriental medicine (see Chapter 21). Because FBDs are so common and many patients self-refer, it may also be useful for biomedical practitioners to check with their patients to see if they have already begun Chinese medical care.

In most cases, self-referral is reasonable; additionally, Chinese medical practitioners are prepared to refer patients to biomedical practitioners when certain symptoms are prominent. Even so, allopathic practitioners often fear that patients will pursue alternative therapies before adequate diagnostic biomedical work-up, causing delay in the diagnosis of a GI malignancy. The likelihood of this outcome can be minimized by openness in discussing a patient's self-care efforts and by establishing strong working relationships with professional Chinese medicine practitioners in the neighborhood of one's practice. Coordinated care is most likely to both benefit and protect the patient.

Some symptoms that may represent a more serious condition (even a malignancy of the GI tract) include unintentional weight loss, blood in the stool, jaundice, or prolonged or recurrent vomiting. While observing the progress of Chinese medicine therapy, the referring biomedical practitioner should continue to monitor and objectively judge the patient's response to treatment. Progression of symptoms or appearance of worrisome symptoms such as those listed should prompt a full evaluation if this has not already been done.

Patients with jaundice or significant liver disease require a complete evaluation by a liver specialist before embarking on herbal treatment. The evaluation is mainly used to exclude the presence of a disease process that could be better managed by biomedicine (e.g., obstruction of the common bile duct by either tumor or stones, which can cause jaundice, or hemochromatosis [iron overload in the liver]). Once the decision is made to begin herbal treatment, it is still wise to continue to follow liver function tests.

DIRECTIONS
FOR THE FUTURE

Oriental medicine has a long history of safe and effective use for GI problems. It is currently in wide use in Japan and China for these conditions. In a United States survey of 575 patients in six clinics, Cassidy found that 22.4% were seeking help with digestive symptoms, and 93% reported disappearance or improvement of symptoms.[46]

Recent research is confirming the clinical experience of effectiveness for several conditions. In addition, biomedicine admits to limitations in its management of certain difficult problems. TCM finds its most widespread use for those conditions that allopathic medicine treats less successfully, including FBDs such as IBS, some cases of IBD (UC and Crohn's disease), and chronic liver disease.

To speed up this process, better clinical research and better education of physicians are needed. Research will gradually provide evidence of the true efficacy of the Chinese medicine approach, thus improving our ability to determine which patients are most likely to benefit from it. If these studies confirm the clinical experience of effectiveness, we can expect an expansion of use of Oriental medicine in the care of GI disorders.

References

1. Moss CA: Five elements and medical acupuncture, *AAMA Rev* 3:21-6, 1991.
2. Helms J: *Acupuncture energetics: a clinical approach for physicians,* Berkeley, Calif, 1995, Medical Acupuncture Publishers.
3. Denmai S: *Introduction to meridian therapy,* Seattle, 1990, Eastland Press.
4. Diehl DL: Acupuncture for gastrointestinal and hepatobiliary disorders, *J Altern Complement Med* 5:27-45, 1999.
5. Malik AH, Lee WM: Chronic hepatitis B virus infection: treatment strategies for the next millennium, *Ann Intern Med* 132:723-31, 2000.
6. Batey RG, Bensoussan A, Fan YY, et al: Preliminary report of a randomized, double-blind, placebo-controlled trial of a Chinese herbal medicine preparation CH-100 in the treatment of chronic hepatitis C, *J Gastroenterol Hepatol* 13(3):244-7, 1998.
7. Maciocia G: *Chinese medicine,* Edinburgh, 1997, Churchill Livingstone.
8. Ross J: *Zang Fu: the organ systems of traditional Chinese medicine,* Edinburgh, 1986, Churchill Livingstone.
9. Kaptchuk TJ: *The web that has no weaver: understanding Chinese medicine,* New York, 1983, Congdon & Weed.
10. Beinfield H, Korngold E: *Between heaven and earth: a guide to Chinese medicine,* New York, 1992, Random House.
11. Rogers PAM: *The choice of acupuncture points for acupuncture therapy,* 1990, The medical acupuncture webpage, http://homepage.tinet.ie/~progers/roghome.htm.
12. Hammerschlag R: Methodological and ethical issues in clinical trials of acupuncture, *J Altern Complement Med* 4(2):159-172, 1998.
13. Li Y, Tougas G, Chiverton SG, et al: The effect of acupuncture on gastrointestinal function and disorders, *Am J Gastroenterol* 87:1372-1381, 1992.
14. Qian LW, Lin YA: Effect of electroneedling of Zusanli on kinetic function of the human pylorus, *Int J Clin Acupunct* 5:139-144, 1994.
15. Lux G, Hagel J, Backer P, et al: Acupuncture inhibits basal gastric acid secretion stimulated by sham feeding in healthy subjects, *Gut* 35:1026-1029, 1994.
16. Tougas G, Yuan LY, Radamaker JW, et al: Effect of acupuncture on gastric acid secretion in healthy male volunteers, *Dig Dis Sci* 37:1576-1582, 1992.
17. Jin HO, Zhou L, Lee KY, et al: Inhibition of acid secretion by electrical acupuncture is mediated via beta-endorphin and somatostatin, *Am J Physiol* 271:G542-30, 1996.
18. Zhou L, Chey WY: The effect of electroacupuncture on gastric secretion in dogs, *Chen Tzu Yen Chiu* 10:131-136, 1985.
19. Dundee JW, Ghaly G: Local anesthesia blocks the antiemetic action of P 6 acupuncture, *Clin Pharmacol Ther* 50:78-80, 1991.
20. Dundee JW, McMillan CM: Clinical uses of P 6 acupuncture antiemesis, *Acupunct Electrother* 15:211-215, 1990.
21. Shen J, Wegner N, Glaspy J, et al: Electroacupuncture for control of myeloablative chemotherapy-induced emesis: a randomized, controlled trial, *JAMA* 28:2755-2761, 2000.
22. Al-Sadi M, Newman B, Julious SA: Acupuncture in the prevention of postoperative nausea and vomiting, *Anesthesia* 52:658-661, 1997.
23. Hu SQ, Stern RM, Koch KL: Electrical acustimulation relieves vection-induced motion sickness, *Gastroenterology* 102:1854-1858, 1992.
24. Liu JX, Zhao Q: Effect of acupuncture on intestinal motion and seroenzyme activity in perioperation, *Chung His I Chieh Ho Tsa Chih* 11:156-157, 1991.
25. Xunshi W: Clinical study on the use of second metacarpal holographic acupoints of reestablishing gastrointestinal motility in patients following abdominal surgery, *Am J Acupunct* 22:353-356, 1994.
26. Kabanov AN, Vozliublennyi SI, Platonov NS, et al: Use of acupuncture for restoring motor and transit functions on the stomach and intestines in suppurative peritonitis, *Klin Khir* 1:33-34, 1989.

27. Wu KH, Hsu YS, Kuo WC, et al: Abdominal surgery without routine gastric decompression, intravenous infusing, and fasting: analysis of 250 cases of subtotal gastrectomy, *Chung Hua I Hsueh Tsa Chih (Taipei)* 7:390-393, 1974.

28. Cahn AM, Carayon P, Hill C, et al: Acupuncture in gastroscopy, *Lancet* 1(8057):182-183, 1978.

29. Li CK, Nauck M, Loser C, et al: Acupuncture for lessening pain during colonoscopy, *Deutsche Med Wochenscrift* 116:367-370, 1991.

30. Wang HH, Chang YH, Liu DM: A study in the effectiveness of acupuncture analgesia for colonoscopic examination compared with conventional premedication, *Am J Acupunct* 20:217-221, 1992.

31. Wang HH, Chang YH, Liu DM, et al: A clinical study on physiologic response in electroacupuncture analgesia and meperidine analgesia for colonoscopy, *Am J Chin Med* 25:13-20, 1997.

32. Chu H, Zhao SZ, Huang YJ: Application of acupuncture during gastroscopy with a fiberoptic endoscope, *J Trad Chin Med* 7:279, 1987.

33. Bensoussan A, Talley NJ, Hing M, et al: Treatment of irritable bowel syndrome with Chinese herbal medicine, *JAMA* 280:1585-1590, 1998.

34. Chase C: 120 cases of the use of shan yao che qian zi tang in the treatment of irritable bowel syndrome, *Shanghai J Chin Herb Med* 3:33, 1992 (translation).

35. Chen Z et al: 596 cases of chronic colitis treated with jianpiling tablet, *Shenxi J Tradit Chin Med* 12(9):406, 1991.

36. Chen Z, Nie ZW, Sun QL: Clinical study in treating intractable ulcerative colitis with traditional Chinese medicine, *J Integrat Chin West Med* 14(7):400-2, 1994.

37. Gaeddert A: *Healing digestive disorders: natural treatments for gastrointestinal conditions,* Berkeley, Calif, 1998, North Atlantic Books.

38. Flora K, Hahn M, Rosen H, et al: Milk thistle *(Silybum marianum)* for the therapy of liver disease, *Am J Gastroenterol* 93:139-143, 1998.

39. Shimizu I, Ma YR, Mizobuchi Y, et al: Effects of Sho-saiko-to, a Japanese herbal medicine, on hepatic fibrosis in rats, *Hepatology* 29(1):149-60, 1999.

40. Oka H, Yamamoto S, Kuroki T, et al: Prospective study of chemoprevention of hepatocellular carcinoma with Sho-saiko-to (TJ 9), *Cancer* 76(5):743-9, 1995.

41. Culliton P: Personal communication, 1999.

42. Cohen M: *Hepatitis help area: an East-West comprehensive approach,* http://www.docmisha.com.

43. Dharmananda S: *Institute for traditional medicine,* http://www.itmonline.org.

44. Larrey D, Pageaux GP: Hepatotoxicity of herbal remedies and mushrooms, *Semin Liver Dis* 15(3):183-188, 1995.

45. Woolf GM, Petrovic LM, Rojter SE, et al: Acute hepatitis associated with the Chinese herbal product Jin Bu Huan, *Ann Intern Med* 121:729-735, 1994.

46. Cassidy CM: Chinese medicine users in the United States. Part I: utilization, satisfaction, medical plurality, *J Altern Complement Med* 4(1):17-27, 1998.

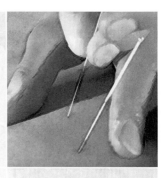

Acupuncture in Women's Reproductive Health

VALENTIN TUREANU
LUMINITA TUREANU

The way of healing is so profound....
How many truly know it?

The Yellow Emperor's Classic of Medicine

More women than men use the health care system in most settings, including alternative medicine.[1-6] The typical private office user of Chinese medicine, as described by Cassidy,[7] is female; she also is of reproductive age, is well-educated, and has a professional or managerial occupation. In Cassidy's study, 17.4% of the sample sought care for women's reproductive-related complaints, and 78.3% of these reported improvement. Attention to women's health forms a large proportion of both training and care delivery in the practice of Chinese medicine. The potential for this type of medicine to improve women's health was recently acknowledged with the establish-ment of the Center for Complementary and Alternative Medicine Research in Women's Health at Columbia University, College of Surgeons and Physicians.[8]

The theory underlying acupuncture care for women's reproductive health can be difficult for biomedical professionals to understand because many concepts and terms have no equivalent in biomedicine. Thus we believe it is so important and eventually so rewarding to develop the necessary background combined with individual inclination to understand Chinese medicine before attempting practice. This chapter provides an introduction to essential concepts, presents some of the problems that can be ad-

310

dressed, and briefly reviews selected research studies on women's reproductive health.

ORIENTAL MEDICAL THEORY AND WOMEN'S REPRODUCTIVE HEALTH

Two points should be emphasized. First, although the focus is on women's reproductive health, Chinese medicine views the woman's health *as a whole*. Second, the theory informing reproductive care is much the same as the theory informing all of Chinese medicine (see Chapter 2).*

Yin and Yang

Women are considered more Yin than Yang in their fundamental characteristics; men the reverse. Yin and Yang are complementary (not opposite), and the woman's Yin tendency is viewed as complementary to and interconnected with the man's Yang tendency. Belonging to Yin implies an important point about the balance of the fundamental substances of Qi and Blood, namely, that women also manifest a preponderance of Blood.

Qi and Blood

Normal physiological behaviors such as menstruation, pregnancy, lactation, menopause, and reproductive system pathological conditions are all manifestations of the balance or imbalance of these two "energetic" entities. Qi is defined as the foundation of all things in the universe and the source of any change and movement. Different categories of Qi have been described and most activity (or function) is attributed to Qi: growing and developing, the moving of Blood and distributing of body fluids, defending, warming, holding,* raising, and regulating.[9] There is neither an equivalent term nor a concept in biomedicine for this complex, nonpalpable ubiquitous foundation. Similarly, although the Chinese concept of Blood *(Xue)* has some overlap with the biomedical concept, it is something rather different than conventional Western thinking. Blood is the nutrient substance that circulates within the vessels (both blood vessels and Meridians/Channels), nourishes the Organs, and provides the foundation for mental activity. Therefore Blood deficiency can manifest as mental disorder.

Qi and Blood have a reciprocal relationship such that a deficiency of one eventually results in a deficiency of the other. For example, in severe Blood loss (as from uterine flooding), it is said that Qi follows the Blood in exhaustion.[9] Thus Qi, also deficient, cannot control the blood, and leaking or further hemorrhages can occur.

The Organs and Women's Reproduction

Chinese medicine identifies 12 Zang-Fu Organs and 6 Curious† Organs. The *Uterus* is one of the Curious Organs. It is also named "Cover of Yin,"‡ and "Palace of the Child" and sometimes is compared with a lotus flower that holds the seeds of a new life. Like other Curious Organs, it stores Essence and Blood.[10]

The Uterus has a strong relationship with the Kidney, since the Kidney Qi commands the reproductive function. The Kidney stores the aspect of Jing Essence that matures at puberty, contributing to the onset of

---

*The perceptions and resulting language of biomedicine and Chinese medicine are considerably different. This chapter uses both terminologies, although readers should note that concepts such as "fetus" and "spermatozoon" do not originate with Chinese medicine, and terms such as "amenorrhea" or "osteoporosis" are biomedical usages applied to conditions long recognized by Chinese medicine. We believe our terminological decision is appropriate since the two medicines are increasingly interacting and Chinese medical texts themselves increasingly use biomedical physiological terms when the underlying concepts are accepted and the terminology is lacking in the traditional phrasing of the medicine.

---

*For example, holding the organs in place; a failure results in prolapse; holding the Blood in the vessels; a failure results in extravasation; and so on.

†Also called Extraordinary Organs, these include the Uterus, Brain, Marrow, Bone, Blood vessels, and Gall Bladder. These resemble Yang Organs in form, but because they store substance instead of passing it through, they are said to perform like Yin Organs. The Gall Bladder is both Yang Organ and Curious Organ because alone among the Yang Organs it stores a pure substance. The Curious Organs function through related Zang-Fu Organs, and are reached and influenced through regular Meridian points.

‡The Uterus is governed by the three *Yin* channels of the foot (Kidney, Spleen, Liver), contains Yin Blood, and has a special relationship to the Ren or *Sea of Yin* Channel.

menstruation and fertility. Classic sources state that in women, it attains its height of development at 28 years of age and then enters a gradual decline. At 49 years of age the classics claim that this Kidney energy is exhausted; therefore menstruation ceases, and the woman loses her ability to conceive.[10]

Because it stores and regulates the volume of circulating Blood, the Liver plays an important role in reproductive health. For example, if the Liver cannot store Blood, amenorrhea or oligomenorrhea (scanty menstrual flow) can occur. The Liver also has an important role in maintaining the free, unobstructed circulation of Qi, thus preventing Qi and Blood stagnation. Liver Qi stagnation caused by anxiety or depression is an etiopathogenic factor in conditions such as premenstrual syndrome (PMS), irregular menstruation, amenorrhea, dysmenorrhea, leukorrhea, pelvic tumor masses, and insufficient lactation. When Liver Qi is excessive, it can attack the Stomach (e.g., causing vomiting in early pregnancy). In severe cases of excess, Liver Fire accumulates and can cause symptoms that biomedicine interprets as psychological, as in preeclampsia, postpartum psychosis, and the mood changes associated with menopause.[9]

The Spleen (together with the Stomach) is the third major Organ with vital links to women's reproductive health. Its functions include transforming food into Qi and Blood and transporting these throughout the body; keeping Blood within the vessels and Organs in their normal positions; and helping to metabolize water and handling excess fluid by transforming and transporting Damp and Phlegm. For example, Spleen deficiency is an important cause of both abnormal uterine bleeding and uterine prolapse. A deficient Spleen also cannot nourish the Channels; when those particularly associated with reproduction are affected, infertility or vomiting during pregnancy may occur.

Although Kidney, Liver, and Spleen are the three Zang-Fu Organs most centrally involved in women's reproductive health, the Heart and Lung also are important. The Uterus is connected with the Heart by way of the Heart Channel.[10] Thus the Heart, which dominates Blood and Vessels, is involved in the control of menstruation. The Heart also has a close relationship with the Kidney; the (Yang) Fire of one warms the (Yin) Water of the other, and vice versa. Heart Yang is likely to become excessive during conditions of Kidney Yin deficiency, such as pregnancy, the postpartum period, and menopause. In this case, expressions of both Heat (e.g., hot flashes) and rising Fire (e.g., irritability, depression) may occur.

The Lung governs the Qi of the entire body. Because Qi rules the Blood, deficiency of Lung Qi can cause hypermenorrhea (excessive menstrual flow). The Lung is connected with the Heart, Spleen, and Kidney and therefore also with the Uterus and the breast; the Lung is thus involved in the onset of lactation.

Channels in Reproductive Health

The 12 Channels that link with the 12 Zang-Fu Organs originate in Eight Extraordinary Channels (see Chapter 2). Three of these Channels begin in the Uterus: the Du, Ren, and Chong Meridians. Of these, the Chong and Ren are particularly important to female reproductive health.

Chong Mai (*mai* means "channel"), referred to as "the Sea of the Twelve Channels" and the "Sea of Blood," is considered to have several functions. Chong Mai coordinates and communicates to maintain the body's balance, and controls body temperature, fluids, fertility, and sexual development. Connected with the Kidney and Stomach Channels, along with the Ren Channel it governs the reproductive function in women; during pregnancy both Ren and Chong support the development of the placenta and nourish the fetus. The classics teach that in women, Chong Mai has more energy than Blood, which is eliminated with menstruation. Injury of the Chong Mai can cause infertility, uterine malpositions and prolapse, vaginitis, miscarriage, intrauterine demise of the fetus, retention of the placenta, and insufficient lactation.

Ren Mai is called the "Conception Vessel" and also "the Sea of the Yin Channels" because it crosses all the Yin Channels. This Channel becomes active at puberty and weakens at menopause.[10] Ren Mai nourishes and regulates the Qi in the Yin Channels, governing Yin as it governs Blood (which is Yin). Dysfunction of the Ren Channel manifests mainly as symptoms of the Yin Channels, especially the Liver and Kidney. Pathological conditions of the Ren are classically associated with infertility, miscarriage and intrauterine demise of the fetus, various menstrual disorders, leukorrhea, menopause symptoms, pelvic tumor masses, and insufficient lactation. Recent biomedical thought has proposed that Ren Mai interacts with several endocrine glands, specifically the thyroid, pancreas, adrenals, and the gonads.

Other Extraordinary Vessels also affect reproductive health. For example, the Du Channel (Governor Vessel) sends a branch to the genitalia and thus can affect menstruation[11] and express dysfunctions as infertility or difficult urination.[10] The Dai (Girdle) Meridian helps hold the Organs in place; weakness in this Meridian may express itself in uterine prolapse and contribute to other conditions such as menstrual irregularity, dysmenorrhea, leukorrhea, and pelvic congestion.

Acupoints in Reproductive Health

Certain acupoints have special applicability in maintaining or treating women's reproductive capacities. For example, Kid 9 *(Zhubin)*, the origin of Yin Wei Meridian, was named "the magical point of pregnancy" by Soulié de Morant, who is often credited with popularizing modern acupuncture in the West.[12] French authors have since used it in the prevention of miscarriages, the therapeutic approach to premature labor, and as prophylactic treatment in cases with a history of hypertension during pregnancy.[13]

Most of the acupoints that are contraindicated during pregnancy are in the abdominal region (front and back), but a few are limb points with unusually strong Qi-moving capabilities.

Menstruation

In both allopathic and Chinese medicine, menstruation is considered the ultimate manifestation of a harmonious female body balance. Normal menstruation is a manifestation of Blood, which is governed by Qi. In this particular case, of utmost importance is the Qi circulation within the Ren and Chong Channels.

Figure 17-1 uses the Yin-Yang symbol to describe the menstrual cycle. In this image, light Yang and dark Yin are contained within a circle separated by a curved line. These features indicate that Yin and Yang are inseparable and in dynamic relationship and that one can transform into the other (see Chapter 2). The bleeding cycle begins on the lower right where Yin energy is relatively low. Blood is Yin, and at this point, blood is being lost. As bleeding subsides and the body rebuilds its substance, Yin increases. At ovulation, Yin

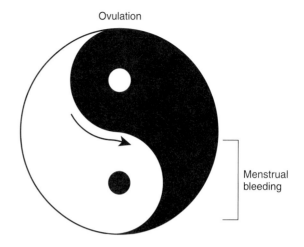

Figure 17-1 Yin-Yang symbol used to describe the menstrual cycle.

reaches its maximum and transforms into Yang, one marker of which is an increase in temperature. In the third quarter, Yang increases. By the fourth quarter, Qi reaches its maximum and as Yang transforms to Yin, Qi moves Blood out of the Uterus. Dysfunction can occur at any point, with characteristic symptoms relating to excessive Qi (i.e., symptoms Western people associate with PMS), abnormal bleeding, and insufficiency or excess of Yin or Yang.

The first part of the menstrual cycle, comprising menstruation, is governed by the Ren Channel. The other three quarters are influenced by the Yin Wei Channel, also called the "Yin Channel of connection," which binds together all the Yin Channels and ensures the distribution of Qi in the Yin areas of the body. Yin Wei starts at the confluent point of all the Yin Channels, the same "miraculous point" of pregnancy previously mentioned, Kid 9 *(Zhubin)*. Moving upward, Yin Wei segments pertain both to each Foot Yin Channel (Spleen, Liver, Kidney) and to each succeeding 7-day period of the menstrual cycle.

When dysfunction of Qi circulation in any of these Channels occurs, disorders can manifest as Qi deficiency (e.g., menorrhagia, blood loss during pregnancy) or Qi stagnation (e.g., amenorrhea, dysmenorrhea, infertility, insufficient lactation). Because Qi and Blood are intimately linked, subsequent Blood dysfunction can manifest as Blood deficiency (e.g., amenorrhea, dysmenorrhea, infertility) or Blood stagnation (e.g., metrorrhagia, eclampsia, afterpains, pelvic inflammatory disease).

The central Organ of menstruation control is the Uterus, which also supervises and nourishes the fetus. The function of the Uterus can be influenced by treating the Ren Mai, Chong Mai, and the three Yin Channels of the foot (Kidney, Liver, and Spleen channels). Important prescription points are located on these Channels (i.e., Ren 4, Ren 6, Sp 6, Sp 9, Kid 3, Kid 6, Liv 3).

As noted earlier, the reproductive function is dominated by the Kidney Qi.[9,10] Normal reproduction, gestation, and labor require strong Kidney Qi. Different causative factors (overstrain, stress, chronic diseases) can weaken the Kidney Qi. Stagnation of Liver Qi (e.g., resulting from disturbance of emotional factors) is commonly associated with irregular menstruation, dysmenorrhea, PMS, threatened abortion, eclampsia, insufficient lactation, and postpartum blues/depression. Finally, a deficient Spleen can manifest as uterine bleeding or uterine prolapse, and during pregnancy, as miscarriage.

Pregnancy

Maintaining an appropriate balance of Qi and Blood is key to a healthy pregnancy and normal development of the fetus. In Chinese medicine, it is believed that the balance shifts in favor of Blood; that Blood accumulates in the pelvis, especially in the uterus. This Blood supports the nourishment and development of the uterus, placenta, and fetus. Normal pregnancy results when several functions and structures interact in harmony: maternal Qi and Blood, fetal Qi and Blood, and free circulation of Qi within the Ren Mai and Chong Mai and maternal Zang organs (especially the Kidney, Liver, and Spleen). Pregnancy begins when the ovum, which is considered to belong to Yin, fuses with the spermatozoon, which is considered to belong to Yang. Classically, it is considered that the fetus establishes its own circulation, starting with Ren 8 *(Shenque)* as point of origin, located at the level of the umbilicus and involving the development of organs starting from the fetal Kidney.[14]

The accumulation of Yin in the lower part of the pregnant woman's body generates a Yang excess in the upper part of the body.[11] Early in pregnancy when the body is not yet fully adapted to its changed state, if excessive, this reversed Qi pattern causes a Liver Yin deficiency expressed in a predilection for sour foods, along with nausea and vomiting (morning sickness).

When pregnancy begins in a body already deficient in Qi or Blood, pathological conditions can occur, including morning sickness (Spleen and Stomach deficiency), abdominal pain and vaginal bleeding in pregnancy (Yang Qi deficiency, Blood deficiency), hypertension (deficiency of the Kidney and Spleen), abnormal presentation of the fetus (deficiency of Qi and Blood, Kidney Qi deficiency, Qi and Blood stagnation), prolonged or difficult labor (deficiency or stagnation of Qi and Blood), retention of the placenta (Qi deficiency), and insufficient lactation (Qi and Blood deficiency). Using acupuncture with or without herbal therapy or other modalities, practitioners can offer prophylactic treatment of imbalances that are known to exist before pregnancy occurs.

Lactation

Pregnancy ends with a great loss of Qi and Blood through labor, delivery, and the postpartum period. Lactation begins in this setting. For lactation to be normal in time of onset and amount of milk and result in eutrophic development of the newborn, several factors play key roles[9,15,16]:

- Adequate feeding and hydration is essential during pregnancy and the postpartum period.
- Qi and Blood must remain balanced especially for the Stomach, Spleen, and Liver.
- Qi must circulate freely. Free circulation can be interrupted by incision (Phannenstiel in cesarean section, episiotomy for vaginal delivery) or can be obstructed by Liver Qi stagnation related to emotional factors in excess or overacting in association with the Blood loss at the end of pregnancy.
- The amount of Blood lost during delivery and the postpartum period must be within normal limits. Not only does the mother need a sufficiency of Blood for her own physiological needs, but the production of milk also demands Blood since milk is interpreted as a form of Blood (with Qi, of course) in Chinese medicine.

Any dysfunction involving these factors can manifest itself as insufficient lactation, pain and inflammation with lactation, or more rarely, no lactation at all.

Menopause

At menopause, the Kidney Qi is said to be exhausted, as are the Ren and Chong Channels. The reproductive function decreases and menstruation ceases. Many symptoms characteristic of menopause, such as hot flashes, facial redness, nervousness, and insomnia, are explained by the relative Yang excess of the Liver and Heart in consequence of the deficiency of the Kidney Yin (the most significant among Kidney deficiencies in this specific period). Kidney Qi deficiency also expresses itself in other ways characteristic of old age. For example, the Kidney is considered to be the Organ that governs the bones[9]; one consequence of Kidney Qi deficiency in women is osteoporosis.

ETIOLOGY AND PATHOGENESIS

According to Chinese medicine, various exogenous causative factors (see Chapter 2) interact with endogenous factors (the seven emotions), the Organs, and Channels to affect the balance between the body and the environment. Some factors, such as a superior diet, enhance adaptability; others, such as excess Heat, social stress, or overwork, increase vulnerability. Although these concepts apply to understanding all forms of pathology in Chinese medicine, some factors play a special role in women's reproductive health. Thus the particularities of female physiology (menstruation, pregnancy, labor, lactation) and the accompanying blood loss easily can cause Blood deficiency, making a woman more vulnerable to the various causative factors. For a woman to be healthy generally, she first must achieve good reproductive health; good reproductive health implies good general health.

Three exogenous factors are particularly important to women's reproductive health. *Cold*—a Yin pathogenic factor that can enter the body by exposure to cold, being in the rain, or wearing inadequate clothing, but also by excessive ingestion of icy, cold, or raw food and drinks—causes contraction and obstruction of the Channels, leading to Qi stagnation and eventually to stagnation of Blood. Women are most vulnerable to Cold during their menstrual period and after childbirth because at those times the Uterus is open. Cold afflictions tend to express as severe fixed pains; cold is a causative factor for dysmenorrhea, amenorrhea, and afterpains. *Heat,* a Yang pathogenic factor, can be caused by constitutional excess of Yang, exogenous pathogenic Heat, internal Heat from an alcohol- or fat-rich diet, severe Yin deficiency, or prolonged Liver Qi stagnation transforming into Fire. Several gynecological conditions are caused by Heat (Table

17-1). The third important factor is *Damp,* which, because it is heavy and viscous, easily obstructs the circulation of Qi and impairs Spleen function. Damp can combine with Heat to form Damp-Heat. Leukorrhea, infertility, and dysmenorrhea are conditions associated with Damp or Damp-Heat.

Diet is considered a very important causative factor in the Chinese medicine view of reproductive health. Inadequate or insufficient nutrition leads to Blood and Qi deficiency; amenorrhea can result. Excessive indulgence in cold foods and drinks (icy sodas, ice cream, raw fruits and vegetables, salads) is believed to injure the Yang of the Spleen; cold accumulates inside the body and can cause amenorrhea or dysmenorrhea. Excessive intake of hot food (spices, alcohol, pasteurized milk, red meats, some drugs, smoking) generates Heat in the Blood, which can manifest as metrorrhagia. Too much sugar, dairy foods, and greasy or fried food cause an excess of Damp to accumulate, eventually leading to Qi obstruction, which can express as leukorrhea, infertility, or pelvic tumors.

Both overstrain and lack of physical exercise also can cause disease. Whereas the former weakens the Kidney Qi, the latter reduces the efficiency of the circulation of Qi and Blood. Excessive sexual activity— defined as beginning too early, too frequent orgasm, or multiple pregnancies—contributes to weakening of the Kidney Essence.

The internal or endogenous causative factors, primarily *emotional,* play an important role and are considered to cause disease primarily when they are in excess. Anger, sadness, and worry—Liver, Heart, and Spleen—are most commonly involved. Each impairs the circulation of Qi, eventually leading to Blood stagnation. For example, stagnation of Liver Qi caused by anger or prolonged depression can manifest as menstrual irregularities or insufficient lactation. Worry and sadness are thought to affect mainly the Spleen, but worry also can affect the Heart.[9] Recalling the complex relationships between the Uterus and the Organs with which it is connected, this influence is easily demonstrated: repercussions of worry easily affect the menstrual cycle, pregnancy, or the ability to lactate successfully.

Pelvic surgery, through the adhesions that sometimes follow, can also function as a causative factor.[17] Although adhesions may be associated only with local symptoms of stagnation of Qi and Blood, because the Uterus has relationships with other Organs, these also may be affected. For example, the Kidney may become deficient after hysterectomy.

TABLE 17-1

Etiologies Related to Chinese Medicine Patterns and Allopathic Manifestations*

Condition	Symptoms	Chinese medicine pattern	Causes
Dysmenorrhea	Distention sensation (abdomen, breast tenderness), irritability, postdated menstruation with scanty flow	Qi stagnation	Emotions (anger, etc.)
	Lower abdominal pain, cold sensation, dark menstrual blood with clots	Blood stagnation	Cold or Wind
	Premenstrual pain, antedated menstruation with excessive flow, dark malodorous menstrual blood	Blood deficiency	Damp-Heat accumulation
	Continuous pain during menstruation, scanty flow with bright blood	Blood deficiency	Malnutrition, excessive blood loss
Amenorrhea	Progressive onset, asthenia, palpitations, dizziness, abdominal distention, depression, anorexia	Qi and Blood deficiency	Stress, inadequate diet, worry
	Sudden onset, irritability, abdominal pain	Qi and Blood stagnation	Anger, Cold or Cold-Damp, Heat-Damp in the Stomach
	Progressive onset, lumbar weakness, asthenia, cold sensation in ankles, pale complexion	Yin deficiency of Liver and Kidney	Sexual abuses, fear, chronic diseases
Menstrual cycle disorders	Antedated menstruation with excessive flow and light red blood	Qi deficiency	Stress, inadequate diet, chronic diseases
	Irregular menstruation, excessive flow, dark blood with clots	Qi stagnation	Emotions (anger, etc.)
	Postdated menstruation with scanty flow and light red blood	Blood deficiency	Worry, blood loss, multiparity
	Postdated menstruation, scanty flow with dark blood and clots	Blood stagnation	Cold
	Excessive flow, malodorous dark blood, preference for cold, dry mouth	Heat in the Blood	Heat; spicy foods, hot drinks
Infertility	Scanty menstrual flow, white, watery leukorrhea, lumbar pain	Kidney Qi deficiency	Congenital, chronic disease, overstrain
	Irregular menstruation, abundant white leukorrhea, obesity	Excess of Phlegm-Damp	Constitutional, excess of greasy foods, alcohol abuse
	Thin, weakened body, nervousness, insomnia	Heat in the Blood	Internal excess of Heat
Leukorrhea	Watery, saliva-like, odorless	Spleen Qi deficiency	Excessive intake of raw fruits, cold drinks
	Abundant, mucous, persistent	Phlegm-Damp accumulation	Constitutional in obese
	Thick, yellow, malodorous	Damp Heat excess	Rich seafood diet, delivery, curettage
	Thick, white, persistent	Liver Qi stagnation	Emotions (anger, etc.)

*As examples only, the table provides the reader with the causative factors involved in some frequent gynecological conditions.

DIAGNOSIS

An important part of the Inquiring section of the diagnostic interview (see Chapter 3) used with women concerns their reproductive health. Most of the questions concern the same issues commonly broached in the biomedical obstetrical and gynecological review. However, some differences of emphasis matter to pattern differentiation in Chinese medicine. For example, women are asked to describe their menstrual, obstetrical, and lactation histories, with the same types of questions about age of menarche, quantity of flow, presence or absence of pain, number of pregnancies, live births or pregnancy losses, lactation history, and so on.

However, some questions are different. Practitioners ask many questions about diet, probe for signs of Cold, Heat, and Damp, and check for evidence of deficiency, excess, or stagnation. For example, patients are asked about the color of their menstrual blood. Dark red blood or blood with clots suggests Blood stagnation or stasis, whereas light, watery blood is a sign of Blood deficiency. Patients with pain are asked to describe it in detail. Pain that is relieved by pressure indicates deficiency, whereas that magnified by pressure suggests excess. Pain that ends with the onset of the menses implies the presence of stagnation, but pain that continues afterward and even through the menstrual cycle suggests a deficiency state. Many other similar details are gathered, and a "most probable" diagnosis is reached based on the balance of symptoms reported.

The condition of the tongue and the pulse diagnosis[9,18] (see Chapter 3) provide more evidence to guide the diagnosis. For example, women entering menopause often present with a red tongue with no coating, suggestive of a deficiency of Yin, which is not unexpected if the Kidney is becoming exhausted. A sticky coating is seen with accumulation of Damp-Phlegm, as in some cases of infertility.

The pulse often shows distinctive patterns in pregnancy. Some patterns are normal, indicating a physiological progression of pregnancy. The most famous of these is the "sliding" or "rolling" pulse, described in the classics as like "pearls rolling on a platter." Other pulses are pathological, such as those indicating threatened abortion, premature labor, or fetal distress. Some authors claim that sex of the fetus can be determined during pulse examination.

In Chinese medicine, the goal is not only to identify the symptoms but also to identify the pattern that is characteristic for a particular patient. A detailed presentation is beyond the purpose of this chapter, but the corresponding etiopathogenic pattern in Chinese medicine is provided for some of the most commonly encountered conditions in obstetrics and gynecology[9,19] (Table 17-2). Although involved in different conditions, some of the patterns are the same as the consequence of the complex relationship between Zang-Fu Organs and the fact that one symptom can be the manifestation of more than one disturbed Organ.

TABLE 17-2

Biomedical Terms Correlated with Chinese Medicine Patterns

General condition	Some etiopathological patterns in Chinese medicine
Premenstrual syndrome	Stagnation of Liver Qi, Yang deficiency of Spleen and Kidney, deficiency of Spleen and Heart
Dysmenorrhea	Qi and Blood stagnation due to Cold-Wind exposure or accumulation of Damp-Heat, Kidney Yin deficiency, Blood deficiency
Abnormal uterine bleeding (ovulatory dysfunction)	Heat in the Blood, Qi deficiency
Menopause symptoms	Kidney deficiency, Yin deficiency of the Liver and Kidney, Yang deficiency of the Spleen and Kidney, imbalance between the Heart and Kidney
Leukorrhea	Spleen Qi deficiency, stagnation of Liver Qi, excess of Damp-Heat, Phlegm-Damp accumulation
Infertility	Kidney Qi deficiency, Blood deficiency, Damp-Phlegm excess, Heat in the Blood, Liver Qi stagnation

Continued

TABLE 17-2

Biomedical Terms Correlated with Chinese Medicine Patterns—cont'd

General condition	Some etiopathological patterns in Chinese medicine
Morning sickness	Stagnation of the Stomach and Liver Qi
Threatened abortion	Deficiency of Qi and Blood, Kidney Qi deficiency, Liver Qi stagnation, Heat in the Blood, Dysfunction of Chong Mai and Ren Mai
Abnormal presentation of the fetus (i.e., breech)	Deficiency of Qi and Blood, Kidney Qi deficiency, Qi and Blood stagnation
Afterpains	Blood stagnation, Blood deficiency, attack of Cold
Insufficient lactation	Qi and Blood stagnation due to Spleen deficiency, Liver Qi stagnation
Urinary tract infections	Excess of Damp-Heat in the Urinary Bladder, Yin deficiency, Qi dysfunction

TREATMENT

The goal of treatment is to restore the energetic balance of the involved structures[9,19,20]: Qi and Blood, Organs, Chong Mai and Ren Mai. The same general therapeutic principles apply to women's reproductive health as throughout Chinese medicine: regulate Qi and Blood, eliminate pathological factors, and increase the body's resistance.[9] However, because Blood is central to women's reproductive health, special attention is directed to the Organs that play major roles in its health: the Spleen and Stomach as sources of Blood, the Liver as storage point for Blood, and the Kidney as governor of the reproductive functions.[21]

Treatment always considers the patient's social status, lifestyle, emotional state, and possible causative environmental factors.[10] Treatment in Chinese medicine has a solid prophylactic side and the woman herself is very much involved. Although no single term was used by Chinese medicine in ancient times to define the concept, the traditional body/spirit/lifestyle/environment approach was "holistic," and so it remains today. Women are engaged in their own treatment and must take responsibility for making many of the changes (diet, lifestyle, avoiding certain environmental factors) recommended by their practitioner. This feature of Chinese medical care contributes to the patient's increased sense of control over the disease; this is what many patients want[7,22] (see Chapter 12).

As one example of treatment, in pregnancy, as more Blood is needed, the practitioner stimulates the Spleen and tonifies the Kidney to help nourish the fe-

tus. As mentioned previously, during pregnancy precautions must be taken not to stimulate uterine contractions unintentionally. The classical Chinese literature advised against using certain "forbidden" points (located mostly on the abdomen[9] and a few on the limbs*); however, modern adaptations mostly advise using precautions.[23] Recently it has been argued that these points also should be avoided during menstruation, considered a time of increased vulnerability, because they might increase loss of Blood, which in turn might lead to Qi and Blood deficiency.[24] Despite these cautions, some of the "forbidden" points are considered very useful in the treatment of several pregnancy-related conditions, such as morning sickness, fainting, and threatened abortion. Appropriate needling technique can overcome some of the limitations of these points.

RESEARCH DATA

The first part of this chapter offered information about the classical Oriental medical approach to women's reproductive health. Although, for purposes of communication of familiar conditions, biomedical terms were frequently used, biomedical explanations were avoided; instead the discussion focused on how

---

*Limb points ST 36, LI 4, SP 6, BL 60, and BL 67 are known for their ability to induce strong uterine contractions. Wang and Liu[24] recommend avoiding points LI 4, CV 2, CV 3, BL 60, GB 21, and ST 25 during both pregnancy and menstruation.

the conditions are interpreted in Chinese medicine (see Table 17-1). This section does not frame the discussion in classical terms but instead reviews studies of acupuncture (and some herb) effectiveness in terms of biomedical physiological understandings. The difference in terminology and perception is important. Chinese medicine achieves its effects through manipulation of the movement of Qi and Blood, and although recent research shows, for example, that acupuncture can affect ovulation or the pituitary-ovarian axis, this does not represent the classical understanding. Most important, however, is that despite differences in physiological perception, classical Chinese treatments result in successful care outcomes, a point that has been clarified by scientific research and is discussed in this section.

Physiology of Acupuncture

Although the mechanisms of acupuncture are not yet fully understood (see the detailed discussion in Chapter 11), reasonably strong evidence exists to support the fact that acupuncture affects the nervous, humoral, vascular, and immune systems.[25] Modern investigation techniques, such as functional magnetic resonance imaging (MRI), ultrasound, and Doppler ultrasound, have been used in several studies[26-28] to quantify the physiological effects of acupuncture. Melzack[29] offered the gate control theory of pain control involving stimulation of δA fibers; recent work has charted the modulation of the neural transmission by endorphins and more recently dynorphin.[30] Endorphins block incoming pain information, whereas serotonin, norepinephrine, and possibly gamma-aminobutyric acid (GABA) also are believed to be involved as mediators in acupuncture analgesia.[20]

Multisystem effects are explained by the fact that acupuncture stimulation is believed to modulate the subcortical structures and limbic system,[31] as shown by functional MRI. A 1998 randomized, controlled clinical trial (RCT)[32] found associated changes in immune parameters: an increase in (1) the numbers of CD3, CD4, and CD8 cells, (2) monocyte phagocytosis, and (3) the percentage of natural killer (NK) cells. This characteristic of acupuncture care provides a starting point for understanding the alleged benefit of acupuncture in the treatment of various inflammatory gynecological conditions.

Physiological Insights on Ovulatory Dysfunction

As a consequence of acupuncture manipulation, specific central nervous system (CNS) neurohormones are evoked through gene expression (detectable effect of a gene).[30,33] This mechanism helps explain the effect of electroacupuncture in the induction of ovulation; that is, acupuncture can regulate the hypothalamic-pituitary-ovarian axis.[34,35] Some evidence also suggests that acupuncture may alter follicle-stimulating hormone (FSH), luteinizing hormone (LH), and estradiol levels and increase progesterone levels.[36] Electroacupuncture also is believed to decrease the blood flow impedance in the uterine arteries of infertile women.[37] Because ovulatory dysfunction is involved in menstrual cycle disorders, infertility, and dysfunctional uterine bleeding, we now have a better understanding of why acupuncture can help in these conditions.

Clinical Research Studies

Review Articles

Two recent articles[38-40] have analyzed clinical studies in obstetrics and gynecology that were present in mainstream medical literature; the common conclusion is that there is an increasing interest in and usage of alternative therapies. For example, Chez and Jonas[38,39] searched the US National Library of Medicine electronic database between January 1966 and March 1997, reviewing articles pertinent to alternative therapies in obstetrical and gynecological care. Use of acupuncture and moxibustion for nausea and vomiting in early pregnancy, breech presentation, premature labor, induction of labor, analgesia during labor, infertility, and dysmenorrhea are critically discussed. These articles provide an opportunity for specialists to increase their awareness of the potential utility of Oriental medicine care and referral in obstetrics and gynecology.

Nausea and Vomiting in Early Pregnancy

One acupoint—Pericardium 6 (PC 6, *Neiguan*)—stands out as the most widely recognized of all acupoints. Used classically to treat nausea and vomiting, it has been tested for the treatment of nausea and vomiting in early pregnancy. As early as 1980, Dundee et al[41] published results on 350 patients who were part of a prospective randomized trial. These patients showed improvement in the frequency of emesis and intensity of nausea. Subsequent studies[42-44] showed the same positive outcome when PC 6 was used for morning sickness and stimulated either with acupressure, sea bands,* or acupuncture. In 1996 Vickers[45] reviewed 33 controlled trials of PC 6. Of these, 11 were randomized, placebo-controlled trials, involving approximately 2000 patients; all demonstrated the significant antiemetic effect of PC 6. Using PC 6 to treat morning sickness has gained wide acceptance as a safe and effective method (see Appendix I).

Nausea and Vomiting After Gynecological Surgery

Recent studies have analyzed the effect of PC 6 on nausea and vomiting after gynecological surgery. In a meta-analysis of 19 studies, including 10 on surgical gynecological patients, Lee and Done[46] found a significant decrease in the incidence of early vomiting in the group with PC 6 stimulation versus placebo groups. Swedish anesthesiologists[47] addressed the issue in outpatient gynecological subjects. In this study, 60 women participated in a double-blind, randomized clinical trial and were divided into three groups (group 1: acupressure on PC 6; group 2: placebo stimulation; group 3: no acupuncture or placebo stimulation). The effect on nausea and vomiting was noted, as was the need for additional antiemetic medication. The authors concluded that both vomiting and the need for antiemetic medication were reduced by acupressure in PC 6, whereas the placebo effect only decreased the incidence of nausea. With statistically significant results ($p <0.05$), acupressure at PC 6 is emerging as a convenient and promising technique for outpatient gynecological patients.

Nausea and vomiting after spinal anesthesia for cesarean section was the subject of another study.[48] This randomized, double-blind study compared the effects of acupressure on PC 6 with intravenous metoclopramide therapy. In the 75 study patients, acupressure proved to be an effective, nonpharmacological alternative for reducing nausea and vomiting after spinal anesthesia for cesarean section. Ho et al[49] also re-

ported positive results using PC 6 to control nausea and vomiting after epidural morphine therapy for pain relief after cesarean section. The prophylactic stimulation of PC 6 in 60 patients significantly ($p <0.05$) reduced the incidence of nausea and vomiting in this particular setting.

Breech Presentation

The use of acupuncture and moxibustion to promote spontaneous fetal version toward cephalic presentation has a long history in Chinese medicine. The traditional point stimulated for this purpose is UB 67 (outer edge of toenail on fifth toe), although other points also have a history of success. Huang[50] reviewed several studies using mostly electroacupuncture. Of the 2736 patients with breech presentation in the reviewed studies, the effectiveness of needling UB 67 was between 71% and 91.3%. Huang also reviewed another study of 82 patients; using acupuncture with warm needle* in Sp 6 (Sanyinjiao) resulted in an 83% success rate in correcting the breech presentation. A similar result of 81.3% is reported by Li and Wang[51] in 39 cases with needling at UB 67. Two control groups, moxibustion and "blank" (no treatment), were used. The authors found that although there was no significant difference in efficacy, patients required fewer sessions of electroacupuncture (average number of sessions 1.41) than of moxibustion (average number of sessions 2.42, $p <0.01$). In 1998 results of the first randomized controlled trial confirmed the efficacy of acupuncture. In this study performed in two hospitals in China, Cardini and Huang[52] described 260 primigravidas with 33-week normal pregnancies and breech presentations confirmed by ultrasound examination; the women were equally divided into one intervention and one control group. Intervention consisted of stimulation by moxibustion of UB 67 (Zhiyin), self-administered by the patient after an instruction session performed by a midwife. The active fetal movements counted by the mother and the number of cephalic presentations at 35 weeks and at delivery were considered as outcome measures. Ninety-eight fetuses (75.4%) from the intervention

---

*Sea bands are commercially available elastic bands with circular metal buttons designed to be centered over PC6.

*"Warm needle" means that once the needle is inserted, moxa is burned on top of it. This carries the needed heat deeper into the body than would occur with moxa burned at the surface. Special apparatus is available to support this treatment. The needle does not become hot.

group were in cephalic presentation at 35 weeks versus 62 fetuses (47.7%) in the control group. No serious side effects were observed. It appears that the mechanism of action is based on the increase in the active fetal movements. The mechanism of moxibustion is not completely clear; however, current data indicate that further clinical research could support the extended use of this simple and effective method for fetal version from breech to cephalic presentation.

Labor

Acupuncture has been used classically to induce uterine contractions and speed up labor. Huang[50] described one study of 771 women with postdated pregnancies in whom electroacupuncture was performed to induce labor, with a 72.1% success rate. These data, together with data from nine other studies representing a sample total of 1225 patients, showed an effectiveness rate of between 60% and 92.7% for labor induction with acupuncture. The most popular point used was SP 6 (Sanyinjiao). Zeisler et al[53] in Austria performed a case-control study of 57 patients who received acupuncture treatment compared with 63 patients in the control group. The authors reported that acupuncture had a positive effect on the duration of labor, shortening the first stage of labor (196 minutes in the acupuncture group versus 321 minutes in the control group). The acupuncture group also required less oxytocin during labor (15% versus 85% in the first stage and 28% versus 72% in the second stage of labor). In a related Austrian study,[54] Tempfer et al found no correlation between the duration of labor and the serum levels of interleukin 8 (IL-8), prostaglandin F_2 alpha ($PGF_2\alpha$), and β-endorphin, which are among the most important biomedical parameters involved in cervical ripening. However, the authors discussed other studies and speculated that the observed beneficial effect of acupuncture on reducing the length of labor might be explained by its action on the thalamic nuclei and hypothalamic-anterior pituitary system, with subsequent increase in oxytocin release or parasympathetic stimulation of the uterus.

Acupuncture also can be used to promote cervical maturation. An RCT conducted by Tremeau et al[55] on 98 subjects aimed to improve cervical maturation (assessed by Bishop score) by acupuncture treatment during the ninth month of pregnancy. A significant difference was noted between cervical maturation in the acupuncture group (2.61 points progression of the

Bishop score) and the placebo and control groups (0.89 points and 1.08 points, respectively).

Abortion

Because acupuncture can be used to induce labor, clearly it also could be used to induce abortion. It is not often used for this purpose; the "forbidden points" earlier mentioned are forbidden precisely to avoid accidentally stimulating the gravid uterus. Acupuncture also can be used to stop uterine contractions, as in threatened abortion, usually supplemented with herbal therapy[11,14,56]; however, extreme caution is necessary when herbal medicine is used during pregnancy. Huang[50] reviewed seven Chinese studies comprising 961 patients in whom acupuncture was used purposefully to induce artificial abortion. Reported effectiveness in the several studies varied from 43.3% to 98.2%. The largest study group (618 patients) used ear acupuncture with a success rate of 43.3%. However, it remains to be seen whether acupuncture has a place in modern obstetrics with regard to its ability to cause dilation of the cervix or stimulate uterine contractions in therapeutic abortions. Nevertheless, this is a field in which less aggressive methods such as acupuncture show potential.

Pain Relief in Childbirth

Acupuncture for pain relief in childbirth has been a popular topic of research, perhaps partly because of a better understanding of the physiology underlying the effects of acupuncture on pain (see Chapter 13). Ternov et al[57] conducted a prospective study of 3317 patients in labor. The intervention group received electroacupuncture, and the control group received standard Western analgesic care (e.g., epidural analgesia, pudendal nerve block, inhalation of nitric oxide, intramuscular meperidine, local infiltration of sterile water) but was not offered acupuncture. The authors concluded that the demand for chemical analgesia was reduced significantly for patients who received acupuncture ($p < 0.01$). Pain relief was reported in 58% of patients, and 78% would consider acupuncture for future deliveries.

Placental Retention

Placental retention is a dangerous situation that carries a risk of severe postpartum hemorrhage. The Western medicine approach—manual extraction of the placenta with the patient under anesthesia—also is not risk-free. Several studies testing the utility of acupuncture treatment for this condition have shown encouraging results. The first Western study was conducted by Chauhan et al[58] in Denmark. Of 75 patients, 30 received acupuncture and 45 had the placenta removed by manual extraction. Of the patients in the acupuncture group, 83% delivered the placenta within 20 minutes with no complications related to acupuncture. In the manual extraction group, the complication rate was 6.6% (usually including hemorrhage, puerperal infection, anesthesia-related complications, and cervical trauma). Furthermore, four of five failures in the acupuncture group were found to have placenta accreta (abnormal adherence to the myometrium), a pathological anatomical condition that explains the failure of acupuncture and requires surgical management. The authors concluded that acupuncture is safe, simple, and effective. Although a number of different acupoints are prescribed for this condition, the Danish study identified two points as especially useful: UB 67 and Ren 3. A randomized clinical trial on a larger population is now needed to establish the efficacy of acupuncture for placental expulsion and encourage its use in everyday obstetrical practice.

Chinese medical literature shows that acupuncture can be used to address most gynecological conditions.[9,21,59] This text has reviewed a number of scientific studies, including RCTs, that tend to support the clinical data, although larger sample sizes and more research are necessary. Current data[25] support the use of acupuncture in the treatment of PMS. The National Institutes of Health (NIH) Consensus Conference[60] concluded that there is good evidence to support the effectiveness of acupuncture in the treatment of menstrual cramps. Other conditions that deserve attention are infertility, hot flashes in menopause, and menstrual irregularities related to hormonal imbalance.[25] Acupuncture also can be beneficial in treating amenorrhea even after oral contraceptives,[61] uterine bleeding, leukorrhea, ovarian cyst, uterine prolapse, sexual dysfunctions such as dyspareunia and vaginismus,[62] and many others.

Premenstrual Syndrome

Although PMS is fertile ground for clinical trials, to our knowledge no RCT using acupuncture or herbs has been conducted. Clinically, acupuncture is expected to help relieve most PMS symptoms, such as irritability, cramping, emotional lability, headache, and bloating. Tables 17-1 and 17-2 show that differentiation of the syndrome is well developed in Chinese medicine. In biomedicine, the etiology of PMS is unknown, and although a variety of therapies have been proposed (hormones, vitamin supplements and evening primrose oil, cognitive-behavioral therapy, and selective serotonin reuptake inhibitors, as well as diet and exercise), to date, no therapy consistently reduces symptoms. Given this lack of effective treatment and based on the need to individualize the treatment approach, acupuncture definitely can contribute to treating the causes and symptoms of PMS. Marwick[63] mentioned acupuncture as an accepted application for PMS because of its possible action on the hypothalamus and pituitary gland.

Dysmenorrhea

Several studies suggest that acupuncture is beneficial in treating dysmenorrhea. Steinberger[64] reported an 80% success rate in treating 48 patients with 6- to 12-month follow-up. In 1987, Helms[65] reported results from one of the first RCTs on dysmenorrhea. Forty-three patients with primary dysmenorrhea were divided into four treatment groups: acupuncture, placebo acupuncture (random points were used), visitation (follow-up only), and control (no treatment). A large majority (90.9%) of the acupuncture group showed improvement, including a 41% decrease in need for analgesic medication. Tsenov[66] gathered data on 24 patients with primary dysmenorrhea and 24 with secondary dysmenorrhea.* Satisfactory relief of pain was obtained in 50% of cases with acupuncture alone. This finding supports the clinical fact that functional disorders (as in primary dysmenorrhea) generally respond better to acupuncture than disorders with developed anatomical changes. Huang[50] reviewed six studies—five by Chinese authors and Helms's study. In these studies, a total of 804 patients received acupuncture, with stimulation of either ear acupoints or Sp 6 *(Sanyinjiao)*. Moxibustion was used in one study. The effectiveness rate varied from 37% to 85.7%. This broad range most likely exists because researchers made no distinction between primary and secondary dysmenorrhea, the latter being presumably a cause when weak results (i.e., 37%) were obtained. Some of

---

*Painful menstruation in the presence of organic disease, such as endometriosis, adhesions secondary to chronic pelvic inflammatory disease, uterine pathological conditions such as fibroids, congenital anomalies, or cervical stenosis, at more than 2 years after menarche.

these patients probably require surgery to address the underlying abnormality, but acupuncture merits a trial in well-selected cases with real expectations.

Infertility

Infertility is one gynecological condition that can benefit from acupuncture or auricular therapy alone or in combination with Chinese herbal medicine. In four Chinese studies reviewed by Huang,[50] a total of 185 patients received either acupuncture or electroacupuncture with various success rates (outcomes were measured as pregnancy occurring after treatment). One study reported 100% effectiveness with the use of acupoint UB 18 (Ganshu). Gerhard and Postneek[67] studied 45 patients (27 with oligomenorrhea and 18 with luteal insufficiency) who received auricular therapy. A control group of 45 patients received hormonal therapy. In the acupuncture group, 22 pregnancies occurred (11 after acupuncture therapy, 7 after medication, and 4 spontaneously). In the control group, 20 pregnancies occurred (5 spontaneous and 15 after treatment).

Other complaints related to the autonomic nervous system (nervous complaints, insomnia, migraine, constipation) normalized during acupuncture treatment. Women who became pregnant after acupuncture more often had menstrual irregularities and hormonal imbalances (luteal insufficiency and decreased levels of estrogen, thyroid-stimulating hormone [TSH], and dehydroepiandrosterone sulfate [DHEAS]). Also, conditions such as endometriosis, adnexitis, or reduced postcoital test were more often present in women with normal menstrual cycles in the acupuncture group. Endometriosis was an important component (35% to 38%, respectively) in women from both groups who did not respond to acupuncture treatment. Multiple factors such as these must be considered if a patient is likely to respond to acupuncture intervention.

Electroacupuncture also has been used to achieve analgesia in oocyte aspiration for in vitro fertilization. A group of Swedish researchers[68] conducted an RCT to assess the effect of electroacupuncture on 75 patients compared with the effect of alfentanil therapy on 74 patients when either treatment method was combined with a paracervical block. Measured as the level of pain related to the surgical procedure, need for anesthesia, or experience of abdominal pain and nausea, no difference was found between the two groups. Although electroacupuncture patients initially showed a higher level of stress (presumably because the procedure was unfamiliar), they had a higher implantation rate (27.2% versus 16.3%; $p < 0.05$), pregnancy rate (45.9% versus 28.3%), and take-home baby rate (41% versus 19.4%). Women who received electroacupuncture also were less tired, more alert during and after the procedure, and experienced less bleeding. Another study by the same authors with a larger group is in progress, aiming to clarify the significantly higher implantation rate in the electroacupuncture group. We believe the published study provides a valuable example of how biomedicine and acupuncture can be integrated for the benefit of the patient.

Male Infertility

Although male infertility is not strictly the topic of this chapter, because the male factor is responsible in 50% of infertile couples, the use of acupuncture to treat certain causes of male infertility is of interest. In a controlled clinical trial of 32 patients equally divided into an acupuncture and a control group, Siterman et al[69] observed a significant increase in the fertility index ($p < 0.05$) due to an increase in total functional sperm fraction, viability, sperm mobility, and the integrity of their axonema in the acupuncture group. Acupuncture also showed promising results in the treatment of low fertility due to reduced sperm activity. A Dutch pilot study[70] of 16 patients with erectile dysfunction used electroacupuncture in a 4-week treatment design. The serum level of several hormones (adrenocorticotropic hormone [ACTH], antidiuretic hormone, cortisol, FSH, LH, and testosterone) was measured. Fifteen percent of the patients showed an improvement in the quality of erection, and 31% experienced an increase in their sexual activity, although no change was detected in hormone levels. Chang and Zhu[71] used acupuncture to treat 500 patients with impotence or ejaculation failure. Treatment was successful in 451 patients (90.2%); those with unsatisfactory results had organic diseases of inflammatory, hormonal, or vascular origin.

Menopausal Symptoms

Women are increasingly interested in choosing an alternative approach to relief from menopausal symptoms. For example, a recent Canadian study[22] found women reporting the following motivations for choosing a nonbiomedical approach: fear of side effects (primarily cancer) from hormone replacement therapy (HRT), dislike of feeling pressured by their physicians to try HRT, increased sense of personal control, and fewer side effects. The choice of an alternative therapy is especially important in patients for whom HRT is not an option.[72] In Chinese medicine, both acupuncture and herbal prescriptions are used to address menopause; however, the latter is considered more effective in nourishing the Kidney Essence.

A recent study[73] found an association between osteoporosis and the sufficiency of Kidney Qi; the researchers also found that Kidney Yin deficiency particularly increases the probability of developing osteoporosis. As the authors concluded, it will be worthwhile to determine whether these deficiency states are correlated with biochemical markers of bone metabolism.

Scientific evidence on this topic is sparse. One Swedish RCT[74] studied 24 patients in natural menopause complaining of hot flushes. Twelve patients received electroacupuncture, and 12 patients received "superficial needle position acupuncture" (shallow insertion) over an 8-week period. In both groups the frequency of the vasomotor symptoms decreased significantly by over 50%. When examined again at a 3-month follow-up, both groups had maintained improvements in vasomotor stability, although the electroacupuncture group had slightly better results than the manual acupuncture group. Because both studies had a small number of patients, further studies are necessary to clarify the uses of acupuncture in menopause. While waiting for the scientific evidence to increase, however, we note that acupuncture can address not only menopausal symptoms but also their primary cause. Because acupuncture can improve general well-being, it is a useful potential tool in contributing to a better quality of life for women in menopause.

Urinary Symptoms

Classical acupuncture regularly treats a variety of urinary symptoms. Several research studies have been published on this topic. Norwegian physicians[75] used acupuncture in an RCT of 67 patients with histories of recurrent lower urinary tract infections (cystitis). Patients were divided into three groups: acupuncture, sham acupuncture, and no treatment, and were followed for 6 months. In the acupuncture group, 85% became free of cystitis symptoms; 58% and 36% achieved relief in the sham acupuncture* and control groups, respectively. One recent study[76] mentions acupuncture among the therapies currently used in the

*Recall from Chapters 13 and 15 how difficult it is to design a true placebo in acupuncture.

management of recurrent urinary tract infections in women; it shows that acupuncture is increasingly recognized as effective therapy in mainstream settings. Chinese authors[77] published a clinical trial of 180 women with urethral syndrome, of whom 128 received acupuncture and moxibustion. Urodynamic parameters (maximal bladder pressure, bladder-neck pressure, and maximal urethral closure during urination) were evaluated before and after treatment in 69 patients from the acupuncture group and 39 from the control group. Nearly 91% of the acupuncture patients achieved short-term improvements, and 80.4% maintained these through follow-up. Only 26.9% of the control group achieved any improvement; this difference is highly significant ($p < 0.001$). Other studies have shown positive results in the treatment of pyelonephritis[78] and glomerulonephritis[79]; in both cases acupuncture provided the advantage of a monotherapeutic option free of the side effects of drugs. Acupuncture for the treatment of renal colic[80] has proved to be a useful alternative, with significantly more rapid onset of the analgesic effect ($p < 0.05$) compared with intramuscular Avafortan. Kelleher et al[81] conducted an RCT of 39 patients with urge incontinence, which was divided into an acupuncture group (20 patients) and an oxybutinin group (19 patients). The authors concluded that acupuncture has comparable effects with the anticholinergic therapy but fewer side effects.

Insufficient Lactation

The treatment of insufficient lactation is also a part of the tradition of Chinese medicine. Useful therapeutic body points are near the breast (e.g., Ren 17 [Tanzhong], St 18 [Rugen]), but two important classical points are distal (SI 1 [Shaoze] on the hand, and GB 21 [Jian Jing] on the shoulder). Ear acupuncture and stronger stimulation using moxa also are used to stimulate milk flow. However, as with all Chinese medicine therapy, a named set of points does not constitute "standard care," and treatment must be individually tailored to the patient.

Clavey[15] reviewed several Chinese studies with a total of 656 patients and found an average of improved lactation in 91.6%. He mentions the importance of proper timing of the acupuncture treatment; the best results are obtained when stimulating the acupoints, especially SI 1, between 1 and 3 PM (the time of maximum Qi on the Small Intestine Channel; see Figure 2-4). Rapidity of response, usually within 24 hours, is a good predictor of ability to sustain the flow; in some cases lactation increased substantially as soon as 4 hours after treatment. Acupuncture to stimulate lactation has been reported to have an effectiveness rate of 70.4%.[16] Although too few studies exist to scientifically support the use of acupuncture for insufficient lactation, there is good evidence that it is an effective and safe technique. Considering that biomedicine has not proved successful in this setting and the need to treat insufficient lactation is great, we believe acupuncture should be offered because it is the only alternative.

Benign Breast Conditions

Acupuncture classically has been used to treat a range of benign breast conditions; however, careful consideration should be given to any breast pathological condition and only after a thorough biomedical evaluation should alternative therapies be considered.

In one study[82] of 43 patients with breast tenderness, a 95% success rate was reported with acupuncture. Huang[50] reviewed five studies with a total of 998 patients; acupuncture was effective in more than 90% of cases. He also reported a study of 110 patients with mastosis (mainly fibrocystic breast disease) in which acupuncture was given with excellent results (disappearance of breast tenderness and lumps) in 30.9% of cases and good results (improvement of symptoms) in 59%. Another Chinese study reviewed by Huang concerned 57 patients with fibrocystic breast disease who received acupuncture. The authors reported effective treatment in 91.2% of cases; 50% had no further symptoms (were "cured").

Breast Cancer

Although Chinese medicine certainly treated breast cancers in the past, today most patients seek biomedical care for cancer. However, acupuncture can play an important supporting role in decreasing postsurgical pain, improving postsurgical mobility, and decreasing the side effects of chemotherapy and radiation therapy.

A recent study conducted in a German university[83] assessed pain relief and movement improvement in 48 patients with breast cancer after mammary ablation and axillary lymphadenectomy. Thirty-two patients from the control group had the same surgical procedure performed but received no acupuncture. Several parameters showed statistically significant improvement in the acupuncture group: maximum abduction angle without pain (80.4 degrees versus 59.1 degrees) and with maximum tolerable pain (92.3 degrees versus 73.6 degrees), and presence of pain in the surgical field on the fifth postoperative day (12.3% versus 50%) and on the seventh postoperative day (8.3% versus 12.5%). The authors consider much of the positive effect to be correlated with individualized acupuncture treatment and with the ability of the patient to feel the de Qi sensation. In another study,[84] acupuncture was given for postradiation edema of the extremity in patients with breast cancer. Acupuncture showed best results in stage I and II edema by improving the lymph flow. Rajan[85] found acupuncture to be beneficial when used in patients with breast cancer after radiotherapy, with rapid pain relief in patients with postradiation brachial plexus neuralgia, healing of ulcers along the scar, and restoration of peripheral sensation.

Also of interest are two review articles in the mainstream medical literature published in early 2000, aiming to quantify the research and use of alternative therapies in patients with breast cancer. Jacobson et al[86] reviewed 51 articles from 1000 citations retrieved from the biomedical literature from 1980 to 1997. Acupuncture is mentioned as especially effective for decreasing nausea, and acupressure is effective for minimizing lymphedema. Lee et al[87] studied the prevalence of use of various alternative therapies in four groups (Latino, white, black, and Chinese) of women with breast cancer. Although acupuncture was again found among the therapeutic choices, the authors emphasize the need for better communication between patients and physicians to achieve a better understanding of patients' choices.

Acupuncture Analgesia

Much has been written about the use of acupuncture in achieving analgesia during surgery, including its use in pelvic and gynecological surgery. Electroacupuncture is usually used, since steady strong stimulation is necessary, but some practitioners also have used ear acupuncture. Acupuncture analgesia has several recognized advantages: the patient remains conscious and awake and is able to respond to the surgeon during the procedure; cardiac and respiratory functions remain stable; there are no drug-related side effects; and the gastrointestinal tract maintains its normal peristalsis.[9,50] Another advantage is that acupuncture analgesia can permit surgery in those sensitive to anesthetics. Among limitations is the fact that approximately 15% of patients do not appear to respond to acupuncture, and muscular relaxation is not as complete as with anesthesia.

Most studies of acupuncture analgesia have been conducted in China. Huang[50] reviewed the use of acupuncture anesthesia for cesarean section in eight studies with a total of 3071 women and found the technique to provide excellent analgesia in 80% of cases. He also reviewed seven studies, with an impressive total of 38,010 patients, and found acupuncture analgesia to be very effective for tubal ligation. Six studies comprising 1071 patients in whom hysterectomies were performed and 1006 patients in whom myomectomies were performed resulted in effectiveness ratings of "excellent" in 22.1% to 82.3% of cases with a total effectiveness rating between 71.2% and 95.7%.[50] Although the results vary markedly among different studies, the large sample sizes support a conclusion that acupuncture can produce sufficient analgesic effect to permit pelvic surgery without anesthetics.

In Western settings, acupuncture is offered as an aid to the chemical anesthetic already in use. The proposed term[30] is "acupuncture-assisted analgesia" (acupuncture given with conventional anesthesia); the combination is valuable in (for example) permitting reduced dosages of anesthetics. A randomized study[88] of 250 patients assessed electroacupuncture as the sole analgesic within standard anesthesia (no other analgesic was used). In the acupuncture group, only 5% required added fentanyl as analgesic drug (the control group received conventional anesthesia). Even more important is the finding that in these intubated patients, the time to spontaneous respiration ($p < 0.02$) and extubation immediately after surgery was decreased in the acupuncture group ($p < 0.001$), and the return to normal self-care also was improved significantly ($p < 0.02$). Grochmal et al[89] successfully used acupuncture anesthesia in office microlaparoscopy and hysteroscopy. Chiang et al[90] studied 40 gynecological patients who received electroacupuncture during elective laparoscopic surgery. Both the study and control group received general anesthesia. The authors found that electroacupuncture decreased the necessary concentration of isoflurane ($p < 0.05$) during surgery and significantly decreased the recovery time after surgery ($p < 0.05$).

REFERRAL

This chapter has reviewed briefly both the theory of women's reproductive health in Chinese medicine and a variety of scientific studies focused on the usefulness of acupuncture in the care of gynecological and obstetrical conditions. These data indicate that acupuncture offers not only a symptom-oriented prescription but also—more powerfully—care based on a variety of fine-tuned etiological causes. An additional advantage is that acupuncture care is associated with few to no side effects. The examples also demonstrated acupuncture working in tandem with biomedicine to reduce adverse effects of radiotherapy, chemotherapy, and surgery.

Because relatively few medical doctors have the requisite training to deliver acupuncture (or herbal) care themselves, those who wish to recommend acupuncture to their patients must consider who is most likely to benefit from referral (see Chapter 21). A first step is establishing a careful biomedical diagnosis. Patients with primarily functional complaints are most likely to benefit from acupuncture alone. Those with conditions such as tumors also can benefit when acupuncture is used in combination with biomedical therapy.

In summary, acupuncture care, or acupuncture care combined with biomedical care, can appropriately be used to optimize the health care provided to our patients.

References

1. Eisenberg DM, Davis RB, Ettner SL, et al: Trends in alternative medicine use in the Unites States: 1990 to 1997, *JAMA* 280(18):1569-75, 1998.
2. Zollmann C, Vickers A: ABC of complementary medicine: users and practitioners of complementary medicine, *BMJ* 319:836-8, 1999.
3. Beal MW: Women's use of complementary and alternative therapies in reproductive health care, *J Nurse Midwifery* 43(3):224-33, 1998.
4. Burg MA, Hatch RL, Neims AH: Lifetime use of alternative therapy: a study of Florida residents, *South Med J* 91(12):1126-31, 1998.
5. Coss RA, McGrath P, Caggiano V: Alternative care: patient choices for adjunct therapies within a cancer center, *Cancer Pract* 6(3):176-81, 1998.
6. Drivdahl CE, Miser WF: The use of alternative health care by a family practice population, *J Am Board Fam Pract* 11(3):193-9, 1998.
7. Cassidy C: Chinese medicine users in the Unites States. Part I: utilization, satisfaction, medical plurality, *J Altern Complement Med* 4(1):17-27, 1998.
8. Murphy PA, Kronenberg F, Wade C: Complementary and alternative medicine in women's health: developing a research agenda, *J Nurse Midwifery* 44(3):192-204, 1999.

9. Cheng X, editor: *Chinese acupuncture and moxibustion,* Beijing, 1987, Foreign Language Press.

10. Maoshing NI: *The Yellow Emperor's classic of medicine,* Boston, 1995, Shambhala.

11. *Concise of traditional Chinese gynecology,* Nanjing College of Traditional Chinese Medicine, 1988, Jiangsu Science and Technology Publishing House.

12. Eckman P: *In the footsteps of the Yellow Emperor: tracing the history of traditional acupuncture,* San Francisco, 1996, Cypress Book.

13. Rinker G, Prat D, Mares P, et al: *Menace d'accouchement premature: interet du point Rein 9. Actualites 1991—acupuncture et gynecologie obstetrique.* Nimes, France, 1991, CHRU de Nimes.

14. Staebler FE: Clinical acupuncture in childbirth, *Br J Acupunct* 8(2):3-12, 1985.

15. Clavey S: The use of acupuncture for the treatment of insufficient lactation (Que Ru), *Am J Acupunct* 24(1):35-46, 1996.

16. Tureanu L, Tureanu V: A clinical evaluation of the effectiveness of acupuncture for insufficient lactation, *Am J Acupunct* 22(1):23-7, 1994.

17. Maciocia G: *Obstetrics and gynecology in Chinese medicine,* London, 1998, Churchill Livingstone.

18. Borsarello JF: *Pulsologie chinoise traditionelle,* Paris, 1961, Masson.

19. Tureanu V, Tureanu L: *Acupuncture in obstetrics and gynecology,* St Louis, 1999, Warren H. Green.

20. Filshie J, White A: *Medical acupuncture: a western scientific approach,* London, 1998, Churchill Livingstone.

21. Liu YC, Fang TY, Chen L, et al: *The essential book of traditional Chinese medicine: theory and clinical practice,* New York, 1988, Columbia University Press.

22. Seidl M, Stewart PE: Alternative treatments for menopausal symptoms, *Can Fam Physician* 44:1272-305, 1998.

23. Dale RA: The contraindicated (forbidden) points of acupuncture for needling, moxibustion, and pregnancy, *Am J Acupunct* 25(1):51-6, 1997.

24. Wang C, Liu X: The side effects of elective acupuncture treatment during menstruation, *Am J Acupunct* 26(1):81-2, 1998.

25. Birch SJ, Felt RL: *Understanding acupuncture,* London, 1999, Churchill-Livingstone.

26. Litscher G, Yang NH, Schwarz G, et al: Computer-controlled acupuncture: a new construction for simultaneous measurement of blood flow velocity of the supratrochlear and middle cerebral arteries, *Biomed Tech (Berl)* 44(3):58-63, 1999.

27. Litscher G, Wang L, Yang HN, et al: Ultrasound-monitored effects of acupuncture on brain and eye, *Neurol Res* 21(4):373-7, 1999.

28. Wu MT, Hsieh JC, Xiong J, et al: Central nervous pathway for acupuncture stimulation: localization of processing with functional MR imaging of the brain-preliminary experience. *Radiology* 212(1):133-41, 1999.

29. Melzack R, Wall PD: Pain mechanisms: a new theory, *Science* 150(699): 971-79, 1965.

30. Ulett GA, Han JS, Han S: Traditional and evidence-based acupuncture: history, mechanism, and present status, *South Med J* 91(12):1115-20, 1998.

31. Hui KK, Liu J, Makris N, et al: Acupuncture modulates the limbic system and subcortical gray structures of the human brain: evidence from fMRI studies in normal subjects, *Hum Brain Mapp* 9(1):13-25, 2000.

32. Petti F, Bragazi A, Liguori A, et al: Effects of acupuncture on immune response related to opioid-like peptides, *J Tradit Chin Med* 18(1):55-63, 1998.

33. Ulett GA, Han S, Han JS: Electroacupuncture: mechanism and clinical application, *Biol Psychiatry* 44(2):129-38, 1998.

34. Chen BY, Yu J: Relationship between blood radioimmunoreactive beta-endorphin and hand skin temperature during the electroacupuncture induction of ovulation, *Acupunct Electrother Res* 16(1-2):1-5, 1991.

35. Chen BY: Acupuncture normalizes dysfunction of hypothalamic-pituitary-ovarian axis, *Acupunct Electrother Res* 22(2):97-108, 1997.

36. Mo X, Li D, Pu Y, et al: Clinical studies on the mechanism for acupuncture stimulation of ovulation, *J Tradit Chin Med* 13(2):115-9, 1993.

37. Stener-Victorin E, Waldenstrom U, Andersson SA, et al: Reduction of blood flow in the uterine arteries of infertile women with electroacupuncture, *Hum Reprod* 11(6): 1314-7, 1996.

38. Chez RA, Jonas WB: Complementary and alternative medicine. I: Clinical studies in obstetrics, *Obstet Gynecol Surg* 52(11):704-08, 1997.

39. Chez RA, Jones WB: Complementary and alternative medicine. II. Clinical studies in gynecology, *Obstet Gynecol Surg* 52(11):709-16, 1997.

40. Beal MW: Acupuncture and acupressure: applications to women's reproductive health care, *J Nurse Midwifery* 44(3):217-30, 1999.

41. Dundee JW, Sourial FB, Ghaly RG, et al: P 6 acupressure reduces morning sickness, *J R Soc Med* 81(8):456-7, 1988.

42. Hyde E: Acupressure therapy for morning sickness, *J Nurse Midwifery* 34(4):171-8, 1989.

43. de Aloysio D, Penacchioni P: Morning sickness control in early pregnancy by Neiguan point acupressure, *Obstet Gynecol* 80(5):852-4, 1992.

44. Belluomini J, Litt RC, Lee KA, et al: Acupressure for nausea and vomiting of pregnancy: a randomized, blinded study, *Obstet Gynecol* 84(2):245-8, 1994.

45. Vickers AJ: Can acupuncture have specific effects on health? a systematic review of acupuncture antiemesis trials, *J R Soc Med* 89(6):303-11, 1996.

46. Lee A, Done ML: The use of nonpharmacologic techniques to prevent postoperative nausea and vomiting: a meta-analysis, *Anesth Analg* 88:1362-9, 1999.

47. Alkaissi A, Stalnert M, Kalman S: Effect and placebo effect of acupressure (P 6) on nausea and vomiting after outpatient gynaecological surgery, *Acta Anaesthesiol Scand* 43(3):270-4, 1999.

48. Stein DJ, Birnbach DJ, Danzer BI, et al: Acupressure versus intravenous metoclopramide to prevent nausea and vomiting during spinal anesthesia for cesarean section, *Anesth Analg* 84(2):342-5, 1997.

49. Ho CM, Hseu SS, Tsai SK, et al: Effect of P 6 acupressure on prevention of nausea and vomiting after epidural morphine for post-cesarean section pain relief, *Acta Anaesthesiol Scand* 40(3):372-5, 1996.

50. Huang CK: *Acupuncture: the past and present,* New York, 1996, Vantage Press.

51. Li Q, Wang L: Clinical observation on correcting malposition of fetus by electroacupuncture, *J Tradit Chin Med* 16(4):260-62, 1996.

52. Cardini F, Huang W: Moxibustion for correction of breech presentation: a randomized controlled trial, *JAMA* 280(18):1580-4, 1998.

53. Zeisler H, Tempfer C, Mayerhofer K, et al: Influence of acupuncture on duration of labor, *Gynecol Obstet Invest* 46(11):22-5, 1990.

54. Tempfer C, Zeisler H, Heinzl H, et al: Influence of acupuncture on maternal serum levels of interleukin-8, prostaglandin F_2-alpha, and beta-endorphin: a matched pair study, *Obstet Gynecol* 92(2):245-8, 1998.

55. Tremeau ML, Fontaine-Ravier P, Teurnier F, et al: Protocol of cervical maturation by acupuncture, *J Gynecol Obstet Biol Reprod (Paris)* 21(4):375-80, 1992.

56. Zharkin NA: Acupuncture in obstetrics: part one, *J Chin Med* 33:10-3, 1990.

57. Ternov K, Nilsson M, Lofberg L, et al: Acupuncture for pain relief during childbirth, *Acupunct Electrother Res* 23(1):19-26, 1998.

58. Chauhan PA, Gasser FJ, Chauhan AM: Clinical investigation on the use of acupuncture for treatment of placental retention, *Am J Acupunct* 26(1):19-25, 1998.

59. Tureanu V, Tureanu L: Acupuncture in gynecological disease. In *Encyclopedia of complementary health practice,* New York, 1999, Springer.

60. Anonymous: NIH Consensus Conference. Acupuncture, *JAMA* 280(17):1518-24, 1998.

61. Tureanu L, Tureanu V: An evaluation of the effectiveness of acupuncture for the treatment of post-oral contraceptive menstrual irregularities and amenorrhea, *Am J Acupunct* 22(2):117-21, 1994.

62. Tureanu V, Tureanu L: Acupuncture in sexual dysfunctions: dyspareunia and vaginismus, *Clin Bull Myofascial Ther* 2(1):25-33, 1997.

63. Marwick C: Acceptance of some acupuncture applications, *JAMA* 278(21):1725-6, 1997.

64. Steinberger A: The treatment of dysmenorrhea by acupuncture, *Am J Chin Med* 9(1):57-60, 1981.

65. Helms JM: Acupuncture for the management of primary dysmenorrhea, *Obstet Gynecol* 69(1):51-6, 1987.

66. Tsenov D: The effect of acupuncture on dysmenorrhea, *Akush Ginekol (Sofia)* 35(3):24-5, 1996.

67. Gerhard I, Postneek F: Auricular acupuncture in the treatment of female infertility, *Gynecol Endocrinol* 6(3):171-81, 1992.

68. Stener-Victorin E, Waldenstrom U, Nilsson L, et al: A prospective randomized study of electroacupuncture versus alfentanil as anesthesia during oocyte aspiration in in-vitro fertilization, *Hum Reprod* 14(10):2480-4, 1999.

69. Siterman S, Eltes F, Wolfson V, et al: Effect of acupuncture on sperm parameters of males suffering from subfertility related to low sperm quality, *Arch Androl* 39(2):155-61, 1997.

70. Kho HG, Sweep CG, Chen X, et al: The use of acupuncture in the treatment of erectile dysfunction, *Int J Impot Res* 11(1):41-6, 1999.

71. Chang Q, Zhu LX: Male sexual dysfunction treated by acupuncture; an observation of 500 cases, *Int J Clin Acupunct* 9(3):265-70, 1989.

72. Waldman TN: Menopause: when HRT is not an option. Part II, *West J Health* 7(6):673-83, 1998.

73. Chen YY, Hsue YT, Chang HH, et al: The association between postmenopausal osteoporosis and kidney-vacuity syndrome, *Am J Chin Med* 27(1):25-35, 1999.

74. Wyon Y, Lindgren R, Hammar M, et al: Acupuncture against climacteric disorders? Lower number of symptoms after menopause, *Lakartidningen* 91(23):2318-22, 1994.

75. Aune A, Alraek S, LiHua H, et al: Acupuncture in the prophylaxis of recurrent lower urinary tract infection in adult women, *Scand J Prim Health Care* 16(1):37-9, 1998.

76. Madersbacher S, Thalhammer F, Marberger M: Pathogenesis and management of recurrent urinary tract infection in women, *Curr Opin Urol* 10(1):29-33, 2000.

77. Zheng H, Wang S, Shang J, et al: Study on acupuncture and moxibustion therapy for female urethral syndrome, *J Tradit Chin Med* 18(2):122-7, 1998.

78. Darenkov AF, Balchii-ool AA, Shemetov VD, et al: Acupuncture in the combined treatment of pyelonephritis, *Urol Nefrol* 2:10-2, 1993.

79. Holub TI: The clinico-laboratory effects of acupuncture in patients with glomerulonephritis, *Lik Sprava* 4:157-61, 1999.

80. Lee YH, Lee WC, Chen MT, et al: Acupuncture in the treatment of renal colic, *J Urol* 147(1):16-8, 1992.

81. Kelleher CJ, Filshie J, Burton G, et al: Acupuncture in the treatment of irritative bladder symptoms, *Acupunct Med* 2:9-12, 1994.

82. Ceffa GC, Chio C, Gandini G: Acupuncture in breast diseases: how, when, and why, *Minerva Med* 72(33):2239-42, 1981.

83. He JP, Friedrich M, Ertan AK, et al: Pain-relief and movement improvement by acupuncture after ablation and axillary lymphadenectomy in patients with mammary cancer, *Clin Exp Obstet Gynecol* 26(2):81-4, 1999.

84. Bardychev MS, Guseva LI, Zubova ND: Acupuncture in edema of the extremities following radiation or combination therapy of cancer of the breast and uterus, *Vopr Onkol* 34(3):319-22, 1988.

85. Rajan S: Post radiotherapy acupuncture, *Acupunct Med* 17(1):64-5, 1999.

86. Jacobson JS, Workman SB, Kronenberg F: Research on complementary/alternative medicine for patients with breast cancer: a review of the biomedical literature, *J Clin Oncol* 18(3):668-83, 2000.

87. Lee MN, Lin SS, Wrensch MR, et al: Alternative therapies used by women with breast cancer in four ethnic populations, *J Natl Cancer Inst* 92(1):42-7, 2000.

88. Poulain P, Leandri EP, Montagne F, et al: Electroacupuncture analgesia in major abdominal and pelvic surgery: a randomized study, *Acupunct Med* 15(1):10-3, 1997.

89. Grochmal SA, Ostrzenski A, Connant C, et al: Seven-year experience with office microlaparoscopy and hysteroscopy, *J Am Assoc Gynecol Laparosc* 3(4 suppl):S16-7, 1996.

90. Chiang Mh, Wong JO, Chang DP, et al: The effect of needleless electroacupuncture in general anesthesia during laparoscopic surgery, *Acta Anesthesiol Sin* 33(2):107-12, 1995.

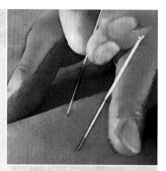

18

Acupuncture in Depression and Mental Illness

R O S A N. S C H N Y E R

J O H N J. B. A L L E N

*P*ractitioners of Chinese medicine are frequently called on to acknowledge and address the wide range of emotional complaints experienced by their patients, including such specific mental illnesses as depression, manic depression, anxiety disorders, and eating disorders, and to assist in the management of more serious mental illnesses such as schizophrenia or schizoaffective disorder. In Western cultures, people do not easily divorce their emotional experience from their physical symptoms when they are ill. However, patients present their illness to an acupuncturist in diverse ways. This spectrum ranges from an exclusively somatic account to strongly defined emotional symptoms and many combinations between these extremes.

Depending on the training and style of the practitioner, the nature of the patient's complaints, and the patient's own background and belief system, the focus of the acupuncture treatment may be reframed in either somatic or psychoemotional terms. One of the greatest strengths of Chinese medicine, however, is the ability to provide a framework for identifying and interrelating physical and emotional symptoms. The organism is considered as a body-mind continuum; therefore somatic and psychological symptoms are equally important.

Many branches of allopathic medicine separate and distinguish mental or emotional disturbances from physical disease. Although fields such as neurology and psychiatry clearly acknowledge the relationship between brain and behavior, these and many other fields offer little explanation of the link between emotional symptoms and *apparently* unrelated physical complaints.

Chinese medicine focuses on disharmonies of Qi and, strictly speaking, it does not address the treatment of diseases as defined by the allopathic medical model. When a practitioner of Chinese medicine evaluates the symptoms presented by a patient, information is gathered by conducting an interview and performing palpation and observation. The data then are viewed and organized primarily through five different "filters."* Each filter underscores an aspect of Chinese medical theory and assists the practitioner in making an evaluation and designing a treatment plan for the patient. The five filters are (1) the Eight Guiding Criteria; (2) the Organs; (3) Qi, Blood, and Body Fluids; (4) the Five Phases; and (5) the Channels and Network Vessels or Meridians.

Varied acupuncture treatment styles incorporate one filter or a combination of several filters through the course of treatment or use different filter combinations at different times. Each filter emphasizes a different aspect of the theoretical framework that helps identify, evaluate, and treat the imbalance presented by the patient.

Chinese medicine postulates a physiology that clearly connects physiological and psychological symptoms that are usually considered unrelated in the allopathic medical model. A patient may consult an acupuncturist specifically for the treatment of an emotional condition or a mental illness (e.g., depression). In the majority of cases, however, the patient has a wide constellation of symptoms that includes, among others, symptoms that define clinical depression. Even when patients may not fully meet Western criteria for a mental illness, they may still interpret their distress in primarily emotional terms. At other times, patients may seek treatment for a biomedical condition or for well-defined physical symptoms yet exhibit a significant element of emotional distress in their configuration.

Health is commonly defined in Chinese medicine as the balance between Yin and Yang. This balance depends on the capacity of an organism to adapt to change and maintain equilibrium. Sickness is the result of *vacuity* or *deficiency* (hypofunction, diminished capacity of a physiological process, decreased resistance) or *repletion* or *excess* (hyperfunction, obstruction of a physiological function, increased reactivity). Vacuity and repletion are both imbalances between Yin and Yang.[1] The following text

presents an overview of each of the five filters and the Chinese medical concepts essential to understanding mental, emotional, and spiritual disorders. Subsequently, a review of research of acupuncture and depression is provided with a focus on research methods appropriate for determining whether acupuncture has efficacy for treating depression and emotional disorders.

ORIENTAL MEDICINE APPROACH TO DEPRESSION AND MENTAL ILLNESS

Yin/Yang and the Eight Guiding Criteria

The theory of Yin and Yang is expanded into four sets of categories that assist in differentiating and interpreting the information gathered during the evaluation.[1] These bipolar categories help the practitioner organize the relationship between clinical signs and symptoms and Yin and Yang; these categories are also known as the Eight Principles (vacuity/repletion, internal/external, hot/cold, Yin/Yang).

When an acupuncturist evaluates a patient using the Eight Guiding Criteria as the filter, all relevant information is woven into a "pattern of disharmony," a description in Chinese medicine terms of the dynamics that portray an imbalance. Physical and emotional symptoms are part of this imbalance, which is reflected in other aspects of the patient's life and behavior.[2]

The patterns of disharmony can be considered as reaction patterns that develop along two continua: Yin Vacuity–Yang Repletion (hyperactivity and increased metabolic response) or Yang Vacuity–Yin Repletion (hypoactivity or decreased metabolic response).[1] From this perspective, when confronted with an emotional stressor or a perceived threat, the organism would tend to react in one of two ways: by activating sympathetic response in preparation for "flight or fight" (Yang) or by withdrawing from external activity and parasympathetically attending to internal demands, thus allowing the organism to "rest and digest" (Yin).[3] A parallel can be established between these two reaction tendencies and the various symptoms presented by a patient. For example, in the case of major depression the clinical symptoms as defined by the *Diagnostic and Statistical Manual of Mental Disorders* (DSM-IV) can be overlapped with patterns of disharmony related to depression, thus drawing a parallel between clinically

---

*The idea of viewing the areas that encompass energetic theory as five "filters" was first expressed by Dr. Mark Seem in his lectures.

defined symptoms and tendencies toward energetic imbalances. One of the defining symptoms of clinical depression, depressed mood, can be experienced either as depressed mood with lethargy and weakness (Yin features/tendency toward Qi or Yang vacuity–Yin repletion) or as depressed mood with anxiety, irritability, and agitation (Yang features/tendency toward Yin vacuity–Yang repletion; see columns 2 and 3 of Table 18-1).

Using the Eight Principles as the framework, mental illness and emotional disorders are generally *internal* in nature; they can arise from either *vacuity (deficiency)* or *repletion (excess)* or a combination of both; they can be either *hot* or *cold,* and they may pres-

ent either *Yin* or *Yang* characteristics. Furthermore, in the context of the Eight Principles, mental illness and emotional disorders can be conceptualized, for example, as stemming from Yang vacuity and Dampness accumulation (repletion of Yin), or from Yin vacuity and Empty Heat. In the first instance, the person may feel fatigued, frozen in fear, indecisive, and lethargic. This person also may experience lower backache, increased sensitivity to cold and a worsening of symptoms in the winter months, decreased libido, overproduction of phlegm, congestion, and brooding or rumination. Conversely, if the mental illness or emotional complaint is characterized by Yin vacuity and Empty Heat, the patient may experience anxiety, agitation, insom-

TABLE 18-1

Expressions of Depression in Oriental Medicine

DSM-IV symptoms	Yin features (tendency toward *deficiency of Qi or Yang* with possible Yin excess)	Yang features (tendency toward *deficiency of Yin* with possible Yang excess)	Qi Stagnation	Shen disturbance
Depressed mood	Depressed mood with lethargy and weakness, lower libido, decreased motivation	Depressed mood with irritability, uneasiness, anxiety, violent outbursts of anger, aggression	Depressed mood with emotional lability, periodic outbursts of anger, frustration, erratic physical complaints, migratory pains, distention of breast and abdomen, sighing	Depressed mood characterized by flat affect
Appetite disturbance	Appetite disturbance characterized by loss of appetite with weak digestion; tendency toward loose stools or diarrhea	Appetite disturbance characterized by excessive appetite, bitter taste in the mouth, thirst	Appetite disturbance characterized by indigestion with belching, nausea, bloating, flatulence, belching; erratic elimination	
Sleep disturbance	Hypersomnia	Dream-disturbed sleep; nightmares		Insomnia with difficulty falling or staying asleep or waking up early
Psychomotor agitation/ psychomotor retardation	Decreased energy level, slow body movements, no desire to move or talk	Inability to sit still, pacing, agitation, nervousness, wiriness		Incessant, nervous talking; slow, soft, monotonous speech; muteness or decreased speech; increased pauses

nia, night sweats, hot flushes, dry throat, tinnitus, and dizziness.

The Organs (Viscera and Bowels)

The homeostasis of an organism is defined by the balance of Yin and Yang, which is sustained by the proper circulation of Qi along energetic pathways known as Channels or Meridians. The Meridians connect the surface of the body with the internal Organs. The Organs in Chinese medicine are traditionally known as Viscera and Bowels and are defined by their functions and interrelations rather than by their somatic structures or specific anatomical locations. The Organs represent a complete set of functions that reflect energetic relationships among physiological and psychological events. Each Organ has a specific responsibility for maintaining the physical and emotional health of the organism. Mental-emotional symptoms may indicate an imbalance in the functioning of an Organ or in the interaction among several Organs. Because each Organ corresponds to a specific set of physiological and psychological functions, the practitioner can assess the imbalance on the basis of this correspondence. For example, in Chinese medicine the Liver Organ is associated with anger; therefore an emotional imbalance characterized by volatility and outbursts of anger may indicate a disturbance in the functions associated with this Organ. Furthermore, because the pathway of the Liver Channel traverses the pelvic region, chest, throat, vertex of the head, and diaphragm, symptoms along these areas would indicate a disturbance in the flow of Qi associated with the Liver Channel, and possibly with the Liver Organ.

In addition to physiological and psychological functions, each Yin Organ houses a specific mental or spiritual aspect of the human mind, known in Chinese medicine as the Five Spirits: *Hun, Shen, Yi, Po,* and *Zhi.* Specific acupuncture points address imbalances in each one of these mental-spiritual aspects (Table 18-2).

Any mental illness or emotional disorder can be a manifestation of an imbalance in any Organ network. Emotions are considered manifestations of the life energy or Qi that, if not expressed or transformed, become stagnant; they only become a cause of disease, however, when they are experienced excessively, for a prolonged period, or both.[4] When Qi does not circulate properly, it becomes "toxic" and generates an imbalance. This concept, known in Chinese medicine as Stagnation, is key to understanding the cause and physiology of mental illness and emotional problems. Stagnation means that the Qi, the Blood, or Body Fluids are not flowing or being transformed properly, therefore they are accumulating and causing a condition of repletion or excess.

Next, consider the five Yin Organs—Liver, Heart, Spleen, Lung, and Kidney—in the context of mental illness and emotional disorders. (See Chapter 2 for a more detailed explanation of the Organs and their functions.)

The Liver's main function is to regulate the flow of Qi by gathering and releasing both the Qi and the Blood, in this way modulating the intensity of all motion and process.[1] The Liver's job is to ensure that the movement of Qi is smooth and free-flowing to prevent

TABLE 18-2

Mental-Spiritual Aspect of the Five Yin Viscera

Viscera (Yin organ)	Mental-spiritual aspect	Translation and correspondence	Acupuncture points
Lung	Po	*Corporeal Soul* Organizational principle of body	UB 42
Heart	Shen	*Spirit* Consciousness	UB 44
Liver	Hun	*Ethereal Soul* Intuition, insight, courage	UB 47
Spleen	Yi	*Thought*	UB 49
Kidney	Zhi	*Will*	UB 52

Stagnation. According to Dr. Leon Hammer,[5] prominent psychiatrist and acupuncturist, the Liver is the first line of emotional defense for the entire organism: the organism's first choice for coping with a stressor. Any experience that thwarts the capacity for growth, development, expression, and change inhibits the Liver's ability to spread the Qi and maintain free flow. Liver Qi stagnation may affect other functions of the Liver Organ, such as storing the Blood, or may manifest as a blockage along its corresponding Channel. However, it also may cause stagnation in other Organs, such as the Lung and the Heart, or affect the functions of other Organs such as the Spleen or the Stomach. Depending on the viability of the Organ systems of a particular individual, Liver Qi stagnation tends to combine with or aggravate preexisting tendencies to imbalances in other Viscera and Bowels, in this way varying the constellation of signs and symptoms. For example, if Liver Qi stagnation affects the Stomach, it may manifest as nausea or vomiting; if it affects the Large Intestine, it can cause irritable Bowel. Coughing and wheezing can be manifestation of Liver Qi stagnation affecting the Lung, whereas agitation and insomnia may indicate Liver Qi stagnation affecting the Heart. Because the first effect of the emotions as causative factors of disease is to upset the movement and transformation of Qi and its proper circulation and direction, the Liver Organ network always is involved to some extent in mental illnesses and emotional problems.

Anger is the emotion corresponding to the Liver. The Liver is said to store the *Hun*. One of the Five Spirits, the *Hun* is sometimes translated as *Ethereal Soul*[6] and is the mental-spiritual aspect of the mind related to intuition and inspiration, insight, and courage. The *Hun* provides a sense of direction and the capacity for planning; it influences sleep and dreaming.

The Heart is said to be the emperor of the body-mind. The Heart governs the Blood (moves it within its vessels) and stores the *Shen* or Spirit, which in Chinese medicine is considered to have a material basis and represents the capacity of the mind to form ideas. *Shen* indicates consciousness and memory, mental and emotional faculties; it maintains our awareness and expresses the integration of our being. Rather than having a religious or spiritual meaning, *Shen* refers to the accumulation of Qi and Blood in the Heart. The *Shen* and the *Hun* complement each others' functions. Several symptoms seen in mental illness and emotional disorders, such as confusion and disorientation,

incoherent speech, sleep disturbances, palpitations, and anxiety, correspond to an imbalance in the Heart's function of housing the *Shen*. Mental illnesses and emotional disorders generally affect the Heart but rather than originating in the Heart, emotional disturbances may begin in some other Organ eventually affecting the Heart.[7] The emotion associated with the Heart is joy. A mental-emotional disorder characterized by total lack of joy or uncontrolled, inappropriate elation may indicate a disturbance of the *Shen*.

The Spleen in Chinese medicine plays an essential role in the creation of Qi and Blood and in the circulation and transformation of Body Fluids. When the Spleen becomes diseased, it may not be able to create and transform Qi and Blood properly, which may result in insufficient Blood to nourish the Heart and insufficient Qi to perform the functions of the body-mind. When the Liver loses its capacity to maintain the smooth flow of Qi, the Qi becomes stagnant, backs up, and accumulates, generating a surplus; this surplus may then counterflow to the Spleen, which is deficient and weak as a result. Therefore the Spleen is the first Organ to become imbalanced after the Liver Qi becomes stagnant. The Spleen houses the *Yi* or thought, our verbally expressed thoughts, our capacity for applied thinking, studying, memorizing, focusing, concentrating, and generating ideas. The emotion associated with the Spleen is worry. Brooding and rumination, for example, are manifestations of an imbalance in the functions of the Spleen.

The Lungs move and circulate the Qi of the body out to the edges and from the top downward; they assist the metabolism of Body Fluids and help protect the body from invasion of external pathogens. Mental illnesses and emotional disorders usually do not originate in the Lungs, but like the Heart, the Lungs are often affected by the disease processes initiated in other Organs.[7] For example, when Liver Qi stagnation moves on to affect the Lungs, it can create a sense of constriction in the chest, weeping, breathlessness, and a feeling of a lump in the throat. The *Po,* commonly translated as the *Corporeal Soul,* is stored in the Lungs; the *Po* gives the body its capacity for movement and coordination. It can be linked to the physical expression of the *Hun* or the organizational principle of the body.[4]

The Kidney stores the *Jing* or Essence, the source of life, the potential for differentiation into Yin and Yang. The *Jing* is the most fundamental material the body uses for its growth, maturity, and reproduction.

It is a very important constituent of the body; all bodily functions depend on it. Overall health and well-being are determined by the *Jing*.[7] The Kidney holds the foundation for the Yin and Yang of all other Organs. Each Organ is considered to have a Yin (storing, nourishing, cooling) component and a Yang (activating, protective, warming) component. Enduring diseases affect the Kidney, including mental illnesses and emotional disorders. The mental-spiritual aspect stored by the Kidney is the *Zhi,* which corresponds to our will, drive, and determination; it provides us with the capacity to store information and is therefore related to long-term memory. The emotion associated with the Kidney is fear. A mental-emotional disorder manifesting with fear and loss of will and determination may point to an imbalance in the Kidney.

When evaluating a mental illness or an emotional complaint on the basis of the Organs, the practitioner determines which aspect of the Organ's function is affected, in what way, and to what extent. For example, a person with depression characterized by irritability and frustration, lack of appetite, difficulty falling asleep, heart palpitations, and lack of concentration (who in addition has a pulse that is wiry in some positions and very weak and thin overall and a pale tongue that is slightly darker on the tip and sides), presents with *Liver* Qi stagnation, *Spleen* Qi and *Heart* Blood vacuity.

Qi, Blood, and Body Fluids

Qi is the capacity of life to transform and maintain itself.[8] Qi motivates all movement, transformation, and change and grants us the qualities of action and self-expression. Blood nourishes and moistens and provides the material foundation for the Shen or Spirit. As explained earlier, in the Chinese medical sense, Shen refers to the accumulation of Qi and Blood in the Heart; if enough Qi and Blood accumulates in the Heart, it gives rise to consciousness, which is called Shen or Spirit in Chinese medicine.[7] The presence of Shen requires sufficient Qi. For the Shen to be calm and settled, sufficient Blood is needed to nourish it; because the Shen is Yang in nature, it tends to become restless. Body fluids, such as saliva, sweat and tears, are in a continuum with Yin, which moistens, softens, stabilizes, and grants us the qualities for rest, tranquility, and quiescence.[9] Vacuity or deficiency of Blood, Yin, or both, are very important in both the cause and the effects of mental emotional problems.

The Qi, Blood, and Body Fluids are part of the Yin and Yang of the body; Qi is Yang and Blood is Yin. When evaluating an imbalance in the context of Qi, Blood, and Body Fluids, the practitioner assesses the relative insufficiency (vacuity or deficiency) and accumulation (repletion or excess) of either Yin or Yang.

If Qi is vacuous because of nervous or physical exhaustion, it affects the capacity to express emotions and enjoy life. If there is not enough Qi transforming and activating the life process (a Yang function), the Yin becomes relatively replete. Mental illness and emotional symptoms that arise from Qi vacuity are characterized by fatigue, apathy, excessive desire to sleep, and slowed movements or speech. If Qi vacuity persists or worsens, it may precipitate Yang vacuity. In such cases, the capacity to engage life and to react and respond is impaired. We may feel bogged down, fearful, confused, or indecisive, unable to express what we want, and hopeless.[9] When Qi and Yang are insufficient, body fluids tend to accumulate, giving rise to Dampness and later to Phlegm.

Conversely, if Yin is vacuous, we tend to feel agitated, unsettled, and confused. If there is not enough Yin to stabilize and nurture, Yang becomes more prevalent, giving rise to psychomotor agitation, anxiety, and insomnia, which are predominantly Yang features. Blood vacuity or deficiency manifests as a lack of sense of direction, fear of making decisions, confusion, and lack of concentration.

Stagnation of Qi may manifest mentally and emotionally as irritability, moodiness, feeling "wound up," snapping easily, frustration, aggression, and outbursts of anger. Because the Liver stores the Blood, Qi stagnation may lead to Blood stasis, manifesting in mental illness and emotional disorders such as anxiety, insomnia, oppression in the chest, restlessness, and agitation. Qi stagnation impedes the proper transformation and circulation of Blood and Body Fluids, causing excess or accumulation.

Within the framework of Qi, Blood, and Body Fluids, a mental illness or emotional disorder may be evaluated as stemming from *Qi* vacuity, *Blood* stasis, *Phlegm* blocking the orifices of the Heart, *Dampness* accumulation, or *Yin* vacuity.

Traditional Chinese Medicine (TCM), uses the three areas previously discussed—Eight Principles, Organs (Viscera and Bowels), and Qi, Blood, and Body Fluids—as the basis for evaluation and treatment. TCM is a specific style of Chinese medicine developed and taught in China over the past 40 years. TCM follows a specific, rational, and step-by-step methodology based on *pattern differentiation*. When assessing a mental illness or an emotional disorder using TCM, the patterns of disharmony are determined by all three areas as appropriate. A practitioner of TCM assessing a patient presenting with depression weaves together the constellation of signs and symptoms to determine a *pattern* or combination of patterns, develops a set of *treatment principles* to address these patterns, and designs a *treatment plan* that may include both acupuncture and Chinese herbal medicine, as well as dietary and lifestyle recommendations. Pattern differentiation is specific to the TCM style of acupuncture treatment. As described later, each acupuncture treatment style is based on its own particular way of using the Chinese medicine theoretical framework.

A Case Example

Let us further develop the example of Liver Qi Stagnation and Spleen Qi–Heart Blood vacuity previously presented. Our patient, Rebecca, is a woman in her twenties who has been experiencing depression for several months. It began after the breakup of a relationship and has become exacerbated by the pressure of trying to complete her master's thesis while working full-time. She feels exhausted and lethargic, yet she is restless. She feels oppression in her chest, sighs frequently, and has a feeling of constriction in her throat. Her appetite is poor, and she has indigestion and difficult elimination. Her menses are scant and pale; she feels confused and cannot concentrate; she is tense and irritable and has bouts of crying for apparently no reason. She has trouble falling asleep. She experiences premenstrual breast and lower abdominal distention and pain; lately her periods have become delayed. She lacks a sense of direction in her life and feels insecure about herself and abilities. Her tongue is pale with a thin white coat and it is slightly darker around the tip and along the edges; her pulse is wiry in the second position on the left, but overall it lacks force.

As noted previously, emotional stress and frustration may cause the Liver to lose its ability to maintain the free flow of Qi, hence Rebecca's irritability, premenstrual symptoms, and crying spells. The oppression in her chest, frequent sighing, and constriction in the throat indicate that the stagnation of Liver Qi is rising and disturbing the descending function of the Lung. As noted, when the Liver becomes stagnant, the Qi of the Spleen becomes vacuous, which manifests as lack of appetite, exhaustion, and lethargy. When the

Spleen becomes deficient and weak, it is unable to create and transform Qi and Blood properly; the Blood also becomes vacuous and cannot nourish the Heart and calm the Shen, giving rise to restlessness and insomnia. The treatment principles are to *course* (or move) *the Liver and rectify the Qi, supplement the Spleen, and nourish the Blood.* A classical point combination to address this pattern includes Liver 3 to course the Liver and rectify the Qi, Pericardium 6 to free the flow of Qi in the chest and calm the Shen, Ren 17 to stimulate the descendence of Lung Qi and relieve fullness and stagnation in the chest, and Ren 4 to supplement the Spleen. A traditional Chinese herbal formula, such as *Xiao Yao San* (Free and Easy Powder), which courses the Liver, rectifies the Qi, nourishes the Blood, and fortifies the Spleen, could be modified by adding ingredients that further nourish the Heart and calm the Shen, such as *Euphoria Longana* (Long Yan Rou), *Semen Ziziphy Spinosa* (Suan Zao Ren), and *Radix Polygalae Tenuifoliae* (Yuan Zhi). Diet and lifestyle recommendations for Rebecca may include eliminating all cold and raw foods, which damage the Spleen, from her diet and a routine of daily relaxation and exercise to help relieve Liver Qi Stagnation and calm the Shen.

The Five Phases

The relationship between Yin and Yang is further differentiated into identifiable stages that describe the process of change between situations and across time. These Stages—Wood, Fire, Earth, Metal, and Water—are known as the Five Phases and reflect the transformation of Yin into Yang and vice versa. Change is a process that occurs gradually as the energy moves around the cycle represented by the Five Phases.[1] The interaction among the Five Phases is described by two patterns, one of generation and the other of restraint, which are commonly known as the Generation *(Sheng)* and Control *(Ke)* Cycles, respectively (see Chapter 2). These Cycles represent the tendencies toward transformation within the Five Phase framework. Along the Generation Cycle, each phase nurtures and promotes the growth of the subsequent phase, counterbalanced by the Control Cycle, which sets limits, inhibits, and restrains.[6] Water creates Wood, Wood creates Fire, Fire creates Earth, Earth creates Metal, and Metal creates Water. On the other hand, Water controls Fire, Fire controls Metal, Metal controls Wood, Wood controls Earth, and Earth controls Water (Figures 18-1 and 18-2).

Clinically, the Five Phases constitute a system for understanding the movement of Qi through the various Organ functions, helping explain some of the physiological interactions among them and the etiology and nature of energetic imbalances. Each Phase corresponds to a set of Meridians and two Organ functions paired by their Yin-Yang relationship. Each paired system is commonly identified by the name of the Yin function. Every Phase characteristically influences physiological and psychological functions that in turn correspond to the particular Organ networks associated with them. The Five Phase theory describes the relationship of human beings to the seasons and to their physical environment; the seasons represents the cyclical nature of the Five Phases. The Generation Cycle of the Five Phases follows the sequence of Spring (Wood), Summer (Fire), Midsummer (Earth), Fall (Metal), and Winter (Water). Water nourishes Wood by moistening; within the body, Kidney essence *(Jing)* generates the Blood stored in the Liver; Wood generates Fire by providing fuel for combustion, whereas the Blood of the Liver nurtures the spirit of the Heart *(Shen)* by providing the foundation for mental functions. In the Control Cycle, Water restrains Fire by extinguishing it, whereas the Yin moisture of the Kidneys counterbalances the Yang Fire of the Heart. Fire restrains Metal by burning and melting it, whereas the Heart's capacity to rule the Blood complements the Lungs' capacity to govern the Qi.[1]

When using the Five Phase model, the practitioner aims to attend to the root of the patient's energetic imbalance while paying attention to the harmony of interaction within the phases. A system of correspondences is used to identify constitutional tendencies and to determine the configuration presented by the interaction of signs and symptoms. For example, suppose that Rebecca is extremely sensitive to wind, experiences an exacerbation of her symptoms (including depression) during the Spring, and has a peculiar aversion to the color green (all Wood correspondences). Through observation, palpation of the pulse and the abdomen, listening, and questioning, the practitioner assesses the relative preponderance or absence of other influences and the relative strength or weakness of the other Phases based on Rebecca's complete presentation. Of special importance are the *Mother* Phase (in this case Water), which nurtures the primary one, and the *Child* Phase (in this case Fire), which is nurtured by it (Generation Cycle). Earth, the Phase controlled by Wood, and Metal, the Phase that controls it (Control Cycle), have special significance as well.

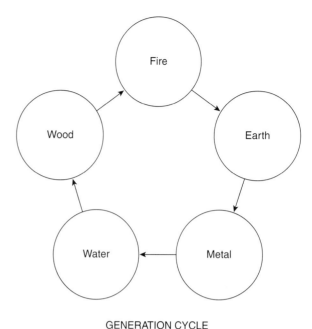

GENERATION CYCLE

Figure 18-1 The Generation Cycle of the Five Phases.

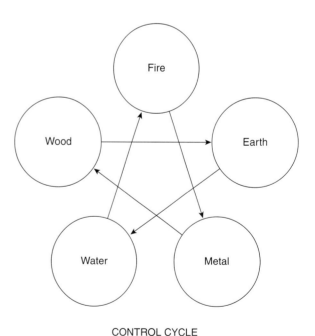

CONTROL CYCLE

Figure 18-2 The Control Cycle of the Five Phases.

The practitioner seeks to develop a profound insight into the nature of the patient, to cultivate the intuitive ability to understand the patient's imbalance, and to design a treatment structure that addresses the patient's orientation. In Rebecca's case, Wood is the primary Phase, Water is its Mother, Fire is its Child, Earth is controlled by the primary Phase, and Metal controls the primary Phase. When Rebecca talks about her depression, she describes herself as a hard worker, highly motivated, goal-oriented, and extremely accomplished. She says that her depression feels like she has run out of steam, but rather than give into the fatigue and apathy, she tries to push herself yet seems unable to focus. Fatigue, lack of appetite, general apathy, and lassitude (Earth), chest oppression, frequent sighing, and throat constriction (Metal) combine with signs and symptoms characteristic of Wood imbalance (irritability and premenstrual abdominal and breast distention and pain). On examination, the Spleen (Earth) pulse is the weakest, whereas the Liver (Wood) pulse feels replete. Because the Spleen (Earth) is deficient, it cannot perform its function of controlling Water, and the Kidney pulse also feels a bit replete.

The points needled aim at reestablishing the balance in the interaction between the Liver (Wood) and Spleen (Earth) and between the Liver (Wood) and Lungs (Metal). The selection may include points for dispersing the Liver (Lv 2) or tonifying the Spleen (Sp 2). Point selection using the Five Phase model is quite complex; there are Wood, Fire, Earth, Metal, and Water points in every Meridian. Based on the clinical indications, the clinician may treat deficiency or excess in the different Phases in a variety of ways. To reestablish the balance of the organism, energy can be moved around and transferred as needed from one Phase to another, using the tendency of transformation as represented by the cycles of Generation and Control. For example, the classical sayings "if the Child is deficient, tonify the Mother" (the Phase that precedes the primary Phase) and "if the Mother is excess, disperse the Child" (the Phase that follows the primary Phase), provide the basis for choosing a treatment approach; one may choose to address excess in the Liver by dispersing the Fire point in the Liver Meridian (Liver 2) because Fire is the Child of Wood, or one may emphasize treating Spleen deficiency by tonifying the Fire point on the Spleen Meridian (Spleen 2) because Fire is the Mother of Earth, and excess Wood causes Earth deficiency. The practitioner also may choose to treat a Phase within a Phase by needling the Earth points (Liver 3, Gall Bladder 34) or the Metal points (Liver 4, Gall Bladder 44) on the Wood Meridians, for example.

Other points may be chosen either in the context of their functions and indications to complement the effect of the treatment or on the basis of their "spirit"— the resonance that a specific point may have with the person and with what the practitioner is trying to accomplish. For example, suppose Rebecca feels numb and frozen internally, as if her spirit was dead, and she tells the practitioner about the experience that precipitated this feeling. On the basis of the "spirit of the point," the practitioner may choose to needle the acupuncture point Kidney 24, translated as *Spirit Burial Ground,* to reawaken her spirit. The two main acupuncture treatment styles based on the Five Phase framework currently practiced in this country are those stemming from the Japanese tradition and from the school developed by Dr. J.R. Worsley (see Chapter 2).

The Meridian System: The Channels and Network Vessels

The Meridians form a network that connects the surface of the body with the internal Organs, serving as a two-way communication system that both conveys messages to the surface about internal malfunctioning and alerts the internal functions about surface phenomena that might be threatening to move deeper into the system.[3] The Meridians are the surface manifestations of the Organs and act as an irrigation system that regulates the supply of Qi and Blood and prevents accumulations. The Channels and Network Vessels (smaller Channels) system is a complex web of pathways that allow the different parts of the body to work as a whole and interact. The network of Channels in the human body is composed by four major systems: the *Twelve Regular Channels,* six Yin and six Yang, which correspond to the Viscera and Bowels*; the *Eight Extraordinary Vessels,* which are thought to develop prenatally before the development of the regular

---

*Recall, there are five Viscera (or Yin Organs): Heart, Spleen, Lung, Kidney, and Liver, and six Bowels (Yang Organs): Small Intestine, Stomach, Large Intestine, Urinary Bladder, San Jiao, and Gall Bladder; for each, there is a corresponding Channel or Meridian. In addition, there is a sixth Yin Channel, the Pericardium/Heart Protector, which within the theory of the Viscera and Bowels is subsumed under the functions of the Heart, and it is seen as an extension that helps carry the functions of the Heart and that also acts as a buffer.

Channels and connect Meridians of the same polarity, whether Yin or Yang; the *Secondary Vessels,* which are situated more superficially than the other Meridians; and the *Divergent Channels,* which connect the Yin and Yang paired Organ functions. Each of these systems represents a different level, and a different type of energy travels through each of them. For example, the Tendinomuscular Channels, which are part of the Secondary Vessels, carry Defensive (Wei) Qi, whereas Jing or Essence travels through the Extraordinary Vessels and Nourishing (Ying) travels in the Regular Channels. Depending on which energetic level is affected (Defensive, Nourishing, or Ancestral), one aims at treating the corresponding energetic network.[10] When using the Meridian system as a framework, the practitioner considers all three levels and may provide a treatment that includes points and techniques that address different Meridian levels.

Let us continue with the case of Rebecca. The Liver rules, among other things, the area of the diaphragm and the region of the ribs. When confronted with a stressor, Rebecca tightens up the diaphragm, the musculature of the chest and the upper back, the throat, the jaw, and the head. Given that her stressor is severe and that her exposure to stress has been prolonged, this constriction of the musculature has begun to develop into a chronic stress response, literally cutting off the circulation of Qi and eventually obstructing the movement of Blood. This stagnation affects not only the pathway of the Liver Channel (which traverses the pelvic region, chest, throat, and vertex of the head in addition to the diaphragm,) but also the Pericardium Channel (which is part of the same greater Channel as the Liver and transverses the chest and upper back) and the Gall Bladder Channel (which is its Yang pair and transverses the sides of the body, neck, shoulders, and temples of the head). The chronic constriction of the diaphragm causes the upper and lower regions of Rebecca's body to "split" apart, so to speak, as if she has been cut off at the diaphragm. The excess of energy generated by the stagnation is beginning to rise to the upper part of her body, creating restlessness and insomnia. At the same time, the lower part of her body has become depleted and cold, giving way to decreased metabolic response manifesting in her case as fatigue; this mechanism is known as *Counterflow Qi.*

According to Oriental medical theory, in addition to storing the Viscera and Bowels, the abdominal cavity is considered to be the energetic center of the human being; it corresponds to the Middle and Lower

Jiao* and is commonly known in the Japanese tradition as *Hara.* Life springs from the lower abdominal area, where the "root" of the Qi is stored and where the Kidney resides; it is therefore regarded with utmost importance in Eastern cultures. Any obstruction in the flow of Qi resulting from diaphragmatic tension may affect the rooting of the Qi in the lower abdomen, allowing the Qi to become entrapped and replete in the upper parts of the body.[11] Many of the symptoms associated with Counterflow Qi are mental and emotional in nature; when a pattern of Counterflow Qi becomes chronic, this energetic blockage (usually at the level of the diaphragm) affects the mental, emotional, and spiritual aspects of the human being, while at the same time manifesting physically in the body.[11] The foundation for diagnosis and treatment is based on palpation of the Hara and the Meridian pathways rather than on a list of signs and symptoms. Careful observation about sensitive points and other physical findings lead the practitioner to search in corresponding areas.

On palpation, the practitioner identifies the areas of constriction and needles them superficially to free up obstruction. By releasing energy that is bound up on the surface, the Qi is made available for strengthening deeper functions.[10] The practitioner may then choose, for example, to open an Extraordinary Vessel or to balance a Divergent Channel on the basis of the findings by palpation, the Channel's clinical indications, and the patient's clinical presentation. In Rebecca's case, the practitioner finds constriction along Chong Mai, the Penetrating Vessel, one of the Eight Extraordinary Channels that travels upward from the pelvic region, alongside the navel, through the breast, and into the throat. To open the flow of this Channel, the practitioner would needle Sp 4, the opening point for Chong Mai and P 6, its pair; in addition to needling other points along the Channel, such as St 30, Kd 22-27, and Lv 14, and points in the diaphragmatic region, such as Ren 10, 11, or 12. It is interesting to note that the clinical indications for the use Chong Mai Channel match some of Rebecca's symptoms, such as constriction of the chest, breast and abdominal distention, tightness in the throat, and indigestion, and that some of the functions of the Liver, such as storing the

---

*The torso is divided in three *Jiao* (the Chinese word) or *Hara* (the Japanese word). These correspond roughly to the chest above the diaphragm, the middle abdomen, and the lower abdomen.

Blood, are closely related to Chong Mai, which is also known as the Sea of Blood.

One Channel in particular plays a very important role in the cause and treatment of mental-emotional and spiritual disorders. Du Mai, the Governing Vessel, is one of the Eight Extraordinary Meridians and does not have a corresponding Organ; it emerges from the Kidney and it is considered the storehouse of the Yang by gathering the Yang Qi of the whole body. It begins its pathway at the perineum and ascends along the spine, up over the head, and into the mouth. It is said to "nourish" the brain and spinal cord; points along its pathway have been used traditionally to affect mental functions. A repletion of energy along the Channel manifests as an exuberance of Yang—too much energy traveling "upward" toward the head or stuck in the upper part of the body creating irritability, restlessness, and insomnia. A deficiency in the flow of energy along its pathway would render the total Yang energy of the organism unable to circulate, raise, and nourish the brain and spinal cord, resulting in apathy, flat affect, and inability to express enthusiasm or emotion.

Meridian acupuncture is the cornerstone of some of the styles in the Japanese tradition, represented by Shudo Denmai,[12] Kiko Matsumoto,[6] and Miki Shima,[13] to name a few. Similarly, the school of French Meridian-energetics, developed by Soulié de Morant,[14] Dr. Van Ghi, and Yves Requena,[15] among others and the Bodymind Energetics style developed by Dr. Mark Seem[3,10] also follow a Meridian approach.

Integration

In the TCM framework, the use of the Twelve Regular Channels with the addition of Du Mai (Governing Vessel) and Ren Mai (the Conception Vessel) are considered sufficient for diagnosis and treatment, because the aim of these filters primarily is to address dysfunctions of the Organs or the Viscera and Bowels, and the Twelve Regular Channels most directly connect with the Organs.[16] As noted previously, these first three filters provide the foundation for the TCM style of acupuncture in which the selection of points mimics the writing of herbal prescriptions. The rest of the Channels and Network Vessels are given little or no attention in the TCM literature.[12] The Five Phase framework focuses primarily on the interactions among the Yin and Yang Organs within a Phase and the interrelations among them. Therefore when conceptualizing

an imbalance on the basis of the Five Phases, the Twelve Regular Channels also are primarily used. However, some Japanese acupuncture treatment styles combine the use of the Meridian and the Five Phase frameworks.

Although different styles of acupuncture have developed their strengths by emphasizing one filter over the others, each style also is based on the theoretical foundation of Chinese medicine as a whole. Also, although the different theories that serve as a foundation for the filters can artificially be compartmentalized, in reality they all function together and are necessary to understand the etiology and progression of energetic imbalances.

The disease mechanisms of mental illnesses and emotional disorders and their treatment protocols can be conceptualized and developed by using any of these filters. Some styles may prove more beneficial for some conditions than for others, or certain people may derive greater benefit by being treated with a particular style versus another or by a specific style at any given time. Given the complexity of mental and emotional disorders, a multilayered energetic approach that draws from a variety of concepts and techniques may prove most helpful. Within any given style of acupuncture, the foundations of Chinese medicine provide a framework for identifying which particular treatment will likely work best for a given patient's pattern of signs and symptoms. As yet no systematic method exists to predict who will benefit from a particular acupuncture treatment style, for what condition, or when. Comparative studies of the efficacy of each treatment approach for specific conditions may shed some light on this issue. We now address acupuncture research in the treatment of depression.

EMPIRICAL RESEARCH ON THE EFFICACY OF ACUPUNCTURE IN TREATING DEPRESSION

Relatively few well-controlled trials of the efficacy of acupuncture in the treatment of depression have been conducted. Although several clinical observations and a few research studies suggest that acupuncture is helpful in alleviating depressive symptoms, very few studies address the specific scientific question of whether acupuncture has efficacy in the treatment of depression. Studies of the *effectiveness* of a treatment address merely whether it is helpful, whereas studies of the *efficacy* of a treatment address whether the treatment works for the reasons it is purported to work. Various research designs have been used in acupuncture research,[17] but each is only suited to address particular questions and to provide certain kinds of information.

Chinese medicine provides a very clear framework for understanding the diverse presentations of the symptoms of depression and for providing individually tailored treatments to address each person's energetic configuration. This framework clearly indicates that the particular points used in the service of addressing the treatment principles are the active "ingredient" in the treatment package. Although at least one study suggests that the particular points may be the critical component that alleviates depressive symptoms, many other factors also may be therapeutic for the depressed person who receives acupuncture. Such factors include making a commitment to a treatment program designed to alleviate depression, having a relationship with a caring and attentive health care professional, believing that one is receiving an effective treatment, and deliberately breaking one's routine to keep regular appointments outside the home. These factors are often termed "nonspecific" factors[18,19] because they characterize virtually any treatment program and are specific to none. Although such nonspecific factors can exert powerful therapeutic effects, it is incumbent on the researcher interested in efficacy to demonstrate that the treatment under study is effective above and beyond such nonspecific factors. These factors extend beyond the common conception of the placebo effect. The placebo effect is often defined as that portion of treatment response resulting from the mere belief that one is receiving treatment. However, as shown in reviewing the previous list of factors and in considering the treatment milieu, many other *active* factors exist aside from the patient's belief that he or she is receiving a good treatment. Before suggesting a "gold standard" for research designs, the merits and limitations of other research designs used in acupuncture research and summarized recently should be considered.[17,20] These designs include (1) case studies and clinical observations of acupuncture, (2) acupuncture treatment compared with wait list controls, (3) acupuncture compared with placebo controls, (4) acupuncture compared with sham controls, (5) acupuncture compared with standard care, and (6) acupuncture plus standard care compared with standard care only.

Treatment Study Designs

Clinical Observation and Case Studies

Clinical observation and case studies are important because they provide the rudimentary evidence to suggest that further study is warranted. Conversely, clinical observation and case studies do not demonstrate *why* a treatment may appear to work. In such studies, treatment response may be due to the effect of acupuncture, or it may be the result of other therapeutic factors, such as the provider-patient relationship or the patient's belief that he or she is receiving an effective treatment. Moreover, such designs often involve retrospective interpretations that make it likely that data will be incomplete and that the sample may be unrepresentative (e.g., the treatment failures are less likely to be noted or to become the focus of a case study). Case studies are an important starting point but do not provide definitive data.

Wait List Controls

Wait list control studies are an extension of clinical observation and case studies. These studies, which pit acupuncture against time alone (i.e., while people await treatment), are an improvement over clinical observation and case studies because they provide systematic observation of more clients, they are prospective and therefore are not subject to retrospective reporting bias, and they involve randomization to treatment or a waiting list so that the people receiving treatment and those receiving no treatment are likely to be comparable. However, this design has many of the same shortcomings as the previous design; most notably, it does not address what specifically is responsible for any observed treatment benefit in the treatment group. The treatment response may be due to the effect of acupuncture, or it may be the result of other therapeutic factors.

Placebo Controls

Placebo controls, which are popular as controls in pharmaceutical trials, involve an inert treatment. In drug trials, the inert treatment typically is a sugar (or other inactive) pill. However, in acupuncture research, placebo controls are considerably more difficult to implement. Ideally, placebo trials provide a control for the expectation of improvement by both client and provider; neither must know that the placebo treatment is in fact inert. Examples include use of placebo needles that do not penetrate the skin[21] or the use of inactive transcutaneous electrical nerve stimulation (TENS).[22] Although such innovative techniques may provide excellent control in some cases, they do not allow a direct comparison to standard needling techniques and therefore may be limited in their application. Moreover, they may not allow for a blinding of the treatment provider in all cases, which could result in greater improvement in the active treatment group versus the placebo treatment group as a result of the providers' expectations that the active treatment is more effective than the placebo treatment.[23]

Sham Controls

Sham controls involve invasive needling of "inert" or "invalid" acupuncture points, often adjacent to the points that are part of the active treatment. It is often perceived that such studies provide a control for expectations by patients, for the general therapeutic milieu, and for nonspecific physiological effects of needle insertion. On the other hand, this design is quite undesirable because it is impossible to conduct a double-blind study (the importance of double blinding is discussed later in this chapter). Because the treatment provider is not blinded to the provision of sham treatment, the provider necessarily believes that the sham treatment is ineffective or, if the provider is also providing the active acupuncture treatment, believes that the sham treatment is much less effective than the active treatment. Because provider expectations can have profound influences on outcome,[23] this design should be avoided or treated solely as a preliminary investigation.

Comparison with Standard Care

This study design compares acupuncture with a treatment that is currently the standard of care and that ideally has demonstrated efficacy in rigorous clinical trials. In such designs, the merit of acupuncture is assumed if the treatment response of those receiving acupuncture is comparable to that of clients receiving the standard treatment. Ideally, such a design is used only after a strict efficacy study has been undertaken. Moreover, two caveats are noteworthy. The first is a statistical point. The logic of statistical tests is that a significant difference between groups is always sought. Statistical tests allow the inference, provided a significant difference exists between groups, that the difference between treatment groups is unlikely to have occurred by chance or, more precisely, that such a difference between groups would have occurred by chance only 5% of the time. (If the difference would

have occurred by chance only 5% of the time, it is reasonable to assume that the difference did not occur by chance and is therefore a result of the treatment.) Conversely, the finding of no difference between treatment groups does not allow a statistically supported conclusion that the treatments are equivalent. Statistical tests can fail to find a significant difference for many reasons, including lack of an adequate sample size, excessive variability among patient outcomes, and comparable treatments.

The second caveat concerns the impact of the standard treatment. The impact of any treatment in research studies varies considerably, and in some studies, even well-validated treatments can fail to demonstrate a sizeable treatment gain. Simply showing that acupuncture does not differ from the standard of care may not necessarily indicate that either treatment is better than a suitable control because it is possible that in a particular trial using this design, the standard treatment was performed more poorly than usual. Therefore, in designs that compare acupuncture with a standard of care, it is often useful to also include either a wait list control or some form of placebo treatment for a third group. In fact, this can be a powerful design because the placebo can be designed with respect to the standard treatment and not the acupuncture treatment—a considerably easier task in most cases. In this "three-arm" design, the efficacy of acupuncture is indicated by a finding that acupuncture produced a larger treatment response than the placebo, regardless of whether it differed from the standard of care. Of course, a stronger finding is that acupuncture not only produced greater treatment gains than placebo but also provided treatment gains at least as large as standard care.

Acupuncture Plus Standard Care Compared with Standard Care Alone

This study design attempts to determine whether there is any incremental advantage to adding acupuncture to an established treatment regimen. In the simplest form, the design compares standard care plus acupuncture with standard care alone. Such a design is confounded because the former group receives considerably more attention and can hold expectations for considerably greater improvement than the latter group. On the other hand, in situations in which efficacy studies of acupuncture already have been conducted, such a design can address the extent to which acupuncture can assist as a complementary treatment.

A stronger design would involve a double-blind study in which standard treatment plus acupuncture was compared with standard treatment plus another treatment that involved similar time, attention, and expectancy but that lacked efficacy. In such a design, the superiority of the former treatment over the latter treatment would suggest that acupuncture could be an important complementary treatment to established treatments. The best and most powerful example of this design is the recent study examining the addition of fish oil (versus the addition of the placebo of olive oil) to the standard care for manic depressive illness.[24]

The "Gold Standard" in Efficacy Designs

Although each of the previously mentioned designs plays an important role in determining whether acupuncture has merit in the treatment of various conditions, a yet more stringent standard for establishing efficacy exists: establishing that the pure effect of a treatment such as acupuncture, unconfounded by other therapeutic aspects of the treatment delivery, is sufficient to produce clinically significant gains.

Double-Blind, Randomized Control Trials

The double-blind, randomized control trial (RCT) is used to demonstrate clinically significant efficacy. The first critical component of the RCT is that research participants are randomly chosen to receive one of two treatments that are identical in every respect *except* for the purported essential ingredient. Placebo-controlled drug studies are the best example of this principle. Patients in both groups receive identical-looking pills and dosing schedules; the only difference is the actual content of the pills. All other nonspecific factors, such as the nature of and quantity of contact with the treatment staff, are comparable between the groups. However, for the nature of the contact with the staff to be comparable, the second critical aspect of the RCT must be present: both the recipients and the providers of treatment must be blinded as to whether a particular treatment is hypothesized to be effective. If either the recipients or the providers discerned which treatment was hypothesized to be more effective, this knowledge would change the nature of the relationship and the expectations regarding the effectiveness of the treatment. Such expectations can exert powerful influences on treatment response; for example,

on average, placebo responses were about 75% as large as drug responses using fluoxetine (Prozac) to treat depression.[25]

Issues in Blinding

Although a double-blind study is challenging to perform, in double-blind research on mental disorders it is often assumed that the study is double-blind in two senses. The first is that neither the patient nor the person rating the outcome is aware of what treatment the patient has received. The second is that neither the patient nor the treatment provider knows what treatment the patient has received. Thus in some sense, the highest standard for treatment should entail a triple-blind study in which the patient, provider, and outcome assessor are unaware of the treatment received by the patient.

In conducting efficacy trials of acupuncture in Western cultures, blinding the patient is relatively easy, provided the patient perceives some needling. Few individuals in Western society know where any acupuncture points are located, much less which points might aid in their particular presentation of depression. It is much more difficult to blind the treatment provider. Using inactive (sham) acupuncture does not adequately blind the treatment provider because the provider is fully aware of which treatments are valid and which are invalid. Such awareness leads the provider to different expectations of outcome for sham versus active treatments. These expectations can and should be assessed in any efficacy study.

The thorny issue of blinding the acupuncture treatment provider is difficult, but not impossible, to resolve. As described previously, the allopathic condition "depression" can be viewed as an imbalance in the person's energetic configuration and can be interpreted using different frameworks based on the Chinese medicine model. Because treatments need to be tailored to each individual to provide the maximum benefit, any two depressed individuals are likely to receive rather different constellations of points in their treatment. Thus if any acupuncture treatment provider were only to receive a set of points to administer, it would not be immediately obvious whether such points would be designed to address an energetic imbalance underlying a particular patient's depression. Following this logic further, it is therefore possible to separate two traditionally integrated functions of the acupuncturist treatment provider: assessment versus treatment. If assessors served only to conceptualize the treatment principles and devise the treatment strategy and associated points, and a different group of treating acupuncturists were provided with these points to administer to clients, then there is a reasonable chance that these treating acupuncturists would be blinded as to whether a treatment would be the most effective for a given client. *Thus although the providers would not be blinded as to which points were used, they may well be blinded as to the particular intent of the treatment.* This strategy presumes that two important restrictions are used: (1) that the treating acupuncturists are prohibited from using assessment procedures (including the interview, palpation, taking of pulses, and examination of the tongue), and (2) that the treating acupuncturists are not fully aware of which theoretical framework (i.e., combination of filters) is being used to conceptualize the patient. Although this strategy would not guarantee that the treating acupuncturist would remain blinded, the effectiveness of this strategy in producing a double blind can be monitored simply by administering questionnaires that tap the expectations and beliefs of the provider and recipient.[26]

Treatment Fidelity

Implicit in the foregoing discussion is that any acupuncture treatment should be faithfully derived from the framework of Chinese medicine. As Hammerschlag[17] has noted, it is clearly inappropriate to implement an invariant treatment for all patients in a study based solely on Western biomedical diagnoses. Because considerable heterogeneity exists, in energetic terms, among those who share a common allopathic diagnosis, any single set of acupuncture points applied to all patients would be absurd from the perspective of Chinese medicine. Instead, careful differential diagnosis from the perspective of Chinese medicine is required to derive individually tailored treatments that Chinese medicine would predict to address the underlying pattern of imbalance. At first glance, such individual tailoring may appear to be in conflict with the scientific need to standardize the treatment approach, but it is possible to deliver manualized, replicable, and standardized treatments that are nonetheless tailored to each patient on the basis of that patient's pattern of disharmony.[26]

Ethical Sensitivity

Many acupuncture practitioners and researchers have worried about whether various research designs are ethical because some designs may not necessarily provide a

treatment known to be (or thought to be) effective to all patients. This concern can be allayed by ensuring that, in any design, all patients ultimately receive the treatment hypothesized to be most effective. For example, in wait list, placebo, or sham designs, patients who first receive one of these treatments instead of the active acupuncture treatment could then be assigned to receive the active acupuncture treatment after the completion of the control treatment. If subjects are provided with informed consent that they may first receive a control treatment and are given information that adequately describes any risks associated with the active or the control treatment, they can decide with full knowledge of the risks and anticipated benefits whether they wish to participate in the clinical trial instead of seeking standard care. It is worth noting that, especially in the case of depression, it is important to select case subjects in the research study who can be ethically subjected to a control treatment. Case subjects with acute risk (e.g., active suicidal potential in the case of depressed patients) should not be included in clinical trials necessitating a potentially ineffective control condition.

The Ideal Progression of Research

Each of the aforementioned designs may have an important role in programmatic research designed to answer the question of whether acupuncture has merit in the treatment of a particular condition. Clinical observation and case studies provide the first evidence that a treatment may merit research, and wait list control studies provide an opportunity to more systematically detail those observations. Controlled trials can then follow that may vary in the degree to which all possible confounding factors are controlled. Placebo control and sham control trials can control some of the confounding factors, but only a blinded (possibly a *triple*-blinded) RCT can provide unequivocal evidence of efficacy. After positive results in a blinded RCT, trials that examine how acupuncture compares with the standard of care or how acupuncture can augment treatment response when used in addition to the standard of care can then provide evidence assessing the use of acupuncture in everyday patient care. The advantage of the latter designs is that because they may not require blinding—if conducted *after* efficacy has been established in a tightly controlled trial—they may provide a better estimate of the magnitude of the treatment response in the typical clinical setting.

With the preceding discussion in mind, we now review the literature examining acupuncture in the treatment of depression. Unfortunately, many studies fall short of the desideratum of the double-blind RCT.

Studies of Acupuncture in the Treatment of Depression and Conditions Involving Depression

Aside from our pilot study,[26] which is detailed in the following text, the only studies of acupuncture as a treatment for depression or syndromes involving depression have been conducted and published in China[27,28] and in Eastern Europe and the former Soviet Union.[29-32] Full evaluation of these studies is difficult because the diagnostic criteria used differ from those used in Western psychiatry and because most of these studies have not been translated into English (other than the abstracts). Collectively, however, these studies suggest that acupuncture can be effective in the treatment of depression and depressive symptoms and may be as effective as tricyclic antidepressant medication is some cases. The following review summarizes these studies, with a focus on the range of depressive symptoms for which acupuncture may or may not be effective.

In a sample of 167 depressed patients, Polyakov[30] found that acupuncture reduced the principal symptoms of depression. The best results were obtained in patients with melancholic depression; poor results were obtained in patients with anxious and apathetic depressions. Acupuncture was almost as effective as antidepressant therapy in cyclothymic depressions and was notably inferior to tricyclic antidepressant therapy in patients with psychotic features. Moreover, Polyakov and Dudaeva[31] report that follow-up studies over 1 to 2 years indicate that adequate maintenance therapy produces results comparable to drug therapy, although inadequate information is provided to evaluate this claim. In this study, acupuncture was performed using a standardized treatment method consisting of five acupuncture points located in the traditional Meridians (St 36, P 5, P 6, Lu 7, and LI 4) plus three ear acupuncture points (AT affect, AT Shen-men, and AT Zero). From the perspective of energetic differential diagnosis (the assessment method of Chinese medicine), the finding of poor treatment response in anxious and apathetic depressions is not surprising because this set of points does not specifically address the features present during anxious or apathetic depressions. This finding highlights the importance of considering individual differences in symptom presentation and tailoring points accordingly.

Other studies provide only abstracts in English. Chengying[27] used points on the Du channel (which runs along the spine) to treat a mix of psychiatric disorders including anxiety, depression, hypochondria, neurasthenia, obsessive-compulsive disorder, aphasia, alexia, and hysterical paralysis. One hundred fifteen patients with a course of disease ranging from 2 months to 8 years were treated with points selected from the Du channel. Points were selected by pressing the points one by one, observing and comparing sensitivity to the points, and choosing to needle the one or two points with the maximum response. Among the 115 patients, 61 experienced complete disappearance of psychoneurotic and somatic symptoms with no recurrence at 6-month follow up; 31 experienced a significant improvement, and 23 had no significant improvement after treatment. Although Chengying[27] studied a heterogeneous group, the comparability of the diagnoses neurasthenia and major depression is noted by Chang.[33] Commenting on the observations of Dunner and Dunner,[34] Chang indicates that almost 50% of psychiatric outpatients in China have a diagnosis of neurasthenia, and that many of these patients would have a diagnosis of major depression according to the DSM-IV. Moreover, Chang[33] notes that antidepressants were as effective for neurasthenia diagnosed by Chinese psychiatrists as with cases of DSM-IV-defined depression.

An additional 103 patients with neurasthenia (with disease courses ranging from 3 months to 20 years; average 4.5 years) were observed clinically at the Academy of Traditional Chinese Medicine.[35] Principal points (Du 14, Du 13, GB 20, the first line on the Bladder channel, bilateral to the spine and the Huatuo paravertebral points [Extra 21]) were used in combination with other points chosen according to symptoms. After treatment, 45 patients experienced total relief of all symptoms and were considered clinically cured; 29 experienced improvement of their main symptoms but some secondary symptoms remained; 21 patients experienced a noticeable improvement; and 8 cases experienced no improvement.

None of these studies would qualify as double-blind RCTs because no provisions were made for blinding, and no control groups existed. The following studies, although not double-blinded, did provide a control group. The first study, also a Chinese study, by Luo et al of the Institute of Mental Health, Beijing Medical College, examined electroacupuncture and amitriptyline treatment of DSM-III–defined major depression. This study, summarized by Han,[28] found comparable decreases in depression severity scores as a function of electroacupuncture and amitriptyline treatments across a 5-week interval. Moreover, fewer side effects were reported for patients who received electroacupuncture. Unfortunately, this study used only two points (Du 20 and Yintang), and it is unclear whether standard needling, as opposed to electroacupuncture, would provide comparable results. Another Chinese study[36] also found comparable decreases in depressive symptoms for patients receiving electroacupuncture and those receiving amitriptyline.

Although far from definitive, the combined results of these studies suggest that favorable results are possible using acupuncture to treat mood-related symptoms, including depression. Thus these studies partly address the effectiveness question, but the efficacy question remains unanswered. These findings encouraged us to undertake a study to examine the efficacy of acupuncture as a treatment for depression.

A Study Examining the Efficacy of Acupuncture in the Treatment of Depression

Our pilot study[26] involved an RCT with blind outcome ratings to assess women with major depression who were randomly assigned to one of three treatment groups for 8 weeks. *Specific treatment* involved acupuncture treatments for symptoms of depression; *nonspecific treatment* involved acupuncture treatment for symptoms that were not clearly part of the depressive episode; a *wait list* condition involved waiting without treatment for 8 weeks. Nonspecific and wait list conditions were followed by crossover to specific treatment.

A community volunteer sample was used with 33 women who met DSM-IV[37] criteria for current Major Depressive Episode of less than 2 years' duration. Thirty-eight women between the ages of 18 and 45 years were recruited through newspaper advertisements. Advertisements mentioned treatment for depression but not acupuncture. Participants were excluded if they had complicating factors such as other mental disorders, uncontrolled medical conditions, or medical conditions that might be a physiological basis

for the depressive symptoms. Five (13%) women terminated partipation before completion of the study,* resulting in a final sample of 33 women who received treatment specifically for depression (and 34 who completed the first 8 weeks and were used in the comparison of specific, nonspecific, and wait list conditions). This final sample had mild-to-moderate depression, with a mean duration of the current episode of 9.2 months (±6.9 SD) and a history of 2.5 (±2.9) prior episodes. In addition, 82% of the participants reported previously psychotherapy, 53% reported previous trials of antidepressants, and 11% reported no previous treatment. Fifty-nine percent of these participants reported that one or more first-degree relatives also had depression of comparable severity.

To control for nonspecific therapeutic factors, the study design provided for the development of two types of acupuncture treatments for each patient: (1) a treatment individually tailored to treat the patient's specific symptoms of depression (specific treatment), and (2) a treatment designed to treat an aspect characteristic of the individual's energetic configuration but not related to the individual's depression (nonspecific treatment; e.g., targeting a structural imbalance). The specific and nonspecific treatment were similar from the perspective of the patients, each involving points in the same general body regions. Moreover, patients were unaware of which treatment they were receiving.

The specific and nonspecific treatment plans were developed by an assessing acupuncturist and were administered by four trained and board-certified acupuncturists other than the assessing acupuncturist. Because the nonspecific treatments involved valid acupuncture points, treating acupuncturists perceived that they were providing a valid treatment, a belief that they would not have held if sham points had been used as a control. The treating acupuncturists were blinded to experimental hypotheses and the nature by which the specific and nonspecific treatments were devised, and they were not informed of which treatment

---

*Two subjects terminated participation for reasons unrelated to treatment (pregnancy and moving out of state), two terminated because of discomfort with the treatment, and one terminated because she was not losing weight and believed that she would lose weight with a pharmacological treatment. This last participant terminated participation after she completed nonspecific treatment but before the commencement of specific treatment and therefore was included in analyses involving the nonspecific treatment. Among these five patients, two terminated from specific treatment, two terminated from nonspecific treatment, and one terminated from the wait list.

plan they were providing. The acupuncturists rated their beliefs about the efficacy of the treatment after the first treatment session for each patient; these ratings did not differ between specific and nonspecific treatments ($F[1,22] < 1$, *ns*), suggesting that the blinding strategy was effective.

The efficacy question was addressed by comparing the effect of the three 8-week treatment conditions, specific, nonspecific, and wait list (Figure 18-3). Clients receiving specific acupuncture treatments demonstrated significantly ($p < 0.05$) greater reduction in depression scores than those receiving the nonspecific acupuncture treatments, and showed marginally ($p < 0.12$) more improvement than wait list controls. Figure 18-3 summarizes the reduction in depression severity for women in each of the three groups. It was also possible to address the effectiveness question in the context of this study because every woman eventually received the specific treatment. After treatments specifically designed to address symptoms of depression, nearly two thirds of women experienced full remission according to DSM-IV criteria. This rate of remission is similar to that reported

in studies of psychotherapy and antidepressant drugs, which show that 50% to 70% of those who complete treatment meet criteria for remission.

In summary, based on this small outpatient sample of women with Major Depressive Episode, it appears that acupuncture has sufficient efficacy to justify a larger clinical trial and that it can provide significant symptom relief at rates comparable to standard treatments, such as psychotherapy or pharmacotherapy.

SUMMARY

Persons who work in the field of mental health know that no easy answers exist in the treatment of mental illnesses and emotional disturbances. Vulnerability to biological imbalances is usually triggered by specific life events that are processed psychologically. At the same time, psychological factors precipitate a complex series of biological symptoms, which are an important part of many mental illnesses. The complexity of the human bodymind cannot be overlooked. Chinese medicine postulates a framework that may help integrate the apparent disparity between the psychological and physiological basis of mental illnesses. In this respect, Chinese medicine may assist in classifying heterogeneous presentations of a single allopathic disorder such as depression. Although allopathic physicians, psychiatrists, and psychologists acknowledge that depression presents very differently for different individuals, currently no clear method exists to specify a priori which treatment will likely work for whom. By contrast, the framework of Chinese medicine provides a basis for individually tailored treatments for a given individual's symptom configuration. At least one well-controlled study[34] suggests that this approach is efficacious in the treatment of depression.

It is not uncommon for practitioners of Chinese medicine to treat patients who are currently undergoing treatment for mental illness or emotional disturbances. One study[38] found that nearly two thirds of patients receiving acupuncture in community clinics reported that they did so for "mood care," among other reasons. Frequently patients begin acupuncture or Chinese herbal treatment when they have just started standard treatment for major depression, when they are struggling to regulate a lifelong history of manic depression, or when they are desperately trying to break the sleeping pill habit. At other times, patients seek acupuncture care first because they want to

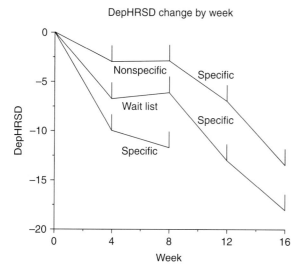

Figure 18-3 Mean (±SE) change on the depression items from the Hamilton Rating Scale for Depression *(DepHRSD)* for patients in the Specific (*N* = 12), Nonspecific (*N* = 11), and Wait list (*N* = 11) groups by week. Note that after 8 weeks, patients in the Nonspecific and Wait list groups began receiving specific treatment. (From Allen JJB, Schnyer RN, Hitt SK: The efficacy of acupuncture in the treatment of major depression in women, *Psychol Sci* 9:397-401, 1998.)

avoid taking prescription drugs or because they refuse to undergo psychotherapy for personal reasons. Experience, observation, and in some cases controlled studies suggest that Chinese medicine can help people with anxiety, depression, or insomnia; it can help reduce or minimize the need for psychotropic medications in more serious disorders; and it can assist to overcome dependency to prescription drugs. However, currently insufficient scientific evidence exists concerning the efficacy of Chinese medicine as a complete alternative to standard psychiatric care, and concerning the efficacy of treatments derived from Chinese medicine for many emotional conditions. Therefore judicious practitioners of Chinese medicine are always most comfortable working in conjunction with mental health professionals when treating patients with serious mental illnesses, patients at risk of suicide, those who are a danger to themselves or others, or patients who do not respond quickly enough to treatment. Mental, emotional, and spiritual well-being is generally an added benefit of acupuncture therapy.

For patients who do not meet psychiatric criteria yet suffer from deep emotional uneasiness, Chinese medicine also can be of great benefit. For patients who present a wide range of symptoms that appear to be totally disconnected from the biomedical perspective or for those who require a very broad combination of prescription drugs, Chinese medicine can help clarify the clinical picture and make allopathic treatment more effective.

References

1. Beinfield H, Korngold E: *Between heaven and earth: a guide to Chinese medicine,* New York, 1991, Ballantine Books.
2. Kaptchuk TJ: *The web that has no weaver: understanding Chinese medicine,* New York, 1983, Congdon & Weed.
3. Seem M: *Bodymind energetics towards a dynamic model of health,* Rochester, Vt, 1987, Thorsons.
4. Maciocia G: *The practice of Chinese medicine: the treatment of diseases with acupuncture and Chinese herbs,* London, 1994, Churchill Livingstone.
5. Hammer L: *Dragon rises, red bird flies: psychology and Chinese medicine,* New York, 1990, Station Hill Press.
6. Matsumoto K, Birch S: *Five elements and ten stems: Nan Ching theory, diagnostics, and practice,* Brookline, Mass, 1983, Paradigm.
7. Flaws B: *Curing insomnia naturally with Chinese medicine,* Boulder, Colo, 1998, Blue Poppy Press.
8. Kaptchuck TJ: Class notes: course in Chinese herbology, New York, 1981, Tri-State College of Acupuncture.
9. Kaptchuk TJ: *Jade pharmacy clinical manual,* Soquel, Calif, 1987, Ming Meu Design. Available from Crane Enterprises.
10. Seem M: *Acupuncture imaging: perceiving the energy pathways of the body,* Rochester, Vt, 1990, Healing Arts Press.
11. Matsumoto K, Birch S: *Hara diagnosis: reflections of the sea,* Brookline, Mass, 1988, Paradigm.
12. Denmai S: *Introduction to meridian therapy,* Seattle, 1989, Eastland Press.
13. Shima M: Seminars and lectures, 1992, Corte Madera, Calif.
14. Soulié de Morant G: *Chinese acupuncture,* Brookline, Mass, 1994, Paradigm.
15. Requena Y: *Terrains and pathology in acupuncture,* ed 2, Brookline, Mass, 1994, Paradigm.
16. Flaws B: Foreword. In Seem M: *Acupuncture imaging: perceiving the energy pathways of the body,* Rochester, Vt, 1990, Healing Arts Press.
17. Hammerschlag R: Methodological and ethical issues in clinical trials of acupuncture, *J Altern Complement Med* 4:159-71, 1998.
18. Arkowitz H: A common factors therapy for depression. In Norcross JC, Goldfried MR, editors: *Handbook of psychotherapy integration,* New York, 1992, Basic Books, pp. 404-32.
19. Grencavage L, Bootzin R, Shoham V: Specific and nonspecific effects of therapy. In Costello CG, editor: *Basic issues in psychopathology,* New York, 1993, Wiley.
20. Ernst E: The case for case studies, *Int J Altern Complement Med* 29-30, 1998.
21. Streitberger K, Kleinhenz J: Introducing a placebo needle into acupuncture research, *Lancet* 352:364-5, 1998.
22. Petrie JP, Hazleman BL: A controlled study of acupuncture in neck pain, *J Rheumatol* 25:271-5, 1986.
23. Berman JS: Social bases of psychotherapy: expectancy, attraction, and the outcome of treatment, *Dissertation Abstracts International* 40:5800-1, 1980 (dissertation abstract).
24. Stoll AL, Severus EW, Freeman MP, et al: Omega 3 fatty acids in bipolar disorder: a preliminary double-blind, placebo-controlled trial, *Arch General Psychiatry* 56:407-12, 1999.
25. Kirsch I, Sapirstein G: Listening to Prozac but hearing placebo: a meta-analysis of antidepressant medication, *Prevention and Treatment* 1, June 26, 1998 (www.apa.org/prevention).
26. Allen JJB, Schnyer RN, Hitt SK: The efficacy of acupuncture in the treatment of major depression in women, *Psychol Sci* 9:397-401, 1998.
27. Chengying Y: Mind-regulating acupuncture treatment of neurosis, using points of Du channel, *Int J Clin Acupunct* 3:193-6, 1992.

28. Han JS: Electroacupuncture: an alternative to antidepressants for treating affective diseases? *Int J Neurosci* 29:79-92, 1986.

29. Frydrykowski A: An attempt at applying acupuncture in the treatment of depressive symptoms, *Psychiatr Pol* 18:247-50, 1984.

30. Polyakov SE: Acupuncture in the treatment of endogenous depressions, *Soviet Neurol Psychiatr* 21:36-44, 1988.

31. Polyakov SE, Dudaeva KI: Neurophysiological changes in reflex therapy for endogenous depression, *Zh Nevrol Psikhiatr Im S S Korsakova* 90:99-103, 1990.

32. Toteva S: Reflexotherapy of patients with associated alcoholism and depressive syndrome, *Zh Nevrol Psikhiatr Im S S Korsakova* 19:83-4, 1991.

33. Chang W: Electroacupuncture and ETC, *Biol Psychiatry* 19:1271-2, 1984.

34. Dunner DL, Dunner PZ: Psychiatry in China: some personal observations, *Biol Psychiatry* 18:799-801, 1983.

35. Suobin K: Clinical observation on 103 cases of neurasthenia treated with plum-blossom needle tapping, *Int J Clin Acupunct* 2:419-21, 1991.

36. Hechun 1988: Summarized by Brewington et al, 1994.

37. American Psychiatric Association: *Diagnostic and statistical manual of mental disorders: fourth edition,* Washington, DC, 1994, The Association.

38. Cassidy CM: Chinese medicine users in the United States. Part I. Utilization, satisfaction, medical plurality, *J Altern Complement Med* 4:17-27, 1998.

19

Acupuncture and Laser Acupuncture to Treat Paralysis in Stroke, Cerebral Palsy, Spinal Cord Injury, and Bell's Palsy

MARGARET A. NAESER

ORIENTAL MEDICINE CONCEPTS OF PARALYSIS

Oriental medicine (OM) is familiar with the same central nervous system (CNS) dysfunctions as biomedicine, although as might be expected, OM interprets and treats the associated physiological conditions differently. This chapter discusses four neurological disorders with paralysis for which some scientific research data are available regarding the efficacy of acupuncture intervention. These four disorders include stroke (cerebrovascular accident [CVA]), cerebral palsy (CP) in infants and children, paralysis/spasticity in spinal cord injury (SCI), and peripheral facial paralysis (Bell's palsy).

Clinically, however, many other CNS conditions are known from classical texts and are currently treated by OM practitioners. For these four selected disorders with paralysis, the number of OM categories exceeds the number of biomedical categories (Table 19-1). These OM categories are discussed briefly for each of the four CNS disorders.

Stroke, or *Wind Stroke* in OM parlance, is well recognized in OM. When a patient presents with symptoms of stroke, the stroke may be further subdivided into *tense* or *flaccid* types.[1] In the former, the patient experiences a collapse of Yin and thus shows extreme Yang symptoms such as grimace, clenched hands and teeth, convulsion, and eyes strained open. The more serious flaccid type, which is a result of Yang collapse, presents with coma, limpness, and partially closed eyes, among other symptoms. Those who survive the acute stage of serious stroke may have residual sequelae, such as hemiplegia, paresis of the lower extremity

TABLE 19-1

Four Neurological Disorders with Paralysis and Their Oriental Medicine Diagnoses

Neurological Disorder	Oriental medicine diagnoses
Stroke[1]	Tense or flaccid type Root cause: Kidney deficiency, Spleen deficiency, or weakness in Channels Branch types: Liver Wind, Phlegm-Fire, Blood stasis, Wind in Channels
Cerebral palsy[2]	Spastic or flaccid type Root cause: Kidney deficiency Cold pattern may be present Stagnation of Qi and Blood in Channels
Paralysis in spinal cord injury[5]	Damage to Du Channel (Governing Vessel) Yang deficiency Kidney deficiency Stagnation of Qi and Blood in Channels

Bell's palsy[1,6]	Stomach Qi deficiency
	  Wind Damp
	  Wind Cold
	Liver Qi stagnation
	Liver excess

(LE), upper extremity (UE), or only the hand, sensory disturbances or numbness, visual field restriction, language problems including aphasia, or other specific cognitive deficits, such as inability to name pictures, recall words, perform calculations, or inability to read or write, depending on the specific locus of the lesion in the brain.

Wind stroke is considered a late expression of a long history of disharmony associated with such factors as overwork, excess stress, irregular diet, and sexual indulgence. Earlier deficiencies of Kidney or Spleen, or weakness in the Channels, if not resolved, allow the development of more serious imbalances of either Yin and Yang or Qi and Blood. For example, in the presence of Kidney Yin deficiency, Liver Yang is insufficiently controlled, allowing a condition labeled Liver Wind to develop. The character of Wind is to rise; hence symptoms develop in the head. A severe case of Liver Wind can express as Wind Stroke, characterized by symptoms such as sudden attack, coma, mental cloudiness, and paralysis.[1]

Paralysis in infants and children that is associated with the biomedical term *cerebral palsy* has been reviewed in OM terminology by Scott and Barlow.[2] They comment that some infants can withstand more prenatal or perinatal birth trauma than others, depending on their inherent Kidney Qi or Jing (Essence)

Qi. If Kidney deficiency is present, the deficiency is usually caused by a prenatal deficiency of Essence (Jing Qi). However, CP can manifest either as Excess type (spastic) or Deficient type (flaccid); often some overlap occurs. To determine whether the case belongs more to one type or the other, Scott and Barlow suggest two questions to ask[2]: (1) Are the limbs in spasm, or are they floppy and flaccid? (2) Is the child deficient in energy overall, or is there evidence of a strong Cold interior condition? This differential diagnosis is important because if strong signs of Cold exist, then moxa should be used. In the spastic type, a quite strong reducing technique can be used, whereas a much gentler treatment is indicated for the flaccid type of CP.

Scott and Barlow[2] stress that the underlying root cause of stroke in adults is similar to the root cause of CP in infants—Kidney deficiency. Although each condition has a spastic and a flaccid type, this is their only similarity. Although a common Kidney deficiency pattern exists in each, instead of a Liver Yang rising pattern (with accompanying heat) in adult stroke, a full Cold pattern may exist in infants and children. In addition, Phlegm is rarely a major contributing factor in CP.

From the OM viewpoint, the treatment of CP requires treatment of both the root cause (Kidney deficiency) and the symptoms in the Channels (limbs). Scott and Barlow[2] stress that the CP cases need many treatments, perhaps more than a hundred, for optimum success. Although obvious results may be noticed after the first five treatments or so, additional treatment of both the root cause and the Channels in the limbs is necessary for acupuncture to be successful in bringing Qi to the limbs. They cite Chinese sources that recommend 10 days of treatment (including weekends) followed by 5 days off as 1 treatment course for Channels/limbs; a minimum of 5 to 15 courses is recommended (e.g., 50 to 150 treatments).

Scott and Barlow[2] recommend following the Chinese schedule of 10 days on with 5 days off. They do not recommend compromised treatment schedules. If patients cannot obtain daily treatments, they recommend weekly treatments only, aimed at both the root cause and the Channels. They stress that treatment of the Channels necessitates the strong daily treatment schedule, whereas the "energetic or root treatment" requires only a weekly treatment. In their experience, a treatment schedule that includes more daily treatments on the Channels/limbs plus a weekly root treatment yields the best results. They suggest that because treatment of CP requires intensive, daily treatments, a need exists for special CP centers where acupuncture can be provided on a daily basis. The notion of continued, intensive treatment of the limbs is addressed in the research section on CP in this chapter, in which the possibility of home treatments with low-level laser acupuncture on the Channels is suggested.[3,4]

Gao et al[5] have reviewed paralysis associated with *spinal cord injury* (SCI) in OM terminology. They note that traumatic paraplegia is the consequence of damage to the Du Channel (Governing Vessel, or Meridian that traverses the midline of the back, extending from the crotch area to the center of the philtrum above the upper lip). The Du Channel is considered to govern the Yang Qi of the whole body; thus injury to the Du Channel results in Yang deficiency. In addition, because the Kidney Qi is located in the loin area, energy to the Kidneys is often disturbed with SCI, resulting in problems with urination and defecation. Overall, the OM diagnosis in SCI includes obstruction of the Channels and Collaterals with sudden stagnation of Qi and Blood circulation, resulting in limb paralysis with dystrophic changes.

The OM treatment strategy with SCI is as follows: (1) clear and activate the Channels and Collaterals, (2) promote blood circulation to dissipate Blood Stasis,

(3) reinforce the Kidney Qi, and (4) support the overall Yang Qi. As with adult stroke cases and infants and children with CP, many treatments are recommended; the sooner the treatments are initiated, the better is the outcome.

In OM terminology, *peripheral facial paralysis (Bell's palsy)* is associated primarily with Wind and Cold of External origin, which invade the Channels traversing the face,[6] disrupting the flow of Qi and Blood and preventing the Vessels and muscles from receiving necessary moistening and nourishment. The OM treatment principle is to spread Qi through the Channels of the face.

ACUPUNCTURE THERAPIES INCLUDING SCALP NEEDLE ACUPUNCTURE TO TREAT CENTRAL NERVOUS SYSTEM DISORDERS

Treatment of CNS disorders in OM includes both the classic forms of body acupuncture, herbology, bodywork techniques, dietary manipulation, and newer interventions, including both auricular and scalp acupuncture. Combined therapy has been the norm in OM care of CNS patients for millennia, including bodywork techniques that closely resemble neuromuscular reprogramming, now becoming recognized as important in rehabilitation in Western nations. Auricular points associated with the CNS and with parts of the anatomy affected in CNS disorders, such as the upper or lower extremities, can be needled.[7] An advantage of auricular acupuncture is that dermal tacks or seeds can be left in place and self-stimulated by the patient, allowing continued acupuncture therapy outside the treatment room.

Chinese scalp acupuncture is a relatively new technique that involves stimulation of points on the scalp located over known cortical regions of the brain associated with a specific activity (motor, sensory, visual, auditory). For example, in the case history on stroke blindness (see Chapter 8), points over the visual areas of the occiput were stimulated using the Chinese scalp acupuncture method. The patient also received treatment at traditional body points.

The Chinese scalp acupuncture method, especially for stroke cases, was developed by Shun-Fa Jiao, MD, at the Jishan County People's Hospital, Shanxi Province, during the Cultural Revolution.[6,8] The scalp area to be treated must be carefully delineated (e.g., the motor cortex line on the side of the scalp overlying the area where the stroke occurred, which is the side of the brain opposite to the paralyzed upper and lower extremities). Traditionally, larger Chinese needles are used (26- to 28-gauge filiform needles between 2.5 and 3 inches in length). The needle is inserted almost horizontally to the scalp (not touching the bone) and slowly rotated until the requisite portion of the needle has been inserted. Once in place, the needle should not be further raised or thrust. Instead, it is rapidly twirled (200 times/minute) with two or three rotations forward and two or three rotations backward, until the characteristic needle sensation (Qi) is obtained. The twirling may continue for 3 to 4 minutes, is followed by 5 to 10 minutes of rest, then begins again. After this pattern is repeated two or three more times, the needle is withdrawn. Electrical stimulation on the needle handles sometimes is used instead of the twirling.[9] The most common response to needling is a hot sensation, usually on the limbs opposite the needling site. Generally, if sensory responses accompany the needling, the result is good, although in some cases treatment is effective despite their absence.[6]

Another technique, *Yamamoto scalp acupuncture from Japan,* is entirely different from the Chinese system, including point locations and treatment method. Yamamoto New Scalp Acupuncture (YNSA) was developed by Toshikatsu Yamamoto, MD, PhD, from Nichinan, Miyazaki, Japan; it was first reported in 1973.[10] With YNSA, the body representation areas are located primarily along the front hairline. (The entire body has a representation here, similar to the concept of whole body representation in ear, hand, or foot acupuncture; see Chapter 4.) The specific somatic areas near the hairline are treated based on location of the patient's somatic problem with careful palpation of the hairline area. In addition, the internal organs are represented in the temporal areas on each side of the scalp. The points in the temporal areas are stimulated based on results from palpation in the lateral triangle of the neck area with additional palpation of these temporal areas. Dr. Yamamoto uses this method to treat many specific disorders, including poststroke paralysis, tremors in Parkinson's disease, and many types of pain, including acute migraine headaches, angina pectoris, postherpetic neuralgia, sciatica, postoperative pain, arthritis, sports injury, and asthma and sinusitis.

The primary advantage of YNSA is that when applied correctly, improvement may begin to occur within a minute, especially in acute severe migraine and in chronic stroke patients with hemiparesis. The YNSA technique uses only half-inch Japanese needles

(usually only 32- or 34-gauge). The needles may be left in place for several hours, and stroke patients can undergo a physical therapy session with the small scalp needles left in place. Because increased range of motion can begin within a few minutes after YNSA needle insertion, the stroke patient begins the physical therapy session with greater range of motion, thus allowing more progress during that session. Patients with migraine headache retain the needles until complete relief is obtained, usually within a few hours.

RESEARCH DATA

Although research on this topic is still in its infancy, some excellent research has been published and is reviewed in the following text. Although these studies focus on acupuncture treatment, readers should remember that in clinical settings, herbal and bodywork treatments also are typically provided. The latter issues and integrated treatment have received less research attention and are not reviewed.*

Acupuncture and Laser Acupuncture to Treat Poststroke Paralysis

Acupuncture care can help to treat acute stroke, but in Western nations, biomedical care is the usual option during the acute stages. Acupuncture care, where available, is often used to treat the sequelae of stroke. However, research showing improved response when acupuncture is added during the acute stage provides good reason for beginning acupuncture as soon as possible poststroke, assuming the patient does not have active bleeding (acute cerebral hemorrhage).

Stroke is the major cause of disability among adults in the United States.[11] Every day, more than 1200 Americans have a stroke, and 400 of these patients are disabled permanently. Today more than 2 million Americans have long-term disabilities from stroke; stroke costs more than $25 billion each year.[12]

Results for 10 studies in which acupuncture was used to treat paralysis in stroke patients are presented in Table 19-2. Sham acupuncture (insertion of needles

---

*Herbal safety and herb-drug interactions are discussed in Chapter 5. Readers with further interest can contact John Chen, PharmD, LAc, pharmacologist, through http://www.Lotusherbs.com.

TABLE 19-2

Acupuncture or Laser Acupuncture to Treat Paralysis in Stroke

Authors	Cases real acupuncture (no.)	Control cases (no.)		Significance level between groups and/or no. of cases with outcome level of good response/markedly effective
		Sham	No acupuncture	
Naeser et al[13] (1992) VA Boston Healthcare System	10 acute arm/leg, starting at 1-3 mo after stroke, 20 real tx, 4 wk	6 acute arm/leg control, 1-3 mo after stroke, 20 sham tx, 4 wk		$p < 0.13$ with CT scan lesion site as a variable 4/10 good response, real acupuncture 0/6 good response, sham acupuncture
Naeser et al[9] (1994a) VA Boston Healthcare System	10 acute, 10 chronic arm/leg, Starting: Acute: 1-3 mo; Chronic: 4 mo to 6 yr after stroke; 20-40 tx, 2-4 mo	Acute arm/leg control; see above study with sham acupuncture	3 chronic arm/leg, no acupuncture	$p < 0.003$ (chronic), with CT scan lesion site as variable 3/10 good response, chronic, real acupuncture 0/3 good response, chronic, no acupuncture 5/10 good response, acute, real acupuncture Isolated active ROM for 8 good response After 20 tx p level Shoulder abd +7% <0.04 Knee flexion +19% <0.02 Knee extens +19% NS After 40 tx p level Shoulder abd +12% <0.04 Knee flexion +22% <0.03 Knee extens +28% <0.01
Naeser et al[14] (1994b) VA Boston Healthcare System	3 acute, 8 chronic hand Acute: 1-3 mo Chronic: 4 mo-8 yr 20-40 tx		2 chronic, no acupuncture	$p < 0.022$ (chronic) All acupuncture, good response, 11/11 = 100% 0/2 Good response, chronic, no acupuncture Finger strength testing for 8 chronic acupuncture Tip pinch +3 lb, 40 tx, $p < 0.04$ Palmar pinch +3 lb, 20 tx, $p < 0.01$

Study	Treatment	Control	Results
Johansson et al[13] (1993) Lund University, Sweden	38 acute, 4-10 days after stroke, 20 tx (twice/wk, 10 wk) plus PT	40 acute, 4-10 days after stroke, PT only	Savings of $26,000/acupuncture patient due to reduced no. of days in rehabilitation facilities $p < 0.01$ and beyond for: Walking and balance at 1 mo and 3 mo; Activities of daily living at 3 mo and 12 mo; Quality of life, mobility, and emotion at 3, 6, and 12 mo
Magnusson et al[17] (1994) Lund University, Sweden	21 acute from Johansson et al[15] study above	21 acute from above study	Follow-up on postural control 2 yr later: $p < 0.01$, greater postural control for cases treated with acupuncture beginning 4-10 days after stroke
Sallstrom et al[18] (1995) Oslo, Norway	24 subacute, 40 days after stroke, 18-24 tx, 6 wk	21 subacute, 40 days after stroke, PT only	Patients who received acupuncture were better after 6 wk on following measures: Motor function, $p = 0.002$; Activities of daily living, $p = 0.02$; Quality of life, Nottingham Health Profile, $p = 0.009$
Hu et al[19] (1993) Taipei, Taiwan	15 acute, acupuncture tx started within 36 hr after stroke	15 acute, no acupuncture	Neurological outcome better at 1 mo ($p = 0.02$) and 3 mo ($p = 0.009$) for acute treated with acupuncture within 36 hr after stroke. Results significant for severe subgroup at 1 mo ($p = 0.009$) and 3 mo ($p = 0.013$), but not significant for mild-moderate subgroup
Zhang et al[20] (1987) Shanghai Medical University, China	53 acute and chronic, 24 tx, 6 tx/wk for 6 wk	41 acute and chronic	Acupuncture group: 44/53 (83%) increased muscle strength by 1-2 grades at 6 joints (shoulder, elbow, wrist, hip, knee, ankle); No acupuncture group: 26/41 (63%); Difference between groups: $p < 0.05$

Abd, abduction; *CT*, computed tomography; *extens*, extension; *J*, joules; *NS*, not significant; *PT*, physical therapy; *tx*, treatment.
*Overall, good response after acupuncture: 128/193 (66.3%).

Continued

TABLE 19-2

Acupuncture or Laser Acupuncture to Treat Paralysis in Stroke*—cont'd

| Authors | Cases real acupuncture (no.) | Control cases (no.) | | Significance level between groups and no. of cases with outcome level of good response/markedly effective |
		Sham	No acupuncture	
Li et al[21] (1989) Shanxi College of Traditional Chinese Medicine, China	Acute cerebral hemorrhage, 2 groups received 2 types of acupuncture: Group 1: ($N = 46$), midline, base of skull, GV 16, GV 15, plus body points Group 2: ($N = 46$), body points only 42-56 tx, daily			Were treated within 24 hr-1 wk after hemorrhage. Most bleeding completed within 4 hr in acute cerebral hemorrhage cases Group 1: 38/46, 82.6%, markedly effective Group 2: 17/46, 37%, markedly effective Difference between groups: $p < 0.01$ Acupuncture pts GV 15 and GV 16 highly recommended in acute cerebral hemorrhage
Naeser et al[22] (1995) VA Boston Healthcare System	Laser acupuncture: 5 arm/leg, 2 hand (6 chronic, 10 mo-6.5 yr after stroke; and 1 acute); 20-60 tx over 2-4 mo; 20 mW, 780 nm, 1 J/point or 101 J/cm²/point			5/7 (71%) good response Results similar to results with needle acupuncture where similar CT scan lesion sites were observed

Abd, abduction; *CT,* computed tomography; *extens,* extension; *J,* joules; *NS,* not significant; *PT,* physical therapy; *tx,* treatment.
*Overall, good response after acupuncture: 128/193 (66.3%).

into nonacupuncture points on the limbs) was performed in only one study.[13] In that study, significantly more acute stroke patients with arm or leg paralysis had "good response" after real acupuncture than sham acupuncture if computed tomography (CT) scan lesion site was a variable ($p < 0.013$). When the lesion occupied less than half of the motor pathway areas on CT scan, especially the periventricular white matter area adjacent to the body of the lateral ventricle (PVWM area, Figure 19-1), acupuncture effectively increased range of motion (ROM) in these patients with mild-to-moderate paralysis. Good response after acupuncture was defined as an increase of at least 10% in isolated active ROM, on at least two of seven arm/leg tests (e.g., shoulder abduction, knee flexion, or knee extension, etc.) No patients who received sham acupuncture had good response regardless of the location of the lesion. All patients in this study were treated with acupuncture beginning 1 to 3 months after the stroke.

Patients who had acute or chronic strokes with arm/leg paralysis of mild-to-moderate severity, with lesion in less than half of the motor pathway areas on CT scan, were observed to have significant increase in shoulder abduction +12%, knee flexion +22%, and/or knee extension +28% ($p < 0.04$ and beyond) after 20 to 40 acupuncture treatments over a 2- to 3-month period.[9] Patients with some isolated finger movement have the best prognosis for improvement in UE ROM after acupuncture treatments.

All patients with chronic or acute strokes who had no major arm/leg paralysis but only a milder hand paresis (all with lesion in less than half of the motor pathway areas on CT scan) had significant improvement in finger and hand strength and dexterity tests ($p < 0.04$ and beyond), even if acupuncture was initiated as late as 6 to 8 years after the stroke.[14] Figure 19-2 provides graphs showing the change in finger and hand strength and dexterity testing before and after 20 acupuncture treatments in cases of acute and chronic hand paresis. Figure 19-3 shows a CT scan and handwriting samples before and after 20 acupuncture treatments in a stroke patient when acupuncture was initiated as late as 5 years after the stroke.

In the three studies by Naeser et al,[9,13,14] 19 of 31 (61%) stroke patients had good response, and all patients who had lesions in less than half of the motor pathway areas on CT scan ($N = 18$) had good responses. (The final borders of an area of infarction, especially near the ventricle, are only well visualized on

CT scan or magnetic resonance imaging [MRI] scan when the scan is performed 3 months after stroke onset.) Many patients with severe hemiplegia with poor response who had lesions in more than half of the motor pathway areas on CT scan did have a beneficial effect, however, after acupuncture where a decrease in hand, arm, or leg spasticity was observed. On follow-up testing in 11 stroke patients at 2 months after the last acupuncture treatment, 72% to 83% of the improved hand, arm, or leg tests showed stabilization or further improvement.[9,14]

When 20 acupuncture treatments were initiated at 4 to 10 days after stroke onset in patients with acute stroke, significantly better outcome occurred (walking, balance, activities of daily living, quality of life) at 1, 3, and 12 months after stroke in patients receiving acupuncture plus physical therapy than in those receiving physical therapy alone ($p < 0.01$ and beyond; Figure 19-4).[15,16] An estimated savings of $26,000/stroke patient treated with acupuncture was realized due to fewer days in nursing homes and rehabilitation facilities. Follow-up of these cases 2 years later showed significantly better postural control for the acupuncture group ($p < 0.01$).[17]

Acupuncture plus physical therapy (PT) versus PT alone was examined in three additional studies. Each study showed that with acute, subacute, or chronic cases, those who received acupuncture, especially early after stroke onset (within 36 hours) had significantly better outcomes.[18-20] Early adjunctive treatment with acupuncture after stroke was especially important in patients with severe paralysis in the acute stage.[19] A study by Li et al[21] observed that acupuncture could be initiated within 24 hours, even in patients with acute cerebral hemorrhage, after the bleeding is controlled.

Naeser et al[22] used painless, noninvasive, low-level laser light (780 nm, 20 mW) instead of needles to stimulate acupuncture points to treat paralysis in stroke patients. Results generally were similar to those observed when needle acupuncture was used in stroke cases with similar CT scan lesion sites. Laser acupuncture is especially desirable for patients with hand paresis because patients can be trained to perform additional home treatment under the supervision of a licensed acupuncturist trained in laser acupuncture.[3] Laser acupuncture is considered investigational by the United States Food and Drug Administration (FDA), similar to the classification of acupuncture needles before 1997. Many US states, such as Massachusetts,

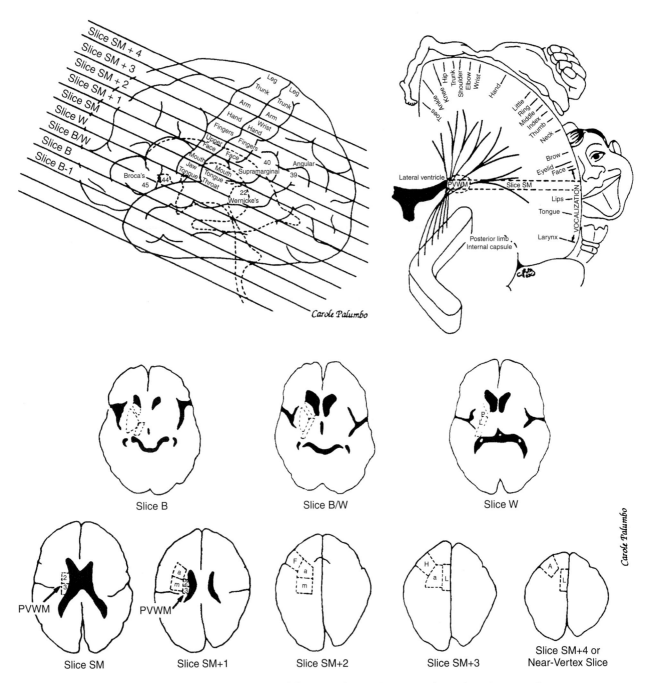

Figure 19-1 Location of descending pyramidal tract pathways (motor pathways) on CT scan. The extent of damage in these motor pathway areas was related to the level of response following acupuncture treatment in the studies by Naeser et al[9,13,14,22] with stroke patients with paralysis. The deep, subcortical periventricular white matter (PVWM) is outlined in the upper right coronal diagram and shown below on CT scan slices SM and SM+1, *arrows.* The total extent of lesion in the second and third quarters of the PVWM area was related to good response versus poor response after acupuncture treatments. *2,* Second quarter PVWM; *3,* third quarter PVWM; *A,* arm cortex area; *F,* fingers cortex area; *H,* hand cortex area; *L,* leg cortex area; *a,* anterior white matter area; *m,* middle white matter area; *PL,* posterior limb, internal capsule (continues on slices B and B/W); *PVWM,* periventricular white matter area; *CT,* computed tomography. (From Naeser MA, Alexander MP, Stiassny-Eder D, et al: *J Neurol Rehab* 6:163-73, 1992.)

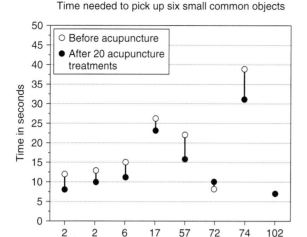

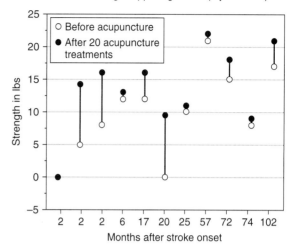

Figure 19-2 Hand dexterity and strength data obtained before and after 20 acupuncture treatments in stroke patients where acupuncture was initiated, ranging from 2 months after stroke to 102 months after stroke.

Florida, Wisconsin, Arkansas, and New Mexico, consider the use of low-level lasers on acupuncture points to be within the scope of acupuncture practice.*

A study by Wong et al[23] was conducted in Taiwan with stroke patients who, at 10 to 14 days after stroke onset, were randomly assigned to PT alone ($N = 59$) or to PT plus electrical acupuncture ($N = 59$), in which mA transcutaneous electrical nerve stimulation (TENS) pads were used on acupuncture points without any acupuncture needle stimulation. After 2 weeks of treatment (5 days/week), the patients who received PT plus TENS on acupuncture points had shorter hospital stays and better neurological and functional outcomes than the control group, with a significant difference in scores for self-care and locomotion.

In 1998 Gosman-Hedstrom et al[24] in Sweden randomly assigned 104 consecutive acute stroke patients to three groups: deep needle, superficial needle, and no acupuncture treatment. Acupuncture treatments were initiated at 4 to 10 days after stroke onset and administered by four physiotherapists twice a week for 10 weeks. All patients also underwent conventional stroke rehabilitation. Two occupational therapists, blinded to the patients' allocation, evaluated the treat-

ment effects. No differences existed between the groups with reference to changes in the neurological score and the Barthel and Sunnaas activities of daily living index scores after 3 and 12 months. No differences in health care and social services were found between the groups.

Shiflett[25] commented on the study by Gosman-Hedstrom et al[24] and criticized aspects of the experimental design compared with other published acupuncture research studies of stroke patients and the study by Johansson et al,[15] also from Sweden. Shiflett[25] observed differences in the acupuncture protocol and the lack of control for severity of paralysis at entry and recommended application of additional statistical procedures. For example, patients in the no-acupuncture control group had substantially less impairment than those in either of the acupuncture groups (deep or superficial needling) at randomization (perhaps as much as 3 standard error of the mean [SEM]), even though the authors indicated that these differences were not significant, resulting in a substantial confounding of impairment severity with treatment condition. The deep-needle acupuncture group had a steeper slope of improvement at 3 months than either the shallow-needle or the no-acupuncture group. In addition, 73% of patients in the deep-needle acupuncture group were living at home after 1 year, in contrast to only 53% of those in the

*For more information on laser acupuncture, including some FDA regulations, see www.Acupuncture.com/acup/laser.htm and www.Acupuncture.com/acup/Naeser.htm.

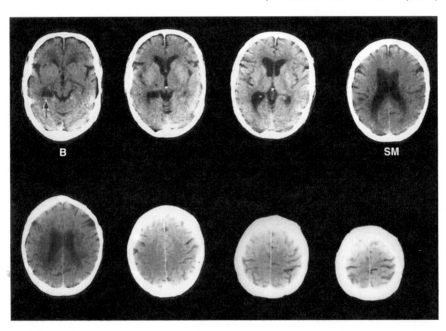

(F) *Fish Take air out of the water.*

Time required to write: 32.5 seconds

Five years following stroke onset
Pre-acupuncture

(R) *Fish take air out of the water.*

Time required to write: 16.5 seconds

Five years following stroke onset
Post-acupuncture
(20 treatments over a 1-month period)

Figure 19-3 Handwriting samples obtained before and after 20 acupuncture treatments and CT scan for a stroke patient treated with acupuncture beginning at 5 years after stroke. (From Naeser MA, Alexander MP, Stiassny-Eder D, et al: *Clin Rehabil* 8:127-41, 1994b.)

shallow-needle acupuncture group and 82% in the no-acupuncture group (Figure 19-5).

Additional problems with the Gosman-Hedstrom et al[24] study and factors to consider in designing future acupuncture research studies with stroke patients with paralysis include the following points:

1. Although all stroke patients were required to be older than 40 years of age at study entry, the mean age was mid-70s to early 80s (standard deviation [SD] and age ranges were not provided). In general, older stroke patients have more complex medical problems and may progress more slowly after a series of treatments than younger patients. Thus it would be better to stratify the study groups by age (e.g., under 60 years of age, between 61 to 80 years of age, and older than 80 years of age). The elderly

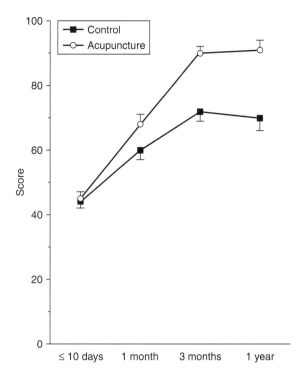

Figure 19-4 Activity of Daily Living Scores (Barthel Index) in stroke patients treated with acupuncture plus physical therapy (acupuncture group) or physical therapy alone (control group). Patients received 20 acupuncture treatments twice a week for 10 weeks, beginning at 4 to 10 days after stroke. Those receiving acupuncture plus physical therapy were significantly better than those receiving only physical therapy (controls) at 1 month, 3 months, and 1 year after stroke. (Courtesy Dr. Barbro B. Johansson, Department of Neurology, Lund University Hospital, Sweden.)

can respond very well to acupuncture treatments for various disorders, but it is inappropriate to mix ages in this type of research.

2. Although the exclusion criteria listed "an earlier cerebral lesion, with a documented need of care," 11% to 24% of stroke patients in each treatment group in this study had suffered a previous stroke. For example, all patients in the acupuncture studies by Naeser et al had only one stroke, as shown on CT scan, for better control of the lesion sites involved in each case; hence a better understanding of which chronic stroke patients were likely to benefit from acupuncture was possible.

3. Although the investigators stratified the assignment of patients with left or right hemisphere stroke (and presence or absence of neglect) across the groups, the results for these potentially disparate groups were reported together. It is likely that patients with right hemisphere lesion (and left-sided neglect syndrome) would have a less successful outcome. Was this the case? Thus the published results for these separate subgroups (e.g., right hemisphere lesion with neglect, right hemisphere lesion without neglect, and left hemisphere lesion) would have been helpful.

4. The number of patients with bilateral lesions across the three groups was neither considered nor reported. Patients with bilateral strokes, for example, recover more slowly and should not be included in research studies with patients who have had only a single, unilateral stroke.

5. It is likely that the majority of stroke patients enrolled in this research project had relatively severe paralysis at randomization (less than 1 week after onset). One of the inclusion criteria was, "The extent of the paresis had to be such that the patient could not walk without support and/or could not eat and/or dress without assistance." Hu et al[19] observed that patients with severe stroke appeared to benefit from early acupuncture intervention (e.g., acupuncture performed within 36 hours after stroke). Although most of the stroke patients in the study by Gosman-Hedstrom et al[24] appeared to be severe at entry, their acupuncture treatments were not initiated for at least 4 to 10 days after stroke onset, well beyond the 36 hours recommended in cases of acute, severe stroke in the study by Hu et al.[19] It is possible that early acupuncture intervention, perhaps within 6 hours of occlusive-vascular stroke onset, could reduce the extent of ischemic damage. In cases of early acupuncture intervention, within a few hours after onset, the possibility exists for increasing functional tissue in the lesion penumbra, thus reducing the severity of the stroke sequelae.

6. The data for the mild-to-moderate cases were not analyzed separately from the severe cases in each subgroup (deep needle, shallow needle, or no acupuncture). In the three studies by Naeser et al,[9,13,14] good response occurred in the mild-to-moderate paralysis cases after a series of 20 acupuncture treatments; poor response occurred in the severe cases. It is likely that if the mild-to-moderate cases were separated from the severe cases in each subgroup in the study by Gosman-Hedstrom et al,[24]

the patients who received acupuncture (deep or shallow needles) would have had significantly better improvement than those receiving no acupuncture. It appears, however, that the majority (if not all) cases in this study were more severe cases.

7. The level of acupuncture training of the physiotherapists who performed the treatments was not specified. (For example, licensed acupuncturists in the United States must have at least 1725 hours of acupuncture training.) All studies reviewed in Table 19-2 showed acupuncture to be helpful in the majority of stroke patients who were treated for paralysis. Most of these studies, including those conducted in the United States by Naeser et al and China and Taiwan, used only fully trained, licensed acupuncturists to perform the treatments.

8. The acupuncture treatment protocol did not include Chinese or Japanese scalp needle acupuncture, a technique often used with stroke patients.[6,9,10,19,26]

Thus there were several confounding factors that could have influenced the negative outcome of this recent acupuncture study with acute (primarily elderly) stroke patients: age, severity, hemispheric side and site of cerebral lesion, possibility of bilateral lesions, level of acupuncture training by the clinician performing the acupuncture treatments, acupuncture protocol used, and statistical analyses. Together these factors suggest that the applicability of this acupuncture study to planning acute stroke care is not generalizable.

Possible Mechanisms for Acupuncture's Effectiveness in Stroke, Blood-Flow Brain SPECT Studies

The mechanism through which acupuncture may produce improvement in motor function or reduce spasticity in stroke patients with paralysis currently is not understood. Acupuncture may increase cerebral blood flow or promote vasodilation.[27-30] A blood-flow brain single photon emission computed tomography (SPECT) scan study is under way in our neuroimaging section at the VA Boston Healthcare System. Blood flow is measured before and immediately after one acupuncture treatment (needles with electroacupuncture and laser acupuncture) on the same day. Four of the five stroke patients examined to date showed an increase in blood flow to the contralateral thalamus and motor cortex area after the acupuncture treatment; increases ranged from +3% and +4% to +24%. The latter increase of +24% was observed in a patient (case WM) who had previous acupuncture (including home treatments with laser acupuncture to reduce hand

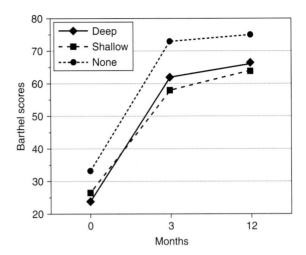

Figure 19-5 Activity of Daily Living Scores (Barthel Index) in three groups of elderly stroke patients treated in the Gosman-Hedstrom et al[24] study with either no acupuncture, shallow needle acupuncture, or deep needle acupuncture by a physiotherapist. All patients received physical therapy. Patients receiving acupuncture were treated twice a week for 10 weeks, beginning at 4 to 10 days after stroke. There were no differences in outcome among the groups. (Courtesy Samuel C. Shiflett, PhD, Kessler Medical Rehabilitation Research and Education Corporation, West Orange, NJ.)

spasticity), whereas for the other cases, this was their first acupuncture treatment (Figure 19-6).

The studies by Alavi et al[27,28] observed a change of approximately 23% in blood flow after acupuncture in the brain stem and thalamus areas in 4 of 5 chronic pain patients who had previously had several weeks of acupuncture treatments. Thus the greater increase of +24% in the stroke patient who had received previous acupuncture versus the smaller increases in the patients for whom this was their first acupuncture treatment requires further research. This result may indicate that acupuncture promotes a greater modulation in blood flow after a series of treatments.

Cho et al[31] showed in 12 normal control volunteers that stimulation of the eye by using direct light (checkerboard 8 Hz light flash) resulted in activation in the occipital lobes as measured with functional MRI (fMRI) similar to stimulation of Bladder 67 (lateral to the fifth toenail), an acupuncture point sometimes used to treat eye disorders. Stimulation of acupoints 2 to 5 cm away (not associated with the treatment of eye disorders) was not associated with activation of the occipital lobes. The level of occipital

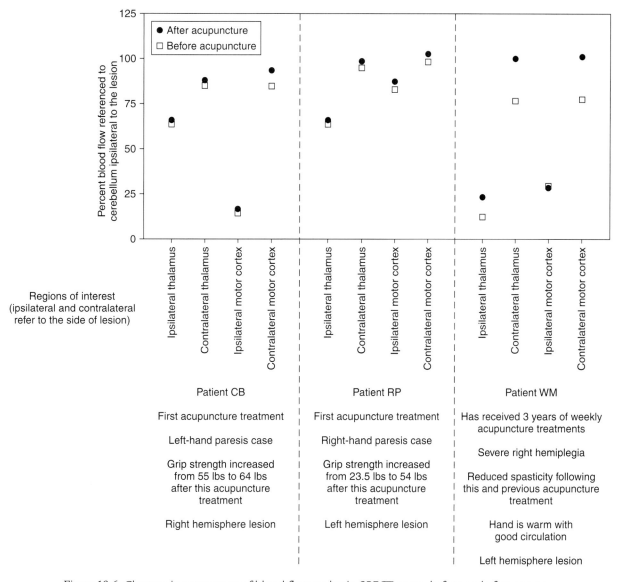

Figure 19-6 Changes in percentage of blood flow on brain SPECT scans, before and after one acupuncture treatment in three chronic stroke patients. (From Naeser MA: *Neurological rehabilitation: acupuncture and laser acupuncture to treat paralysis in stroke and other paralytic conditions and pain in carpal tunnel syndrome.* Paper published in program proceedings: National Institutes of Health consensus development conference on acupuncture sponsored by the Office of Alternative Medicine and the Office of Medical Applications of Research, Bethesda, Md, November 3-5, 1997, pp 93-109.)

lobe activation during stimulation of Bladder 67 was variable across the 12 cases: 4 cases showed an increase in activation, and 8 cases showed a decrease.

In nonacupuncture studies of stroke patients who recovered from paralysis, an increase in blood flow or cerebral metabolism has been observed in the thalamus and motor cortex areas (sometimes bilaterally) in patients with good spontaneous recovery from paral-

ysis within a few months after stroke onset.[32-36] If a series of acupuncture treatments over several weeks does significantly modulate activation in these areas (thalamus and motor cortex) in stroke patients with paralysis, this acupuncture-induced modulation may promote more rapid and improved brain reorganization for motor control after the stroke. Clearly, additional brain imaging studies are needed.

Summary: Poststroke Paralysis and Acupuncture

Acupuncture or laser acupuncture effectively reduced severity of paralysis in 66.3% of the 193 cases reviewed in Table 19-2. The best results were observed when acupuncture treatments were initiated within 24 to 36 hours after stroke onset in ischemic infarct cases and after bleeding was controlled in hemorrhagic cases. The effect of acupuncture in increasing cortisol levels[37,49] may contribute to less brain edema in acute stroke. Patients with acute stroke were treated at least 3 times/week, and chronic stroke patients were treated 2 times/week, for 20 to 40 treatments over a 2- or 3-month period. The Swedish study by Johansson et al[15] reported savings of $26,000/stroke patient when acupuncture was initiated at 4 to 10 days after stroke as a result of fewer days in the hospital and rehabilitation facilities. These patients also had better motor function, activities of daily living, and quality of life measures at 1 and 3 months and 1 year after the stroke, in addition to better postural control at 2 years after the stroke, than patients treated only with PT beginning at 4 to 10 days after the stroke ($p < 0.01$ and beyond).

Acupuncture is beneficial for both chronic and acute stroke patients. Acupuncture is an excellent complementary treatment for stroke patients with paralysis, and use of acupuncture as an adjunctive treatment with current therapies is recommended. Often patients gain greater ROM and benefit from PT and occupational therapy (OT) when acupuncture is administered immediately before a PT or an OT session. With the YNSA method, short acupuncture needles are left in place on the scalp for the duration of the day, including treatment sessions.[10,38]

Severity of paralysis in stroke patients varies. In general, for patients with mild-to-moderate paralysis, improvement in knee flexion and extension and shoulder abduction is expected; and in mild cases in which some isolated finger movement is present (acute or chronic hand paresis), improvement in finger and hand strength and dexterity is expected. Injection of Botox into the wrist area may interfere with a positive acupuncture response for the hand.[39] For patients with severe paralysis and spasticity, a reduction in spasticity is expected after acupuncture but little change in ROM is expected. A reduction in spasticity is expected in almost all cases, acute or chronic, mild-to-moderate, or severe. There are no specific acupuncture studies on stroke patients with flaccid paralysis.

Home treatment programs with laser acupuncture supervised by a licensed acupuncturist trained in laser acupuncture can further help to reduce spasticity and increase finger and hand strength and dexterity.[3] These home treatment programs should be adjunctive and are not intended to replace standard acupuncture treatments, in which scalp needle acupuncture and other methods of treatment with needle acupuncture (electroacupuncture and moxibustion) should be performed weekly or monthly as necessary with chronic stroke patients.

Acupuncture and laser acupuncture may modulate activity in specific areas of the brain, including the thalamus and motor/sensory cortex areas in stroke patients with paralysis. Further research is recommended with acupuncture and neuroimaging studies in which cerebral blood flow and metabolism can be measured after a series of acupuncture treatments. This information will help provide a better understanding of the physiological mechanisms that may underlie the benefits gained from acupuncture to treat paralysis in stroke patients.

Results from neuroimaging studies also may help explain why acupuncture appears to be helpful in the treatment of other paralytic conditions, including CP, SCI, peripheral facial paralysis (Bell's palsy), and others not reviewed in this chapter but included in a previous report for the National Institutes of Health (NIH) Office of Alternative Medicine (OAM) (e.g., head injury, multiple sclerosis, pseudobulbar palsy, and reversal of coma).[40] In all areas reviewed, acupuncture was helpful in the majority of cases, and initiation of acupuncture (with or without laser acupuncture) treatments was recommended as soon as possible after stroke onset.

Acupuncture or Laser Acupuncture to Treat Cerebral Palsy in Infants and Children

CP may be defined as a chronic disability of CNS origin characterized by aberrant control of movement or posture that appears early in life and is not the result of a progressive disease. CP is estimated to occur in 0.1% of births (approximately 250,000 cases in the United States). CP is more frequently observed in infants with a low birthweight (<2500 g).[41]

Results for eight studies are summarized in Table 19-3. Two studies used a control treatment, limb

TABLE 19-3

Acupuncture or Laser Acupuncture to Treat Cerebral Palsy in Infants and Children*

Authors	Cases real acupuncture (no.)	Control cases (no.)		Significance level between groups and/or cases with outcome level of good response/ markedly effective (no.)
		Sham	No acupuncture	
Filipowicz[44] (1991) Warsaw, Poland; Toronto, Canada	65 infants and children, age 40 days–4 yr, acupressure, needle acupuncture, laser acupuncture (2–10 mW, red-beam laser) electroacupuncture, 2-3 tx/wk over 5-yr period			65/65 (100%), considerable improvement 4, "complete recovery" when acupuncture tx starts at less than 6 mo of age. The earlier the acupuncture tx is initiated, the greater the reduction in spasticity Laser acupuncture especially effective to treat contractures of Achilles tendon; after 30-60 sec exposure, "considerable and immediate improvement"
Lao[48] (1992) New York, New York	10-mo-old infant, needle acupuncture, 50 tx over 5-mo period			Before acupuncture: unable to sit up (with or without assistance); Achilles tendons tight, bilaterally After 10 acupuncture tx: able to sit, started to crawl, spasticity alleviated. After 50 acupuncture tx: at 15 mo of age, walking independently, similar to children his age
Shi et al[49] (1992) Shanghai Medical University, China	117 children, age 6 mo-10 yr, 30 acupuncture tx, 4-5 mo			63/117 (53.8%), markedly improved or better
Xiao and Meng[42] (1995) Beijing, China	30 children, age 1-14 yr, 30 tx, 66-day period Ear stimulation plus limb massage		30 children, age 1-14 yr, 30 tx, 66-day period; limb massage only	Ear stimulation plus massage: 16/30 (53%), improved Massage only: 4/30 (13.3%), improved. Difference between groups: $p < 0.01$
Ma and Zhang[43] (1995) Gansu, China	48 children, age 1-6 yr; 12 children, older than 6 yr; acupuncture treatments 1-4 mo		9 children, age 1-6 yr; 3 older than 6 yr; vitamins and herbs, 1-3 mo	Acupuncture group: 39.60 (65%), markedly improved Vitamins plus herbs group: 2/12 (16.6%), markedly improved Difference between groups: $p < 0.01$

CP, Cerebral palsy; *J,* joules; *tx,* treatments.
*Overall, good response after acupuncture: 224/321 (69.8%).

Continued

TABLE 19-3

Acupuncture or Laser Acupuncture to Treat Cerebral Palsy in Infants and Children—cont'd

Authors	Cases real acupuncture (no.)	Control cases (no.)		Significance level between groups and/or cases with outcome level of good response/ markedly effective (no.)
		Sham	No acupuncture	
Spears[54] (1979) Chatham, New Jersey	5 teenagers, 1 child, age 4.8 yr; electroacupuncture, ear stimulation At least 8 tx			6/6 (100%), less spasticity, loosened Achilles tendon, control of drooling
Lidicka and Hegyi[45] (1991) Prague, Czech Republic; Budapest, Hungary	Laser acupuncure: 5 mW, red-beam; 145 children, age 2 wk–5 yr, treated for several mo-yr			Majority: less spasticity, improved motor function for sitting, crawling, and walking Recommend laser acupuncture tx be used with infants likely to develop CP, starting at 2 wk after birth; 2 yr of age considered late to start acupuncture tx
Asagai et al[4] (1994) Shinano Handicapped Children's Hospital, Nagano, Japan	150 CP, age 10 mo–20 yr, all with spastic CP Laser acupuncture (60 mW or 100 mW, CW, 810 nm, near-infrared-beam laser), 86.5 J/cm²–288.3 J/cm² per point; tx schedule not available			"In the majority of the patients, spasm was successfully suppressed . . . with the notable exception of those patients suffering from severe joint contracture. . . . The effect lasted from one to several hours in cases with severe spasticity." 34/42 hand (91%) that were involuntarily clenched before tx, able to open hand with less effort after tx Authors write that low-level laser therapy particularly useful as supplementary of adjunctive therapeutic modality . . . to improve functional training in children with CP

CP, cerebral palsy; *CW,* continuous wave; *J,* joules; *tx,* treatments.

massage only[42] or vitamins and Chinese herbs only.[43] Each study observed better outcome in the acupuncture group ($p <0.01$).

Laser acupuncture was included in three studies.[4,44,45] These studies observed that stimulation of acupuncture points with low-level, red-beam laser reduced spasticity and improved motor function for sitting, crawling, and walking. For example, Asagai et al[4] in Japan used low-level laser therapy (LLLT) on acupuncture points to treat spasticity in 150 cases of CP (ages 10 months to 20 years). Two gallium-aluminum arsenide diode (60 mW or 100 mW, continuous wave, 810-nm wavelength [near infrared]) lasers were used for 15 to 30 seconds/point. Improvement was reported in the majority of the 150 infants and children; exceptions were those with severe joint contracture. In addition, in 42 patients whose hands were normally involuntarily clenched, 34 (81%) were able to open their hands with less effort. The authors quote Kamikawa et al,[46] who hypothesized that LLLT may cause vascular dilatation through the sympathetic nervous system and reduce tonic muscle spasms in muscles that had been in a hypoxemic state. The authors concluded:

Compared with conventional methodology, laser therapy has proved to be a simple, reliable, and noninvasive method which enabled painless suppression of spasm.... The effect of low-level laser therapy lasted from one to several hours in patients with severe spasticity....the authors feel that low-level laser therapy is particularly useful as a supplementary or adjunctive therapeutic modality to improve the overall efficacy of physical rehabilitation and functional training in children with cerebral palsy.

Laser acupuncture may be performed in the home by the mother and supervised by a licensed acupuncturist trained in laser acupuncture.[3] Home laser acupuncture treatment reduced the number of seizures, thus allowing a child with CP to require less medication.[47] CP condition requires lifelong treatment; adjunctive home treatment with laser acupuncture could reduce treatment costs. Studies recommend initiating acupuncture very early (preferably 2 weeks after birth or younger than 1 year of age).[45,48]

As mentioned previously, Scott and Barlow[2] describe specific acupuncture treatment protocols for children with CP (flaccid pattern and spastic pattern). This text provides differential diagnoses within traditional Chinese medicine (TCM) and includes body and scalp needle protocols. They recommend 100 to 150 treatments, recognizing that this is a lifelong condition. The earlier these treatments are started, the better is the outcome.*

The results from these eight studies indicate an outcome level of "good response/markedly effective" in 224 (69.8%) of 321 cases of infants and children treated with acupuncture, laser acupuncture, or both. These treatments are especially helpful in reducing spasticity. Plasma cortisol levels were significantly increased in 77% of the children treated with acupuncture for CP.[49]

Summary: Cerebral Palsy

Acupuncture with or without laser acupuncture treatments effectively reduced spasms and improved motor function in 70% of the 321 cases reviewed. Treatments were especially effective when initiated within a few weeks or 1 year after birth. Initially treatments are administered daily or 3 times/week. Later the frequency may be reduced. CP is a lifelong condition, and acupuncture treatments should be continued over several years as necessary. Laser acupuncture should be considered for adjunctive home treatment programs under the supervision of a licensed acupuncturist trained in laser acupuncture to help reduce the overall treatment cost.

Acupuncture to Treat Paralysis in Spinal Cord Injury

Approximately 200,000 persons in the United States are now permanently confined to wheelchairs because of SCI. Each year, some 10,000 more people are injured, suffering paralysis and loss of sensation. Two thirds of these people are younger than 30 years of age. The required specialized care costs approximately $5 billion each year in the United States.[11]

Results for three acupuncture studies are summarized in Table 19-4; none had a control group. Overall, 340 (94.4%) of 360 cases had an outcome level of beneficial progress, including reduction in muscle spasms, some increased level of sensation, and improved bladder and bowel function. Patients were treated from a period of 5 months to 2 to 3 years. The acupuncture treatments also helped in the treatment of bedsores with these patients. Red-beam laser acu-

---

*Their book also contains a chapter on "Hyperactivity and Attention Deficit Disorder."

TABLE 19-4

Acupuncture to Treat Paralysis in Spinal Cord Injury*

Authors	Cases real acupuncture (no.)	Control cases (no.) Sham	No acupuncture	Cases with outcome level of beneficial progress (no.)
Gao[55] (1984) Yuci City Institute of Paralysis, Shanxi Province, China	17 inpatients, with complete traumatic paraplegia, acute, 1 mo after onset and chronic, 5 yr after onset, tx over 2-3-yr period			15/17 (88%) Includes improvement in the following: Reduction in muscle spasms Increased level of sensation Improved bladder and bowel function Recommends beginning acupuncture as soon as possible after spinal cord injury, even during early stage of spinal cord shock, to reduce occurrence of spasms Younger patients had better outcome
Wang[56] (1992) Institute of Health Preservation, Beijing, China	82, treated with acupuncture/ electroacupuncture, along Bladder Meridian (para-vertebral) for 5 mo			76/82 (93%), effective Includes improvement in the following: Improvement in lower limb paralysis Improved bladder and bowel function
Gao et al[5] (1996) Yuci City Institute of Paralysis, Shanxi Province, China	261, treated beginning at 1 mo after onset-more than 5 yr after onset			249/261 (95%) effective Effective defined as: Basic recovery of functions of nervous system with ability to walk freely and almost voluntary urination (3%) Marked effectiveness with partial recovery of functions of nervous system, with ability to walk on crutches and restoration of urinary bladder reflex (35.2%) Improvement of functions of nervous system with some limb movement, defecation, and/or urination (57.1%) Recommend beginning acupuncture as soon as possible after spinal cord injury

*Overall, beneficial progress after acupuncture, 340/360 (94.4%).

puncture may be used on the hands or feet to help reduce muscle spasms.[3,39] (A low-level laser acupuncture treatment program for SCI cases is available from Dr. Albert Bohbot in France[39]; see www.laserponcture.net or edwige.nault@infonie.fr.) Authors recommend beginning acupuncture as soon as possible after SCI, even during the acute stage of spinal cord shock, to reduce spasm development.

Acupuncture reduced muscle spasms, increased level of sensation, and improved bladder and bowel function in 94.4% of the 360 cases reviewed. Initiation of acupuncture treatment was recommended as soon as possible after SCI with treatments continuing for 2 to 3 years, or even 5 years. Electroacupuncture along the Bladder Meridian (paravertebral) area is especially recommended. Laser acupuncture also can be applied in a home treatment program to help reduce muscle spasms in the hands and feet.

Acupuncture or Laser Acupuncture to Treat Peripheral Facial Paralysis (Bell's Palsy)

Bell's palsy is the most common disease of the facial nerve. Its presumed cause is an inflammatory reaction in or around the facial nerve near the stylomastoid foramen. "Fully 80 percent of patients recover within a few weeks or in a month or two."[50] Improvement in the facial paralysis associated with Bell's palsy may occur sooner, and in a higher number of cases treated with acupuncture and/or laser acupuncture, improvement may occur within 3 days of onset.

Results for five acupuncture studies are summarized in Table 19-5; none had a control group. Overall, 983 (97.4%) of 1009 achieved an outcome level of cured or markedly effective. Patients were treated ranging from 1 day to several years after onset. When

TABLE 19-5

Acupuncture or Laser Acupuncture to Treat Peripheral Facial Paralysis (Bell's Palsy) *

Authors	Cases real acupuncture (no.)	Duration of paralysis	Duration of acupuncture treatment	Cases with outcome level of cured or markedly improved (no.)
Gao and Chen[52] (1991) Beijing College of Traditional Chinese Medicine, China	60 Mild, N = 30 Severe, N = 30	3 days-30 yr <2 mo, N = 40 >2 mo, N = 20	10 tx, every other day	Overall, 59/60 (98%) Mild: cured 93%, excellent 7% Severe: cured 70%, excellent 13%, improved 13%, failed 3% <2-mo duration: cured 92.5%, excellent 5%, improved 2.5% >2-mo duration: cured 60%, excellent 20%, improved 15%, failed 5% Recommend starting acupuncture soon after onset
Cui[57] (1992) Tangshan Hospital of TCM, Hebei Province, China	100, 9 were recurrent	1-5 days, N = 62 6-30 days, N = 3 1-6 mo, N = 6 <6 mo, N = 2	5-40 tx, daily 94/100 received 30 tx over 1-mo period	90/100 (90%), cured or markedly improved
Liu[51] (1995) Shandong College of TCM, Jinan, China	718	All: <4 days	1-2 mo tx	715/718 (99.6%), cured or marked effect <48 hr: 572/572 (100%) 2-3 days: 112/112 (100%) 3-4 days: 31/34 (91.2%)

Tx, Treatments.

*Overall, cured or markedly improved after acupuncture: 983/1009 (97.4%).

Continued

TABLE 19-5

Acupuncture or Laser Acupuncture to Treat Peripheral Facial Paralysis (Bell's Palsy)—cont'd

Authors	Cases real acupuncture (no.)	Duration of paralysis	Duration of acupuncture treatment	Cases with outcome level of cured or markedly improved (no.)
Cheng et al[58] (1991) Chinese Academy of TCM, Beijing, China	31: 3 mild, 6 moderate, 22 severe with spasm of eyelids, cheeks, both mouth corners	1 wk-20 yr 27/31, >1 yr	Acupuncture plus laser acupuncture: Red-beam 15 mW, HeNe laser, 20 min, spasmodic area	26/31 (84%), basically controlled, markedly effective, or improved Basically controlled: 8/31 (25.8%) Markedly effective: 8/31 (25.8%) Improved: 10/31 (32.3%) Ineffective: 5/31 (16.1%)
Wu[53] (1990) Pu Yang City People's Hospital, Henan Province, China	100	<3 days, 39 <10 days, 33 6 mo, 6 <1 yr, 2	Laser acupuncture: red-beam, 6-9 mW, HeNe laser, 2-4 wk	93/100 (93%), cured Completely recovered in 2 wk: 54/100 (54%) Completely recovered in 4 wk: 39/100 (39%) With most severe, needle acupuncture also used

acupuncture was initiated within 3 days of onset in 684 cases, 100% of the patients were cured or experienced a marked effect.[51] Even 80% of cases treated more than 2 months after onset, and 83% of severe cases were cured or had excellent effects.[52] Red-beam laser acupuncture also was effective in mild-to-moderate cases[3]; it was combined with needle acupuncture in severe cases.[53] Most patients were treated for 2 to 4 weeks (up to 8 weeks).

Acupuncture, with or without laser acupuncture, cured or markedly improved peripheral facial paralysis in 97.4% of the 1009 cases reviewed. It was 100% effective when initiated within 3 days after onset of the facial paralysis. Acupuncture also was beneficial in 80% of cases when initiated more than 2 months after onset and in 83% of severe cases.

References

1. Maciocia G: *The practice of Chinese medicine: the treatment of diseases with acupuncture and Chinese herbs,* Edinburgh, 1994, Churchill Livingstone.

2. Scott J, Barlow T: *Acupuncture in the treatment of children,* ed 3, Seattle, 1999, Eastland Press.

3. Naeser MA, Wei XB: *Laser acupuncture: an introductory textbook for treatment of pain, paralysis, spasticity, and other disorders,* Boston, 1994, Boston Chinese Medicine.

4. Asagai Y, Kianai H, Miura Y, et al: Application of low reactive-level laser therapy (LLLT) in the functional training of cerebral palsy patients, *Laser Ther* 6:195-202, 1994.

5. Gao XP, Gao CM, Gao JC, et al: Acupuncture treatment of complete traumatic paraplegia: analysis of 261 cases, *J Tradit Chin Med* 16(2):134-7, 1996.

6. O'Connor J, Bensky D: *Acupuncture: a comprehensive text, Shanghai College of Traditional Chinese Medicine,* Chicago, 1981, Eastland Press.

7. Oleson T: *Auriculotherapy manual: Chinese and Western systems of ear acupuncture,* Los Angeles, 1998, Health Care Alternatives.

8. Yau PS: *Scalp-needling therapy,* Hong Kong, 1980, Medicine & Health Publishing.

9. Naeser MA, Alexander MP, Stiassny-Eder D, et al: Acupuncture in the treatment of paralysis in chronic and acute stroke patients: improvement correlated with specific CT scan lesion sites, *Acupunct Electrother Res* 19:227-50, 1994a.

10. Yamamoto T, Yamamoto H: *Yamamoto new scalp acupuncture-YNSA,* Tokyo, 1999, Axel Springer (English translation).

11. Weinfeld: National survey of stroke, *Stroke* 12:2, 1981.

12. NIH Report: *Progress and promise* 1992: *a status report on the NINDS implementation plan for the decade of the brain,* The National Advisory Neurological Disorders and Stroke Council, National Institute of Neurological Disorders and Stroke, National Institutes of Health, December, 1992.

13. Naeser MA, Alexander MP, Stiassny-Eder D, et al: Real vs. sham acupuncture in the treatment of paralysis in acute stroke patients: a CT scan lesion site study, *J Neurol Rehabil* 6:163-73, 1992.

14. Naeser MA, Alexander MP, Stiassny-Eder D, et al: Acupuncture in the treatment of hand paresis in chronic and acute stroke patients: improvement observed in all cases, *Clin Rehabil* 8:127-41, 1994b.

15. Johansson K, Lindgren I, Widner H, et al: Can sensory stimulation improve the functional outcome in stroke patients? *Neurology* 43:2189-92, 1993.

16. Johansson BB: Has sensory stimulation a role in stroke rehabilitation? *Scand J Rehabil Med Suppl* 29:87-96, 1993.

17. Magnusson M, Johansson K, Johansson BB: Sensory stimulation promotes normalization of postural control after stroke, *Stroke* 25:1176-80, 1994.

18. Sallstrom S, Kjendahl A, Osten PE: Acupuncture therapy in stroke during the subacute phase: a randomized controlled trial, *Tidsskr Nor Laegeforen* 115(23):2884-7, 1995.

19. Hu HH, Chung C, Liu TJ, et al: A randomized controlled trial on the treatment for acute partial ischemic stroke with acupuncture, *Neuroepidemiology* 12:106-13, 1993.

20. Zhang WX, Li SC, Chen GB, et al: Acupuncture treatment of apoplectic hemiplegia, *J Tradit Chin Med* 7:157-60, 1987.

21. Li DM, Li WD, Wei LH, et al: Clinical observation on acupuncture therapy for cerebral hemorrhage, *J Tradit Chin Med* 9(1):9-13, 1989.

22. Naeser MA, Alexander MP, Stiassny-Eder D, et al: Laser acupuncture in the treatment of paralysis in stroke patients: a CT scan lesion site study, *Am J Acupunct* 23(1):13-28 1995.

23. Wong AMK, Su T-Y, Tang F-T, et al: Clinical trial of electrical acupuncture on hemiplegic stroke patients, *Am J Phys Med Rehabil* 78:117-22, 1999.

24. Gosman-Hedstrom G, Claesson L, Klingenstierma U, et al: Effects of acupuncture on daily life activities and quality of life: a controlled, prospective, and randomized study of acute stroke patients, *Stroke* 29:2100-8, 1998.

25. Shiflett S: Commentary on Akupunktur bei Schlaganfall, *Forsch Komplementarmed* 6:272-6, 1999.

26. Yamamoto T: Personal communication, 1993.

27. Alavi A, LaRiccia P, Sadek AH, et al: Objective assessment of the effects of pain and acupuncture on regional brain function with Tc 99m HMPAO SPECT imaging, *J Nucl Med* 37(suppl 5):278, 1996.

28. Alavi A, LaRiccia PJ, Sadek AH, et al: Progress report: SPECT scan imaging of the brain before and after acupuncture, *Acupunct Electrother Res* 22(1):68, 1997.

29. Chen GS, Erdmann W: Effects of acupuncture on tissue-oxygenation of the rat brain, *Comp Med East West* 5(2):147-54, 1977.

30. Omura Y: Pathophysiology of acupuncture treatment: effects of acupuncture on cardiovascular and nervous systems, *Acupunct Electrother Res* 1:51-141, 1975.

31. Cho ZH, Chung SC, Jones JP, et al: New findings of the correlation between acupoints and corresponding brain cortices using functional MRI, *Proc Natl Acad Sci U S A* 95:2670-3, 1998.

32. Frakowiak RJS, Weiller C, Chollet F: *CIBA Found Symp* 164:235-44, 1991.

33. Weiller C, Chollet F, Friston KJ, et al: Functional reorganization of the brain in recovery from striatocapsular infarction in man, *Ann Neurol* 31:463-72, 1992.

34. Weder B, Knorr U, Herzog H, et al: Tactile exploration of shape after subcortical ischaemic infarction studied with PET, *Brain* 117:593-605, 1994.

35. Binkofski F, Seitz RJ, Arnold S, et al: Thalamic metabolism and corticospinal tract integrity determine motor recovery in stroke, *Ann Neurol* 39:460-70, 1996.

36. Bookheimer SY, Cohen MS, Dobkin B, et al: Functional MRI during motor activation following stroke, *Human Brain Mapp* 1(suppl):429, 1995.

37. Cheng R, McKibbin L, Roy B, et al: Electroacupuncture elevates blood cortisol levels in naive horses: sham treatment has no effect, *Int J Neurosci* 10:95-7, 1980.

38. Yamamoto T, Maric-Oehler W: *Yamamoto Neue Schadelakupunktur YNSA,* Freiburg im Breisgau, Germany, 1991, CHUN-JO Verlag.

39. Naeser MA: Personal observation.

40. Naeser MA: Acupuncture in the treatment of paralysis due to central nervous system damage, *J Altern Complement Med* 2(1):211-48, 1996.

41. Cummins SK, Nelson KB, Grether JK, et al: Cerebral palsy in four northern California counties: births 1983 through 1985, *J Pediatr* 123:230-7, 1993.

42. Xiao JH, Meng F: Ear-pressing in treatment of cerebral palsy: a report of 60 cases, *Int J Clin Acupunct* 6(3):275-8, 1995.

43. Ma XP, Zhang YT: Needling three pairs of paravertebral points in treating cerebral palsy: a clinical observation of 72 cases, *Int J Clin Acupunct* 6(3):279-83, 1995.

44. Filipowicz WA: The application of modern acupuncture techniques and methods on children with cerebral palsy, *Am J Acupunct* 19:5-9, 1991.

45. Lidicka M, Hegyi G: Summary of acupuncture and laser acupuncture treatments with brain-damaged babies and children. Presented at the 1991 ICMART (International Council on Medical Acupuncture and Related Techniques) Acupuncture Research Meetings, Munich, Germany, June 14-17, 1991. In Naeser M, Wei XB, *Laser acupuncture: an introductory textbook for treatment of pain, paralysis, spasticity, and other disorders,* Boston, 1994, Boston Chinese Medicine, p 77.

46. Kamikawa K, Ohnishi T, Suzuki M, et al: Laser therapy of pain, *J Jpn Soc Laser Med* 3:345-8, 1982.

47. Colbert A: Personal communication.

48. Lao HH: Case study in the pathogenesis and treatment principles of spastic cerebral palsy in infancy according to traditional Chinese medicine, *Am J Acupunct* 20:113-8, 1992.

49. Shi BP, Bu HD, Lin LY: A clinical study on acupuncture treatment of pediatric cerebral palsy, *J Tradit Chin Med* 12(1):45-51, 1992.

50. Adams R, Victor M: *Principles of neurology,* New York, 1977, McGraw-Hill.

51. Liu YT: A new classification system and combined treatment method for idiopathic facial nerve paralysis: report of 718 cases, *Am J Acupunct* 23(3):205-10, 1995.

52. Gao HB, Chen D: Clinical observation on 60 cases of peripheral facial paralysis treated with acupoint penetration needling, *Int J Clin Acupunct* 2(1):25-8, 1991.

53. Wu XB: 100 Cases of facial paralysis treated with He-Ne laser irradiation on acupoints, *J Tradit Chin Med* 10(3): 300, 1990.

54. Spears CE: Auricular acupuncture: new approach to treatment of cerebral palsy, *Am J Acupunct* 1(7):49-54, 1979.

55. Gao XP: Acupuncture for traumatic paraplegia, *Int J Chin Med* 1(2):43-7, 1984.

56. Wang HJ: A survey of the treatment of traumatic paraplegia by traditional Chinese medicine, *J Chin Med* 12(4):296-303, 1992.

57. Cui YM: Treatment of peripheral facial paralysis by scalp acupuncture: a report of 100 cases, *J Tradit Chin Med* 12(2):106-7, 1992.

58. Cheng ZY, Zhao CX, Zhang YH, et al: Superficial acupuncture combined with He-Ne laser radiation in the treatment of facial spasm, *Int J Clin Acupunct* 2(1):95-7, 1991.

Suggested Readings

Chollet F, DiPiero V, Wise RJS, et al: The functional anatomy of motor recovery after stroke in humans: a study with positron emission tomography, *Ann Neurol* 29:63-71, 1991.

Hyvarinen J, Karlsson M: Low-resistance skin points that may coincide with acupuncture loci, *Med Biol* 55:88-94, 1977.

APPENDIX: ACUPUNCTURE POINTS USED FOR ACUPUNCTURE TREATMENTS OF STROKE

Location of acupoints	List of acupoints
Right arm, paralyzed side*	LI 4, LI 11, LI 15; TW 5, TW 9, three distal Baxie (extra) points
Right leg, paralyzed side*	St 31, St 36; GB 34, GB 39; Liv 3
Left arm, nonparalyzed side	LI 4, LI 11
Left leg, nonparalyzed side	St 36
Right and left ears	Ear Shenmen
Scalp acupuncture on side of hemispheric infarction (left)†	Four or five needles along the Motor Cortex Line of the Scalp

From Naeser MA, Alexander MP, Stiassny-Eder D, et al: *Acupunct Electrother Res* 19:227-250, 1994a.

*Low-pulse repetition rate stimulation (1 to 2 Hz) was used on pairs of needles inserted on the right (paralyzed) arm and leg, using points as listed, for 20 minutes/treatment session. The intensity of stimulation was controlled by the patient and maintained at a comfortable level. Treatments were offered 3 times/week for 20 or 40 treatments. Patients with chronic conditions who reach a plateau in their progress after the series of treatments need follow-up maintenance treatments once or twice a month.

†Low-pulse repetition rate electrical stimulation (1 to 2 Hz) was also used on the scalp needles (20 minutes). Microamps (not milliamps) electrical stimulation is now recommended on the needles.[39]

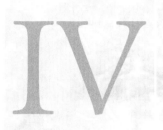

THE PROFESSION
OF ORIENTAL MEDICINE

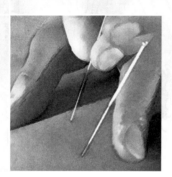

*I*f Oriental medicine is to succeed in large-scale and urban society, it must organize itself and become professionalized. Chapter 20, by Barbara Mitchell, reveals the process of professionalization in the United States by reviewing how Oriental medicine practitioners are trained and how each state licenses them. She also discusses the professional organizations that support Oriental medicine practice, from those that certify practitioners to those that honor high achievement. Sidebars highlight teaching and various professional societies.

The text ends with the highly pragmatic Chapter 21. This chapter on referral is written specifically for biomedical practitioners but contains suggestions that should be valuable to all practitioners and to patients. We hope the information in this chapter makes referral to professional Chinese medicine practitioners easier, efficient, and rewarding for all concerned. ❧

Supplementary Readings

General Texts for Professionals

Bensky D, Barolet R: *Chinese herbal medicine formulas and strategies,* Seattle, 1990, Eastland Press.

Bensky D, Gamble A, Kaptchuk T: *Chinese herbal medicine materia medica,* Seattle, 1993, Eastland Press.

Birch S, Felt R: *Understanding acupuncture,* Edinburgh, 1999, Churchill Livingstone.

Deadman P, Al-Khafaji M: *A manual of acupuncture,* East Sussex, England, 1998, Journal of Chinese Medicine Publications.

Ehling D, Swart S: *The Chinese herbalist's handbook,* revised ed, Santa Fe, NM, 1996, Inword Press.

Ellis A, Wiseman N, Boss K: *Fundamentals of Chinese acupuncture,* Brookline, Mass, 1991, Paradigm.

Larre C, Schatz J, Rochat de la Vallee E: *Survey of traditional Chinese medicine,* Columbia, Md, 1986, Traditional Acupuncture Institute.

Liao SJ, Lee M, Ng LKY: *Principles and practice of contemporary acupuncture,* New York, 1994, Marcel Dekker.

Maciocia G: *The foundations of Chinese medicine: a comprehensive text for acupuncturists and herbalists,* Edinburgh, 1989, Churchill Livingstone.

Maciocia G: *The practice of Chinese medicine: the treatment of diseases with acupuncture and Chinese herbs,* Edinburgh, 1994, Churchill Livingstone.

Manaka Y, Itaya K, Birch S: *Chasing the dragon's tail: the theory and practice of acupuncture in the work of Yoshio Manaka,* Brookline, Mass, 1995, Paradigm.

Ross J: *Acupuncture point combinations: the key to clinical success,* Edinburgh, 1995, Churchill Livingstone.

Scott J, Barlow T: *Acupuncture in the treatment of children,* ed 3, Seattle, 1999, Eastland Press.

Seem M: *A new American acupuncture, acupuncture osteopathy, the myofascial release of the bodymind's holding patterns,* Boulder, Colo, 1993, Blue Poppy Press.

Peer-Reviewed Journals

Acupuncture and Electro-Therapeutics Research
Alternative Medicine Review: A Journal of Clinical Therapeutics
American Journal of Acupuncture
American Journal of Chinese Medicine
European Journal of Oriental Medicine
Guideposts: Acupuncture in Recovery
Journal of Alternative and Complementary Medicine: Research on Paradigm, Practice, and Policy
Journal of Chinese Medicine
Journal of Traditional Chinese Medicine

20

The Professionalization of Acupuncture and Oriental Medicine in the United States

BARBARA B. MITCHELL

*A*cupuncture has been the most rapidly accepted form of alternative/complementary medicine in the United States during the past 25 years. As of November 2000, 41 states and the District of Columbia have enacted statutes or rules establishing standards for acupuncturists.* The US

Department of Education has recognized the Accreditation Commission for Acupuncture and Oriental Medicine to accredit master's level programs in acupuncture and in Oriental medicine.* The National Certification Commission for Acupuncture and Oriental Medicine has certified more than 10,000 practitioners and is accredited by the National Commission for Certifying Agencies. Acupuncture and Oriental medicine colleges have established internships in hospitals and outpatient facilities. Major third-party payers such as Oxford and Blue Cross-Blue Shield reimburse licensed acupuncturists, and health maintenance organizations such as Kaiser Permanente include

---

*The following jurisdictions have passed statutes: Alaska, Arkansas, Arizona, California, Colorado, Connecticut, [District of Columbia], Florida, Georgia, Hawaii, Idaho, Illinois, Indiana, Iowa, Louisiana, Maine, Maryland, Massachusetts, Minnesota, Missouri, Montana, Nevada, New Hampshire, New Jersey, New Mexico, New York, North Carolina, Ohio, Oregon, Pennsylvania, Rhode Island, South Carolina, Tennessee, Texas, Utah, Vermont, Virginia, Washington, West Virginia, and Wisconsin. In Kansas and Michigan, the Board of Medical Examiners has passed rules allowing nonmedical doctors to practice acupuncture. Legislation has been introduced in Alabama, Kansas, Kentucky, Michigan, Nebraska, Oklahoma, and Wyoming.

---

*The master's level program in Oriental medicine includes Chinese herbology and acupuncture.

BOX 20-1

List of United States National Acupuncture Organizations

Accreditation Commission for Acupuncture and
  Oriental Medicine (ACAOM)
7501 Greenway Center Drive, Suite 820
Greenbelt, MD 20770
301-313-0855; fax 301-313-0912

Acupuncture and Oriental Medicine Alliance
  (Acupuncture Alliance)
14637 Starr Road SE
Olalla, WA 98359
253-851-6896; fax 253-851-6883
www.acuall.org

American Academy of Medical Acupuncture (AAMA)
  and Medical Acupuncture Research Foundation
  (MARF)
4929 Wilshire Boulevard, Suite 428
Los Angeles, CA 90010
323-937-5514; fax 213-937-0059
www.medicalacupuncture.org

American Association of Teachers of Oriental
  Medicine (AATOM)
PO Box 9563
Austin, TX 78766-9563
512-451-2866; fax 512-454-7001
www.AATOM.org

American Association of Oriental Medicine (AAOM)
433 Front Street
Catasauqua, PA 18032
610-266-1433; fax 610-264-2768
www.aaom.org

American Organization for the Bodywork Therapy
  of Asia (AOBTA)
Laurel Oak Corporate Center, Suite 408
1010 Haddenfield-Berlin Road
Voorhees, NJ 08043
856-782-1616, fax 856-782-1653
www.aobta.org

Council of Colleges of Acupuncture and Oriental
  Medicine (CCAOM)
7501 Greenway Center Drive, Suite 820
Greenbelt, MD 20770
301-313-0868, fax 301-313-0869
www.ccaom.org

International Veterinary Acupuncture Society (IVAS)
PO Box 1478
Longmont, CO 80502-1478
970-266-0666, fax 970-266-0777
www.ivas.org

North American Acupuncture and Oriental Medicine
  Council (NAAOMC)
(Formerly NAFTA Acupuncture and Oriental
  Medicine Commission)
14637 Starr Road SE
Olalla, WA 98359
253-851-6896; fax 253-851-6883

National Academy of Acupuncture and Oriental
  Medicine (NAAOM)
44 Linden Street
Brookline, MA 02146
914-631-2369
www.naaom.org

National Acupuncture Detoxification Association
  (NADA)
PO Box 1927
Vancouver, WA 98668-1927
888-765-NADA; fax 360-260-8620
www.acudetox.com

National Acupuncture Foundation (NAF)
PO Box 2271
Gig Harbor, WA 98335-4271
253-851-6538; fax 253-851-6883

National Certification Commission for Acupuncture
  and Oriental Medicine (NCCAOM)
11 Canal Center Plaza, Suite 300
Alexandria, VA 22314
703-548-9004; fax 703-548-9079
www.nccaom.org

National Sports Acupuncture Association (NSAA)
PO Box 2271
Gig Harbor, WA 98335-4271
206-374-2505
www.sportsacupuncture.com

Society for Acupuncture Research (SAR)
PMB 106-241
4200 Wisconson Avenue, NW
Washington, DC 20016-2143
301-571-0624
www.acupunctureresearch.org

comprehensively trained acupuncturists in their program. Acupuncture has been so widely accepted that in many circles it is no longer considered as alternative or complementary; it is considered mainstream.

One of the major factors contributing to this rapid acceptance has been the profession's early and strong emphasis on establishing standards according to accepted processes. In the early 1980s, recognizing the value of national standards and a strong infrastructure, the profession developed an accreditation commission for colleges, a national certification agency for practitioners, a voluntary membership council for colleges, and a national professional membership association for practitioners (Box 20-1). Since then several other national organizations have been established, including a teachers' association, a society for acupuncture research, and a national academy modeled after the National Academy of Sciences. Professional membership organizations exist in virtually every state, and both state and national membership associations hold annual meetings and provide continuing education seminars. Although several organizations are in their fledgling stage, their existence is a clear indication of the growing strength of this profession.

These national standards and organizations, combined with the profession's flexibility in dealing with local philosophies and political needs, have paved the way for broad acceptance of this profession.

EDUCATIONAL STANDARDS

Two national acupuncture and Oriental medicine organizations provide direction for education in the United States: the Accreditation Commission for Acupuncture and Oriental Medicine (ACAOM) and the Council of Colleges of Acupuncture and Oriental Medicine (CCAOM).

The ACAOM was established in 1982 and has met the highest standards of recognition for accrediting bodies in the United States. It is recognized by the U.S. Department of Education and the Council on Higher Education Accreditation and is a charter member of the Association of Specialized and Professional Accreditors.

To achieve accreditation, a program must meet 14 essential requirements that set standards regarding (1) educational purpose, (2) legal organization, (3) governance, (4) administration, (5) records, (6) admissions, (7) evaluations processes, (8) program of study, (9) faculty, (10) student services, (11) library and learning resources, (12) physical facilities and equipment, (13) financial resources, and (14) publications and advertising. Accreditation requires that each program examines its goals, activities, and outcomes; considers the criticism and suggestions of a visiting team; determines internal procedures for action on recommendations from the Commission; and maintains continuous self-study and improvement mechanisms.

ACAOM accredits two types of programs. The first is a 3-year master's level program in acupuncture.* An accredited acupuncture program must contain a minimum of 47 semester credits (705 hours) in Oriental medical theory, diagnosis, and treatment techniques in acupuncture and related studies; 22 semester credits (660 hours) of clinical training, and 24 semester credits (360 hours) in biomedical clinical sciences.

The second program accredited by ACAOM is a 4-year master's level program in Oriental medicine. The Oriental medicine program includes Chinese herbology and acupuncture. Both programs usually include other aspects of Oriental medicine, such as bodywork, Qi Gong, and nutritional therapy. The Oriental medicine curriculum must contain at least 47 semester credits (705 hours) of Oriental medical theory, diagnosis, and treatment techniques in acupuncture and related studies; 30 semester credits (450 hours) in Oriental herbal studies; 22 semester credits (660 hours) in clinical training, and 24 semester credits (360 hours) in biomedical clinical sciences.

Both programs require a minimum of 2 years of accredited undergraduate baccalaureate education before entering the program, and both are designed to educate independent health care professionals. The biomedical component of the core curriculum in acupuncture or Oriental medicine educates graduates to interact in the prevailing health care model, to recognize their limitations, and to refer patients appropriately. Biomedical competencies include knowledge of anatomy, physiology, and pathology; biomedical and clinical concepts and terms; clinical relevance of laboratory and diagnostic tests and procedures; infectious diseases, sterilization procedures, and other issues relevant to blood-borne and surface pathogens; and the basis and need for referral or consultation.

---

*The term "master's level" is used because, although all accredited colleges must meet the same requirements, not all state departments of education have authorized colleges to offer a master's degree.

A Teacher Reflects

*Michael A. Phillips, LAc, Center
for Traditional Acupuncture*

Recently a student told me about his excitement at having one of his patients make a discovery about his symptoms. After years of experiencing sinusitis, the patient sought relief from acupuncture and came to our student-faculty clinic. On one occasion, after being needled, he proclaimed, "I understand why I've had this sinusitis. It is the tears I've stuffed back inside me all these years!" This insight into the interrelationship of physical illness and mental/emotional/spiritual life is a most exquisite aspect of this work and a source of great awe and joy for me as a teacher and practitioner.

One of the first lessons I was taught about the practice of acupuncture is that we bring four tools to our patients: (1) education, (2) needles, (3) moxa, and (4) more education. As a teacher and a practitioner, I try to honor the root of the word *educate*—to draw out of—as compared to *instruct*, which suggests putting something into. Drawing out awareness and insight is integral to healing and is a necessary complement to whatever else the physician offers the patient, be it needles, herbs, or advice. Furthermore, it enriches and enhances the practitioner's choice of appropriate acupuncture points. When patients or students discover knowledge inside themselves, it has power for them. When students are instructed in a technique or a theory, they can only embody this knowledge when they integrate it into something that they draw forth from within themselves, which makes that instruction personal and meaningful. I seek a balance of education and instruction with the intention of crafting well-honed practitioners who are in touch with and able to deeply listen to themselves and their patients.

The tradition of acupuncture I practice and teach has its roots in Five Element, Leamington-style acupuncture. As such, a great deal of the learning process concerns the observation of nature. The students learn that "as without, so within." In other words, if we really see the movements of life around us, we will be given insight—the ability to see within ourselves and others. Nature reflects our own natures back to us. Students of this tradition do self-reflective work: learning their own natures, discovering their strengths and challenges, and tuning themselves to be available to the needs of those who will seek their talents. When we have met ourselves with some measure of honest inquiry, we can begin to meet another in service and create partnership in the treatment room.

We purposefully let students build their own practices. In part, this prepares them for making contact with the public and speaking from their hearts and their heads about what they offer. Also, they must cooperate with one another in the operation of the clinic and the accommodation of their patients' scheduling, which prepares them for the practical aspects of clinical practice after training. It also illustrates basic principles of Eastern philosophy that empower them as practitioners, such as selflessness, respect, and harmony.

Students may grumble as their fears about being able to achieve their personal and collective requirements come to the surface, but we teachers, and eventually the students themselves, see much acquired confidence and competence at graduation. Similarly, when supervising their clinical treatments, the faculty does not prescribe treatments and have students carry out the protocols. Rather, the students must persuade us of the design and logic of their treatment plan before they are allowed to execute it. After graduation, these practitioners are able to think on their feet and treat from their heads and hearts. As one who is privileged to teach, seeing such competent, caring graduates satisfies me deeply and offers hope that more and more people will be well served by this rich form of medicine. ❧

As of November 2000, 37 programs have been accredited, and nine programs hold candidacy status.

The second organization in the educational process in the United States, the CCAOM, is a voluntary membership association of accredited and candidate acupuncture and Oriental medicine colleges. Membership in CCAOM requires colleges to meet the 14 essential requirements of the ACAOM. The CCAOM develops academic and clinical guidelines and core curriculum requirements; provides programs in faculty and administrative development; supports research, translation, and other academic work in Oriental medicine; provides guidance in institutional development for member colleges; and supports member and non-member colleges in their work toward accreditation. The CCAOM has developed master's-level programs in acupuncture, Oriental medicine, and Chinese herbology. The CCAOM also developed guidelines and curriculum requirements for doctoral-level programs in Oriental medicine that served as the basis of the new clinical doctorate guidelines adopted by the ACAOM in May 2000.*

When the ACAOM and the CCAOM were established in 1982, the master's level was chosen as the level of education most appropriate to the stage of development of the colleges. At that time, the colleges did not have the infrastructure necessary for doctorate-level programs (e.g., library and facility resources, doctorate-level faculty). Until now there has been no accredited doctorate-level program offered in the United States.† However, now that ACAOM has developed guidelines for a doctorate in Oriental medicine, colleges will be able to offer an approved doctorate that will meet national educational standards. Some colleges are expected to begin offering doctorate programs in the fall of 2001. For the doctorate programs to be approved by the Department of Education, ACAOM must request approval to change its scope of accreditation to include doctorate-level programs. At the state level, colleges need to apply for state approval to offer a doctorate degree.

CERTIFICATION STANDARDS

The National Certification Commission for Acupuncture and Oriental Medicine (NCCAOM) was established in 1982 and is accredited by the National Commission of Certifying Agencies, the agency with the highest standards of voluntary certification in the United States. NCCAOM is a member of the National Organization of Certifying Agencies (NOCA) and, since its inception, has followed NOCA's nationally recognized guidelines for certification of health professionals.

NCCAOM offered its first national certification program in acupuncture in 1984. It now offers three certification programs: acupuncture, Chinese herbology, and Asian bodywork therapy. These certification programs have allowed state regulators to use national standards and avoid the high cost of local examination development and administration. Virtually every state* that licenses acupuncturists recognizes NCCAOM certification or uses the NCCAOM board examination in its licensure process.† NCCAOM examinations reflect the broad range of traditions within the profession and are administered in English, Chinese, and Korean.‡ The eligibility routes for certification also reflect the cross-cultural background of the profession. Applicants for certification in acupuncture and Chinese herbology can qualify on the basis of graduation from a formal college program,§ completion of an apprenticeship of at least 4000 contact hours within 3 to 6 years, 4 years of professional practice at a minimum level,‖ or a combination of the previous.¶ In the Chinese herbology program, provisions are also available for acupuncturists who studied herbs after they completed their acupuncture training.

To be certified in acupuncture, an applicant must pass a written examination on acupuncture, Oriental medical theory, and clean needle technique and a practical examination of point location. An applicant also

---

*For a copy of the doctorate guidelines, see the Acupuncture and Oriental Medicine Alliance Web page at www.AcupunctureAlliance.org.
†Doctorate-level programs in acupuncture and Oriental medicine are rare anywhere in the world. The entry-level program in the People's Republic of China is 5 years after high school. Postgraduate master's and doctorate (PhD) programs are available. However, few individuals attain a doctorate.

---

*Except California, Louisiana, and Nevada.
†States use the NCCAOM in different ways. Some grant licensure based solely on NCCAOM certification through examination or Credentials Documentation Review (grandparenting). Many states have their own eligibility requirements in addition to requiring passage of the national examination administered by NCCAOM. A few states administer the NCCAOM examination under their own testing program, and a handful have additional practical or jurisprudence examinations.
‡The profession has been very careful to respect its roots. Several accredited colleges offer programs in Chinese and/or Korean as well as English.
§Three years for certification in Acupuncture and 4 years for Chinese herbology.
‖This route of eligibility was phased out on December 31, 2000.
¶Graduation from a college is by far the most frequently used basis of eligibility. However, apprenticeship is traditional within Oriental medicine and is allowed by several states. Professional practice was used primarily to qualify for NCCAOM certification several years ago when China did not release college transcripts but individuals were able to document practice. Very few applicants seek certification based on the combination method.

must pass a Clean Needle Technique Course. The latter reflects the strong emphasis, present since the establishment of the national organizations, on clean needle technique in the practice of acupuncture. The certification program in Chinese herbology requires passage of a comprehensive examination in Chinese herbs. The new Oriental bodywork therapy program offered its first examination in 1999.

All NCCAOM diplomates undergo a recertification process every 4 years based on criteria that reflect an individual's competency to practice a health care profession. To maintain active certification, a diplomate must document professional activity, such as teaching, research, or continuing education, and clinical practice within the 4-year period. The NCCAOM investigates any reports of ill health, chemical dependency, and ethical, legal, and disciplinary issues related to the practice of a health care professional. In this way, the NCCAOM ensures states and the public that active diplomates are professionally active and current in their field. The safety record of the profession is remarkable. Since 1984, after certifying more than 10,000 practitioners, NCCAOM has never had reason to take action against a diplomate for negligent or harmful treatment to a patient.*

STATE LEGISLATION

The profession has been very flexible in adapting to local legislative philosophies and needs. This flexibility has resulted in a wide variation in the scopes of practice, titles of practitioners, governing structures, required interface with other health care practitioners, and so on. It also has been one of the profession's greatest strengths in establishing itself.

---

*NCCAOM has taken action against one diplomate for sexual harassment issues.

The Society for Acupuncture Research

Richard Hammerschlag, PhD, FNAAOM, Oregon College of Oriental Medicine

The mission of the Society for Acupuncture Research (SAR) is to promote scientifically sound inquiries into the clinical efficacy, physiological mechanisms, patterns of use, and theoretical foundations of acupuncture, herbal therapy, and other modalities of Oriental medicine. Since its first annual symposium in 1993, SAR has served as a focal point for practitioners, researchers, health care policy makers, and students interested in conducting, improving, and disseminating what is broadly described as Oriental medicine research.

SAR aims to achieve its mission by:

- Offering assistance in study design to those embarking on research in Oriental medicine
- Providing an annual forum for the presentation and discussion of research findings and research design in Oriental medicine
- Educating the broad-spectrum health care community, both practitioners and the people they serve, on research findings and their relevance to clinical practice

In addition to its annual meetings, SAR's accomplishments include responding to a commission from the National Academy of Acupuncture and Oriental Medicine to prepare a summary of positive outcome clinical trials of acupuncture. This project was completed in 1996 by SAR board members Stephen Birch and Richard Hammerschlag, with the publication of *Acupuncture Efficacy: A Compendium of Controlled Clinical Trials.*

SAR also was actively involved in the 1997 Consensus Development Conference on Acupuncture, sponsored by the U.S. National Institutes of Health (NIH). Six members of the SAR Board were among the presenters at the conference that concluded with the NIH panel's endorsement: "... there is sufficient evidence of acupuncture's value to expand its use into conventional medicine and to encourage further study of its physiology and clinical value."

SAR is committed to this conclusion and encourages anyone interested in acupuncture research to become an affiliate member.

For further information, contact SAR at its Web site: www.acupunctureresearch.org. ∾

In most states, acupuncturists are licensed, registered, or certified* as independent health care providers with no need for prior diagnosis or supervision.† The status of independent practitioner is consistent with the training provided by accredited colleges. However, almost one third of the states require some form of allopathic medical intervention or oversight; this usually includes a referral or a prior diagnosis by or collaboration with a medical doctor, doctor of osteopathy, dentist, or chiropractor before treatment. In New York, the statute requires that the acupuncturist advises the patient about the importance of consulting with a licensed physician (Table 20-1 and Figure 20-1).

This terminology has fallen into disfavor for several reasons. First, legislators increasingly view the language as a restriction on consumer access. Second, allopathic medical boards are concerned that this terminology may place their licensees in a legally vulnerable position by requiring them to supervise a practice that is not included within their normal professional training.‡ Finally, the safety record of the profession is so excellent that there does not appear to be any need for this type of oversight.§ Iowa, Maryland, Massachusetts, and Virginia dropped their requirement for supervision or prior diagnosis, and other states are considering doing the same.

The statutory definition of acupuncture, and therefore the scope of practice, also varies substantially from state to state. Every state includes the insertion of acupuncture needles. Many include moxibustion, cupping, and electrical, manual, and thermal stimulation. Several add Oriental bodywork and dietary and lifestyle counseling. One half specifically include the practice of Chinese herbology. A few states include Western herbology, homeopathy, and Western nutritional supplements.

There are also structural variations among the states. Approximately one third have an independent board of acupuncture or Oriental medicine, one third regulate licensed acupuncturists through the Board of Medical Examiners, and the remaining third place acupuncturists, with or without independent or advisory boards, under state agencies such as the Department of Health, Licensing, Professional Regulation, or Education. The latter strategy has been necessary partly because of the increasing resistance of governments to establishing new boards. However, the primary factor has been financial. There are usually too few practitioners in the unregulated states to support an independent board when legislation is first introduced; therefore acupuncturists are usually placed under an existing agency. This practice may change as the number of licensed acupuncturists increases.*

CHALLENGES FOR THE FUTURE

One of the issues facing the profession is the use of the accredited doctoral degree under consideration by the ACAOM. The CCAOM, which developed the curriculum proposal, created the doctorate as an optional degree to provide further education for practitioners, faculty, clinical supervisors, researchers, and administrators, not as an entry level for the profession. This move is supported by the safety record of the profession, which clearly indicates that the current level of education protects the public.

Currently it is unclear whether the acupuncture and Oriental medicine profession in the United States will either move toward a single doctorate level similar to that of chiropractors and naturopaths or develop a multitude of tiers with several levels of education and responsibility as in allopathic medicine. Given the broad scope of Oriental medicine and the

*Although all statutes establish *licensure* (the requirement that individuals must meet state standards of competency in order to practice) states have chosen to use various titles to denote state recognition. Four states grant the title *Doctor;* Arkansas, New Mexico, and Nevada grant the title *Doctor of Oriental Medicine;* and Rhode Island grants the title *Doctor of Acupuncture.* Florida uses the title *Acupuncture Physician.*
†Two states, Florida and New Mexico, provide that acupuncturists are primary care providers. In California, licensed acupuncturists are considered primary care providers under workers' compensation.
‡Although survey courses in complementary medicine are becoming more common, no allopathic medical school has yet incorporated in-depth training in acupuncture or Oriental medicine into its core curriculum. The American Academy of Medical Acupuncture provides a 300-hour postgraduate training for medical doctors.
§See *Safety Record of Acupuncture* published by the National Acupuncture Foundation.

*Maryland and California, both of which formerly placed licensed acupuncturists under the board of medical examiners, have changed their statutes to provide for independent acupuncture boards. Pennsylvania has introduced similar legislation.

TABLE 20-1

States with Acupuncture and Oriental Medicine Practice Acts

State	Governing structure	Title of practitioner	Medical referral, prior diagnosis, or supervision	Specific training required by MDs
Alaska	Division of Occupational Licensing	LAc	None	None
Arizona	Arizona Acupuncture Board of Examiners	LAc	None	None
Arkansas	Board of Acupuncture and Related Therapies	DOM	None	None
California	Acupuncture Board	LAc	None	None
Colorado	Department of Regulatory Agencies	Registered Acupuncturist	None	None
Connecticut	Department of Public Health	Acupuncturist	None	None
District of Columbia	Advisory Committee under Board of Medicine	Acupuncturist	Written authorization from collaborating MD or DO	250 hr
Florida	Board of Acupuncture	Acupuncture Physician	None	"Education and training"
Georgia	Board of Medical Examiners	LAc	None	300 hr
Hawaii	Board of Acupuncture	LAc	Referral by MD or DDS for organic disorders	Must be LAc
Idaho	State Board of Acupuncture	LAc	None	None
Illinois	Department of Professional Regulation	Acupuncturist	Written referral by physician or DDS	None
Indiana	Medical Licensing Board	LAc	Referral, written diagnosis, or written documentation	None
Iowa	Board of Medical Examiners	LAc	None	None
Louisiana	Board of Medical Examiners	Acupuncture Assistant (if 36 mo training)	Employed and supervised by MD	6 mo training, titled LAc
Maine	Board of Complementary Health Care Providers	LAc	None	None
Maryland	State Board of Acupuncture	LAc	None	200 hr
Massachusetts	Acupuncture Committee under Board of Medicine	LAc	None	None
Minnesota	Acupuncture Advisory Council under Board of Medical Practice	LAc	None	None
Missouri	Acupuncturist Advisory Committee under the Board of Chiropractic Examiners	LAc	None	None

State	Regulatory Board	Title	Physician Involvement	Training
Nevada	Board of Oriental Medicine	DOM, DAc, Assistant in Acupuncture	None for DOM or DAc; Acupuncture Assistant must be supervised by DOM or DAc	"Adequate training"
New Hampshire	Board of Acupuncture Licensing	LAc	None	None
New Jersey	Acupuncture Examining Board	Certified Acupuncturist	Referral or diagnosis from physician	300 hr including 150 clinical
New Mexico	Board of Acupuncture and Oriental Medicine	DOM	None	None
New York	Advisory Board under State Board of Regents	LAc	Must advise patient about importance of consulting with licensed physician	300 hr (titled Certified Acupuncturist)
North Carolina	Acupuncture Licensing Board	LAc	None	"Sufficient education and training"
Ohio	State Medical Board	Acupuncturist	Referral and supervision	Unknown
Oregon	Advisory Committee under Board of Medical Examiners	LAc	None	None
Pennsylvania	Board of Medical Examiners and Board of Osteopathic Examiners	Acupuncturist	Supervision by MD, DO, or DS registered as acupuncture supervisor	200 hr
Rhode Island	Department of Health	DAc	None	None
South Carolina	Board of Medical Examiners	Acupuncturist	Supervision and referral by MD or DDS	None
Tennessee	Advisory Committee under Board of Medicine	LAc	None	None
Texas	Board of Acupuncture Examiners under Board of Medical Examiners	LAc	Evaluation by licensed physician or DDS within 6 mo or referral by chiropractor within 30 days	None
Utah	Board of Acupuncture	Acupuncturist	None	None
Vermont	Office of Professional Regulation	LAc	None	None
Virginia	Advisory Committee under Board of Medicine	LAc	Exam by MD or DO	200 hr
Washington	Consulting Group under Department of Health	LAc	Consultation or referral for specific conditions	None
West Virginia	Acupuncture Board	LAc	None	None
Wisconsin	Department of Regulation and Licensing	Acupuncturist	None	None

DAc, Doctor of Acupuncture; DO, Doctor of Osteopathy; DOM, Doctor of Oriental Medicine; DDS, Doctor of Dental Surgery; LAc, Licensed Acupuncturist; MD, Doctor of Medicine. Information reprinted from Acupuncture and Oriental Medicine, 1999 edition, with permission of the National Acupuncture Foundation.

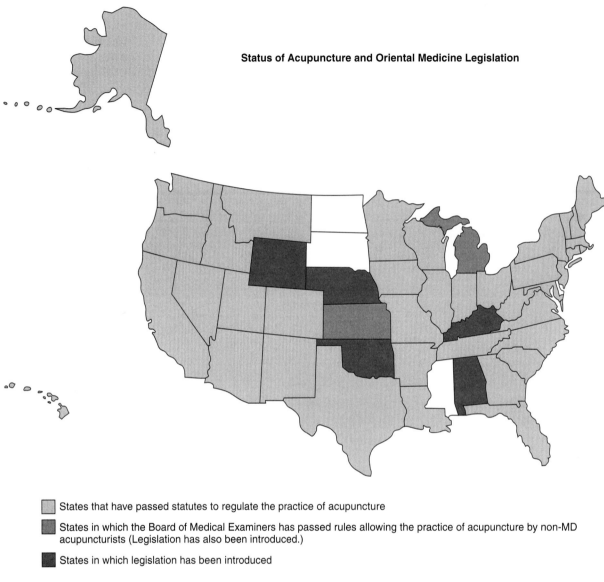

Figure 20-1 Legislative status of acupuncture and Oriental medicine. (Based on information from the Acupuncture and Oriental Medicine Alliance, September 2000.)

variety of schools of thought* and professional tracks around the world,† a multitiered profession is more likely, particularly because a multitiered system already exists in several states. Nevada has a Doctor of

*Some schools of thought incorporate herbology, such as traditional Chinese medicine, and others do not, such as Five Element acupuncture, Nogier auricular acupuncture, Korean hand acupuncture, Korean constitutional acupuncture, French energetics, and Japanese meridian therapy.
†Acupuncturists, Chinese herbalists, Oriental medical doctors, various types of Oriental bodywork, medical Qi Gong practitioners, Chinese herbal pharmacologists, and so on.

Oriental Medicine accreditation and an Assistant in Acupuncture. Arizona, Connecticut, Georgia, Indiana, Missouri, New York, South Carolina, Tennessee, Texas, and Virginia provide for acupuncture chemical dependency specialists. Massachusetts has created an acupuncture assistant accreditation and a separate board certification in Chinese herbology for licensed acupuncturists.

Other challenges facing the profession have been created by the popularity and effectiveness of this type of medicine. Many other health care providers, not understanding that acupuncture is one portion of a com-

National Academy of Acupuncture and Oriental Medicine, Inc

June Brazil, Dipl Ac, PDM, LAc, FNAAOM

Founded in 1993, the NAAOM is an honor society established to recognize and provide a forum for professionals in a variety of fields who have made significant contributions to the advancement of knowledge and the scientific acceptance of acupuncture and Oriental medicine (AOM). Fellows are elected to the Academy for life and are recognized for contributions to the areas of teaching, scholarship, research, and publishing, as well as special recognition for those whose contributions have been in politics and social integration.

The Founding Mission of the Academy expressed the desire of its governors to aid in the establishment of an unbiased forum that could ensure that open, free, and honest intellectual discussion of crucial issues relating to the advancement of AOM could take place at every level of scientific and professional development. To achieve this end, the Academy has devoted itself to supporting conferences, discussions, and other activities that allow diverse and varied points of view to be heard and discussed.

One of the Academy's principal achievements is the publication of a comprehensive review of the best clinical evidence for the usefulness of acupuncture. *Acupuncture Efficacy: A Compendium of Controlled Clinical Studies,* by Stephen Birch and Richard Hammerschlag, published in 1996, is now in its fourth printing.

Written to provide scientists, students, professionals, lawmakers, and policymakers with sound evidence of acupuncture efficacy in a variety of conditions and clinical situations, the book is presented in a format designed to be accessible to both the lay public and the scientific investigator. The first edition contains abstracts of 70 scientific studies with commentary about their significance in the question of the efficacy of acupuncture as a therapeutic modality. Each study is presented in a standard format, making it easy to absorb and apply. This valuable book is available in libraries throughout the world and is a required text for students in AOM schools in much of the United States.

The Academy also publishes a journal, *The Journal of the National Academy of Acupuncture and Oriental Medicine (JNAAOM),* devoted to the promulgation of scholarly and scientific articles in the field and to providing a forum for information about the activities of the Fellows. In 1998 the NAAOM joined with the Society of Acupuncture Research to become founding partners in the production and publication of *Clinical Acupuncture and Oriental Medicine,* published by Churchill Livingstone.

The Academy remains dedicated to providing a common forum for discussion and development of research, education, and scientific excellence in AOM. Future programs of action include sponsoring postgraduate fellowships in advanced clinical and academic study in AOM and promoting conferences to explore issues that pertain to the development of a strong evidence base for AOM in contemporary health care practice.

For further information, contact the NAAOM by mail: PO Box 62, Tarrytown, NY 10591; voice: 914-332-4576; fax: 914-631-2369; or e-mail: info@naaom.org. ∾

---

plex medical system founded on a different paradigm of the human body, view acupuncture as the simple technique of inserting a needle that can be quickly incorporated into their practice. Given the popularity of "alternative medicine," this perception is a strong lure. This view is enhanced by the fact that most states allow medical doctors to practice acupuncture without any training,* even though acupuncture is not included within the allopathic curriculum and there are no accredited certification programs in acupuncture or Oriental medicine for other health care providers.* In some states, chiropractors,† naturopaths, physician's assistants, and nurses also may practice acupuncture.‡

---

*Ten states have set training requirements for medical doctors to practice acupuncture, ranging from "adequate training" to 300 hours. Hawaii requires all individuals who practice acupuncture to meet the requirements for licensed acupuncturists.

---

*The American Academy of Medical Acupuncture offers a 300-hour course for medical doctors.
†Twenty-eight states consider acupuncture to be within the scope of practice of chiropractors, 18 of which have set training requirements.
‡All information regarding definition of acupuncture, regulatory structure, and practice by other health care providers is based on *Acupuncture and Oriental Medicine Laws* by Barbara B. Mitchell, 2001 edition, published by the National Acupuncture Foundation.

Because acupuncture can be effective in some instances with little understanding of the underlying theory or mechanisms, it is likely that the impetus by other health care providers to incorporate acupuncture into their practice will increase. This movement creates two challenges for the profession of licensed acupuncturists. The first is to work with other health care professions to assist them in developing standards of training necessary to practice acupuncture safely within their scope of practice.* This training must be coupled with the recognition of when to refer patients to the professionals comprehensively trained in this medicine. The second challenge is to establish a national identity that allows consumers to make an informed choice about whether they want to see either a practitioner comprehensively trained in acupuncture and Oriental medicine or a practitioner who uses acupuncture as an adjunct to his or her primary professional training and license. Although the variation in

---

*For example, the minimum education necessary for licensed acupuncturists to treat the full range of medical problems has been set at the 3-year master's level and passage of the NCCAOM examination in acupuncture. The National Acupuncture Detoxification Association program to train acudetox specialists to use five ear points for the treatment of chemical dependency is 80 hours. Educational standards generally are set by establishing the goals of the training, the skills and knowledge necessary to meet those goals, and the curriculum necessary to provide the skills and knowledge. Once this has been established, the number of hours necessary to teach that curriculum may be determined. This process is better than arguing in the halls of the legislature about the number of hours necessary to practice acupuncture.

licensure titles has made the establishment of a national identity difficult, referral services exist that provide the names of comprehensively trained practitioners in the United States.*

LEGISLATIVE STATUS OUTSIDE THE UNITED STATES

Outside the United States, Japan, China, and Korea, the general rule is that acupuncture and Oriental medicine is usually within the scope of practice of biomedical doctors and, in some cases, physical therapists and heilpraktikers.† Generally, comprehensively trained acupuncturists have not been recognized as independent professionals.‡ There are exceptions. For example, in Canada three provinces (Alberta, British Columbia, and Quebec) have established regulatory bodies governing acupuncturists. In England acupuncturists have established an accreditation body for colleges and are seeking government recognition, whereas in Australia acupuncturists have established a strong educational system and national presence.

---

*The Acupuncture and Oriental Medicine Alliance lists more than 10,000 primary-verified, state-licensed, or NCCAOM-certified acupuncturists on its Web page (www.acuall.org).
†A German health care profession similar to naturopathy.
‡See *Acupuncture and Oriental Medicine Laws,* 1997 *edition* and Acupuncture and Oriental Medicine Alliance newsletter, *The Forum,* Fall 2000, on the Alliance Web page: www.acuall.org.

 The Acupuncture Research Resources Centre

Alison Gould, MSc, York, England
History and Aims

The Acupuncture Research Resources Centre (ARRC), the first national acupuncture research resource center, was founded in 1994 to serve as a British research resource centre for acupuncture. Today, ARRC is used by practitioners and researchers from around the world. ARRC serves the needs of acupuncture research by providing information, encouraging the growth of interest in research among practitioners, and supporting the development of research expertise. Begun as a collaborative project between the

Foundation for Traditional Chinese Medicine, a research charity, and the British acupuncture profession's umbrella body, the British Acupuncture Council, ARRC also aims to increase awareness of the use and effectiveness of acupuncture and hence help in promoting the wider use of acupuncture.

Context: Why the ARRC?
By 1994 it was becoming clear that more research on acupuncture was needed. The current emphasis on evidence-based medicine and the market economy approach to health care drove a strong demand for evi-

Continued

The Acupuncture Research Resources Centre—cont'd

dence of effectiveness, particularly in the form of results from clinically based trials. The dearth of extensive high-quality scientific evidence of the effectiveness of Chinese medicine care was cited as a major barrier to being taken seriously by policymakers and biomedical practitioners. Demand for acupuncture treatment also was growing, and patients rightly required more information and pragmatic evidence of the utility of complementary medical approaches to help them make personal health care choices. Finally, every mature profession needs to take a reflective and questioning attitude toward its work to maintain and improve its standards, both in education and the delivery of health care.

Research designs reflect the market at which the research is aimed, and different forms of evidence are seen as relevant and acceptable to different audiences. The initiators of ARRC were clear that the profession needed to play a key role in the planning and execution, particularly of clinical acupuncture research, ensuring that the practice of acupuncture is adequately reflected in trial designs, that well-trained practitioners are used in such trials, and that measures of outcome are relevant to the holistic aims of traditional acupuncture. ARRC represents a significant commitment to meeting these needs from a foundation established within the acupuncture profession. In addition, the initiators recognized the need for a mechanism to store and distribute research data and to inform and train practitioners to support the develop of research expertise within the profession. ARRC represents a significant commitment to meeting these needs from a foundation established within the Chinese medicine profession.

What ARRC Does

Provides an information service based around a computerized database called ARRCBASE. ARRC provides a rapid and expert information service on acupuncture research and practice for registered acupuncturists and other interested persons and organisations. This helps practitioners and researchers access a wide range of Chinese medicine resources, often materials otherwise not easily found.

A computerized database, ARRCBASE, has been constructed to provide for this growing need. ARRCBASE is a computerized resource dedicated to storing information on acupuncture and related practices, such as moxibustion, transcutaneous electric nerve stimulation (TENS), Qi Gong, Tai Chi, and Chinese herbal medicine. The main reference sources are the US National Institutes of Health database (MEDLINE), and the British Library's alternative medicine database (AMED). To date, ARRCBASE holds more than 9000 references that are updated monthly. Gradually more information from unpublished sources such as conference proceedings is being added. The aim is to create a database that incorporates as much of the material written on acupuncture as possible. At present, the major holdings are in English but a variety of European and Oriental language articles also are referenced.

Clarifies the aims of acupuncture and Oriental medicine research. ARRC works to generate interest in research, particularly among Oriental medicine practitioners. With a primarily clinical history, the profession now needs to develop expertise in research methods to help ensure that work is judged by criteria that acupuncture professionals, and our patients, feel are relevant. In addition, practitioners need to address questions internal to the profession; for example, which patients respond best, which conditions is AOM best at treating, what is the pattern of change for patients over time, and how can we improve our practice?

Furthers the aims and supports practitioners by:
• Organising annual acupuncture research symposia that bring together expert speakers from the United Kingdom and abroad and provide opportunities for widening experience and in-depth discussion. Proceedings are available from ARRC.
• Running Study Days, small workshops designed to teach research methods and examine particular research projects in detail.
• Commissioning briefing papers. ARRC is now commissioning a series of briefing papers that will provide information on topics, such as research on the effectiveness of acupuncture in particular conditions and the language of research and research methods.
• Building a library of research tools. ARRC is compiling copies of protocols, questionnaires, outcome measures, and similar materials as a resource to help would-be researchers. This function is also a

Continued

The Acupuncture Research Resources Centre—cont'd

vital part of promoting the growth of a research awareness.

- Maintaining an Acupuncture Research Directory. The directory records practitioners who are involved in or interested in research.

In summary, the existence of a centralized resource providing information, advice, and research expertise has proved of great value in the United Kingdom. Increasing numbers of individuals and organisations use ARRC's services, and ARRC has enabled the development of a small group of practitioner researchers. As the possibility of multicentre research projects arises,

ARRC also offers the obvious potential for becoming a centre for data collection and analysis. The British Chinese medicine profession is committed to its continuing existence as evidenced by its recent relocation to the Centre for Complementary Health Studies at the University of Exeter.

For further information, contact the ARRC by mail: Centre for Complementary Health Studies, University of Exeter, Exeter, Devon EX4 4RJ, United Kingdom; telephone: 0-1392-264459; fax: 0-1392-433828; e-mail: arrc@exeter.ac.uk; or Web site: www.acupuncture-research.org.uk. ∾

SUMMARY

In his introduction to *Medical Ethics in Imperial China—A Study in Historical Anthropology,* Paul Unschuld[1] lists nine dimensions of professionalization: (1) the acceptance of remuneration of services rendered, (2) the use of technical terminology, (3) the wearing of professional symbols, (4) the passing of formal training, (5) the emphasis on a professional ethics, (6) monopoly and licensing, (7) autonomy of the profession, (8) internationalization, and (9) social status. He states, "The relative development of these dimensions in a group indicates its degree of professionalization compared to other groups."* Since the James Reston *New York Times* article in 1971 regarding his experience with acupuncture in China, acupuncture has gained a

firm foothold in the American consciousness and has established an independent and respected profession by all of Unschuld's indicators.[2] Although challenges remain, such as increased third-party coverage and greater acceptance into health care networks and hospitals, acupuncturists are rapidly being accepted into these systems. If the profession advances as rapidly during the next 25 years as it has in the last, we soon can look forward to a health care system in which various types of practitioners, Eastern and Western, work side by side for the optimum care of the patient.

References

1. Unschuld P: *Medical ethics in imperial China—a study in historical anthropology,* Berkeley, Calif, 1979, University of California Press.
2. Reston J: Now about my operation in Peking, *New York Times* July 26, 1971, pp 1, 6.

---

*Quoted on www.acuall.org.

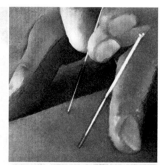

Referral

CLAIRE M. CASSIDY

oday it is clear that the future of health care includes a wide variety of options from which patients and practitioners can choose. In this situation, practitioners who view medicine as a cooperative endeavor and develop a wide referral network will not only be better able to serve their patients but will probably find their practices more satisfying.

This book has shown that the practice of Oriental medicine (OM) offers an important option for referral. OM includes a comprehensive theory of disorder and of care developed from an extraordinarily long and detailed clinical experience. This clinical experience is supported by a rapidly increasing fund of scientific research knowledge. Most practitioners today are trained in professional schools according to demanding standards. Surveys also have shown that patients report being remarkably satisfied with OM care. Accessibility to this care is rising rapidly in terms of

increasing numbers of practitioners, greater availability of third-party remuneration for care, and legal support for its practice. Finally, OM interventions are extremely safe. These days it should be relatively easy for biomedical practitioners—medical doctors, nurse practitioners, psychologists, dentists, and others—to refer patients successfully to OM care.

This short chapter offers guidance both in selecting appropriate patients for referral and developing collegial relationships with professional OM practitioners.

REFERRING PATIENTS FOR ORIENTAL MEDICINE CARE

Several previous chapters have ended with brief suggestions concerning referral. Box 21-1 summarizes several features to use in deciding whether to refer a pa-

BOX 21-1

Selecting Patients to Refer for Oriental Medical Care

1. Patients with acute conditions who may benefit from coordinate biomedical and Oriental care
   - Examples: Nausea of pregnancy; trauma; presurgery immunological strengthening; postsurgical acute recovery period; poststroke acute recovery period; acute pain conditions
2. Patients with recurrent or chronic conditions or complex medical histories who may benefit from coordinate biomedical and Oriental care
   - Examples: Chronic pain conditions, such as lower back pain, neck pain, headaches; chronic neurological conditions, such as poststroke and epilepsy; chronic digestive complaints, such as irritable bowel syndrome and hepatitis; chronic respiratory complaints, such as sinusitis, rhinitis, and asthma; reproductive complaints, such as dysmenorrhea, infertility, and symptoms of menopause; nausea and fatigue associated with radiation or chemotherapy treatments; immunocompromised conditions, such as lupus and multiple sclerosis, or frequent infections (e.g., urinary, respiratory, Lyme disease); and mental illness conditions, such as depression and anxiety syndromes
3. Patients whose conditions have not responded to biomedical care or those who present unique problems of intervention
   - Those with multiple drug sensitivities
   - Those who by biomedical standards "have nothing wrong" yet continue to complain of discomfort
   - Those with multiple complaints that "do not make sense" within a biomedical analytic framework
   - Those who have "tried everything" in biomedical medicine without sufficient benefit
   - Former drug abusers who need to to minimize use of pharmaceuticals
   - Those with fragile conditions that preclude biomedical interventions such as surgery
4. Patients who dislike, fear, or resist the options offered within biomedicine
   - Those who do not wish to take pharmaceuticals
   - Those who wish to try other options before resorting to surgery or other forms of tertiary biomedical care
   - Those who have had numerous "bad experiences" within biomedicine
   - Those with energetic imbalances
5. Patients who can benefit from a high relational health care setting
   - Those who like to spend time talking and understanding their health and health care
   - Those who express a desire to be more in charge of their own bodies, health care, or both
   - Those who express an interest in nonbiomedical alternatives
   - Those who appear committed to changing their lives around a specific health issue, especially one that has not responded to standard care

tient for OM care; the points in the box are developed below.

Acute and Chronic Care

Just as many patients are treated by both a biomedical internist or family practitioner and another biomedical specialist (e.g., psychologist, physical therapist, dentist, ophthalmologist, cardiologist), so many patients see both biomedical and OM practitioners. Chapter 12 reviewed data showing that a majority of OM patients continue to consult biomedical practitioners; however, it also has been reported that many do not *tell* their biomedical practitioners when they see alternative practitioners.[1] This situation requires remediation because good medical care benefits from open communication. The first step a biomedical practitioner can take is to become alert to the patient's wants and practices. The second is served by this book (and others): to become informed about the alternatives, in our case OM, which is probably the fastest growing* of the alternatives.

---

*This remark is based on the fact that the number of practitioners and schools in Western nations has increased rapidly in the past 30 years; however, in terms of numbers of practitioners, chiropractic and massage therapy still outweigh OM.

The entries in Box 21-1 concerning acute and chronic care are listed on the assumption that most patients with these complaints and conditions will benefit from care provided by both biomedical and OM practitioners. Chapters 13 to 19 reviewed bodily systems and clusters of conditions that respond well to OM interventions. Each author has emphasized conditions with particularly good research track records. A series of case histories in Chapter 8 provide additional clinical data. However, this book is not all-inclusive. Because OM is a comprehensive medicine,* other conditions can also respond, and biomedical practitioners need not limit referral recommendations to those conditions discussed in this book.

A useful guideline is this: consider recommending OM if the condition has a significant "functional" component, physical changes, or both that have not progressed beyond a level that can "self-correct" with appropriate energetic intervention. However, even in cases that do require surgery or other tertiary care, OM can still serve. For example, acupuncture care and herbs can speed recovery from trauma (from automobile accidents to surgery) and can improve energy and control nausea in patients receiving chemotherapy or radiation treatment.

The history of OM in the United States has somewhat biased views of the practice, particularly toward its recommendation for pain syndromes. OM can be extremely effective in reducing or abolishing pain—in arthritis, headaches, phantom limb syndromes, muscular complaints such as fibromyalgia, and so forth (see Chapter 13). In addition, it effectively deals with a wide range of other conditions as emphasized throughout this book.

One condition merits particular emphasis. Previously, little research was done to test the clinical findings of the effectiveness of OM in patients with abnormal immune responses. Chapter 11 discusses the bimodal response pattern to acupuncture: it tends to return the body to a state of homeostasis. Thus both conditions of immune deficiency (e.g., frequent respiratory, urinary, or skin infections) and of immune hyperreactivity (e.g., allergies, lupus, rheumatoid arthritis, multiple sclerosis) can respond positively to OM care.

Acupuncture intervention in stroke care has seen rapid growth. Currently, stroke care in biomedicine focuses primarily on supportive care while waiting for the body to self-correct. Acupuncture care offered in the acute and recovery stages provides an active intervention option, one that apparently helps neurons recover from shock and thus permits a more rapid and complete recovery of the patient. Although few hospitals currently offer or even permit acupuncture intervention in acute conditions, within a few years the benefits of such intervention will be widely understood.

Patients Who Do Not Respond Well to Biomedical Care

Although the majority of patients do respond well to biomedical care, inevitably some do not. This situation is equally true for OM. This section reviews several situations in which referral is appropriate because the patient either does not respond to biomedical care, should not receive biomedical care, or resists biomedical care. In each case, a trial* of OM care may benefit the patient.

Responsiveness Issues

Some patients are difficult to treat within the biomedical framework because their complaints are multiple, subtle, do not "make sense," or are not detectable on examination or laboratory tests. Practitioners try many ways to serve such patients, but eventually both parties to the medical process become frustrated. Practitioners may conclude that the patient is psychologically abnormal. Patients may express frustration by becoming "noncompliant," by expressing resentment and anger, or by whining and making excessive demands on the practitioner.

A biomedical practitioner who believes that little more can be done for a particular patient yet senses that the patient may indeed benefit from another form

*Technically, a *comprehensive* medicine is one that treats all conditions based on a developed theory of cause and a multiplicity of interventional modalities and strategies. Only a few comprehensive medicines exist (see Chapter 1); others (e.g., chiropractic, homeopathy) are more limited in their theory, intervention strategies, and goals. Despite the breadth of the definition, however, no comprehensive medicine is equally successful in addressing all forms of malfunction. For example, biomedicine is unusually strong in its ability to treat extremes of illness with pharmaceuticals and malformations by surgery, whereas other practices of medicine emphasize early intervention, illness avoidance, and health maintenance.

*A *trial* should consist of at least eight treatment sessions because the effects of acupuncture care are additive.

of intervention may consider recommending OM to that patient. Symptoms that are irrelevant or do not "make sense" within biomedicine often make very good sense within OM, and this fact opens the treatment option anew. Patients with multiple chemical sensitivities who must avoid pharmaceuticals may respond well to acupuncture, herbs, or other OM modalities.

Some patients must actively avoid the two major interventional modalities of biomedicine. One such group is former drug abusers who must minimize use of all drugs, including pharmaceuticals and usually herbs. However, such patients may fare well with acupuncture or Qi Gong. Another group is patients who are too fragile to receive surgery. In some cases, OM may help such individuals to recover sufficient strength either to avoid surgery* or become strong enough to undergo it. A case of the latter type was presented in Chapter 8 under the title, "An Excruciating Lesion: A Case of Nonhealing Ulcerations" by Carol Kari.

Resistance to Biomedical Care

Some patients resist the standard interventions of biomedicine, sometimes for moral or ethical reasons, sometimes because they fear them, and sometimes because of previous bad experiences. Others may want to try every option short of surgery or a pharmaceutical on which they may become dependent (e.g., thyroid hormone, insulin, steroids). Such patients often may be receptive to other medical options, such as OM. Except in extreme cases, it makes sense to encourage efforts to avoid both surgery and strong pharmaceuticals.

As noted in Chapter 12, one of the most important reasons why people independently seek OM care is that they want to stop using a pharmaceutical drug. Numerous patient reports and lengthy clinical experience show that patients who have mild or early expressions of many conditions (e.g., mild hypothyroidism or hyperthyroidism, hypoglycemia, incipient type II diabetes) can recover normal function with OM. Other patients with a long dependence on various drugs, such as patients with asthma or depression,

often can reduce or end their use of these pharmaceuticals with appropriate OM care.

Referring Patients Who May Benefit from a High Relational Health Care Setting

Biomedicine is particularly successful in delivering rapid condition-specific care. Over the past generation, the amount of time spent by biomedical practitioners with their patients has steadily decreased. As a result, today few patients and practitioners can develop meaningful relationships. Patients especially do not like this feature of biomedical care, which is a point of discussion in many studies and is frequently the focus of efforts to improve the delivery of biomedicine.

Meanwhile, most OM practitioners spend 30 to 60 minutes with each patient, using this time to listen in depth to the patient, to deliver care, and to educate and guide the patient (see Chapter 7). This extended time and the associated ability to develop a warm relationship with the practitioner were the twin features of OM care most valued by patients in a 1999 study of OM (see Chapter 12).

Therefore biomedical practitioners whose patients demand a degree of relationship that they cannot provide may wish to refer them for OM care. To identify patients who fit this criterion, physicians should look for those who like to control their own care, who seek to educate themselves about their own health conditions, who appear committed to making health-enhancing changes in their lives and need guidance to do so, or who seek a high level of wellness.

Many such patients may actually present themselves in a somewhat negative light; for example, they may like to challenge the practitioner's knowledge, argue, or question biomedical recommendations while presenting conflicting evidence gleaned from the Internet. Other patients may eagerly request interventions that biomedical practitioners do not feel able to provide, such as acupuncture analgesia during surgery, nutriceutical therapy, meditation guidance, or nonpharmaceutical interventions.

Patients who seek high relationship care may be very grateful for a referral to a competent nonbiomedical practitioner such as an acupuncturist, and such a referral may help to cement their relationship with their biomedical practitioner.

---

*As noted in Chapter 12 (Table 12-7), two surveys showed that slightly more than 50% of patients for whom surgery was recommended for a variety of conditions avoided it after receiving OM care.

Cost-Effectiveness of Acupuncture

Richard Hammerschlag, PhD, and Patricia Culliton, MA, LAc, Co-Presidents of the Society for Acupuncture Research

The cost of acupuncture care is relatively low compared with the cost of biomedical care. There are several reasons for this, including low need for costly equipment, delivery in settings consisting primarily of the practitioner and patient (only sometimes including a receptionist), charges assessed by treatment rather than by technique, and (commonly, but changing) lack of insurance coverage, which reduces the paperwork load and need for accessory personnel. Although to date there has been little formal cost-effectiveness research on acupuncture care,[2] patient reports indicate that users feel they are saving money (see Chapter 12), and some studies have reported cost savings as summarized below.[3]

Avoidance of Surgery. Twenty-nine patients with severe osteoarthritis of the knee, each awaiting arthroscopic surgery, were randomly assigned to receive 6 weeks of acupuncture treatment or be placed on a waiting list to receive similar acupuncture treatment starting 9 weeks later. Of the 29 patients, 7 were able to cancel their scheduled surgeries at a cost savings of $9000/patient. (See Christensen BV, Iuhl IU, Vilbeck H, et al: Acupuncture treatment of severe knee osteoarthritis: a long-term study, *Acta Anaesthesiol Scand* 36:519-25, 1992.)

Fewer Days in Hospital and Rehabilitative Nursing Home. One half of 718 stroke patients receiving standard in-hospital rehabilitative care (initiated within 10 days of stroke) were randomly assigned to receive adjunctive acupuncture treatment. Patients given standard care plus acupuncture recovered faster and to a greater extent. Those receiving acupuncture spent an average of 88 days per patient in the hospital and nursing homes compared with 161 days/patient receiving standard rehabilitative care alone. Cost savings averaged $26,000/patient. (See Johansson K, Lindgren I, Wilder H, et al: Can sensory stimulation improve the functional outcome in stroke patients? *Neurology* 43:2189-92, 1993.)

Quicker Return to Physical Labor. Fifty-six patients at a workers' compensation clinic were randomly assigned to receive physical therapy, occupational therapy, and/or exercise with or without acupuncture. Of the 29 patients treated with acupuncture, 18 were able to return to their original or equivalent jobs, and 10 returned to lighter employment. Of the 27 patients who received only the standard therapy, 4 were able to return to their original or equivalent jobs, and 14 returned to lighter employment. (See Gunn CC, Milbrandt WE, Little AS, et al: Dry needling of muscle motor points for chronic low-back pain: a randomized clinical trial with long-term follow-up, *Spine* 5:279091, 1980.)

Avoidance of Surgery. One hundred five patients with angina pectoris had acupuncture and self-care education added to their pharmaceutical treatment. Seventy-three participants had been recommended for invasive procedures. The treatment protocol consisted of 12 visits over a 4-week period that included an acupuncture treatment and an education session. A 90% reduction in hospitalization and a 70% reduction in surgery resulted in an estimated cost savings of $32,000/patient. (See Ballegaard S, Johannessen A, Karpatschof B, et al: Addition of acupuncture and self-care education in the treatment of patients with severe angina pectoris may be cost beneficial: an open, prospective study, *J Altern Complement Med* 5:405-13, 1999.)

Avoidance of Surgery, Fewer Hospital Visits, and Greater Return to Employment. Sixty-nine patients with severe angina received 12 acupuncture treatments in 4 weeks. Patients also were instructed in performing shiatsu 2 times/day and received counseling in stress reduction, exercise, and diet. At the 2-year follow-up, of the 49 patients who had been candidates for coronary artery bypass or balloon angioplasty surgery, 30 postponed surgery because of clinical improvement. The cost savings from avoided surgery was $13,000/patient. The number of in-hospital days decreased for all 69 patients, averaging 79% reduction in the first year of postoperative treatment and 95% in the second year. Outpatient visits decreased by 60% and 87%, respectively. Additional cost savings resulted from the increase in percent of patients able to work, from 11% before treatment to 60% at 2 years after treatment. Estimated savings in annual sick pay was $9,000/patient. (See Ballegarrd S, Norrelund S, Smith DF: Cost-benefit of combined use of acupuncture, Shiatsu, and lifestyle adjustment for treatment of patients with severe angina pectoris, *Acupunct Electrother Res* 21:187-97, 1996.)

Continued

Cost-Effectiveness of Acupuncture—cont'd

Reduction of Inpatient Alcohol Detoxification Episodes. Eighty severe recidivist alcoholics received ear acupuncture for 2 months at points specific to the treatment of substance abuse (treatment group) or at nonspecific points (control group). Participants were asked to attend follow-up interviews at 1, 3, and 6 months after acupuncture. Detoxification admissions were examined for all participants regardless of whether they attended the follow-up interviews. The total cost of admissions to detoxification centers over the 6-month follow-up period was $20,424 higher in the control group than in the treatment group. (See Bullock ML, Culliton PD, Olander RT: Controlled trial of acupuncture for severe recidivist alcoholism, *Lancet* 1:1435-9, 1989.)

Reduction in Days of Missed Work. One hundred twenty patients with migraine without aura were randomly assigned to an acupuncture group (AG) or a conventional drug therapy group. AG patients received acupuncture twice/week for a maximum of 30 treatments. Four sites in Italy (two hospitals and two university public centers) provided the acupuncture; the two university sites also provided the pharmacological therapy. Severity and frequency of headache and days of missed work were evaluated 12 months after admission. The AG had an absence rate of 1120 working days/year, and the drug therapy group had a total absence rate of 1404 working days/year. This resulted in a cost savings of $35,480/year for the 60 patients receiving acupuncture compared with those in conventional drug therapy. (See Liguori A, Petti F, Bangrazi A, et al: Comparison of pharmacological treatment versus acupuncture treatment for migraine without aura: analysis of socio-medical parameters, *J Trad Chin Med* 20:231-40, 2000.)

ESTABLISHING COLLEGIAL RELATIONSHIPS WITH ORIENTAL MEDICINE PRACTITIONERS

One task of referral is to determine which patients can benefit from OM care. The linked task is to know to whom to refer them. These two tasks are as inseparably united as Yin and Yang. This section reviews methods to assess, meet, and establish collegial relationships with OM practitioners in one's region.

Assessing the Training and Skills of Oriental Medicine Practitioners

Training

The first step in assessing an OM practitioner is to determine the completeness of his or her education. A wide range of people claim skills in acupuncture, fewer in herbology, and fewer yet in the other Oriental modalities of diet, moving meditation, and massage. This book has focused on the work of professional practitioners who have received a full range of school training, usually 3 to 4 years plus an extensive internship (see Chapter 20). Such professional practitioners are recommended to biomedical practitioners as referral colleagues. Practitioners who have completed this extensive training often have additional background skills in biomedicine, nursing, massage therapy, dietetics, psychology, and so on.

The following are two basic traits of the well-trained OM practitioner:

- Completion of a minimum of 3 years of acupuncture and OM training. In the United States and other Western nations, students study at accredited schools. In Asia, not all schools are accredited.
- Licensure to practice in one's state, province, or country. In the United States, licensure for an licensed acupuncturist is abbreviated *LAc*. Currently no separate licensure to identify skill in herbs or other modalities exists.

OM practitioners receive a number of different titles when they finish their education, depending on the form of accreditation of their institution (see Chapter 20). Despite the multiplicity, *legally speaking and in terms of adequacy and character of education, all these titles are equivalent.* The most common equivalent labels include Dipl Ac (Diplomate of Acupuncture), MAc (Master's of Acupuncture), MOM (Master's of Oriental Medicine), OMD (Oriental Medical Doctor), and DOM (Doctor of Oriental Medicine). The latter two titles are used primarily in Asia or among Asian-trained practitioners elsewhere; no separate doctorate-level program yet exists in the United States or in European countries, although such programs are under discussion.

The OM practitioner's business card or patient brochure may offer further technical information. For example, many OM practitioners are also board certified. In the United States, those who have passed the U.S. national examination are likely to display this on their business card as *NCAAOM* Board Certified*. Those who have achieved high recognition among their peers may add other initials after their names. For example, fellowship in the U.S. National Academy of Acupuncture and Oriental Medicine is indicated with the initials *FNAAOM*.

Two other issues are of interest. First, although most OM practitioners are generalists similar to family practitioners, some do specialize. This specialization is likely to be listed on the business card or will be noted in discussion. Common specializations include pediatrics, gerontology, stroke and neurological care, obstetrics and gynecology, sports and musculoskeletal care, and asthma and allergy. Second, increasing numbers of practitioners also are involved in research, a point that is likely to be learned only through conversation.

Skills

In the United States and elsewhere in the Western world, OM practitioners usually have primary skills in acupuncture and moxibustion, have secondary skills in herbs, and have received varying amounts of training in dietetics, bodywork, and moving meditation. Many have additional skills gained through specialized training (e.g., scalp acupuncture, detoxification [auricular] acupuncture, hand acupuncture, allergy elimination techniques), and in other areas not connected with OM.

Because acupuncture and moxibustion are the baseline skills, they may not be mentioned on a business card. Herbology is likely to be listed, especially if the practitioner emphasizes its use in his or her practice and has received advanced training in this modality. Similarly, those with advanced skills in bodywork

or in dietetics are likely to list these specialties separately on business cards or in brochures describing their practice.

One modality that tends to be practiced independently of the others is moving meditation, which includes Qi Gong and Tai Chi. Training for these modalities is specialized and lengthy for those who wish to develop deep skills. Although training usually begins in a school situation, in advanced stages it involves an apprenticeship (see Chapter 6). Therefore biomedical practitioners who wish to recommend moving meditation as a self-care modality or medical Qi Gong as a specialty intervention should not seek regular OM practitioners but specialists. However, local acupuncturists can help in this search. Teachers of moving meditation usually are listed in the Yellow Pages of the telephone book (refer to *martial arts*). However, practitioners of medical Qi Gong are rare and are best identified by learning about their local reputations.

Meeting Oriental Medicine Practitioners

It is easy to meet OM practitioners at health fairs, at alternative medicine conventions, and in office settings in which practitioners from a number of backgrounds work together. Colleagues are also a useful source, since increasing numbers of biomedical practitioners are making working contacts with nonbiomedical practitioners. Acupuncturists often offer public lectures—at churches, holistic health centers, schools, and so forth—providing another setting in which to listen and consider the potential of meeting. Others write for alternative health newspapers; most large cities have at least one of these publications readily available. Major newspapers usually also feature a health section, and OM practitioners may be profiled or insert publicity as do other health providers.

Another possibility is for local medical societies to invite acupuncturists and herbalists as speakers. Patients are often a rich source of information. Finally, the Yellow Pages of the telephone directory provide a listing. Practitioners with ads that attract the eye might be worth a cold call, perhaps followed by with a meeting for coffee or lunch. Many practitioners also offer "observation" training to students; established biomedical practitioners could probably also arrange to observe care sessions with OM practitioners with whom they wish to establish collegial relationships.

---

*National Certification Commission for Acupuncture and Oriental Medicine.

The practice of OM is heterogeneous, and so (of course) are its practitioners. For this reason, it is wise to get to know each practitioner as an individual and not as a representative of OM. Ask questions of the person you are meeting to learn what types of patients or conditions they particularly like to treat. Perhaps this person prefers to work with patients who are experiencing severe pain or who have had a stroke. Someone else may focus on the spiritual and emotional health of patients. Clearly, the biomedical practitioner would wish to refer a different set of patients to these two practitioners. Patients also should be reminded of this phenomenon: a person who had a bad experience with a medical doctor would likely shrug and seek another; this same behavior applies to the receipt of OM care. Sometimes a relationship simply does not develop, but the whole practice should not be avoided on the basis of one bad experience.

POTENTIAL BARRIERS

In some ways, the practice of OM is very similar to that of biomedicine. For example, OM practitioners have the same intention of serving and helping the patient and abide by similar ethics of care and delivery as do biomedical practitioners. In addition, the OM office setting differs only slightly from that of the biomedical practitioner. Features such as sliding-fee scales are normative in both OM and biomedicine.

In other ways, the practice of OM is different, both for historical reasons and because the underlying theory that guides practice is different. These points were developed in Chapter 7. The next few paragraphs are devoted to identifying potential barriers to creating collegial contacts.

The issue of OM fee structure differs from that of biomedicine. Most OM practitioners not only bill patients directly but are paid directly by their patients, very often without employing intermediary personnel. OM practitioners ordinarily bill by the treatment rather than by task or time spent, so a 1-hour treatment costs the same as a half-hour treatment. The number of needles used, the use of moxibustion, the addition of electrostimulation, or the use of other modalities such as tuina (massage) usually does not change the cost of a treatment (some practitioners do charge separately, but this is unusual). On the other hand, when herbs are prescribed, patients must pay separately for them. Many herbs and compound herbal formulas are not readily available in Western pharmacies. Therefore many OM practitioners compound their own herbal mixtures and sell both purchased OTC formulas and compound herbal formulas directly to their patients. This practice was formerly common in biomedicine but became legally controlled (at least in the United States) in an effort to protect patients from inflated drug prices. Obviously, this problem also could occur in OM. However, most reputable OM practitioners clearly explain their herb fee structure to their patients. A common pattern is to charge "at cost" prices for herbs, plus a fee for creating the prescription. The practitioner's pricing of herbs is one question the biomedical practitioner might wish to discuss with an OM practitioner with whom he or she is getting acquainted.

The use of needles in acupuncture often initially seems like a barrier to both practitioners and patients. However, as shown in this book, needles are safe (clean needle technique is discussed in Chapter 4), and most patients readily adjust to needling, even coming to enjoy the sensations associated with them (Chapters 4 and 12). Finally, acupuncturists quickly develop skill in making patients feel at ease around acupuncture needles by using transitional techniques, showing them exactly what they are going to do, and training patients to distinguish pain from the *da qi* sensation.

Related potential barriers are language and culture. Asian practitioners, even those with many years of experience in OM, may not speak English well, or may speak with an accent that requires practice to understand. A more subtle issue is that of cultural difference. For example, patterns of self-presentation, politeness, and recognition tend to differ in East Asian settings from those in Eurocentric societies. Culturally, Asian practitioners may be punctilious about titles, greetings, and putting patients at ease in a quiet and restrained setting, whereas culturally Western practitioners may prefer a more extroverted style of practice and self-presentation. Asian practitioners may emphasize every form of training they have received and list every honor and connection; many Western practitioners, in contrast, underreport the extent of their training and the breadth of their networks. These differences matter only occasionally, but they merit consideration if a contact begins to seem puzzling.

The issue of quality of care and its down side are other concerns. By working with OM practitioners who are well trained, have good reputations, and are convincing in their self-presentation, most trouble in this area can be avoided. However, some OM practitioners, like their counterparts in biomedicine, may not be particularly gifted healers, or they may have unattractive personality characteristics. Rarely a practitioner may be found who promises more than he or she can deliver. In all these cases, it is wise not to refer patients. At the same time, it is important not to generalize from a few unfortunate experiences. Without doubt, the majority of professional OM practitioners are capable, personable, and appropriate referral resources.

Another barrier is structural, and it concerns access to OM. In large cities in many parts of the world, a range of OM practitioners can be found; in many areas, OM practitioners are also working in smaller cities and towns. However, outside Asia, most practitioners work independently and are not affiliated with institutions such as hospitals where they could be called on to deliver acute care. This situation is changing. However, the current structure of hospitals, with their nearly unilineal emphasis on biomedicine, has so far kept OM from becoming readily available to seriously ill patients. This situation is entirely different in Asia, where hospitals devoted to Oriental care serve the full range of patients.

SUMMARY

In many situations, the biomedical practitioner will profit by establishing collegial relationships with OM practitioners and referring selected patients for OM care. Because both OM and biomedicine are comprehensive medicines, the two are parallel. Collegial relationships can be equilateral and cooperative, a feature that should serve both practitioners and patients. As OM increasingly develops its voice in Western nations, the usefulness of integrating biomedical and OM care is becoming ever clearer.

References

1. Eisenberg DR, Kessler D, Foster F, et al: Unconventional medicine in the United States, prevalence, costs, and patterns of use, *N Engl J Med* 328:246-52, 1993.
2. Society for Acupuncture Research: Available at: www.acupunctureresearch.org. Accessed 2001.
3. White A: Economic evaluation of acupuncture, *Acupunct Med* 14:109-13, 1996.

NIH Consensus Statement on Acupuncture*

NATIONAL INSTITUTES OF HEALTH, CONTINUING MEDICAL EDUCATION, OFFICE OF THE DIRECTOR

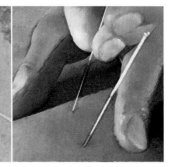

DISCLOSURE STATEMENT

All of the panelists who participated in this conference and contributed to the writing of this consensus statement were identified as having no financial or scientific conflict of interest, and all signed conflict of interest forms attesting to this fact. Unlike the expert speakers who present scientific data at the conference, the individuals invited to participate on NIH consensus panels are selected specifically because they are not professionally identified with advocacy positions with respect to the conference topic or with research that could be used to answer any of the conference questions.

ABSTRACT

OBJECTIVE

The objective of this NIH Consensus Statement is to inform the biomedical research and clinical practice communities of the results of the NIH Consensus Development Conference on Acupuncture. The statement provides state-of-the-art information regarding the appropriate use of acupuncture and presents the conclusions and recommendations of the consensus panel regarding these issues. In addition, the statement identifies those areas of study that deserve further investigation. On completion, the reader should possess a clear working clinical knowledge of the state-of-the-art information regarding this topic. The target audience of physicians for this statement includes, but is not limited to, family practitioners, medical acupuncturists, psychiatrists, and specialists in pain medicine.

PARTICIPANTS

The NIH Consensus Statement was composed by a nonfederal, nonadvocate, 12-member panel representing the fields of acupuncture, pain, psychology, psychiatry, physical medicine and rehabilitation, drug abuse, family practice, internal medicine, health policy, epidemiology, statistics, physiology, biophysics, and the public. In addition, 25 experts from these same fields presented data to the panel and a conference audience of 1200.

EVIDENCE

The literature was searched through MEDLINE, and an extensive bibliography of references was provided to the panel and the conference audience. Experts prepared abstracts with relevant citations from the literature. Scientific evidence was given precedence over clinical anecdotal experience.

CONSENSUS PROCESS

The panel, answering predefined questions, developed their conclusions based on the scientific evidence presented in open forum and the scientific literature. The panel composed a draft statement, which was read in its entirety and circulated to the experts and the audi-

---

*Date of original release: November 5, 1997; volume 15, number 5; November 3-5, 1997.

ence for comment. Thereafter, the panel resolved conflicting recommendations and released a revised statement at the end of the conference. The panel finalized the revisions within a few weeks after the conference. The draft statement was made available on the World Wide Web immediately after its release at the conference and was updated with the panel's final revisions.

CONCLUSIONS

Acupuncture as a therapeutic intervention is widely practiced in the United States. Although there have been many studies of its potential usefulness, many of these studies provide equivocal results because of design, sample size, and other factors. The issue is further complicated by inherent difficulties in the use of appropriate controls, such as placebos and sham acupuncture groups. However, promising results have emerged, showing efficacy of acupuncture in adult postoperative and chemotherapy nausea and vomiting and in postoperative dental pain. There are other situations, such as addiction, stroke rehabilitation, headache, menstrual cramps, tennis elbow, fibromyalgia, myofascial pain, osteoarthritis, low back pain, carpal tunnel syndrome, and asthma, in which acupuncture may be useful as an adjunct treatment or an acceptable alternative or may be included in a comprehensive management program. Further research is likely to uncover additional areas where acupuncture interventions will be useful.

INTRODUCTION

Acupuncture is a component of the health care system of China that can be traced back for at least 2500 years. The general theory of acupuncture is based on the premise that there are patterns of energy flow (Qi) through the body that are essential for health. Disruptions of this flow are believed to be responsible for disease. Acupuncture may correct imbalances of flow at identifiable points close to the skin. The practice of acupuncture to treat identifiable pathophysiological conditions in American medicine was rare until the visit of President Nixon to China in 1972. Since that time, there has been an explosion of interest in the United States and Europe in the application of acupuncture to Western medicine.

Acupuncture describes a family of procedures involving stimulation of anatomical locations on the skin by a variety of techniques. There are a variety of approaches to diagnosis and treatment in American acupuncture that incorporate medical traditions from China, Japan, Korea, and other countries. The most studied mechanism of stimulation of acupuncture points employs penetration of the skin by thin, solid, metallic needles, which are manipulated manually or by electrical stimulation. The majority of comments in this report are based on data that came from such studies. Stimulation of these areas by moxibustion, pressure, heat, and lasers is used in acupuncture practice, but because of the paucity of studies, these techniques are more difficult to evaluate.

Acupuncture has been used by millions of American patients and has been performed by thousands of physicians, dentists, acupuncturists, and other practitioners for relief or prevention of pain and for a variety of health conditions. After reviewing the existing body of knowledge, the U.S. Food and Drug Administration recently removed acupuncture needles from the category of experimental medical devices and now regulates them just as it does other devices, such as surgical scalpels and hypodermic syringes, under good manufacturing practices and single-use standards of sterility.

Over the years, the National Institutes of Health (NIH) has funded a variety of research projects on acupuncture, including studies on the mechanisms by which acupuncture may produce its effects, as well as clinical trials and other studies. There is also a considerable body of international literature on the risks and benefits of acupuncture, and the World Health Organization lists a variety of medical conditions that may benefit from the use of acupuncture or moxibustion. Such applications include prevention and treatment of nausea and vomiting; treatment of pain and addictions to alcohol, tobacco, and other drugs; treatment of pulmonary problems such as asthma and bronchitis; and rehabilitation from neurological damage such as that caused by stroke. To address important issues regarding acupuncture, the NIH Office of Alternative Medicine and the NIH Office of Medical Applications of Research organized a 2½ day conference to evaluate the scientific and medical data on the uses, risks, and benefits of acupuncture procedures for a variety of conditions. Cosponsors of the conference were the National Cancer Institute, the National Heart, Lung, and Blood Institute, the National Institute of Allergy and Infectious Diseases, the National Institute of

Arthritis and Musculoskeletal and Skin Diseases, the National Institute of Dental Research, the National Institute on Drug Abuse, and the Office of Research on Women's Health of the NIH. The conference brought together national and international experts in the fields of acupuncture, pain, psychology, psychiatry, physical medicine and rehabilitation, drug abuse, family practice, internal medicine, health policy, epidemiology, statistics, physiology, and biophysics, as well as representatives from the public.

After 1½ days of available presentations and audience discussion, an independent, nonfederal consensus panel weighed the scientific evidence and wrote a draft statement that was presented to the audience on the third day. The consensus statement addressed the following key questions:

- What is the efficacy of acupuncture, compared with placebo or sham acupuncture, in the conditions for which sufficient data are available to evaluate?
- What is the place of acupuncture in the treatment of various conditions for which sufficient data are available, in comparison or in combination with other interventions (including no intervention)?
- What is known about the biological effects of acupuncture that helps us understand how it works?
- What issues need to be addressed so that acupuncture can be appropriately incorporated into today's health care system?
- What are the directions for future research?

WHAT IS THE EFFICACY OF ACUPUNCTURE, COMPARED WITH PLACEBO OR SHAM ACUPUNCTURE, IN THE CONDITIONS FOR WHICH SUFFICIENT DATA ARE AVAILABLE TO EVALUATE?

Acupuncture is a complex intervention that may vary for different patients with similar chief complaints. The number and length of treatments and the specific points used may vary among individuals and during the course of treatment. Given this reality, it is perhaps encouraging that there exist a number of studies of sufficient quality to assess the efficacy of acupuncture for certain conditions.

According to contemporary research standards, there is a paucity of high-quality research assessing

efficacy of acupuncture compared with placebo or sham acupuncture. The vast majority of papers studying acupuncture in the biomedical literature consist of case reports, case series, or intervention studies with designs inadequate to assess efficacy.

This discussion of efficacy refers to needle acupuncture (manual or electroacupuncture) because the published research is primarily on needle acupuncture and often does not encompass the full breadth of acupuncture techniques and practices. The controlled trials usually have involved only adults and did not involve long-term (i.e., years) acupuncture treatment.

Efficacy of a treatment assesses the differential effect of a treatment when compared with placebo or another treatment modality using a double-blind controlled trial and a rigidly defined protocol. Papers should describe enrollment procedures, eligibility criteria, description of the clinical characteristics of the subjects, methods for diagnosis, and a description of the protocol (i.e., randomization method, specific definition of treatment, and control conditions, including length of treatment and number of acupuncture sessions). Optimal trials should also use standardized outcomes and appropriate statistical analyses. This assessment of efficacy focuses on high-quality trials comparing acupuncture with sham acupuncture or placebo.

Response Rate

As with other types of interventions, some individuals respond poorly to specific acupuncture protocols. Both animal and human laboratory and clinical experience suggest that the majority of subjects respond to acupuncture, with a minority not responding. Some of the clinical research outcomes, however, suggest that a larger percentage may not respond. The reason for this paradox is unclear and may reflect the current state of the research.

Efficacy for Specific Disorders

There is clear evidence that needle acupuncture is efficacious for adult postoperative and chemotherapy nausea and vomiting and probably for the nausea of pregnancy.

Much of the research is on various pain problems. There is evidence of efficacy for postoperative dental pain. There are reasonable studies (although sometimes only single studies) showing relief of pain with acupuncture on diverse pain conditions such as menstrual cramps, tennis elbow, and fibromyalgia. This suggests that acupuncture may have a more general effect on pain. However, there are also studies that do not find efficacy for acupuncture in pain.

There is evidence that acupuncture does not demonstrate efficacy for cessation of smoking and may not be efficacious for some other conditions.

Although many other conditions have received some attention in the literature and the research suggests some exciting potential areas for the use of acupuncture, the quality or quantity of the research evidence is not sufficient to provide firm evidence of efficacy at this time.

Sham Acupuncture

A commonly used control group is sham acupuncture, using techniques that are not intended to stimulate known acupuncture points. However, there is disagreement on correct needle placement. Also, particularly in the studies on pain, sham acupuncture often seems to have either intermediate effects between the placebo and "real" acupuncture points or effects similar to those of the "real" acupuncture points. Placement of a needle in any position elicits a biological response that complicates the interpretation of studies involving sham acupuncture. Thus there is substantial controversy over the use of sham acupuncture in control groups. This may be less of a problem in studies not involving pain.

WHAT IS THE PLACE OF ACUPUNCTURE IN THE TREATMENT OF VARIOUS CONDITIONS FOR WHICH SUFFICIENT DATA ARE AVAILABLE, IN COMPARISON OR IN COMBINATION WITH OTHER INTERVENTIONS (INCLUDING NO INTERVENTION)?

Assessing the usefulness of a medical intervention in practice differs from assessing formal efficacy. In conventional practice, clinicians make decisions based on the characteristics of the patient, clinical experience,

potential for harm, and information from colleagues and the medical literature. In addition, when more than one treatment is possible, the clinician may make the choice taking into account the patient's preferences. Although it is often thought that there is substantial research evidence to support conventional medical practices, this is frequently not the case. This does not mean that these treatments are ineffective. The data in support of acupuncture are as strong as those for many accepted Western medical therapies.

One of the advantages of acupuncture is that the incidence of adverse effects is substantially lower than that of many drugs or other accepted medical procedures used for the same conditions. As an example, musculoskeletal conditions, such as fibromyalgia, myofascial pain, and tennis elbow, or epicondylitis, are conditions for which acupuncture may be beneficial. These painful conditions are often treated with, among other things, antiinflammatory medications (e.g., aspirin, ibuprofen) or with steroid injections. Both medical interventions have a potential for deleterious side effects but are still widely used and are considered acceptable treatments. The evidence supporting these therapies is no better than that for acupuncture.

In addition, ample clinical experience, supported by some research data, suggests that acupuncture may be a reasonable option for a number of clinical conditions. Examples include postoperative pain and myofascial and low back pain. Examples of disorders for which the research evidence is less convincing but for which there are some positive clinical trials include addiction, stroke rehabilitation, carpal tunnel syndrome, osteoarthritis, and headache. Acupuncture treatment for many conditions such as asthma or addiction should be part of a comprehensive management program.

Many other conditions have been treated by acupuncture; the World Health Organization, for example, has listed more than 40 for which the technique may be indicated.

WHAT IS KNOWN ABOUT THE BIOLOGICAL EFFECTS OF ACUPUNCTURE THAT HELPS US UNDERSTAND HOW IT WORKS?

Many studies in animals and humans have demonstrated that acupuncture can cause multiple biological responses. These responses can occur locally (i.e., at or close to the site of application) or at a distance, mediated mainly by sensory neurons to many structures within the central nervous system. This can lead to activation of pathways affecting various physiological systems in the brain and the periphery. A focus of attention has been the role of endogenous opioids in acupuncture analgesia. Considerable evidence supports the claim that opioid peptides are released during acupuncture and that the analgesic effects of acupuncture are at least partially explained by their actions. That opioid antagonists such as naloxone reverse the analgesic effects of acupuncture further strengthens this hypothesis. Stimulation by acupuncture may also activate the hypothalamus and the pituitary gland, resulting in a broad spectrum of systemic effects. Alteration in the secretion of neurotransmitters and neurohormones and changes in the regulation of blood flow, both centrally and peripherally, have been documented. There is also evidence of alterations in immune functions produced by acupuncture. Which of these and other physiological changes mediate clinical effects is at present unclear.

Despite considerable efforts to understand the anatomy and physiology of the acupuncture points, the definition and characterization of these points remain controversial. Even more elusive is the scientific basis of some of the key traditional Eastern medical concepts such as the circulation of Qi, the meridian system, and other related theories, which are difficult to reconcile with contemporary biomedical information but continue to play an important role in the evaluation of patients and the formulation of treatment in acupuncture.

Some of the biological effects of acupuncture have also been observed when sham acupuncture points are stimulated, highlighting the importance of defining appropriate control groups in assessing biological changes purported to be due to acupuncture. Such findings raise questions regarding the specificity of these biological changes. In addition, similar biological alterations, including the release of endogenous opioids and changes in blood pressure, have been observed after painful stimuli, vigorous exercise, and/or relaxation training; it is at present unclear to what extent acupuncture shares similar biological mechanisms.

It should be noted also that for any therapeutic intervention, including acupuncture, the so-called "nonspecific effects" account for a substantial proportion of its effectiveness and thus should not be casually discounted. Many factors may profoundly determine therapeutic outcome, including the quality of the relationship between the clinician and the patient, the degree of trust, the expectations of the patient, the compatibility of the backgrounds and belief systems of the clinician and the patient, as well as a myriad of factors that together define the therapeutic milieu.

Although much remains unknown regarding the mechanism(s) that might mediate the therapeutic effect of acupuncture, the panel is encouraged that a number of significant acupuncture-related biological changes can be identified and carefully delineated. Further research in this direction not only is important for elucidating the phenomena associated with acupuncture but also has the potential for exploring new pathways in human physiology not previously examined in a systematic manner.

WHAT ISSUES NEED TO BE ADDRESSED SO THAT ACUPUNCTURE CAN BE APPROPRIATELY INCORPORATED INTO TODAY'S HEALTH CARE SYSTEM?

The integration of acupuncture into today's health care system will be facilitated by a better understanding among providers of the language and practices of both the Eastern and Western health care communities. Acupuncture focuses on a holistic, energy-based approach to the patient rather than a disease-oriented diagnostic and treatment model.

An important factor for the integration of acupuncture into the health care system is the training and credentialing of acupuncture practitioners by the appropriate state agencies. This is necessary to allow the public and other health practitioners to identify qualified acupuncture practitioners. The acupuncture educational community has made substantial progress in this area and is encouraged to continue along this path. Educational standards have been established for training of physician and nonphysician acupuncturists. Many acupuncture educational programs are accredited by an agency that is recognized by the U.S. Department of Education. A national credentialing agency exists for nonphysician practitioners and provides examinations for entry-level competency in the field. A nationally recognized examination for physician acupuncturists has been established.

A majority of states provide licensure or registration for acupuncture practitioners. Because some acupuncture practitioners have limited English proficiency, credentialing and licensing examinations should be provided in languages other than English where necessary. There is variation in the titles that are conferred through these processes, and the requirements to obtain licensure vary widely. The scope of practice allowed under these state requirements varies as well. Although states have the individual prerogative to set standards for licensing professions, consistency in these areas will provide greater confidence in the qualifications of acupuncture practitioners. For example, not all states recognize the same credentialing examination, thus making reciprocity difficult.

The occurrence of adverse events in the practice of acupuncture has been documented to be extremely low. However, these events have occurred on rare occasions, some of which are life-threatening (e.g., pneumothorax). Therefore appropriate safeguards for the protection of patients and consumers need to be in place. Patients should be fully informed of their treatment options, expected prognosis, relative risk, and safety practices to minimize these risks before their receipt of acupuncture. This information must be provided in a manner that is linguistically and culturally appropriate to the patient. Use of acupuncture needles should always follow FDA regulations, including use of sterile, single-use needles. It is noted that these practices are already being done by many acupuncture practitioners; however, these practices should be uniform. Recourse for patient grievance and professional censure are provided through credentialing and licensing procedures and are available through appropriate state jurisdictions.

It has been reported that more than 1 million Americans currently receive acupuncture each year. Continued access to qualified acupuncture professionals for appropriate conditions should be ensured. Because many individuals seek health care treatment from both acupuncturists and physicians, communication between these providers should be strengthened and improved. If a patient is under the care of an acupuncturist and a physician, both practitioners should be informed. Care should be taken to ensure that important medical problems are not overlooked. Patients and providers have a responsibility to facilitate this communication.

There is evidence that some patients have limited access to acupuncture services because of inability to pay. Insurance companies can decrease or remove financial barriers to access depending on their willingness to provide coverage for appropriate acupuncture services. An increasing number of insurance companies are either considering this possibility or now provide coverage for acupuncture services. Where there are state health insurance plans, and for populations served by Medicare or Medicaid, expansion of coverage to include appropriate acupuncture services would also help remove financial barriers to access.

As acupuncture is incorporated into today's health care system, and further research clarifies the role of acupuncture for various health conditions, it is expected that dissemination of this information to health care practitioners, insurance providers, policymakers, and the general public will lead to more informed decisions in regard to the appropriate use of acupuncture.

WHAT ARE THE DIRECTIONS FOR FUTURE RESEARCH?

The incorporation of any new clinical intervention into accepted practice faces more scrutiny now than ever before. The demands of evidence-based medicine, outcomes research, managed care systems of health care delivery, and a plethora of therapeutic choices make the acceptance of new treatments an arduous process. The difficulties are accentuated when the treatment is based on theories unfamiliar to Western medicine and its practitioners. It is important, therefore, that the evaluation of acupuncture for the treatment of specific conditions be carried out carefully, using designs that can withstand rigorous scrutiny. To further the evaluation of the role of acupuncture in the management of various conditions, the following general areas for future research are suggested.

What Are the Demographics and Patterns of Use of Acupuncture in the United States and Other Countries?

There is currently limited information on basic questions, such as who uses acupuncture, for what indications is acupuncture most commonly sought, what variations in experience and techniques used exist among acupuncture practitioners, and are there differences in these patterns by geography or ethnic group. Descriptive epidemiologic studies can provide insight into these and other questions. This information can in turn be used to guide future research and to identify areas of greatest public health concern.

Can the Efficacy of Acupuncture for Various Conditions for Which It Is Used or for Which It Shows Promise Be Demonstrated?

Relatively few high-quality, randomized, controlled trials have been published on the effects of acupuncture. Such studies should be designed in a rigorous manner to allow evaluation of the effectiveness of acupuncture. Such studies should include experienced acupuncture practitioners to design and deliver appropriate interventions. Emphasis should be placed on studies that examine acupuncture as used in clinical practice and that respect the theoretical basis for acupuncture therapy.

Although randomized controlled trials provide a strong basis for inferring causality, other study designs, such as those used in clinical epidemiology or outcomes research, can also provide important insights regarding the usefulness of acupuncture for various conditions. There have been few such studies in the acupuncture literature.

Do Different Theoretical Bases for Acupuncture Result in Different Treatment Outcomes?

Competing theoretical orientations (e.g., Chinese, Japanese, French) currently exist that might predict divergent therapeutic approaches (i.e., the use of different acupuncture points). Research projects should be designed to assess the relative merit of these divergent approaches and to compare these systems with treatment programs using fixed acupuncture points.

To fully assess the efficacy of acupuncture, studies should be designed to examine not only fixed acupuncture points but also the Eastern medical systems that provide the foundation for acupuncture therapy, including the choice of points. In addition to assessing the effect of acupuncture in context, this would also provide the opportunity to determine if Eastern medical theories predict more effective acupuncture points.

What Areas of Public Policy Research Can Provide Guidance For the Integration of Acupuncture Into Today's Health Care System?

The incorporation of acupuncture as a treatment raises numerous questions of public policy. These include issues of access, cost-effectiveness, reimbursement by state, federal, and private payers, and training, licensure, and accreditation. These public policy issues must be founded on quality epidemiologic and demographic data and effectiveness research.

Can Further Insight Into the Biological Basis for Acupuncture Be Gained?

Mechanisms that provide a Western scientific explanation for some of the effects of acupuncture are beginning to emerge. This is encouraging and may provide novel insights into neural, endocrine, and other physiological processes. Research should be supported to provide a better understanding of the mechanisms involved, and such research may lead to improvements in treatment.

Does an Organized Energetic System That Has Clinical Applications Exist in the Human Body?

Although biochemical and physiologic studies have provided insight into some of the biologic effects of acupuncture, acupuncture practice is based on a very different model of energy balance. This theory might or might not provide new insights to medical research, but it deserves further attention because of its potential for elucidating the basis for acupuncture.

CONCLUSIONS

Acupuncture as a therapeutic intervention is widely practiced in the United States. There have been many studies of its potential usefulness. However, many of these studies provide equivocal results because of design, sample size, and other factors. The issue is further complicated by inherent difficulties in the use of appropriate controls, such as placebo and sham acupuncture groups.

However, promising results have emerged, such as efficacy of acupuncture in adult postoperative and chemotherapy nausea and vomiting and in postoperative dental pain. There are other situations, such as addiction, stroke rehabilitation, headache, menstrual cramps, tennis elbow, fibromyalgia, myofascial pain, osteoarthritis, low back pain, carpal tunnel syndrome, and asthma, for which acupuncture may be useful as an adjunct treatment or an acceptable alternative or be included in a comprehensive management program. Further research is likely to uncover additional areas where acupuncture interventions will be useful.

Findings from basic research have begun to elucidate the mechanisms of action of acupuncture, including the release of opioids and other peptides in the central nervous system and the periphery and changes in neuroendocrine function. Although much needs to be accomplished, the emergence of plausible mechanisms for the therapeutic effects of acupuncture is encouraging.

The introduction of acupuncture into the choice of treatment modalities readily available to the public is in its early stages. Issues of training, licensure, and reimbursement remain to be clarified. There is sufficient evidence, however, of its potential value to conventional medicine to encourage further studies.

There is sufficient evidence of acupuncture's value to expand its use into conventional medicine and to encourage further studies of its physiology and clinical value.

Consensus Development Panel

Keh-Ming Lin, MD, MPH
Professor of Psychiatry, UCLA
Director, Research Center on the Psychobiology of Ethnicity
Harbor-UCLA Medical Center
Torrance, California

Daniel E. Moerman, PhD
William E. Stirton Professor of Anthropology
University of Michigan, Dearborn
Ypsilanti, Michigan

Sidney H. Schnoll, MD, PhD
Chairman, Division of Substance Abuse Medicine
Professor of Internal Medicine and Psychiatry
Medical College of Virginia
Richmond, Virginia

Marcellus Walker, MD
Honesdale, Pennsylvania

Christine Waternaux, PhD
Associate Professor and Chief, Biostatistics Division
Columbia University and New York State Psychiatric Institute
New York, New York

Leonard A. Wisneski, MD, FACP
Medical Director, Bethesda Center
American WholeHealth
Bethesda, Maryland

David J. Ramsay, DM, DPhil
Panel and Conference Chairperson
President, University of Maryland, Baltimore
Baltimore, Maryland

Marjorie A. Bowman, MD, MPA
Professor and Chair, Department of Family Practice and Community Medicine
University of Pennsylvania Health System
Philadelphia, Pennsylvania

Philip E. Greenman, DO, FAAO
Associate Dean, College of Osteopathic Medicine
Michigan State University
East Lansing, Michigan

Stephen P. Jiang, ACSW
Executive Director, Association of Asian Pacific Community Health Organizations
Oakland, California

Lawrence H. Kushi, ScD
Associate Professor, Division of Epidemiology
University of Minnesota School of Public Health
Minneapolis, Minnesota

Susan Leeman, PhD
Professor, Department of Pharmacology
Boston University School of Medicine
Boston, Massachusetts

Speakers

Abass Alavi, MD
"The Role of Physiologic Imaging in the Investigation
    of the Effects of Pain and Acupuncture on Regional
    Cerebral Function"
Professor of Radiology
Chief, Division of Nuclear Medicine
Hospital of the University of Pennsylvania
Philadelphia, Pennsylvania

Brian M. Berman, MD
"Overview of Clinical Trials on Acupuncture for Pain"
Associate Professor of Family Medicine
Director, Center for Complementary Medicine
University of Maryland School of Medicine
Baltimore, Maryland

Stephen Birch, LAc, PhD
"Overview of the Efficacy of Acupuncture in the
    Treatment of Headache and Face and Neck Pain"
Anglo-Dutch Institute for Oriental Medicine
The Netherlands

Hannah V. Bradford, MAc
"Late-Breaking Data and Other News From the Clinical
    Research Symposium (CRS) on Acupuncture
    at NIH"
Acupuncturist, Society for Acupuncture Research
Bethesda, Maryland

Xiaoding Cao, MD, PhD
"Protective Effect of Acupuncture on
    Immunosuppression"
Professor and Director, Institute of Acupuncture
    Research
Shanghai Medical University
Shanghai, China

Daniel C. Cherkin, PhD
"Efficacy of Acupuncture in Treating Low Back Pain:
    A Systematic Review of the Literature"
Senior Scientific Investigator, Group Health Center
    for Health Studies
Seattle, Washington

Patricia D. Culliton, MA, LAc
"Current Utilization of Acupuncture by United States
    Patients"
Director, Alternative Medicine Division
Hennepin County Medical Center
Minneapolis, Minnesota

David L. Diehl, MD
"Gastrointestinal Indications"
Assistant Professor of Medicine, UCLA Digestive
    Disease Center
University of California, Los Angeles
Los Angeles, California

Kevin V. Ergil, LAc
"Acupuncture Licensure, Training, and Certification
    in the United States"
Dean, Pacific Institute of Oriental Medicine
New York, New York

Richard Hammerschlag, PhD
"Methodological and Ethical Issues in Acupuncture
    Research"
Academic Dean and Research Director, Yo San
    University of Traditional Chinese Medicine
Santa Monica, California

Ji-Sheng Han, MD
"Acupuncture Activates Endogenous Systems
    of Analgesia"
Professor, Neuroscience Research Center
Beijing Medical University
Beijing, China

Joseph M. Helms, MD
"Acupuncture Around the World in Modern Medical
    Practice"
Founding President, American Academy of Medical
    Acupuncture
Berkeley, California

Kim A. Jobst, DM, MRCP
"Respiratory Indications"
University Department of Medicine and Therapeutics
Gardiner Institute
Glasgow, Scotland, United Kingdom

Gary Kaplan, DO
"Efficacy of Acupuncture in the Treatment
    of Osteoarthritis and Musculoskeletal Pain"
President, Medical Acupuncture Research Foundation
Arlington, Virginia

Ted J. Kaptchuk, OMD
"Acupuncture: History, Context, and Long-Term
    Perspectives"
Associate Director, Center for Alternative Medicine
    Research
Beth Israel Deaconess Medical Center
Boston, Massachusetts

Janet Konefal, PhD, EdD, MPH, CA
"Acupuncture and Addictions"
Associate Professor, Acupuncture Research
    and Training Programs
Department of Psychiatry and Behavioral Sciences
University of Miami School of Medicine
Miami, Florida

Lixing Lao, PhD, LAc
"Dental and Postoperative Pain"
Assistant Professor of Family Medicine
Department of Family and Complementary Medicine
University of Maryland School of Medicine
Baltimore, Maryland

C. David Lytle, PhD
"Safety and Regulation of Acupuncture Needles
    and Other Devices"
Research Biophysicist, Center for Devices
    and Radiological Health
U.S. Food and Drug Administration
Rockville, Maryland

Margaret A. Naeser, PhD, LAc, DiplAc
"Neurological Rehabilitation: Acupuncture and Laser
    Acupuncture to Treat Paralysis in Stroke
    and Other Paralytic Conditions and Pain in Carpal
    Tunnel Syndrome"
Research Professor of Neurology, Neuroimaging
    Section
Boston University Aphasia Research Center
Veterans Affairs Medical Center
Boston, Massachusetts

Lorenz K.Y. Ng, MD
"What Is Acupuncture?"
Clinical Professor of Neurology, George Washington
    University School of Medicine
Medical Director, Pain Management Program
National Rehabilitation Hospital
Bethesda, Maryland

Andrew Parfitt, PhD
"Nausea and Vomiting"
Researcher, Laboratory of Developmental
    Neurobiology
National Institute of Child Health and Human
    Development
National Institutes of Health
Bethesda, Maryland

Bruce Pomeranz, MD, PhD
"Summary of Acupuncture and Pain"
Professor, Departments of Zoology and Physiology
University of Toronto
Toronto, Ontario, Canada

Judith C. Shlay, MD
"Neuropathic Pain"
Assistant Professor in Family Medicine
Denver Public Health
Denver, Colorado

Alan I. Trachtenberg, MD, MPH
"American Acupuncture: Primary Care, Public Health,
    and Policy"
Medical Officer, Office of Science Policy
    and Communication
National Institute on Drug Abuse
National Institutes of Health
Rockville, Maryland

Jin Yu, MD
"Induction of Ovulation With Acupuncture"
Professor of Obstetrics and Gynecology
Obstetrical and Gynecological Hospital
Shanghai Medical University
Shanghai, China

Planning Committee

Alan I. Trachtenberg, MD, MPH
Planning Committee Chairperson
Medical Officer, Office of Science Policy
    and Communication
National Institute on Drug Abuse
National Institutes of Health
Rockville, Maryland

Brian M. Berman, MD
Associate Professor of Family Medicine
Director, Center for Complementary Medicine
University of Maryland School of Medicine
Baltimore, Maryland

Hannah V. Bradford, MAc
Acupuncturist, Society for Acupuncture Research
Bethesda, Maryland

Elsa Bray
Program Analyst, Office of Medical Applications
    of Research
National Institutes of Health
Bethesda, Maryland

Patricia Bryant, PhD
Director, Behavior, Pain, Oral Function,
  and Epidemiology Program
Division of Extramural Research
National Institute of Dental Research
National Institutes of Health
Bethesda, Maryland

Claire M. Cassidy, PhD
Director, Paradigms Found Consulting
Bethesda, Maryland

Jerry Cott, PhD
Head, Pharmacology Treatment Program
National Institute of Mental Health
National Institutes of Health
Rockville, Maryland

George W. Counts, MD
Director, Office of Research on Minority and Women's
  Health
National Institute of Allergy and Infectious Diseases
National Institutes of Health
Bethesda, Maryland

Patricia D. Culliton, MA, LAc
Director, Alternative Medicine Division
Hennepin County Medical Center
Minneapolis, Minnesota

Jerry M. Elliott
Program Management and Analysis Officer, Office
  of Medical Applications of Research
National Institutes of Health
Bethesda, Maryland

John H. Ferguson, MD
Director, Office of Medical Applications of Research
National Institutes of Health
Bethesda, Maryland

Anita Greene, MA
Public Affairs Program Officer, Office of Alternative
  Medicine
National Institutes of Health
Bethesda, Maryland

Debra S. Grossman, MA
Program Officer, Treatment Research Branch
Division of Clinical and Services Research
National Institute on Drug Abuse
National Institutes of Health
Rockville, Maryland

William H. Hall
Director of Communications, Office of Medical
  Applications of Research
National Institutes of Health
Bethesda, Maryland

Richard Hammerschlag, PhD
Academic Dean and Research Director, Yo San
  University of Traditional Chinese Medicine
Santa Monica, California

Freddie Ann Hoffman, MD
Deputy Director, Medicine Staff, Office of Health
  Affairs
U.S. Food and Drug Administration
Rockville, Maryland

Wayne B. Jonas, MD
Director, Office of Alternative Medicine
National Institutes of Health
Bethesda, Maryland

Gary Kaplan, DO
President, Medical Acupuncture Research Foundation
Arlington, Virginia

Carol Kari, RN, LAc, MAc
President, Maryland Acupuncture Society
Member, National Alliance
Kensington, Maryland

Charlotte R. Kerr, RN, MPH, MAc
Practitioner of Traditional Acupuncture
The Center for Traditional Acupuncture
Columbia, Maryland

Thomas J. Kiresuk, PhD
Director, Center for Addiction and Alternative
  Medicine Research
Minneapolis, Minnesota

Cheryl Kitt, PhD
Program Officer, Division of Convulsive, Infectious,
  and Immune Disorders
National Institute of Neurological Disorders
  and Stroke
National Institutes of Health
Bethesda, Maryland

Janet Konefal, PhD, EdD, MPH, CA
Associate Professor, Acupuncture Research
  and Training Programs
Department of Psychiatry and Behavioral Sciences
University of Miami School of Medicine
Miami, Florida

Sung J. Liao, MD, DPH
Clinical Professor of Surgical Sciences, Department
    of Oral and Maxillofacial Surgery
New York University College of Dentistry
Consultant, Rust Institute of Rehabilitation Medicine
New York University College of Medicine
Middlebury, Connecticut

Michael C. Lin, PhD
Health Scientist Administrator, Division of Heart
    and Vascular Diseases
National Heart, Lung, and Blood Institute
National Institutes of Health
Bethesda, Maryland

C. David Lytle, PhD
Research Biophysicist, Center for Devices
    and Radiological Health
U.S. Food and Drug Administration
Rockville, Maryland

James D. Moran, LAc, DAc, CAAP, CAS
President Emeritus and Doctor of Acupuncture,
    American Association of Oriental Medicine
The Belchertown Wellness Center
Belchertown, Massachusetts

Richard L. Nahin, PhD
Program Officer, Extramural Affairs
Office of Alternative Medicine
National Institutes of Health
Bethesda, Maryland

Lorenz K.Y. Ng, MD, RAc
Clinical Professor of Neurology, George Washington
    University School of Medicine
Medical Director, Pain Management Program
National Rehabilitation Hospital
Bethesda, Maryland

James Panagis, MD
Director, Orthopaedics Program
Musculoskeletal Branch
National Institute of Arthritis and Musculoskeletal
    and Skin Diseases
National Institutes of Health
Bethesda, Maryland

David J. Ramsay, DM, DPhil
Panel and Conference Chairperson
President, University of Maryland, Baltimore
Baltimore, Maryland

Charles R. Sherman, PhD
Deputy Director, Office of Medical Applications
    of Research
National Institutes of Health
Bethesda, Maryland

Virginia Taggart, MPH
Health Scientist Administrator, Division of Lung
    Diseases
National Heart, Lung, and Blood Institute
National Institutes of Health
Bethesda, Maryland

Xiao-Ming Tian, MD, RAc
Clinical Consultant on Acupuncture for the National
    Institutes of Health
Director, Academy of Acupuncture and Chinese
    Medicine
Bethesda, Maryland

Claudette Varricchio, DSN
Program Director, Division of Cancer Prevention
    and Control
National Cancer Institute
National Institutes of Health
Rockville, Maryland

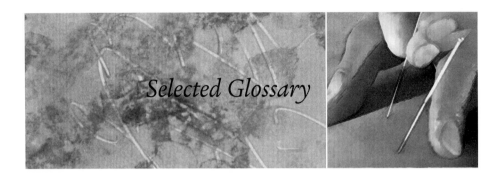

Selected Glossary

This short glossary offers a limited set of words that are used distinctively either in this text or in Chinese or Oriental medicine generally.

Acupoint Specific points on the body through which the bodily energy can be accessed and used to deliver acupuncture care to patients.

Anatomical Organs Physical organs that have specific locations and shapes and are described materialistically, as well as physiologically in the theory and practice of biomedicine. These are identified in this text with small initial letters: lung, heart, stomach, and so forth. Compare to *Functional Organs*.

Channel Alternative word for *Meridian*.

Comprehensive Health Care System A health care system that offers a complete theory of the body, what constitutes health and what makes people sick, a wide range of interventive modalities, formal schooling of practitioners, formal delivery locales, support systems in the form of legal and professional mandates, economic and social acceptability, and productive delivery systems for the interventive modalities. Few of the hundreds of medicines in the world meet all these criteria. Some that do are ayurveda, biomedicine (allopathy), and Chinese (Oriental) medicine. Compare to *Limited Health Care System*.

Conception Vessel A Meridian that runs along the anterior midline of the body. Also called the *Ren Meridian*.

Du Meridian A Meridian that runs along the posterior midline of the body. Also called the *Governing Vessel*.

Functional Organs Aspects of the body-person that are physiologically linked in the theory and practice of Chinese/Oriental medicine; also called *Zang-Fu*. Despite their mostly familiar names, these Organs are not limited in scope to the anatomical organs of similar name but include multiple aspects and components, including the physical, physiological, emotional, mental, and spiritual, as described in Chapter 2. In this text the Functional Organs are distinguished from the anatomical organs by the use of an initial capital letter. The more Yin or Interior (vital) of these include the Lung, Heart, Pericardium (Heart Protector), Spleen, Liver, and Kidney. The more Yang and Exterior of these include the Large Intestine (Colon), Small Intestine, San Jiao (Triple Heater, Triple Burner), Stomach, Gall Bladder, and Urinary Bladder. There are additional Extraordinary (Curious) Organs as well (see Chapter 2). Compare to *Anatomical Organs*.

Governing Vessel A Meridian that runs along the posterior midline of the body. Also called the *Du Meridian*.

Heart Protector The first line of defense of the Heart. Also called the *Pericardium Organ*.

Limited Health Care System A health care system that offers a focused and limited approach to care based on a focused theory of the body and its ills; a limited health care system may have a well-developed legal and professional mandate, schooling system, and delivery system. Examples of such systems include chiropractic, Christian Science healing, massage therapy, naturopathy, and shamanic healing.

Medicine A large-scale complex of theory and methods of intervention and practice that together result in a distinctive approach to understanding the body-person in health and illness and in knowing how to deliver health care. Chinese or Oriental medicine, as well as ayurveda, allopathy/biomedicine, chiropractic, naturopathy, and osteopathy, are examples of Medicines. Compare to *Practice, Style, Modality.*

Meridian   A line that links acupoints into energetic groups, each of which is given a distinct name according the Organ to which it most closely relates. Also called a Channel or in Chinese, *Mai.* Thus the Lung Meridian relates to the Lung Organ; in addition, it is partnered with the Large Intestine (Colon) Meridian (see Chapter 2). By current understanding, Meridian lines are not anatomical structures. Nevertheless, when an acupoint is appropriately stimulated, patients often feel energy move to specific distant regions as if it were moving in a Channel; even naive patients can accurately map the Meridians by describing this pattern of the passage of energy.

Modality   A particular way of intervening to improve health. It subsumes much more than a mere technique. For example, acupuncture is a modality comprising a multitude of types of needles or other stimulating devices, moxibustion, and related techniques, plus theory and methods of use. Pharmacy is a modality in biomedicine, again comprising a great deal more than merely the giving of drugs. Medical systems usually offer several modalities of intervention (e.g., Oriental medicine offers acupuncture, herbs, massage, diet, and Qi gong). Compare to *Medicine, Practice, Style.*

Pericardium Organ   The first line of defense of the Heart. Also called the *Heart Protector Organ.*

Practice   A verb describing what an individual actually does when she or he delivers health care. This word can also be used as a noun to mean the place and content of (scope of) practice of an individual. Compare to *Medicine, Modality, Style.*

Professional Oriental or Chinese Medicine Practitioner   A licensed practitioner of Oriental medicine, acupuncturist, or herbalist, who has received at least 3 years of professional training at an accredited school of Chinese or Oriental medicine and who practices Oriental medicine as his or her primary health care profession. Such a person may have any of the following equivalent degrees: Diplomate of Acupuncture, Master's of Acupuncture, Doctor of Oriental Medicine, or Oriental Medicine Doctor (see Chapter 20).

Ren Meridian   A Meridian that runs along the anterior midline of the body. Also called the *Conception Vessel.*

San Jiao Organ   An "organ without a shape" that is concerned with water metabolism within the body. Also called *Triple Heater* or *Triple Burner Organ.*

Style   A particular approach to practicing a Medicine that shares general aspects of its theory and method but has also evolved distinctive explanations, approaches, or interventions that make it different from other styles within that Medicine. In the case of Oriental medicine, some well-known styles include TCM ("Traditional Chinese Medicine"), Worsley or Leamington style Five Element Acupuncture, Toyo Hari Japanese style, or French Energetics style; there are many others. A parallel within biomedicine is the multiple styles of practice within the larger approach called psychotherapy. In chiropractic, two well-known styles are called "straight" and "mixer." Compare to *Medicine, Modality, Practice.*

Triple Burner, Triple Heater   An "organ without a shape" that is concerned with water metabolism within the body. Also called *San Jiao Organ.*

Zang-Fu   See *Functional Organs.*

Index

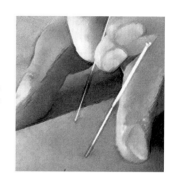

About the Author

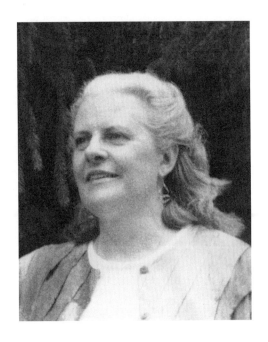

Claire Monod Cassidy, PhD, Dipl Ac, LAc, FNAAOM, is a medical anthropologist, human biologist, and acupuncturist with over 25 years of experience in the study of alternative and integrative medicine. As a researcher, she focuses her skills on analysis and comparison of urban or large-scale medical systems and on developing research methodologies that accurately reflect the character of the health care system being studied. Her recent research has emphasized collecting experiential and perceptual data from both practitioners and patients, including the design of appropriate questionnaires and the analysis of the resulting data; in the 1990s she completed two multiclinic outcomes surveys of patient experience of acupuncture care.

Dr. Cassidy served on the Editorial Board of the NIH Office of Alternative Medicine (1992 to 1995), which culminated in the publication of the multiedited text, *Alternative Medicine, Expanding Medical Horizons,* and on the NIH Planning Committee for the Consensus Conference on Acupuncture (1997).

For 6 years (1991 to 1997), she served as Research Director at a leading acupuncture school. In 1998 she entered acupuncture school, and in 2001 she received her Diplomate of Acupuncture. Currently, she continues to teach and write about comparative medical issues and methodological concerns, serves on the boards of two leading alternative medicine journals, and has opened her own acupuncture office, Windpath Healing Works.